NEUROENDOCRINE AND IMMUNE CROSSTALK

ANNALS OF THE NEW YORK ACADEMY OF SCIENCES
Volume 1088

NEUROENDOCRINE AND IMMUNE CROSSTALK

Edited by George P. Chrousos, Gregory A. Kaltsas, and George Mastorakos

Published by Blackwell Publishing on behalf of the New York Academy of Sciences
Boston, Massachusetts
2006

Library of Congress Cataloging-in-Publication Data

International Society for Neuroimmunomodulation. Meeting
(6th : 2005 : Athens, Greece)
   Neuroendocrine and immune crosstalk / edited by
George P. Chrousos, Gregory A. Kaltsas, and George Mastorakos.
      p. ; cm. – (Annals of the New York Academy of Sciences,
ISSN 0077-8923 ; no. 1088)
   Includes bibliographical references.
   ISBN-13: 978-1-57331-623-1
   ISBN-10: 1-57331-623-7
   1. Neuroendocrinology–Congresses. 2. Neuroimmunology–
Congresses. 3. Immune response–Regulation–Congresses.
I. Chrousos, George P. II. Kaltsas, Gregory A. III. Mastorakos,
George. IV. New York Academy of Sciences. V. Title. VI. Series.
   [DNLM: 1. Neuroimmunomodulation–Congresses. W1 AN626YL
v.1088 2006 / WL 102 I619275n 2006]

   QP356.4.I565 2006
   612.8–dc22

                                                    2006029677

The *Annals of the New York Academy of Sciences* (ISSN: 0077-8923 [print]; ISSN: 1749-6632 [online]) is published 28 times a year on behalf of the New York Academy of Sciences by Blackwell Publishing, with offices located at 350 Main Street, Malden, Massachusetts 02148 USA, PO Box 1354, Garsington Road, Oxford OX4 2DQ UK, and PO Box 378 Carlton South, 3053 Victoria Australia.

Information for subscribers: Subscription prices for 2006 are: Premium Institutional: $3850.00 (US) and £2139.00 (Europe and Rest of World).
Customers in the UK should add VAT at 5%. Customers in the EU should also add VAT at 5% or provide a VAT registration number or evidence of entitlement to exemption. Customers in Canada should add 7% GST or provide evidence of entitlement to exemption. The Premium Institutional price also includes online access to full-text articles from 1997 to present, where available. For other pricing options or more information about online access to Blackwell Publishing journals, including access information and terms and conditions, please visit www.blackwellpublishing.com/nyas.

Membership information: Members may order copies of the *Annals* volumes directly from the Academy by visiting www.nyas.org/annals, emailing membership@nyas.org, faxing 212-298-3650, or calling 800-843-6927 (US only), or +1 212-298-8640 (International). For more information on becoming a member of the New York Academy of Sciences, please visit www.nyas.org/membership.

Journal Customer Services: For ordering information, claims, and any inquiry concerning your institutional subscription, please contact your nearest office:
UK: Email: customerservices@blackwellpublishing.com; Tel: +44 (0) 1865 778315; Fax +44 (0) 1865 471775
US: Email: customerservices@blackwellpublishing.com; Tel: +1 781 388 8599 or 1 800 835 6770 (Toll free in the USA); Fax: +1 781 388 8232
Asia: Email: customerservices@blackwellpublishing.com; Tel: +65 6511 8000; Fax: +61 3 8359 1120
Members: Claims and inquiries on member orders should be directed to the Academy at email: membership@nyas.org or Tel: +1 212 838 0230 (International) or 800-843-6927 (US only).

Printed in the USA.
Printed on acid-free paper.

Mailing: The *Annals of the New York Academy of Sciences* are mailed Standard Rate.
Postmaster: Send all address changes to *Annals of the New York Academy of Sciences*,
Blackwell Publishing, Inc., Journals Subscription Department, 350 Main Street, Malden,
MA 01248-5020. Mailing to rest of world by DHL Smart and Global Mail.

Disclaimer: The Publisher, the New York Academy of Sciences, and the Editors cannot
be held responsible for errors or any consequences arising from the use of information
contained in this publication; the views and opinions expressed do not necessarily reflect
those of the Publisher, the New York Academy of Sciences, or the Editors.

Annals are available to subscribers online at the New York Academy of Sciences and also at
Blackwell Synergy. Visit www.annalsnyas.org or www.blackwell-synergy.com to search the
articles and register for table of contents e-mail alerts. Access to full text and PDF downloads
of *Annals* articles are available to nonmembers and subscribers on a pay-per-view basis at
www.annalsnyas.org.

The paper used in this publication meets the minimum requirements of the National Standard for Information Sciences Permanence of Paper for Printed Library Materials, ANSI
Z39.48-1984.

ISSN: 0077-8923 (print); 1749-6632 (online)
ISBN-10: 1-57331-623-7 (paper); ISBN-13: 978-1-57331-623-1 (paper)

A catalogue record for this title is available from the British Library.

Digitization of the *Annals of the New York Academy of Sciences*

An agreement has recently been reached between Blackwell Publishing and the New York
Academy of Sciences to digitize the entire run of the *Annals of the New York Academy of
Sciences* back to volume one.

The back files, which have been defined as all of those issues published before 1997, will
be sold to libraries as part of Blackwell Publishing's Legacy Sales Program and hosted on
the Blackwell Synergy website.

Copyright of all material will remain with the rights holder. Contributors: Please contact
Blackwell Publishing if you do not wish an article or picture from the *Annals of the New
York Academy of Sciences* to be included in this digitization project.

ANNALS OF THE NEW YORK ACADEMY OF SCIENCES

Volume 1088
November 2006

NEUROENDOCRINE AND IMMUNE CROSSTALK

Editors
GEORGE P. CHROUSOS, GREGORY A. KALTSAS, AND
GEORGE MASTORAKOS

This volume is the result of a meeting entitled **the 6th Meeting of the International Society for Neuroimmunomodulation: Neuroendocrine and Immune Crosstalk**, held on September 25–28, 2005 in Athens, Greece.

CONTENTS

Dedication to Samuel M. McCann. *By* GEORGE P. CHROUSOS xiii

Preface. *By* GREGORY A. KALTSAS xv

An Overview of the Volume. *By* GEORGE P. CHROUSOS, GREGORY A. KALTSAS, AND GEORGE MASTORAKOS xvi

Part I. Introduction

Chronology of Advances in Neuroendocrine Immunomodulation. *By* SAMUEL M. MCCANN, ANDREA DE LAURENTIIS, AND VALERIA RETTORI ... 1

The Mitochondrion as a Primary Site of Action of Regulatory Agents Involved in Neuroimmunomodulation. *By* A.M.G. PSARRA, S. SOLAKIDI, AND C.E. SEKERIS 12

Immunomodulatory Properties of Substance P: The Gastrointestinal System as a Model. *By* HON WAI KOON AND CHARALABOS POTHOULAKIS 23

Part II. The Neuroendocrine Immune Basis for Autoimmune and Allergic Disorders

Hypothalamic-Pituitary-Adrenal Axis Function in Sjögren's Syndrome: Mechanisms of Neuroendocrine and Immune System Homeostasis. *By* ELIZABETH O. JOHNSON, MARIA KOSTANDI, AND HARALAMPOS M. MOUTSOPOULOS 41

The Role of Chaperone Proteins in Autoimmunity. *By* JOHN G. ROUTSIAS AND
ATHANASIOS G. TZIOUFAS 52

The Role of Stress in Asthma: Insight from Studies on the Effect of Acute and
Chronic Stressors in Models of Airway Inflammation. *By*
RATTANJEET S. VIG, PAUL FORSYTHE, AND HARISSIOS VLIAGOFTIS 65

The Critical Role of Mast Cells in Allergy and Inflammation. *By*
THEOHARIS C. THEOHARIDES AND DIMITRIOS KALOGEROMITROS 78

Immunomodulation: The Future Cure for Allergic Diseases. *By*
DAPHNE C. TSITOURA AND YANNIS TASSIOS 100

Neural Correlates of IgE-Mediated Allergy. *By* FREDERICO AZEVEDO
COSTA-PINTO, ALEXANDRE SALGADO BASSO, LUIZ CARLOS DE SÁ-ROCHA,
LUIZ ROBERTO GIORGETTI BRITTO, MOMTCHILO RUSSO, AND
JOÃO PALERMO-NETO 116

Dialogue between the Brain and the Immune System in Inflammatory
Arthritis. *By* DIMITRIOS VASSILOPOULOS AND
DIMOSTHENIS MANTZOUKIS 132

Part III. Neuroimmunoendocrinology in Aging and Pain

Neurosteroids as Endogenous Inhibitors of Neuronal Cell Apoptosis in
Aging. *By* IOANNIS CHARALAMPOPOULOS, VASSILIKI-ISMINI ALEXAKI,
CHRISTOS TSATSANIS, VASSILIS MINAS, ERENE DERMITZAKI,
IAKOVOS LASARIDIS, LINA VARDOULI, CHRISTOS STOURNARAS,
ANDREW N. MARGIORIS, ELIAS CASTANAS, AND ACHILLE GRAVANIS 139

Role of Thymulin or Its Analogue as a New Analgesic Molecule. *By*
MIREILLE DARDENNE, NAYEF SAADE, AND BARED SAFIEH-GARABEDIAN ... 153

Therapeutic Management of Chronic Neuropathic Pain: An Examination of
Pharmacologic Treatment. *By* ATHINA VADALOUCA, IOANNA SIAFAKA,
ERIPHYLLI ARGYRA, EVI VRACHNOU, AND ELENI MOKA 164

Part IV. Neural and Neuroendocrine Regulation of
Dendritic Cell Function

Regulation of Dendritic Cell Differentiation by Vasoactive Intestinal Peptide:
Therapeutic Applications on Autoimmunity and Transplantation. *By*
ALEJO CHORNY, ELENA GONZALEZ-REY, AND MARIO DELGADO 187

Neuroendocrine Regulation of Skin Dendritic Cells. *By* KRISTINA SEIFFERT AND
RICHARD D. GRANSTEIN 195

PPARγ, a Lipid-Activated Transcription Factor as a Regulator of Dendritic
Cell Function. *By* ISTVAN SZATMARI, EVA RAJNAVOLGYI, AND
LASZLO NAGY 207

Part V. Novel Functions of Cytokines in the Nervous System

Roles of Glia-Derived Cytokines on Neuronal Degeneration and
Regeneration. *By* AKIO SUZUMURA, HIDEYUKI TAKEUCHI, GUIQIN ZHANG,
REIKO KUNO, AND TETSUYA MIZUNO 219

Brain Cytokines and the 5-HT System during Poly I:C-Induced Fatigue. *By* TOSHIHIKO KATAFUCHI, TETSUYA KONDO, SACHIKO TAKE, AND MEGUMU YOSHIMURA 230

Participation of the Endocannabinoid System in the Effect of TNF-α on Hypothalamic Release of Gonadotropin-Releasing Hormone. *By* JAVIER FERNANDEZ-SOLARI, JUAN P. PRESTIFILIPPO, STEFAN R. BORNSTEIN, SAMUEL M. MCCANN, AND VALERIA RETTORI 238

Part VI. Neuroimmunomodulation in Chronic Infectious and Inflammatory Diseases

Low-Grade Inflammation in Chronic Infectious Diseases: Paradigm of Periodontal Infections. *By* NIKI M. MOUTSOPOULOS AND PHOEBUS N. MADIANOS 251

Local Amplification of Glucocorticoids by 11β-Hydroxysteroid Dehydrogenase Type 1 and Its Role in the Inflammatory Response. *By* KAREN E. CHAPMAN, AGNES COUTINHO, MOHINI GRAY, JAMES S. GILMOUR, JOHN S. SAVILL, AND JONATHAN R. SECKL 265

Immunoneuroendocrine Interactions in Chagas Disease. *By* ELIANE CORRÊA-DE-SANTANA, FERNANDA PINTO-MARIZ, AND WILSON SAVINO 274

Thymus-Dependent T Cell Tolerance of Neuroendocrine Functions: Principles, Reflections, and Implications for Tolerogenic/Negative Self-Vaccination. *By* VINCENT GEENEN 284

Part VII. The Adrenal Connection in Neuroimmunoendocrinology

Molecular Understanding of Cytokine–Steroid Hormone Dialogue: Implications for Human Diseases. *By* JIMENA DRUKER, ANA C. LIBERMAN, MATÍAS ACUÑA, DAMIANA GIACOMINI, DAMIÁN REFOJO, SUSANA SILBERSTEIN, MARCELO PAEZ PEREDA, GÜNTER K. STALLA, FLORIAN HOLSBOER, AND EDUARDO ARZT 297

The Role of Toll-like Receptors in the Immune–Adrenal Crosstalk. *By* S.R. BORNSTEIN, C.G. ZIEGLER, A.W. KRUG, W. KANCZKOWSKI, V. RETTORI, S.M. MCCANN, M. WIRTH, AND K. ZACHAROWSKI 307

Adrenocortical Tumorigenesis. *By* FELIX BEUSCHLEIN AND MARTIN REINCKE . . . 319

Alpha 2-Adrenergic Receptors Decrease DNA Replication and Cell Proliferation and Induce Neurite Outgrowth in Transfected Rat Pheochromocytoma Cells. *By* G. KARKOULIAS, O. MASTROGIANNI, I. ILIAS, A. LYMPEROPOULOS, S. TARAVIRAS, N. TSOPANOGLOU, N. SITARAS, AND C.S. FLORDELLIS 335

Pheochromocytoma: Physiopathologic Implications and Diagnostic Evaluation. *By* EVANGELIA ZAPANTI AND IOANNIS ILIAS 346

Part VIII. The Stress System: Activators, Mediators, Effectors, and Counterregulators

Beyond Heart Rate Variability: Vagal Regulation of Allostatic Systems. *By* JULIAN F. THAYER AND ESTHER STERNBERG 361

Interleukin-6: A Cytokine and/or a Major Modulator of the Response to
    Somatic Stress. *By* GEORGE MASTORAKOS AND IOANNIS ILIAS 373

The Role of Stress in the Clinical Expression of Thyroid Autoimmunity. *By*
    AGATHOCLES TSATSOULIS 382

Annexin 1, Glucocorticoids, and the Neuroendocrine–Immune Interface. *By*
    JULIA C. BUCKINGHAM, CHRISTOPHER D. JOHN, EGLE SOLITO,
    TANYA TIERNEY, RODERICK J. FLOWER, HELEN CHRISTIAN, AND
    JOHN MORRIS 396

Index of Contributors 411

Financial assistance was received from:

- Novartis
- Ipsen PC

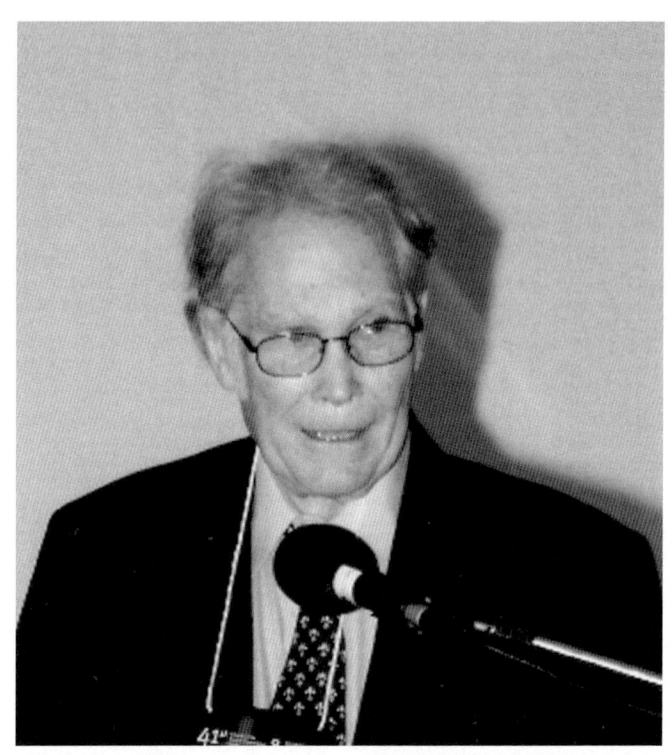

SAMUEL M. MCCANN

Dedication to Samuel M. McCann

Samuel M. McCann was born in Houston, Texas on September 8, 1925, the only son of intellectual parents. His father was a faculty member and registrar at Rice University in Houston, Texas. McCann took an early interest in science and was number one in both his high school class and at Culver Military Academy. With the onset of World War II he entered an accelerated program at Rice University and was once again at the head of his class. He completed his medical degree in three years at the University of Pennsylvania, School of Medicine, also number one in the class, where he also carried out research. Two papers were published in the *American Journal of Physiology*, pointing to a role for stress and adrenal corticol hormones in hypertension. While an intern and assistant resident in medicine at Massachusetts General Hospital (MGH), with two other residents, he ran the second artificial kidney in the United States. After two years at MGH, he returned to the University of Pennsylvania as an instructor in physiology. Shortly afterward, he received his draft notice and spent 20 months in the Army Medical Corps at Walter Reed Hospital, also working in building and formation at the National Institutes of Health.

These early experiences helped determine the course for McCann's research throughout his professional career. With Farell he showed that epinephrine would increase blood ACTH in rats within a minute, indicating neural control, presumably by a factor reaching the pituitary by the portal vessels. He went on to show that destruction of the median eminence, the site of origin of the portal vessels, blocked ACTH release in both the rat and cat. These lesions were often associated with gonadal failure caused by decreased gonadotrophin release.

With the end of the war, McCann returned to the University of Pennsylvania and initiated research to look for peptidergic transmitters to stimulate the various anterior pituitary hormones. His work rapidly attracted international recognition, which led to numerous invitations to speak at meetings throughout the United States and abroad. Many international postdoctoral fellows were attracted to McCann's laboratory, where subsequently they were the first to discover the ACTH-releasing action of vasopressin, followed by peptides CRF, LHRF, FSHRF, GHRF, and GHIF. He was promoted through the ranks and became full professor in 1964 after one year as acting chairman.

In 1965 McCann was simultaneously offered the chairmanship of the physiology department at Tulane University in New Orleans and at the University of Texas Southwestern Medical School in Dallas. He decided on Dallas, where he built an excellent department. At the age of 70 years he was awarded an

Ann. N.Y. Acad. Sci. 1088: xiii–xiv (2006). © 2006 New York Academy of Sciences.
doi: 10.1196/annals.1366.035

endowed chair from Pennington Biomedical Research Center, Louisiana State University in Baton Rouge, gaining ample research support from the NIH.

Dr. McCann is a member of many societies and has sat on the councils of the American Physiological Society and the Endocrine Society. He was president of the International Neuroendocrine Federation, the Society for Experimental Biology and Medicine, the International Society of Neuroendocrinology, and the International Society of Neuroimmunomodulation. He also served as editor-in-chief of *Neuroendocrinology*.

We take particular pleasure in honoring Samuel M. McCann, knowing that he has influenced, in a most positive way, everyone associated with this volume.

GEORGE P. CHROUSOS
University of Athens, Medical School
11527 Athens, Greece

Preface

The publication of the proceedings of the 5th International Congress of the International Society for Neuroimmunomodulation marks the continuation of an ongoing successful relationship between the society and the *Annals of the New York Academy of Sciences* that began in 1990, with the purpose of bringing the most recent advances in the field of neuroimmunomodulation to the global scientific community. Whereas in previous volumes there was a strong focus on the hypothalamic-pituitary-adrenal (HPA) axis and the role of its key hormones, corticotropin-releasing hormone (CRH) and glucocorticoids in inflammation, the intent of this volume is to purposefully focus on the role of neural and neuroendocrine factors in autoimmune, inflammatory, allergic, and infectious diseases. This is, in part, because of the exponential growth and diversity of the field, but also to emphasize the susceptibility of humans to certain infectious and noninfectious inflammatory disorders, which is profoundly affected by neural and neuroendocrine factors.

The central nervous system (CNS) alters the immune response through activation of the HPA axis and the sympathetic nervous system (SNS). In this context, the immune system functions as a sensory system alerting the CNS to the presence of pathogenic inducers through the secretion of cytokines. The immune system's response to neuroendocrine factors released by activation of the CNS may result in increased immunity and/or immunosuppression, depending on the time and timing of the stressor in relation to the exposure to the immune agent. Stress-induced "immunosuppression" may cause increased susceptibility to infections, resulting in more severe diseases, or might also allow the establishment of persistent infections leading to autoimmunity. An in-depth understanding of the cytokine and neuroendocrine networks involved in these interactions may lead to the development of targeted therapies for a variety of diseases. In the current volume, there is extensive coverage of the cross-talk between the neuroimmunoendocrine systems and the effect this may have on the pathophysiology of aging, pain perception, sleeping patterns, and the development of several infectious, allergic, and autoimmune disorders.

GREGORY A. KALTSAS
University of Athens, Medical School
Athens, Greece

Ann. N.Y. Acad. Sci. 1088: xv (2006). © 2006 New York Academy of Sciences.
doi: 10.1196/annals.1366.033

An Overview of the Volume

GEORGE P. CHROUSOS, GREGORY A. KALTSAS,
AND GEORGE MASTORAKOS

University of Athens, Medical School, 11527 Athens, Greece

In the Introduction, Professor Samuel McCann and his colleagues provide a very detailed description of many of the major developments that have taken place in the field of neuroimmunomodulation over the last 50 years. Through this article, the reader becomes familiar not only with many of the scientific achievements in the field, but also with some of its major players. In the same section, Psarra and colleagues highlight the important roles of the mitochondria in neuroimmunomodulation, as these cellular organelles represent a major target for glucocorticoids and cytokines, whereas Koon provides evidence for the immunomodulatory properties of substance P.

The Neuroendocrine Immune Basis for Autoimmune and Allergic Diseases

Johnson and colleagues explore possible common pathophysiologic and genetic mechanisms that may operate in inflammatory and stress-related disorders, particularly endocrine and metabolic factors. They demonstrate that hypothalamo-pituitary-adrenal axis hypoactivity characterizes the majority of patients with Sjögren's syndrome and fibromyalgia. The potential role of heat-shock proteins in the induction of autoimmune disorders is raised by Routsias and Tzioufas. The increased production of host and microbial heat-shock proteins at the site of infection may provide a critical link between infection and autoimmunity. Vassilopoulos presents an overview of recent information regarding the regulation of complex pathways of neuroendocrine response during the different phases of rheumatoid arthritis. The effects of the recently introduced biological therapies on neuroendocrine function in patients with rheumatoid arthritis are discussed.

Asthma, a common chronic allergic/inflammatory disorder, is influenced by psychologic factors and stress. Vig and his colleagues extensively review major clinical and animal studies that provide evidence of close links between these factors and the development/severity of asthma, and they try to identify potential mechanisms for such interactions. Palermo-Neto and colleagues also

Ann. N.Y. Acad. Sci. 1088: xvi–xix (2006). © 2006 New York Academy of Sciences.
doi: 10.1196/annals.1366.034

provide novel experimental information exploring neuroimmune interactions during allergic responses. Furthermore, Theoharides and Kalogeromitros examine the involvement of mast cells in allergic and anaphylactic reactions and expand on the other potential roles of these cells in a variety of inflammatory disorders. Tsitoura and Tassios discuss the role of immunomodulation in the development of a future cure for allergic disorders through downmodulation of the immune mechanisms that initiate and maintain the allergic cascade.

Neuroimmunoendocrinology in Aging and Pain

Gravanis and colleagues describe the beneficial neuroprotective role of the neuroactive steroids, dehydroepiandrosterone (DHEA) and its sulfate ester DHEAS and allopregnanolone (Allo), and suggest that the decline of neurosteroid levels during aging may leave the brain unprotected against neurotoxic challenges. Dardenne discusses in detail the role of the thymic peptide thymulin and its direct and/or indirect interactions with the nervous system, particularly as an inducer of hyperalgesia through its action on afferent nerve terminals. Modulation of this action may lead to reduction of inflammatory pain and expression of proinflammatory cytokines and may represent a potential future therapeutic option. Vadalouka's article provides the latest information regarding the management of chronic neuropathic pain based on the results of recent randomized controlled trials and personal experience.

Neural and Neuroendocrine Regulation of Dendritic Cell Function

Seiffert and Granstein expand on the neuroendocrine regulation of skin dendritic cells, suggesting that although they originally evolved to defend the organism against invading pathogens and thus maintain immune homeostasis, may, under certain conditions, become unbalanced, exacerbating cutaneous inflammation. Alejo Chorny and colleagues provide evidence on the expanding regulatory role of the neuropeptide vasoactive intestinal peptide (VIP) on dendritic cell regulation, which might be of particular interest in autoimmunity and transplantation, whereas Nagy and colleagues provide new evidence on the expanding role of PPAR-γ, which, besides being a key component of adipose tissue development and a target of insulin-sensitizing drugs, also has a role in immune cell differentiation and function. PPAR-γ is likely to be a regulator of dendritic cell function, altering antigen uptake, processing, and presentation, as well as cell maturation, activation, migration, and cytokine production, making this receptor a relevant target for pharmacologic intervention in immune diseases.

Novel Functions of Cytokines in the Nervous System

Suzumura and colleagues describe the accumulation of activated microglia and astrocytes in a variety of inflammatory and degenerative disorders in the central nervous system. They suggest that glial cell–derived cytokines may function synergistically with other local factors in causing neuronal degeneration, either directly or by altering the production of neurotrophic factors. Katafuchi and colleagues deal with the pathophysiology of a very common and occasionally devastating symptom, fatigue. They provide evidence supporting the idea that a decrease in serotonin in an immunologically induced fatigue model may be an important underlying mechanism of this condition. In addition, Rettori and colleagues describe a model that provides evidence for a key role of the endocannabinoid system in the effects that inflammatory signals have on the function of the reproductive system.

Neuroimmunomodulation in Chronic Infectious and Inflammatory Diseases

Moutsopoulos and colleagues provide evidence implicating periodontitis, a chronic inflammatory disease of the tooth-supporting structures, as a potential risk factor for increased morbidity and/or mortality from cardiovascular disease (atherosclerosis, heart attack, and stroke), pregnancy complications (spontaneous preterm birth), and diabetes mellitus. Although further research is required, they suggest that periodontal therapy may improve surrogate cardiovascular outcomes, such as endothelial function, and may reduce by four- to fivefold the incidence of premature birth. Seckl's team provides evidence of the effect that prereceptor binding glucocorticoid metabolism may exert on acute inflammatory reactions in several different tissues. They suggest that enzymes involved in glucocorticoid metabolism may be engaged early in the inflammatory response and its subsequent resolution. Savino and colleagues describe the particular immunoneuroendocrine interactions that occur following infection by *Trypanosoma cruzi*, the causative agent of Chagas disease, which are characterized by structural and functional changes in infected individuals. In another very interesting article, Geenen provides basic principles of thymic development and function and elegantly describes the presentation of neuroendocrine self-antigens to the thymus, the primary role of a defect in central tolerance in the development of autoimmune endocrinopathies, and the theoretical principles of negative self-vaccination, particularly for type 1 diabetes mellitus.

The Adrenal Connection in Neuroimmunoendocrinology

Arzt's team examines in detail the molecular mechanisms of immunoendocrine interactions. They suggest that the functional cross-talk at the molecular level between immune and steroid signals constitutes the final integrative level of interaction between the immune and neuroendocrine systems. Expanding further on this field, Bornstein and colleagues demonstrate the crucial role toll-like receptors play in the immune adrenal cross-talk and suggest potential novel therapeutic interventions. Flordellis's team describes a newer role for the α_2-adrenergic receptors, different from that in neurotransmission, showing that they may also exhibit neurotrophic actions. On a clinical level, Beuschlein and Zapanti provide new evidence in the pathogenesis, investigation, and treatment of adrenal pathology. In his extensive article, Beuschlein summarizes the molecular aspects of adrenocortical tumorigenesis and discusses some prospects for clinical applications, whereas Zapanti integrates new developments of imaging modalities of the adrenal medulla in the diagnostic evaluation of pathologic lesions of this region.

The Stress System: Activators, Mediators, Effectors, and Counterregulators

Sternberg and Thayer describe how the autonomic nervous system is involved in many somatic and mental disorders, using a model of neurovisceral interaction. They suggest that vagal activity exhibits an inhibitory role in the regulation of homeostatic systems and that the identification of regulatory components of this system may help illuminate the way psychologic factors may influence health and disease. Tsatsoulis elegantly describes how stress hormones, acting on antigen-presenting immune cells, may influence the differentiation of bipotential T helper (Th) cells away from a Th1 and toward a Th2 phenotype and how this effect applies in the development of several autoimmune diseases in the thyroid gland. Buckingham and colleagues have provided evidence on annexin and glucocorticoids and their neuroendocrine–immune interface. Mastorakos and Ilias describe the way glucocorticoids and proinflammatory cytokines (particularly interleukin-6) are involved in somatic stress and affect health and disease. They also provide evidence of current therapeutic interventions that target interleukin-6 and/or its soluble receptor in a variety of autoimmune and inflammatory disorders.

Chronology of Advances in Neuroendocrine Immunomodulation[a]

SAMUEL M. McCANN, ANDREA DE LAURENTIIS, AND VALERIA RETTORI

Centro de Estudios Farmacológicos y Botánicos, Consejo Nacional de Investigaciones Científicas y Técnicas (CEFYBO-CONICET), Facultad de Medicina, UBA, Paraguay 2155, CP 1121, Buenos Aires, Argentina

ABSTRACT: This review documents the remarkable progress over the last 50 years of our knowledge of the control of anterior pituitary hormone release and synthesis by a family of peptidic releasing and inhibiting hormones, synthesized in hypothalamic neurons and released into the hypophysial portal vessels. These vessels transport them to the anterior pituitary, where they stimulate release and synthesis of pituitary hormones or inhibit these processes. In general, there are at least two hypothalamic hormones for each pituitary hormone–vasopressin and corticotrophin-releasing hormone (CRH) for adrenocorticotropin hormone (ACTH) and growth hormone–releasing hormone (GHRH) and growth hormone–inhibiting hormone (GIH) for growth hormone (GH). Some of these hormones have extrapituitary action: for example, luteinizing hormone–releasing hormone (LHRH) stimulates mating behavior. High doses of LHRH have an inhibitory action on the growth of prostate cancer. Proinflammatory and anti-inflammatory cytokines act not only in the brain, but also on the pituitary and peripheral tissues. All of these transmitters are controlled by neuronal transmitters. We anticipate further rapid progress and clinical application of these transmitters and the discovery of new ones.

KEYWORDS: vasopressin; oxytocin; corticotropin-releasing hormone (CRH); LHRH; FSH-RH; GHRH; GH-inhibiting hormone (GHI); somatostatin; prolactin-inhibitory factor

I was fortunate to be on the scene as the dramatic developments in neuroendocrine immunomodulation took place over the last 55 years. Biological science had its birth with the Greeks and the first great physician, Hippocrates; however, his studies were observational, and it remained for Galen

[a]This paper has been modified with permission from an article by Samuel M. McCann in *Physiological Mini-Reviews* (Vol. 1, No. 9, April 2006) published by the Argentina Physiological Society.

Address for correspondence: Samuel M. McCann, Facultad de Medicina, UBA, CEFYBO-CONICET, Paraguay 2155, piso 16, CP 1121, Buenos Aires, Argentina. Voice: 54-11-4508-3680; fax: 54-11-4508-3680.
e-mail: smmccann2003@yahoo.com

Ann. N.Y. Acad. Sci. 1088: 1–11 (2006). © 2006 New York Academy of Sciences.
doi: 10.1196/annals.1366.010

(AD 130–200) to initiate studies employing the experimental method. There were virtually no advances during the subsequent 1,300 years, until Michael Servetus in the 16th century discovered the valves in veins. His reward was to be burned at the stake for heresy by Philip II of Spain.[1] Descartes (1596–1650) speculated on the function of the pituitary, but modern physiology had its birth when Walter Cannon (1871–1945) studied the flight-or-fright response of animals in stress involving activation of the adrenal medulla, which secreted sympathin-excitatory (e) and sympathin-inhibitory (i). Unfortunately, he did not discover the structure of the secreted substances. Presumably, sympathin was epinephrine. It remained for U.S. von Euler to determine this structure, and that this compound was norepinephrine.[1]

Hans Selye discovered the activation of the adrenal cortex by stress, and demonstrated many other changes produced by stress, such as involution of lymph nodes and the thymus that were accompanied by lymphopenia, eosinopenia, and leukocytosis. He believed that these changes were caused by increases in plasma histamine activating adrenocorticotropic hormone (ACTH) release directly from the adenohypophysis. He did not believe that the central nervous system (CNS) was involved. Actually histamine can activate the hypothalamic–pituitary–adrenal axis, but this is not the major pathway.[2]

A means by which the brain could control the anterior pituitary gland was discovered by B. A. Houssay *et al.* (1933).[1] In the living toad, they found that portal vessels drained blood from a primary capillary plexus in the median eminence (ME) down the pituitary stalk to the sinusoids in the anterior pituitary gland. Popa and Fielding[1] found these vessels in dead animals but believed that the blood flow was upward from the pituitary to the ME, a conclusion also reached in the dead rabbit by G. W. Harris.[1] Later, with Green (1947),[1] he found that the flow was downward in the living rat. Because the blood pressure in the portal vessels is very low, it is likely that, depending on the conditions, flow can be either upward or downward. In addition, the short portal vessels carry blood from the neural lobe across the intermediate lobe to the anterior lobe, thus delivering neural lobe hormones directly in high concentrations to the anterior lobe of the gland. This fact has been largely neglected.[1]

Dwight Ingle (1938) carried out pioneering studies that indicated that the adrenal cortical hormones had a negative feedback at the pituitary gland to suppress ACTH secretion.[3] It was thought at that time that the response of the cortical hormones to stress was slow; however, Ingle showed that following unilateral adrenalectomy there was an increase in weight of the remaining adrenal within 6 h caused by decreased secretion of adrenal steroids. This decreased negative feedback of these steroids resulted in increased ACTH secretion, which produced enlargement of the remaining gland.[3]

In 1943 Li *et al.*[4] and Sayers *et al.*[5] almost simultaneously isolated ACTH, facilitating studies with this important stress hormone. Sayers[6] had shown that stress caused a decrease in adrenal ascorbic acid concentration within 1 h, which could also be produced by ACTH. The stress-induced decline was blocked by hypophysectomy. Farrell and I decided to see whether we could measure ACTH in blood by etherizing rats and withdrawing blood from the external jugular vein, which was then injected into the external jugular vein of a hypophysectomized rat. Indeed, detectable ACTH was found. A further significant increase was induced within 1 min by intravenous (i.v.) injection of 5 μg of epinephrine. This ACTH was purified by the acid acetone method of Lyons. These studies convinced us that there was a hypothalamic–pituitary axis under minute-to-minute control by hypothalamic releasing factors, which we named corticotrophin-releasing factors (CRFs).[7] This term was coined by my roommate Al Rothballer, who showed that stress caused a depletion of the Gomori-positive material from the neurohypophysis. He gave the name CRF to Murray Saffran, who never acknowledged its origin.

I set about to determine whether ME lesions would block the adrenal cortical stress response in both cats and rats. I knew that unilateral adrenalectomy in etherized rats led to a dramatic depletion of adrenal ascorbic acid within 1 h and showed that ME lesions completely blocked this response (1953).[8] With Walle Nauta, we also showed that arcuate nucleus lesions caused testicular and accessory sex organ atrophy, an indication that gonadotropin secretion had been blocked.[8] There was atrophy of the neural lobe of the pituitary accompanied by diabetes insipidus, indicative of deficiency of the neurohypophysial hormone, vasopressin, and hypertrophy of the intermediate lobe— suggesting augmentation of intermediate lobe hormone secretion, which was later proven. The anterior lobe was usually moderately decreased in size and was well vascularized, suggesting that portal blood flow was intact. Plasma and pituitary ACTH was drastically lowered in etherized rats with ME lesions, providing further evidence for hypothalamic control of synthesis and release of ACTH.[9]

Bogdanove (1954)[1] did similar studies that were reported later, but did not study ACTH secretion. Ganong showed that ME lesions blocked compensatory adrenal hypertrophy in dogs (1954).[1] ME lesions also blocked ACTH secretion in the cat, as evidenced by decreased cortisol in adrenal venous blood and histological changes in adrenals similar to those following hypophysectomy (1955).[10]

We hypothesized that the anterior pituitary was controlled by a family of releasing factors, one for each pituitary hormone. The assay animal for these factors would be the rat with ME lesions. Obviously we could not perform histologic studies to determine whether the lesions were complete, but in the process of making many such lesions in rats that were allowed to recover for 10–14 days, we noticed that rats that drank 200 mL or more of water per day (those with severe diabetes insipidus), roughly seven times of the normal intake, did not respond to stress or unilateral adrenalectomy with ascorbic acid depletion 1 h later. Histologic examination of the brains of these rats indicated that the supraoptic hypophyseal tract had been interrupted in the ME, which was itself destroyed.

Interestingly, as the water intake increased up to 150 mL/day, the adrenal weight decreased to a minimum. Some rats with ME lesions had much higher water intakes, as a result of which the adrenal weight increased from the minimum to a maximum. We still do not know the cause of this.[11] Ascorbic acid depletion was still blocked.[12] ME lesions increase αMSH secretion from the pars intermedia and prolactin release[11,13] by obliterating dopaminergic inhibitory control of prolactin because ME lesions would destroy the tuberoinfundibular DA neurons.

Therefore, we used these rats with ME lesions and H_2O intake of 200 mL or more per day as an assay animal to screen for possible CRFs. Pitressin, a commercial arginine vasopressin preparation, decreased adrenal ascorbic acid significantly in a dose-dependent manner in rats with ME lesions. Commercial oxytocin had no effect. There was no action of epinephrine (1954).[12] Probably because of the long period between operation and testing, it occurred to us that testing only 48 h after lesions might yield a more sensitive preparation. Indeed, if these rats had a water intake of 100 mL or more 24 h after lesions were made, they were much more sensitive to vasopressin but did not respond to nonspecific stimuli. We used these rats to demonstrate the CRF activity of synthetic lysine vasopressin given to us by du Vigneaud,[14,15] who had just received the Nobel Prize for synthesizing vasopressin as well as oxytocin.

Using this more sensitive assay, we demonstrated the CRH activity of rat stalk median eminence (SME) extracts and SME extracts from sheep. These were contaminated with ACTH and vasopressin, and we quantified their ascorbic acid–depleting activity in our animals; roughly 80% of the activity was due to CRF (1959).[16] Royce and Sayers obtained similar results.

Our major competitors were the first to use incubation of quartered anterior pituitaries and confirmed the ability of vasopressin to release ACTH, but claimed that there was a CRF activity contaminating the vasopressin that could also stimulate secretion of ACTH. This was also demonstrated in the presence of norepinephrine. Guillemin and Hearn and Saffran and Schally used paper chromatographic systems to separate vasopressin from CRF. Using our assay we found vasopressin with CRF activity, but no CRF using their chromatographic systems. Subsequently Guillemin and Schally claimed to isolate α1 and α2 and βCRF. These CRFs were part of the prophetic literature and soon disappeared from the literature. A major problem of these researchers' work was that they used pituitary and not hypothalamic extracts. Also they did not preincubate the pituitaries, so that the hormones that leaked from the cut glands made it very difficult to see a small increment of ACTH possibly released by neural lobe extracts. Joe Meites was the first to preincubate hemi-anterior pituitaries to wash out the hormones from the cut glands, which made it possible to use hemipituitaries as a bioassay for releasing factors. Later both Guillemin and Schally extracted hypothalami. Schally used porcine and Guillemin used ovine hypothalami.

Our CRF was purified and separated on Sephadex G-25 followed by CMC chromatography[17,18] from other releasing and inhibiting factors (1959–1965). Because it was a much larger peptide (40 aa [amino acids]) than the other releasing factors, it defied structural characterization for many years. As late as the late 1960s, the President of the American Endocrine Society drew a diagram of the hypophysial–adrenal axis leaving out the hypothalamus and CRF. Later we found that vasopressin potentiates the action of CRFs on the pituitary.[19]

Evidence that oxytocin might be a prolactin-releasing factor was provided by Benson and Foley (1959). We confirmed their finding that oxytocin delayed the histological involution of mammary glands of rats from which the litter had been removed. Much later we obtained evidence for a physiological role of oxytocin in the control of prolactin secretion.[20]

Reflection made it seem odd that oxytocin, one of the three most abundant peptides in the body (the others being vasopressin and atrial natriuretic peptide) would have so little function. As I was flying down to Rio de Janeiro, this obvious idea occurred to me. Furthermore, I guessed that it was involved in cardiovascular system function. When I arrived at the office of José Antunes Rodrigues, one of my long-term collaborators, his assistant jumped at the idea and lo and behold, oxytocin has a physiologically significant role in physiology of the cardiovascular system to decrease the rate and force of contraction of the heart and to dilate blood vessels (1997).[21] It is present in the heart and blood vessels and plays a role in the development of the circulation. Oxytocin can convert stem cells into a sheet of synchronously beating cardiomyocytes (2002).[22] These studies complemented our studies of the role of ANP in the cardiovascular system and the body fluid homeostasis (1997).[23]

I felt that there should be both a follicle-stimulating hormone-releasing factor (FSHRF) and a luteinizing hormone-releasing hormone (LHRH) to control secretion of follicle-stimulating hormone (FSH) and luteinizing hormone (LH), respectively, from the anterior pituitary. What we needed was an assay animal. Because the gonads are steroid-secreting glands like the adrenal, I hypothesized that LH might cause a depletion of ascorbic acid in the testis or from the corpus luteum obtained from pseudopregnant rats. I found little if any effect. That year (1958), the Federation Meeting was held in Philadelphia, a stone's throw away from my office. Amazingly, Al Parlow presented the assay for LH in young pregnant mare's serum (PMS) and human chorionic gonadotropin (HCG) hormone–injected female rats. I was amazed and immediately set out to verify his results. I also injected a 0.1 N HCl extract of rat SMEs, the exact method used to extract CRF.

There was a dose-related effect of SME extract, in that it depleted ovarian ascorbic acid, whereas similar extracts from cerebral cortex had no effect. There was no effect of epinephrine, norepinephrine, serotonin, or substance P. To rule out LH in the hypothalamic extracts, I had the people at the Hormone Assay Lab inject PMS followed by HCG either before or after hypophysectomy and then send the rats to me by air mail. To my chagrin, hypophysectomy caused a 2–3-fold decline in ovarian ascorbic acid and a loss of sensitivity to LH.

I was going to the International Congress of Physiology in Buenos Aires in 1959 and had planned to give the results. Instead, after meeting Bernardo Houssay and Luis Leloir, the first a Nobel laureate, and the second as stated by Houssay to become one (for Chemistry, in 1970), I met Samuel Taleisnik (director of the Institute in Cordoba), who was to join me in Philadelphia on the recommendation of Houssay. We took the night train to Cordoba. I asked him if he could do hypophysectomy in baby rats. He said he could. I showed him the data and told him that he would be doing hypophysectomy in Philadelphia. He came to Philadelphia and was working on nine papers in 1 year. We ruled out LH as a factor in the ascorbic acid depletion and published the first paper on LH-RF.[24] I asked Taleisnik to stay, but he could not because he was director of the Institute. After he left, I showed that if you inject hypothalamic extract i.v. into ovariectomized, estrogen-primed rats, blood LH increases. Also, LH-RF was a peptide according to enzymatic degradation studies.

At this time (1963), Masao Igarashi came from Japan. He brought with him a new, more sensitive assay for FSH, the mouse uterine weight augmentation assay. The Steelman-Pohley assay was too insensitive for our studies. I told him that after a few improvements, his assay would be suitable and we would discover the FSH-RF. He presented the discovery of FSH-RF at the Endocrine Meeting in Atlantic City in 1963 and we published in full shortly after in 1964.[25] I had no experience and had no luck trying to recruit peptide chemists. Gel filtration on Shephadex G-25 appeared to be an ideal technique to separate small peptides. Therefore, I set up a small column of Shephadex G-25 and collected the fractions overnight in the cold room. The peaks of FSH-RF and LHRH overlapped completely.

Fortunately, Anand Dhariwal arrived at this point (1965). He set up a tall skinny Shephadex G-25 column. There was a clear separation of the FSH-RF eluting just prior to the LHRH. Schally confirmed these results using the FSH assay, shown to him on the way back to Japan by Igarashi. Now, Schally does not quote his own work, which was doing severe damage to this field! Not only did we separate FSH-RF from LHRH but also from other releasing factors.[17,26]

We believe FSH-RF is lamprey GnRH III. Antibodies against it block the action of FSH-RF. It is localized to the dorsomedial preoptic area, an area that controls FSH release and not LH release.[27] Mass spectroscopy of purified FSH-releasing hypothalamic extracts reveals a peptide with its molecular weight (unpublished data). Biotinylated L-GnRH III binds selectively to FSH gonadotropes, whereas biotinylated LHRH binds selectively to LH gonadotropes.[27] FSH-RF mediates separate pulses of FSH.[27]

It occurred to me that since mating behavior occurred in the rat shortly after LH was released to induce ovulation, LHRH might induce mating behavior. I had no experience with mating studies, but Lady Luck came to my aid. I needed an electrophysiologist for the physiology department. I indicated this to my friend Barry Cross at poolside at a meeting at the Santa Ines Inn off Sunset Boulevard, looking on the sea. He said Bob Moss, an American, had shown that oxytocin had a positive feedback on oxytocin neurons and wanted to come back to the USA. When I saw his CV, I discovered that he had obtained his degree for sex behavior studies in rats. When he came, I told him my idea and said that when the structure of LHRH broke we would test it for mating behavior. It was not long until the structure was elucidated in Schally's laboratory by Matsuo. I called Schally and asked if we could have some synthetic LHRH. He said it already was being provided to people in 40 laboratories around the world. Fortunately, we got it quite without his help soon. I gave some to Moss and asked him to try it. Several months went by. Finally I called him in. He said he was sure it would not work, so he had not tried it. I said I think it will work, so try a high dose in ovariectomized estradiol-primed rats. If it does not work, you will be finished with it, but if it works, you will be working with it for the rest of your life. It worked like a charm,[28] and he worked on it until his premature death.

We had earlier studied the effect of cAMP on hypothalamic pituitary function and since cGMP had no known functions and was a major cyclic nucleotide, we wondered whether cGMP might have a role to play. Indeed, we found that cGMP mediated the action of GnRHs on the pituitary.[2,29,30] Now we know that nitric oxide (NO) stimulates gonadotropin release by cGMP.[27]

Lad Krulich from Prague had been working with us for some years. We decided to see whether our hypothalamic extracts would stimulate GH release from the pituitary. He would inject the SME extract intravenously and then measure the depletion of GH from the pituitary assayed by widening of the tibial epiphyseal plate of hypophysectomized rats. He quickly found a hypothalamic GH-RF and then switched to a better assay studying the effect of purified hypothalamic extracts on GH release from rat pituitaries *in vitro*. With Dhariwal, he purified the growth hormone–inhibitory factor (GIF) by gel filtration and carboxymethylcellulose ion exchange chromatography (CMC), separating it from the other releasing factors.[31,32]

Several years later, Guillemin's group purified this peptide and synthesized it, renaming it somatostatin (1972). In the original version of this manuscript he didn't mention our work. The referees complained, and it was changed to say that we had found it in crude extracts. That was incorrect because crude extracts had a GH-releasing action. Somatostatin is a tetradecapeptide that has never been shown to have growth inhibitory action. The name is a misnomer but is still used.

We purified and separated all of these peptides, one from another that we worked on. Gel filtration on Sephadex G-25 separated more or less according to molecular weight. The larger peptide is the one eluted earlier—the largest CRF eluted followed by GRF, GIF, FSH-RF, LHRH, and vasopressin.[17] We discovered a peptidic prolactin-inhibiting factor (PIF), but did not pursue this further since dopamine turned out to be a powerful PIF.[27]

By cutting frozen sections horizontally and frontally we localized the various releasing factors in the preoptic and hypothalamic areas,[33] results later confirmed by immunocytochemistry. Martini postulated that pituitary hormones would have a short-loop negative feedback and that hypothalamic hormones would have an ultrashort negative feedback. We have found many examples of these actions,[27] which probably act for all transmitters.

In the ovariectomized estrogen-primed female rat, the negative feedback of estrogen to decrease LHRH release is reversed and becomes positive to increase LHRH release by NO, which stimulates LH release from the adenohypophysis but also acts in the brain stem to augment mating behavior by inducing lordosis. It also activates pelvic neurons, which act by releasing NO in the corpora cavernosa of the penis to cause penile erection.[27] This is but one example of the ubiquitous role of NO as a synaptic transmitter.

Acetylcholine, dopamine, NE, serotonin, glutamic acid, gamma amino butyric acid, and NO interact in complex ways to participate in the hypothalamic control of hormone release and inhibiting hormone release.[27]

In 1966, we published our first study on neuroimmunomodulation, which was a comparison of the effect of environmental and preoptic heating with that of fever induced by purified bacterial lipopolysaccharide (LPS), which caused an increase in the cortisol release in dogs.[34] Twenty years later we determined the ability of proinflammatory cytokines to induce the pattern of pituitary hormone release during infection.[35] With Valeria Rettori and Les Dees we showed with immunocytochemistry that there were some neurons containing IL-1 α among the dorsomedial preoptic temperature-sensitive neurons and that they were dramatically induced by LPS.[36] Ma Li Wong showed that IL-1 βmRNA could be induced in neurons in the paraventricular and arcuate nucleus by LPS.[37]

With Omid Khoram and Jim Lipton we showed that alpha melanocyte-stimulating hormone (αMSH) had an antipyretic effect on LPS-induced fever. Indeed α-MSH is an anti-inflammatory cytokine.[38]

With Tibor Wenger and Valeria Rettori we studied the hypothalamic action of δ9-tetrahydrocannabinol, the active ingredient of marijuana.[39] We believed that there must be an endogenous cannabinoid with appropriate receptors. We were pleased to see the discovery of an endogenous ligand, anandamide (AEA) with two receptors, CB1r and CBb2r. With Valeria Rettori and her group we have carried out extensive studies indicating that many drugs act by endocannabinoids' activating CB1r or CB2r. For example the action of alcohol to suppress LHRH release can be blocked by a CB1r blocker.[40]

With Ramirez, we found that immature rats were excruciatingly sensitive to the negative feedback of gonadal steroids. After puberty the sensitivity declined several-fold.[41] Some time later Coleman discovered dwarfed obese sterile mice. The defect was in a single gene named obese (*Ob*). Only homozygous *Ob-Ob* mice showed the defects. Coleman parabiosed a thin mouse to an *Ob-Ob* mouse, resulting in the fat mouse's becoming thin. It was hypothesized that there was a hormonal defect in the fat mouse. People looked in vain for the hormone in the blood and in the urine. Nothing happened until Zhang and Friedmann obtained its structure by positional cloning, making possible the synthesis of leptin.

With Wen Yu we determined that leptin acted in the basal tuberal region to release LHRH via NO. It also acted on the anterior pituitary to stimulate LH and to a lesser extent FSH with the same potency as LHRH. Surprisingly, leptin was present in adipocytes in large amounts and secretion could be stimulated within 10 min. There was a circadian rhythm of plasma leptin with a peak at 1:30 AM and a nadir at 7:30 AM in man and rats. Finally, plasma leptin throughout the 24 h paralleled that of NO_2-NO_3, suggesting that leptin stimulated NO. Indeed, leptin stimulated NO_2-NO_3 and TNF-α release from incubated epididymal fat pads.[42] Finally, Julio Licinio demonstrated that *Ob-Ob* humans failed to go into puberty, but that it could be induced by leptin, indicating that leptin is the major inducer of puberty.[43]

In conclusion, it has been a wonderful ride. I believe scientists can be increasingly productive in the next 50 years if we continue to provide money to productive people. Money should be provided on the basis of merit and not age. When productivity declines, money should be reallocated. We must be open to new ideas. Almost every new idea we had met with a barrier. One must take time to go over a problem considering all the possibilities for its solution. This is the way to get new ideas. The most important thing for progress is the new idea. Without it progress ceases.

REFERENCES

1. McCANN, S.M., A.P.S. DHARIWAL & J.C. PORTER. 1968. Regulation of the adeno-hypophysis. Annu. Rev. Physiol. **30:** 589–640.
2. LIBERTUM, C. & S.M. McCANN. 1976. The possible role of histamine in the control of prolactin and gonadotropin release. Neuroendocrinology **20:** 110–120.
3. INGLE, D.J. 1938. Science **86:** 245.
4. LI, C.H., H.M. EVANS & M.E. SIMPSON. 1943. J. Biol. Chem. **149:** 413–424.
5. SAYERS, G., A. WHITE & C.N.H. LONG. 1943. J. Biol. Chem. **149:** 425–436.
6. SAYERS, G. 1950. The adrenal cortex and homoestasis. Physiol. Rev. **30:**241–320.
7. FARREL, G.L. & S.M. McCANN. 1952. Detectable amounts of adrenocorticotropic hormone in blood following epinephrine. Endocrinology **50:** 274–276.
8. McCANN, S.M. 1953. Effect of hypothalamic lesions on the adrenal cortical responses to stress in the rat. Am. J. Physiol. **175:** 13–20.
9. McCANN, S.M. & K.L. SNYDOR. 1954. Blood and pituitary adrenocorticotrophin in adrenalectomized rats with hypothalamic lesions. Proc. Soc. Exp. Biol. Med. **87:** 369–373.
10. LAQUEUR, G.L., S.M. McCANN, L.H. SCHREINER, *et al.* 1955. Alterations of adrenal cortical and ovarian activity following hypothalamic lesions, based on eosinophile response, hormone assay and histological examination. Endocrinology **57:** 44–54.

11. MARUBAYASHI, U., S.M. MCCANN & J. ANTUNES RODRIGUES. 1987. Factors controlling adrenal weight and corticosterone secretion in male rats as revealed by median eminence lesions and pharmacological alteration of prolactin secretion. Brain. Res. Bull. **19:** 511–518.
12. MCCANN, S.M. & J.R. BROBECK. 1954. Evidence for a role of the supraoptico-hypophyseal system in regulation of adrenocorticotrophin secretion. Proc. Soc. Exp. Biol. Med. **87:** 318–324.
13. BISHOP, W., L. KRULICH, C.P. FAWCETT & S.M. MCCANN. 1971. The effect of median eminence (ME) lesions on plasma levels of FSH, LH and prolactin in the rat. Proc. Soc. Exp. Biol. Med. **136:** 925–927.
14. MCCANN, S.M. & A. FRUIT. 1957. Effect of synthetic vasopressin on release of adrenocorticotrophin in rats with hypothalamic lesions. Proc. Soc. Exp. Biol. Med. **96:** 566–567.
15. MCCANN, S.M. 1957. The ACTH-releasing activity of extracts of the posterior lobe of the pituitary *in vivo*. Endocrinology **60:** 664–676.
16. MCCANN, S.M. & P. HABERLAND. 1959. Relative abundance of vasopressin and corticotrophin-releasing factor in neurohypophyseal extracts. Proc. Soc. Exp. Biol. Med. **102:** 319–325.
17. MCCANN, S.M., A.P.S. DHARIWAL & J.C. PORTER. 1968. Regulation of the adeno-hypophysis. Annu. Rev. Physiol. **30:** 589–640.
18. MCCANN, S.M. 1988. Saga of the discovery of releasing and inhibiting hormones. *In* People and Ideas in Endocrinology, S.M. McCann, Ed.: 41–62. American Physiological Society.
19. YATES, F.E., S.M. RUSSELL, M.F. DALLMAN, *et al.* 1987. Potentiation by vasopressin of corticotropin release induced by corticotropin-releasing factor. Endocrinology **88:** 3–15.
20. SAMSON, W.K., M.D. LUMPKIN & S.M. MCCANN. 1986. Evidence for a physiological role for oxytocin in the control of prolactin secretion. Endocrinology **119:** 554–560.
21. ANTUNES RODRIGUES, J., M. DE CASTRO, L.L. ELIAS, *et al.* 2004. Neuroendocrine control of body fluid metabolism. Physiol. Rev. **84:** 169–208.
22. PAQUIN, J., B.A. DANALACHE, M. JANKOWSKI, *et al.* 2002. Oxytocin induces differentiation of P19 embryonic stem cells to cardiomyocytes. Proc. Natl. Acad. Sci. USA **99:** 9550–9555.
23. ANTUNES RODRIGUES, J., S.M. MCCANN & W.K. SAMSON. 1986. Central administration of atrial natriuretic factor inhibits salt intake in the rat. Endocrinology **118:** 1726–1729.
24. MCCANN, S.M., S. TALEISNIK & H.M. FRIEDMAN. 1960. LH-releasing activity in hypothalamic extracts. Proc. Soc. Exp. Biol. Med. **104:** 432–434.
25. IGARASHI, M. & S.M. MCCANN. 1964. A hypothalamic follicle stimulating hormone releasing factor. Endocrinology **74:** 446–452.
26. DHARIWAL, A.P.S., R. NALLAR, M. BATT & S.M. MCCANN. 1965. Separation of FSH-releasing factor from LH-releasing factor. Endocrinology **76:** 290–294.
27. MCCANN, S.M., S. KARANTH, C.A. MASTRONARDI, *et al.* 2002. Hypothalamic control of gonadotropin secretion. *In* Progress in Brain Research, Volume 141, Gonadotropin-Releasing Hormone: Molecules and Receptors. I.S. Parhar, Ed.: 153–166. Elsevier Science. Amsterdam, the Netherlands.
28. MOSS, R.L. & S.M. MCCANN. 1973. Induction of mating behavior in rats by luteinizing hormone-releasing factor. Science **181:** 177–179.

29. NAKANO, H., C.P. FAWCETT, F. KIMURA & S.M. McCANN. 1978. Evidence for involvement of cGMP in regulation of gonadotropin release. Endocrinology **103:** 1527–1533.
30. NAOR, Z., C.P. FAWCETT & S.M. McCANN. 1978. The involvement of cGMP in LHRH stimulated gonadotropin release. Am. J. Physiol. **235:** 586–690.
31. KRULICH, L., A.P. DHARIWAL & S.M. McCANN. 1968. Stimulatory and inhibitory effects of purified hypothalamic extracts on growth hormone release from rat pituitary *in vitro*. Endocrinology **83:** 783–790.
32. KRULICH, L. & S.M. McCANN. 1969. Effect of GH-releasing factor and GH-inhibiting factor on the release and concentration of GH in pituitaries incubated *in vitro*. Endocrinology **85:** 319–324.
33. WHEATON, J.E., L. KRULICH & S.M. McCANN. 1975. Localization of LHRH in the preoptic area and hypothalamus of the rat using RIA. Endocrinology **97:** 30–38.
34. CHOWERS, I., H.T. HAMMEL & S.M. McCANN. 1964. Comparison of effect of environmental and preoptic cooling on plasma cortisol levels. Am. J. Physiol. **207:** 577–582.
35. McCANN, S.M., M. KIMURA, W.H. YU, *et al.* 2001. *In* Vitamins and Hormones, Vol 63. G. Litwack, Ed.: 29–62. Academic Press, San Diego.
36. RETTORI, V., W.L. DEES, J.K. HINEY, *et al.* 1994. An IL-1 α-like neuronal system in the preoptic hypothalamic region and its induction by LPS in concentrations which alter pituitary hormone release. Neuroimmunomodulation **1:** 251–258.
37. WONG, M.L., V. RETTORI, A. AL-SHEKLEE, *et al.* 1996. Inducible NO synthase gene expression in the brain during systemic inflammation. Nat. Med. **2:** 581–584.
38. SHIH, S.T., O. KHORRAM, J.M. LIPTON & S.M. McCANN. 1986. Central administration of α-MSH antiserum augments fever in the rabbit. Am. J. Physiol. **250:** 803–806.
39. WENGER, T., V. RETTORI, G.D. SNYDER, *et al.* 1987. Effects of delta 9-tetrahydrocannabinol (THC) on the hypothalamic-pituitary control of LH and FSH secretion in adult male rats. Neuroendocrinology **46:** 488–493.
40. FERNANDEZ SOLARI, J., C. SCORTICATI, C. MOHN, *et al.* 2004. Alcohol inhibits luteinizing hormone-releasing hormone release by activating the endocannabinoid system. Proc. Natl. Acad. Sci. USA **101:** 3256–3268.
41. RAMIREZ, V.D. & S.M. McCANN. 1963. A comparison of the regulation of luteinizing hormone (LH) secretion in immature and adult rats. Endocrinology **72:** 452–464.
42. McCANN, S.M., S. KARANTH, W.H. YU & C.A. MASTRONARDI. 2003. Neuroendocrine regulation of leptin secretion and its role in nitric oxide secretion. *In* Leptin and Reproduction. Henson & Castracane, Eds.: Kluwer Academic Plenum Publishers. New York.
43. LICINIO, J., S. CAGLAYAN, M. OZATA, *et al.* 2004. Phenotypic effects of leptin replacement on morbid obesity, diabetes mellitus, hypogonadism, and behavior in leptin-deficient adults. Proc. Natl. Acad. Sci. USA **101:** 4531–4536.

The Mitochondrion as a Primary Site of Action of Regulatory Agents Involved in Neuroimmunomodulation

A.M.G. PSARRA,[a] S. SOLAKIDI,[b] AND C.E. SEKERIS[b]

[a]*Foundation for Biomedical Research of the Academy of Athens, Center for Basic Research, 11527 Athens, Greece*

[b]*National Hellenic Research Foundation, Institute of Biological Research and Biotechnology, Laboratory of Molecular Endocrinology, 11635 Athens, Greece*

ABSTRACT: A major system of neuroimmunomodulation is the hypothalamic-pituitary-adrenocortical (HPA) axis, acting through glucocorticoids and their intracellular signaling components, exerting both stimulatory and inhibitory effects on the immune reaction. Glucocorticoids inhibit the production of proinflammatory cytokines by interacting with nuclear transcription factors (nuclear factor [NF]-κB, activated protein [AP]-1) and induce the production of several anti-inflammatory cytokines by gene activation. In some cells and/or in extreme stress conditions, apoptosis is evoked. In most processes related to neuroimmunomodulation a prominent role is emerging for mitochondria. These organelles generate more than 90% of the cell's energy requirements through oxidative phosphorylation (OXPHOS), which is regulated by several agents, including steroid and thyroid hormones. These hormones are inducers of nuclear and mitochondrial OXPHOS gene transcription and they exert a primary action not only on nuclear but also on mitochondrial genes by way of cognate receptors. Recently, additional nuclear transcription factors involved in neuroimmunomodulation have been detected in mitochondria (NF-κB, AP-1, p53, calcium/cAMP response element binding protein [CREB]), and binding sites of these and putative binding sites of other nuclear transcription factors have been identified in the mitochondrial genome. The interaction of these factors with mitochondrial regulatory proteins, with receptors and with the genome has been shown and, in some cases, modulation of mitochondrial transcription was observed with possible effects on energy yield. The mitochondria store a host of critical apoptotic activators and inhibitors in their intermembrane space and the release of these factors could be another possible mode of action of the mitochondrially translocated regulatory agents and receptors.

Address for correspondence: Prof. CE Sekeris, 48 Vas Constantinou Ave, 11635 Athens, Greece. Voice: 0030-210-7273767; fax: 0030-210-7273677.
e-mail: csekeris@eie.gr

Ann. N.Y. Acad. Sci. 1088: 12–22 (2006). © 2006 New York Academy of Sciences.
doi: 10.1196/annals.1366.019

KEYWORDS: neuroimmunomodulation; mitochondrion; transcription factors; steroid/thyroid receptors; oxidative phosphorylation; apoptosis

INTRODUCTION

The modulation of the immune response by neuronal and hormonal agents is currently receiving strong experimental support. In this context, the autonomic nervous system, the hypothalamic-pituitary-adrenocortical (HPA) axis, and the sympathetic-neural-adrenomedullary systems exert both stimulatory and inhibitory effects on the immune reaction, through hormones, other regulatory agents, and their intracellular signaling components.[1,2]

Glucocorticoids represent major regulatory agents of the immune and inflammatory response, inhibiting the production of proinflammatory cytokines and chemokines (such as tumor necrosis factor (TNF)-α, interleukin (IL)-2, IL-6, IL-1β, IL-8, and RANTES [regulated on activation normal T cell expressed and secreted]), as well as cytokine receptors, whereas they induce the synthesis of anti-inflammatory cytokines (such as IL-10, IL-4, and TGF-β) by activating transcription of respective genes.[3,4] The inhibitory effects of glucocorticoids on the proinflammatory elements are exerted by crosstalk with nuclear transcription factors and signaling pathways, such as nuclear factor (NF)-κB and activated protein (AP)-1. Glucocorticoids thus lead to negative effects on the transcription of immunoregulatory genes, containing the respective NF-κB and AP-1 binding sites on their promoters or regulatory regions.[5] Glucocorticoids also regulate thymocyte and lymphocyte selection and survival and some of their functions.[6]

In addition to the important nuclear events, recent findings point to the emerging role of mitochondria in neuroimmunomodulation. Mitochondria represent the principal energy source of the cell, providing more than 90% of its needs by way of oxidative phosphorylation (OXPHOS). Furthermore, mitochondria contain the enzymes needed for free fatty acid metabolism, the Krebs cycle, and the key steps of heme biosynthesis and hormone synthesis. Additionally, the mitochondria generate the majority of cellular reactive oxygen species (ROS), have specialized scavenging systems to protect themselves and the cell from these toxic byproducts, and host key machinery for programmed cell death, serving, therefore, as gatekeepers of apoptosis.[7] The energy requirements of the cell fluctuate depending on the physiological state, are higher in metabolically demanding developmental conditions and lower when the cell initiates a series of steps leading to apoptosis, the attenuation of energy production being one of the early events in this process.

Steroid and thyroid hormones are major regulators of energy yield, by exerting rapid, nongenomic effects, as well as by inducing nuclear and mitochondrial OXPHOS genes.[8] These hormones exert their actions not only at the nuclear, but also at the mitochondrial level, by way of cognate receptors localized both in cell nucleus and mitochondria.[8]

In addition to hormone receptors, other nuclear transcription factors known to play a major role in neuroimmunomodulation, such as NF-κB, AP-1, p53, and calcium/cAMP response element binding protein (CREB), have been detected in mitochondria. The role of these nuclear transcription factors on mitochondrial physiology and their potential crosstalk with nuclear emanating processes in neuroimmunomodulation is now beginning to receive due consideration.

STEROID AND THYROID HORMONE RECEPTORS IN MITOCHONDRIA

In the past decade, steroid and thyroid hormone receptors have been detected in mitochondria of animal cells. Glucocorticoid receptors were first detected in rat liver mitochondria by the Western blotting of mitochondrial extracts, using specific antibodies to the receptor and by immunogold electron microscopy.[9] Subsequently, glucocorticoid receptors were found in mitochondria from various sources, such as HeLa cells,[10] rat brain cells,[11] C_2C_4 mouse glial cells,[12] salamander retina Mueller cells,[13] and recently in human hepatocarcinoma HepG2 and osteosarcoma SaOS-2 cell lines.[14] Estrogen receptors have also been detected in mitochondria of various cells.[15–20] Recently, androgen receptors were also found in mitochondria of human spermatozoa and human prostate cancer LnCap cells.[20] The mitochondria-specific thyroid hormone receptor p46, a truncated form of TR-α, was also detected[21] and its importance in transcription regulation was demonstrated.[8] Thyroid hormone receptor was also demonstrated in HeLa cells by immunofluorescence confocal microscopy.[8,22] Other members of the nuclear receptor family present in mitochondria are the retinoic acid receptor (RAR),[23,24] the retinoic X receptor (RXR), and the orphan receptor Nur70.[25]

OTHER NUCLEAR TRANSCRIPTION FACTORS PRESENT IN MITOCHONDRIA

NF-κB

The presence of NF-κB in mitochondria was reported in 2001.[26] An interaction of the inhibitory protein IκB-α with the mitochondrial ATP/ATP translocator ANT1, using a two-hybrid system in yeast was shown. This led to the detection of an IκB-α/p65-NF-κB complex in mitochondria and the demonstration of the p65 molecule in mitochondria of Jurkat cells, by immunogold electron microscopy. The p65 molecule was found in the intermembrane space and was shown to be released together with IκB-α after induction of apoptosis in Jurkat cells, upon engagement of the Fas surface molecule with the specific CH11 antibody. In a subsequent report,[27] a mitochondrial localization of

NF-κB and IκB-α was also demonstrated in U937 cells, by immunogold electron microscopy and immunoprecipitation in rat liver mitochondria by respective antibodies. Cytokine treatment of the cells led to reduction of expression of the mitochondrially encoded cytochrome oxidase III and cytochrome *b* mRNAs, whereas inhibition of the activation prevented the loss of expression of COXIII and cyt *b* mRNAs, pointing to a negative role of NF-κB on mitochondrial mRNA expression. Recently, NF-κB (p65 and p50) with DNA-binding activity was detected in mitochondria of human prostate cell lines.[28] By electrophoresis mobility shift analysis (EMSA) it was also shown that treatment of the cells with the TNF-related apoptosis-inducing ligand (TRAIL) increased DNA binding of NF-κB without changing the amount of p65 in mitochondria, suggesting activation of NF-κB without additional translocation of NF-κB subunits to mitochondria. TRAIL treatment also led to decreased mitochondrial-genome-encoded mRNA levels, which was prevented by inhibition of NF-κB, suggesting a role of NF-κB in the mitochondrial genome transcription process.[28]

Overexpressed ANT1 in HeLa cells led to a recruitment of the IκB-α/NF-κB complex into mitochondria with a coincidental decrease in nuclear NF-κB DNA-binding activity and downregulation of the antiapoptotic genes Bcl-X_L, MnSoD$_2$, and cIP$_2$.[29] It was proposed that mitochondrial recruitment of NF-κB following ANT1 overexpression was correlated to the proapoptotic activity of ANT1.

AP-1

The presence of AP-1 in mitochondria was demonstrated in studies investigating the effects of glutamic acid and its agonist kainate on brain function.[30] The excitatory amino acid L-glutamate participates in various neuronal processes, ranging from transient signal communication to long-term plasticity and immunomodulation. This is accomplished through the interaction of glutamic acid with ionotropic and metabotropic receptors in the central nervous system (CNS), the former classified into NMDA, alpha-amino-3-hydroxy-5-methyisoxazole-4-propionate, and kainate receptors. Glutamic acid signals lead to increased expression of both the c-fos gene and the c-Fos protein in mice and potentiation of DNA-binding activity of AP-1. In particular, the glutamic acid agonist kainate, known to induce the expression of c-Fos, c-Jun, JunB, and JunD, was administered to mice and 1–3 h later an enhanced AP-1 binding to DNA was detected in both mitochondrial and nuclear extracts of cerebral cortex and hippocampus. c-Fos was detected within mitochondria of subfield CA pyramidal and dental granular cells in hippocampus, by immunogold electron microscopy. DNA binding was inhibited by oligonucleotides containing sequences similar to the AP-1 binding site detected in the noncoding region of mitochondrial DNA. It was suggested that kainate may facilitate the expression of the AP-1 complex and its subsequent translocation into mitochondria, where it could participate in mechanisms associated with transcriptional regulation of mitochondrial DNA.[30] In a follow-up article, the potential binding sites of AP-1, corresponding to its nuclear binding sites, were identified in the noncoding region of the mitochondrial DNA (sequences MT1 to MT10).[31] Enhanced binding of AP-1 to sequences MT-3 and MT-9 was demonstrated by electrophoretic mobility shift analysis with mitochondrial extracts from hippocampi 2–6 h after kainate administration. In a recent article reporting the presence of NF-κB in prostate carcinoma cell mitochondria,[26] mitochondrial DNA-binding activity to AP-1 binding sequences was detected and it was significantly increased after TRAIL treatment of these cells.[26]

CREB

In studies concerning the possible importance of CREB in synaptic transmission, retrograde memory and brain function, this transcription factor was detected in mitochondria of rat brain and particularly in the inner mitochondrial membrane, by immunoblotting and immunogold electron microscopy.[32] It was also shown that mitochondrial CREB can be phosphorylated by protein kinase A and, as demonstrated by EMSA, can bind to double-stranded DNA containing the calcium-cycle AMP-responsive element consensus sequence. In a recent article that confirmed the previous findings, it was demonstrated that CREB is located in the matrix of the inner mitochondrial membrane of rat brain cells and that a calcium-dependent phosphatase regulates its phosphorylation state.[33]

p53

p53 was detected in membranes of mitochondria of fibroblasts of primary cultures of human skin and in cytoplasmic organelles, presumably mitochondria, of PHA-stimulated peripheral blood mononuclear cells.[34] Other research groups working with human HT1080 and murine C3H10T1/2 cells demonstrated, by immunoprecipitation using p53 and GRP75 (heat shock protein) antibodies, the presence of a p53-heat shock protein complex in mitochondrial extracts.[35] They also demonstrated the presence of p53 in mitochondria by immunogold electron microscopy. At the onset of p53-dependent apoptosis, after either DNA damage or hypoxia, a small, but significant, p53 fraction of stress-induced p53 was detected in the inner membrane fraction but also within the mitochondria of human cell lines, which was not the case during p53-independent apoptosis or during p53-mediated cell arrest.[36] The translocation of p53 into mitochondria was rapid, preceding the release of cytochrome c and procaspase activation, and was blocked by overexpression of the antiapoptotic protein Bcl-2. Targeting of p53 to mitochondria, using a mitochondrial import leader sequence, was sufficient to induce apoptosis in p53-deficient cells. Later, it was shown that the wild-type p53 protein directly induces mitochondrial permeabilization and cytochrome *c* release by forming inhibitory complexes with protective BclXL and Bcl2 proteins.[37] Some authors did not find a p53 consensus DNA-binding site by mitochondrial genome computer search.[36] Others, however, identified a putative p53 binding sequence in mitochondrial DNA, implying a direct effect of p53 on mitochondrial transcription/replication.[38] A role of p53 in mitochondrial transcription and translation processes in stress-related conditions has been proposed.[39-43] In cell lines conditionally immortalized with SV40, the proliferative potential is temperature-dependent. At the restrictive temperature, heat inactivation of the large T antigen caused p53 release, growth arrest, and apoptosis. A lower mitochondrial membrane potential ($\Delta \Psi$m) was observed, which correlated with an uncoupling of electron transport from ATP production. This was linked to the induction of apoptosis and associated with a decrease in the rate of mitochondrial translation.[39]

During early-stage response of HA-1 fibroblasts to oxidative stress, when extensive growth arrest and moderate apoptosis was observed, degradation of mitochondrial, but not nuclear, DNA took place,[40] accompanied by downregulation of mitochondrial, but not nuclear, RNA, encoding OXPHOS. Yoshida *et al.*[41] observed, corroborating previous findings, that at the onset of p53-dependent apoptosis, a fraction of p53 localized in mitochondria and could interact with the mitochondrial transcription factor mtTFA, enhancing its capacity to bind to cis-platin-damaged DNA, which indicated the involvement of p53 in the mitochondrial transcription process. A direct role of p53 in mitochondrial transcription has been suggested.[42] Treatment of NIH3T3 cells with a dominant negative p53 mutant led to decreased mitochondrial 16s rRNA and decreased staining of the mitochondria with the mitochondria-specific dye Mitotracker Red CMXRos. Altered expression of mitochondrial 16s rRNA has also been shown by differential RNA display in p53 knockout mouse embryos at the neurulation stage.[38]

NUCLEAR TRANSCRIPTION FACTORS IN MITOCHONDRIA: MODULATORS OF MITOCHONDRIAL TRANSCRIPTION AND APOPTOSIS

The detection of numerous transcription factors in mitochondria that are involved in immunomodulation, metabolic growth, developmental processes, and apoptosis, raises the question of the role of these factors in mitochondrial physiology and mitochondrial-linked processes. Practically all steroid and thyroid hormones affect some of these processes, not only by way of cognate receptors, which modulate gene activity, but also by initiating rapid hormonal effects through signal transduction pathways. The same nuclear receptors, in some cases in a variant form, have also been detected in mitochondria. The other nuclear transcription factors localized in mitochondria, are activators or inhibitors of transcription of several nuclear genes, either by direct interaction with the nuclear genome or indirectly by interaction with other DNA-binding proteins, such as the nuclear receptors. Many of the affected genes are involved in immunomodulation, including genes encoding cytokines, chemokines, and cytokine receptors.

The role within the confines of mitochondrion of nuclear transcription factors translocating into the organelle, particularly after the action of agents involved in immunomodulation and stress induction, is therefore in the center of interest. Regarding the nuclear receptor superfamily, experimental evidence has accumulated supporting an action in transcription within the confines of the mitochondrion, in a similar way as within the confines of the nucleus.[8,43]

Effects on mitochondrial RNA metabolism—transcription, processing, turnover, and translation—have been experimentally supported, regarding the action of NF-κB and p53 found in mitochondria.[27,42] Consensus sequences for these and other nuclear transcription factors have been determined in a computer search of the mitochondrial genome.[44] In this context, the interaction of steroid hormone receptors with NF-κB and AP-1, which is observed in the extramitochondrial space and plays a major role in modulating gene transcription, could also take place within the mitochondria.[5,45] The mitochondrial genome is totally devoted to energy production, as it solely encodes components of the OXPHOS complexes and RNA translation machinery. All cell-regulatory actions, including those involved in neuroimmunomodulation, are energy-dependent and are coupled to mitochondria. Depending on the degree of energy requirement, the mitochondria can respond to lower energy needs by allosteric activation of the OXPHOS chain and, in case of high demands, by increased expression of the OXPHOS enzymes. Steroid and thyroid hormones are known to exert their effects on energy metabolism by both genomic and nongenomic mechanisms.[8] Transcription factors localized in mitochondria could, therefore, also exert such a dual action. DOK-4 is a member of the downstream kinase family of adaptor proteins, an anchoring molecule for the tyrosine kinase c-src (also found in mitochondria), which enhances the production of TNF-α-mediated ROS, TNF-α-mediated NF-κB activation, and effects on complex I of the respiratory chain.[46] The presence of DOK-4 in mitochondria of endothelia points to the participation of src-kinase in mitochondrially mediated inflammatory responses and to mitochondrial NF-κB action on immunomodulation by rapid nongenomic effects.

Concerning apoptosis and the role of mitochondria and the mitochondrial transcription factors in this process it seems that these organelles store in their intermembrane space a panel of critical apoptotic activators and effectors of cell death, including cytochrome c, Smart/diabolo, AIF, and procaspase 2, and 9. A growing list of proapoptotic proteins that translocate to mitochondria and exert their proapoptotic functions interacting with the apoptotic agents stored in the organelles has been observed. Some of the effects of the translocating transcription factors on apoptosis could be exerted through nongenomic mechanisms, as described for the action of NF-κB[27] and p53.[47] The factors determining the choice between transcription-dependent and -independent mechanisms are still poorly understood.

EPILOGUE

Mitochondria are the main energy providers of the cell by way of OXPHOS, but also perform a series of other important functions. Their role in development, particularly in connection with muscle differentiation and pathophysiology of neuromuscular diseases, in aging and apoptosis is now being recognized. In addition to proteins involved in these processes, several translocating proteins not previously associated with mitochondrial functions and belonging to other biochemical classes are now being detected in mitochondria. Emerging categories of such proteins are the nuclear hormone receptors and the transcription factors NF-κB, AP-1, CREB, and p53. These proteins serve known developmental, growth, metabolic and neuroimmunomodulatory functions by way of genomic and nongenomic molecular mechanisms of action. Their presence in mitochondria, after translocation from the cytoplasm under diverse conditions, such as neuroimmunomodulation, suggests that these molecules in the mitochondria are involved in similar regulatory events as exerted in the nucleus, thus complementing and amplifying them. The experimental results supporting this concept are still mainly fragmentary and of a descriptive nature. However, the growing interest in this emerging field and the increasing rate of relevant research papers heralds rapid progress in our in-depth understanding of the role of mitochondria and the mitochondrially translocated nuclear transcription factors in neuroimmunomodulation.

ACKNOWLEDGMENTS

We thank the Bodossaki Foundation for financial support.

REFERENCES

1. CHROUSOS, G.P. 1995. The hypothalamic-pituitary-adrenal axis and immune-mediated inflammation. N. Engl. J. Med. **332:** 1351–1362.
2. WATKINS, L.R. & S.F. MAIER. 2005. Immune regulation of central nervous system functions: from sickness responses to pathological pain. J. Intern. Med. **257:** 139–155.
3. CATO, A.C., H. SCHACKE, W. STERRY & K. ASADULLAH. 2004. The glucocorticoid receptor as target for classic and novel anti-inflammatory therapy. Curr. Drug Targets Inflamm. Allergy **3:** 347–353.

4. SMOAK, K.A. & J.A. CIDLOWSKI. 2004. Mechanisms of glucocorticoid receptor signaling during inflammation. Mech. Ageing Dev. **125:** 697–706.
5. DE BOSSCHER, K., W. VANDEN BERGHE & G. HAEGEMAN. 2003. The interplay between the glucocorticoid receptor and nuclear factor-kappa B or activator protein-1: Molecular mechanisms for gene repression. Endocr. Reviews **24:** 488–522.
6. MANN, C.L., F.M. HUGHES, Jr. & J.A. CIDLOWSKI. 2000. Delineation of the signaling pathways involved in glucocorticoid-induced and spontaneous apoptosis or rat thymocytes. Endocrinology **141:** 528–538.
7. WALLACE, D.C. 1999. Mitochondrial diseases in man and mouse. Science **283:** 1482–1488.
8. SCHELLER, K., P. SEIBEL & C.E. SEKERIS. 2003. Glucocorticoid and thyroid hormone receptors in mitochondria of animal cells. Int. Rev. Cytol. **222:** 1–61.
9. DEMONACOS, C., N.C. TSAWDAROGLOU, R. DJORDJEVIC-MARKOVIC, et al. 1993. Import of the glucocorticoid receptor into rat liver mitochondria *in vivo* and *in vitro*. J. Steroid Biochem. Mol. Biol. **46:** 401–413.
10. SCHELLER, K., C.E. SEKERIS, G. KROHNE, et al. 2000. Localization of glucocorticoid hormone receptors in mitochondria of human cells. Eur. J. Cell Biol. **79:** 299–307.
11. MOUTSATSOU, P., A.-M.G. PSARRA, A. TSIAPARA, et al. 2001. Localization of the glucocorticoid receptor in rat brain mitochondria. Arch. Biochem. Biophys. **386:** 69–78.
12. KOUFALI, M.M., P. MOUTSATSOU, C.E. SEKERIS & K.C. BREEN. 2003. The dynamic localization of the glucocorticoid receptor in rat C6 glioma cell mitochondria. Mol. Cell. Endocrinol. **209:** 51–60.
13. PSARRA, A.-M.G., M.L. BOCHLATON-PIALLAT, G. GABBIANI, et al. 2003. Mitochondrial localization of glucocorticoid receptor in glial (Müller) cells in the salamander retina. Glia **41:** 38–49.
14. PSARRA, A.-M.G., S. SOLAKIDI, I.P. TROUGAKOS, et al. 2005. Glucocorticoid receptor isoforms in human hepatocarcinoma HepG2 and SaOS-2 osteosarcoma cells: Presence of glucocorticoid receptor alpha in mitochondria and of glucocorticoid receptor beta in nucleoli. Int. J. Biochem. Cell Biol. **37:** 2544–2558.
15. MONJE, P. & R. BOLAND. 2001. Subcellular distribution of native estrogen receptor alpha and beta isoforms in rabbit uterus and ovary. J. Cell. Biochem. **82:** 467–479.
16. CHEN, J.Q., M. DELANNOY, C. COOKE & J.D. YAGER. 2004. Mitochondrial localization of ERalpha and ERbeta in human MCF7 cells. Am. J. Physiol. Endocrinol. Metab. **286:** E1011–E1022.
17. YANG, S.H., R. LIU, E.J. PEREZ, et al. 2004. Mitochondrial localization of estrogen receptor beta. Proc. Natl. Acad. Sci. U.S.A. **101:** 4130–4135.
18. CAMMARATA, P.R., S. CHU, A. MOOR, et al. 2004. Subcellular distribution of native estrogen receptor alpha and beta subtypes in cultured human lens epithelial cells. Exp. Eye Res. **78:** 861–871.
19. SOLAKIDI, S., A.-M.G. PSARRA & C.E. SEKERIS. 2005. Differential subcellular distribution of estrogen receptor isoforms: Localization of ERalpha in the nucleoli and Erbeta in the mitochondria of human osteosarcoma SaOS-2 and hepatocarcinoma HepG2 cell lines. Biochim. Biophys. Acta **1745:** 382–392.
20. SOLAKIDI, S., A.-M.G. PSARRA, S. NIKOLAROPOULOS & C.E. SEKERIS. 2005. Estrogen receptors {alpha} and {beta} (ER{alpha} and ER{beta}) and androgen receptor (AR) in human sperm: localization of ER{beta} and AR in mitochondria of the midpiece. Hum. Reprod. **20:** 3481–3487.

21. WRUTNIAC, C., I. CASSAR-MALEK, S. MARCHAL, *et al.* 1995. A 43-kDa protein related to c-Erb A alpha 1 is located in the mitochondrial matrix of rat liver. J. Biol. Chem. **270:** 16347–16354.

22. SCHELLER, K., C.E. SEKERIS, R. HOCK & U. SCHEER. 1998. Localization of glucocorticoid and thyroid hormone receptors in mitochondria of human cells. Biol. Cell **90:** 116.

23. BERDANIER, C.D., H.B. EVERTS, C. HERMOYIAN & C.E. MATHEWS. 2001. Role of vitamin A in mitochondrial gene expression. Diabetes Res. Clin. Pract. **54** (Suppl 2): S11–S27.

24. CASAS, F., L. DAURY, S. GRANDEMANGE, *et al.* 2003. Endocrine regulation of mitochondrial activity: involvement of truncated RXRalpha and c-Erb Aalpha1 proteins. FASEB J. **17:** 426–436.

25. JEONG, J.H., J.S. PARK, B. MOON, *et al.* 2003. Orphan nuclear receptor Nur77 translocates to mitochondria in the early phase of apoptosis induced by synthetic chenodeoxycholic acid derivatives in human stomach cancer cell line SNU-1. Ann. N. Y. Acad. Sci. **1010:** 171–177.

26. BOTTERO, V., F. ROSSI, M. SAMSON, *et al.* 2001. IkappaB-alpha, the NF-kappaB inhibitory subunit, interacts with ANT, the mitochondrial ATP-ADP translocator. J. Biol. Chem. **276:** 21317–21324.

27. COGSWELL, P.C., D.F. KASHATUS, J.A. KEIFER, *et al.* 2003. NF-kappaB and Ikappa-Balpha are found in the mitochondria. Evidence for regulation of mitochondrial gene expression by NF-kappaB. J. Biol. Chem. **278:** 2963–2968.

28. GUSEVA, N.V., A.F. TAGHIYEV, M.T. STURM, *et al.* 2004. Tumor necrosis factor-related apoptosis-inducing ligand-mediated activation of mitochondria-associated nuclear factor-kappaB in prostatic carcinoma cell lines. Mol. Cancer Res. **2:** 574–584.

29. ZAMORA, M., C. MERONO, O. VINAS & T. MAMPEL. 2004. Recruitment of NF-kappaB into mitochondria is involved in adenine nucleotide translocase 1 (ANT1)-induced apoptosis. J. Biol. Chem. **37:** 38115–38123.

30. OGITA, K., H. OKUDA, M. KITANO, *et al.* 2002. Localization of activator protein-1 complex with DNA binding activity in mitochondria of murine brain after *in vivo* treatment with kainate. J. Neurosci. **22:** 2561–2570.

31. OGITA, K., Y. FUJINAMI, M. KITANO & Y. YONEDA. 2003. Transcription factor activator protein-1 expressed by kainate treatment can bind to the non-coding region of mitochondrial genome in murine hippocampus. J. Neurosci. Res. **73:** 794–802.

32. CAMMAROTA, M., G. PARATCHA, L.R.M. BEVILAQUA, *et al.* 1999. Cyclic AMP-responsive element binding protein in brain mitochondria. J. Neurochem. **72:** 2272–2277.

33. SCHUH, R.A., T. KRISTIAN & G. FISKUM. 2005. Calcium-dependent dephosphorylation of brain mitochondrial calcium/cAMP response element binding protein (CREB). J. Neurochem. **92:** 388–394.

34. KATSUMOTO, T., K. HIGAKI, K. OHNO & K. ONODERA. 1995. Cell-cycle dependent biosynthesis and localization of p53 protein in untransformed human cells. Biol. Cell **84:** 167–173.

35. MERRICK, B.A., C. HE, L.L. WITCHER, *et al.* 1996. HSP binding and mitochondrial localization of p53 protein in human HT1080 and mouse C3H10T1/2 cell lines. Biochim. Biophys. Acta **1297:** 57–68.

36. MARCHENKO, N.D., A. ZAIKA & U.M. MOLL. 2000. Death signal-induced localization of p53 protein in mitochondria. A potential role in apoptotic signaling. J. Biol. Chem. **21:** 16202–16212.

37. MIHARA, M., S. ERSTER, A. ZAIKA, *et al.* 2003. p53 has a direct apoptogenic role at the mitochondria. Mol. Cell **11:** 577–590.
38. HEYNE, K., S. MANNEBACH, E. WUERTZ, *et al.* 2004. Identification of a putative p53 binding sequence within the human mitochondrial genome. FEBS Lett. **578:** 198–202.
39. GODEFROY, N., S. BOULEAU, G. GRUEL, *et al.* 2004. Transcriptional repression by p53 promotes a Bcl-2-insensitive and mitochondria-independent pathway of apoptosis. Nucl. Acids Res. **32:** 4480–4490.
40. ABRAMOVA, N., K.J.A. DAVIES & D.R. CRAWFORD. 2000. Polynucleotide degradation during early stage response to oxidative stress is specific to mitochondria. Free Rad. Biol. Med. **28:** 281–288.
41. YOSHIDA, Y., H. IZUMI, T. TORIGOE, *et al.* 2003. p53 physically interacts with mitochondrial transcription factor A and differentially regulates binding to damaged DNA. Cancer Res. **63:** 3729–3734.
42. DONAHUE, R.J., M. RAZMARA, J.B. HOEK & T.B. KNUDSEN. 2001. Direct influence of the p53 tumor suppressor on mitochondrial biogenesis and function. FASEB J. **15:** 635–644.
43. DEMONACOS, C.V., N. KARAYANNI, E. HATZOGLOU, *et al.* 1996. Mitochondrial genes as sites of primary action of steroid hormones. Steroids **61:** 226–232.
44. SOLAKIDI, S. & C.E. SEKERIS. 2003. Oligonucleotide sequences similar to transcription factor consensi [*sic*] of nuclear genes are present in the human mitochondrial genome. Anticancer Res. **23:** 1389–1393.
45. WIDEN, C., J.A. GUSTAFSSON & A.C. WIKSTROM. 2003. Cytosolic glucocorticoid receptor interaction with nuclear factor-kappaB proteins in rat liver cells. Biochem. J. **373:** 211–220.
46. ITOH, S., S. LEMAY, M. OSAWA, *et al.* 2005. Mitochondrial Dok-4 recruits Src kinase and regulates NF-kappaB activation in endothelial cells. J. Biol. Chem. **28:** 26383–26396.
47. MOLL, U.M. & A. ZAIKA. 2001. Nuclear and mitochondrial apoptotic pathways of p53. FEBS Lett. **493:** 65–69.

Immunomodulatory Properties of Substance P

The Gastrointestinal System as a Model

HON WAI KOON AND CHARALABOS POTHOULAKIS

Gastrointestinal Neuropeptide Center, Division of Gastroenterology,
Beth Israel Deaconess Medical Center, Harvard Medical School,
Boston Massachusetts 02215, USA

ABSTRACT: Communication between nerves and immune and inflammatory cells of the small and large intestine plays a major role in the modulation of several intestinal functions, including intestinal motility, ion transport, and mucosal permeability. Neuroimmune interactions at intestinal sites have been associated with the pathophysiology of infectious and enterotoxin-mediated diarrhea and intestinal inflammation, including inflammatory bowel disease (IBD). During the past 20 years the neuropeptide substance P (SP) has been identified as an important mediator in the development and progress of intestinal inflammation by binding to its high-affinity neurokinin-1 receptor (NK-1R). This peptide, released from enteric nerves, sensory neurons, and inflammatory cells of the lamina propria during intestinal inflammation, participates in gut inflammation by interacting, directly or indirectly, with NK-1R expressed on nerves, epithelial cells, and immune and inflammatory cells, such as mast cells, macrophages, and T cells. SP-dependent activation of these cells leads to the release of cytokines and chemokines as well as other neuropeptides that modulate diarrhea, inflammation, and motility associated with the pathophysiology of several intestinal disease states. The recent development of specific nonpeptide NK-1R antagonists and NK-1R-deficient mice helped us understand the functional importance of the SP-NK-1R system in mediating intestinal neuroimmune interactions and to identify the particular cells and signaling pathways involved in this response. This review summarizes our understanding on the immunomodulatory properties of SP and its receptor in the intestinal tract with particular focus on their involvement in intestinal physiology as well as in the pathophysiology of several intestinal disease states at the *in vivo* and cell signaling level.

KEYWORDS: inflammation; colon; epithelial; neuropeptide

Address for correspondence: Charalabos Pothoulakis, M.D., Gastrointestinal Neuropeptide Center, Division of Gastroenterology, DANA 601 330 Brookline Avenue, Boston, MA 02215. Voice: 617-667-1259; fax: 617-667-2767.
e-mail: cpothoul@bidmc.harvard.edu

Ann. N.Y. Acad. Sci. 1088: 23–40 (2006). © 2006 New York Academy of Sciences.
doi: 10.1196/annals.1366.024

SUBSTANCE P IN THE INTESTINAL TRACT

Substance P (SP), an 11-amino acid neuropeptide, was originally isolated and purified by Chang and Leeman from bovine pituitary glands on the basis of its sialogogic activity.[1] SP is a member of the tachykinin family of peptides because it induces rapid smooth muscle contraction in guinea pig ileum and rat duodenum.[1] Other members of the tachykinin family, sharing common carboxyl terminal Phe-X-Gly-Leu-met-NH2 sequences in mammals, include neurokinin A and neurokinin B.[2] In mammals, tachykinins are produced by two genes, preprotachykinin-A (PPT-A) and preprotachykinin-B (PPT-B), and SP is a product of the PPT-A gene.[3,4] SP is localized in the central nervous system as well as in several peripheral tissues, including the entire length of the gastrointestinal tract as well as the colon. The main sources of SP in the gut include the myenteric and submucosal plexus, intrinsic sensory neurons, as well as sensory neurons originating from the dorsal root ganglia.[5,6] A newly identified gene, preprotachykinin C gene, encodes for the sequence of a new preprotachykinin protein designated hemokinin (HK) and produced primarily by hematopoietic cells.[7] HK binds with high selectivity to NK-1R and has similar *in vivo* potency to SP.[8] Like SP, HK is an 11-amino acid peptide having $\sim$55% amino acid similarity to SP.[7,9]

SP RECEPTORS AND GUT DISTRIBUTION

The effects of SP are mediated by three different G-protein-coupled receptors (GPCRs), namely neurokinin (NK)-1, 2, and 3. SP binds with high affinity to NK-1 receptor (NK-1R), and with low affinity to NK-2 and 3 receptors. NK-1 receptors are present in both small intestine and colon of animals and humans and are localized in a variety of cells, including nerves, smooth muscle, immune cells, glands, endothelial cells, as well as epithelial cells.[10–15,16] Although NK-1 receptors have been associated with several intestinal pathophysiologic conditions (see below), NK-2 receptors have been linked mostly with circular muscle contraction,[17] and are localized in circular muscle and muscularis mucosae.[18] Although NK-2 receptors are present predominantly on smooth muscle and, like NK-1, can affect gut motility,[19] NK-3 receptors are expressed predominantly in neurons and can stimulate or diminish muscle contraction indirectly following SP binding to neuronal cells in the submucosal and myenteric nerve plexuses of the gastrointestinal tract.[20,21] NK-3 receptors also provide slow excitatory synaptic input to neurons in ganglia of the sphincter of Oddi.[22] Thus, both NK-2 and NK-3 receptors affect motility responses in the GI, but there is very little evidence that they are involved in neuroimmune interactions.

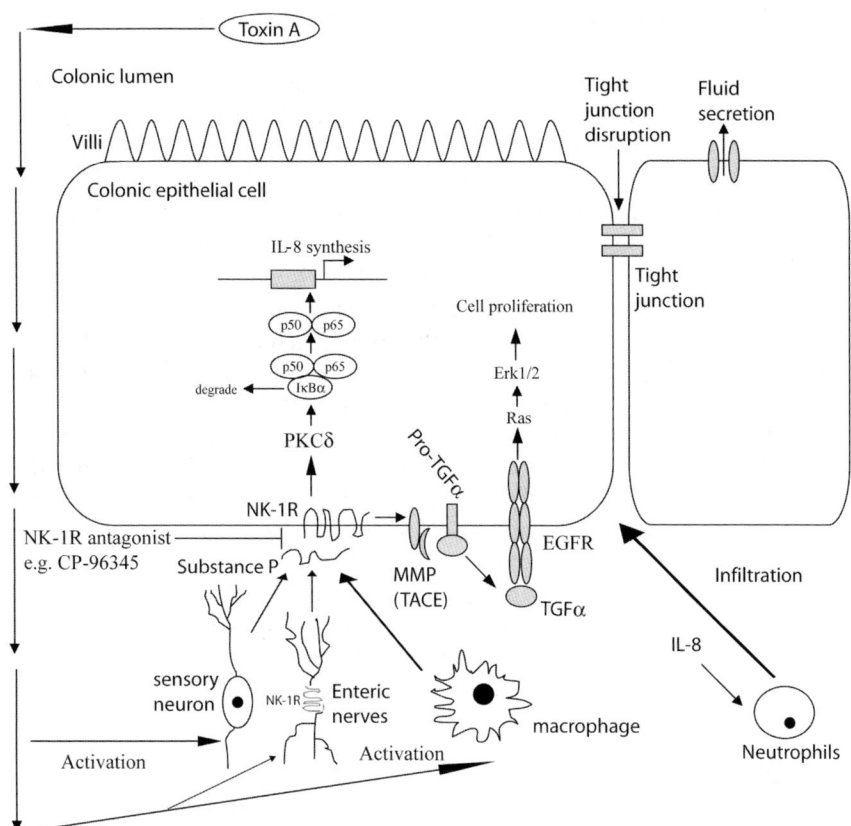

FIGURE 1. Substance P–dependent neuroimmune signaling during *C. difficile* toxin A–induced intestinal inflammation and tissue repair. Toxin A or other pathological stimuli activates substance P (SP) synthesis from sensory neurons and/or macrophages. SP binds to its high-affinity neurokinin-1 receptor (NK-1R) in target cells and activates protein kinase C δ phosphorylation, which activates the NF-κB system, leading to increased synthesis of NF-κB-driven proinflammatory genes, such as interleukin-8 (IL-8). IL-8 and other potent chemoattractants released from epithelial and lamina propria cells cause neutrophil infiltration and release of potent neutrophil mediators. Enteric nerves also express NK-1R as well as SP. During the repair phase of intestinal inflammation, SP binds to NK-1R, and induces matrix metalloproteinase activity that releases TGF-α into the external environment. TGFα binds to epidermal growth factor receptor, which activates ERK and mediates cell proliferation participating in tissue recovery.

SP AND NK-1R IN IMMUNE CELLS: REGULATION DURING AN INFLAMMATORY RESPONSE

Although SP and its receptors have been primarily associated with neurons, both centrally and peripherally, several pieces of evidence indicate that immune cells in several different organs, including the gastrointestinal tract, express SP, or its NK-1 receptor, or both. Thus, SP has been localized in human dendritic cells,[23,24] brain microglia,[25] mononuclear phagocytes,[26] and lymphocytes.[27,28] These immune cells may have SP-related autocrine regulatory pathways as well as influencing other cells containing SP receptors in a paracrine manner. Along these lines, NK-1R is found in T lymphocytes,[29] B lymphocytes,[30] macrophages,[26] dendritic cells,[24] neutrophils,[31] mast cells,[32] and natural killer cells.[33]

Accumulating evidence indicates that the SP-NK-1 receptor system represents a major immunoregulatory circuit involved in several physiological and pathophysiological gut responses and disease states. In the gut, lamina propria macrophages (LPMs) express both SP and NK-1R,[34] while T cells express a functional NK-1R.[35] SP-NK-1 receptor neuroimmune interactions participate in basic colonic responses, such as chloride secretion, gut permeability, and modulation of inflammation. This review will discuss the available evidence for participation of SP-mediated responses in several disease states, including inflammatory bowel disease, enterotoxin-mediated diarrhea and inflammation, and infectious diarrhea of various etiologies. We summarize here evidence showing the importance of SP-NK-1 receptor neuroimmune interactions in intestinal inflammation and we highlight the signaling mechanisms involved in this response. We also attempt to provide information that points to putative new therapeutic approaches in intestinal inflammatory and secretory states where SP appears to play an important role.

ROLE OF SUBSTANCE P IN *CLOSTRIDIUM DIFFICILE*–INDUCED DIARRHEA AND INFLAMMATION

Clostridium difficile is the primary etiologic agent of antibiotic-associated colitis in animals and humans and is an emerging health problem in hospitalized patients in the USA and abroad.[36] *Clostridium difficile* mediates its intestinal effects by releasing two exotoxins, toxins A and B, that bind to colonocytes and initiate a diarrheal response characterized by increased intestinal permeability, destruction of colonocytes, activation of immune cells of the lamia propria, and release of proinflammatory cytokines leading to activation and transmigration of neutrophils.[37] The mechanisms of *C. difficile* toxins can be divided into direct effects on enterocytes and colonocytes and indirect effects on subepithelial cells triggered by cytokines, neuropeptides, and other neuroimmune mediators.

One important characteristic of *C. difficile* toxin A pathophysiology is the dependency of toxin A–associated intestinal secretion and inflammation on activation of intestinal nerves and neuropeptides, and in particular SP. Experiments using anesthetized animals demonstrated that enteric nerves and capsaicin-sensitive sensory neurons mediate toxin A-induced ileal fluid secretion, mucosal permeability, mast cell degranulation, and intestinal inflammation.[38–40] Pretreatment with the capsaicin vanilloid receptor subtype 1 (VR1) antagonist, capsazepine, also significantly inhibited toxin A–induced colitis,[41] indicating a neurogenic inflammatory circuit that signals sensory neurons in the spinal cord. Because SP is the major constituent of primary sensory neurons, our laboratory and that of others examined the possibility that SP is involved in the intestinal effects of toxin A. Parenteral administration of a nonpeptide NK-1 receptor antagonist in rats inhibited all toxin A–associated secretory and inflammatory responses,[39,42] suggesting a proinflammatory role for SP in this enterotoxin model of intestinal inflammation. Toxin A also induces an early (30 min) increase of SP in the cell bodies of dorsal root ganglia followed by increased SP expression in the intestinal mucosa[34] which initiates or propagates the intestinal inflammatory response. In parallel, toxin A administration also stimulates a prompt upregulation in NK-1R expression in the intestinal mucosa, an effect also evident in mucosal biopsies of patients with *C. difficile* colitis.[43] A major role for SP and its NK-1 receptor in the mediation of intestinal inflammation in the toxin A colitis model was directly confirmed by studies demonstrating that mice genetically lacking NK-1 receptors have significantly attenuated intestinal responses to toxin A, including tumor necrosis factor α (TNF-α) expression.[44] *In vivo* evidence also indicates that the peptides neurotensin and corticotropin-releasing hormone, both of which play a proinflammatory role in the ileal loop model of toxin A colitis, mediate their effect, at least in part, by release of SP in the intestinal mucosa.[45,46]

The cell surface enzyme called neutral endopeptidase (NEP) is responsible for degrading SP in extracellular fluid and terminating its proinflammatory effects.[47] The importance of the SP/NEP system was also confirmed in the *C. difficile* toxin A enteritis model. Thus, compared to the wild-type, NEP-deficient mice had exacerbated inflammatory and secretory responses, while pretreatment of recombinant NEP prevented exacerbated inflammation in response to toxin A.[48] In contrast, pretreatment of wild-type mice with the NEP inhibitor phosphoramidon exacerbated toxin A enteritis.[48] Thus, NEP can terminate enteritis induced by toxin A by degrading SP.

SP–Mast Cell Interactions in the Toxin A Model

Several studies indicate that nerve mast cell communication participates in the pathophysiology of intestinal inflammation,[49] and neuronal SP interacts with mast cells in the intestinal mucosa.[50] Early studies indicated that injection of toxin A into ileal loops caused mast cell degranulation, and stimulated release of rat mast cell protease II (RMCPII),[38,51] a specific mucosal mast cell protease. Interestingly, ablation of sensory neurons with capsaicin or administration of the NK-1R antagonist CP-96345 dramatically reduced release of RMCPII upon exposure to toxin A (TxA),[38] indicating SP–mucosal mast cell interactions during toxin A-induced neurogenic gut inflammation. The role of mast cell–SP communication in the development of intestinal inflammation was further confirmed in the toxin A model by use of mast cell–deficient mice and NK-1R antagonists. Results from these studies indicated SP-mast cell–dependent pathways in the regulation of toxin A–induced secretion and neutrophil infiltration.[52] Whether SP can directly stimulate proinflammatory responses in intestinal mast cells and whether mucosal mast cells express SP receptors is still a matter of controversy. Part of this controversy appears to be the difficulty in isolating pure gut mast cell preparations retaining full function. Early studies indicated that human mucosal mast cells isolated from the intestine respond to supraphysiological concentration of SP (10^{-4} M) by releasing histamine.[32] Recent results indicated that, while nonactivated human mast cells do not respond and do not express NK-1R, they do so upon IgE stimulation.[53]

Intestinal Monocytes/Macrophages and SP Responses During Toxin A Enteritis

Macrophages are implicated in the pathophysiology of intestinal inflammation and IBD.[54] SP can also stimulate IL-1β production from human blood monocytes,[55] and activated monocytes have enhanced responses to SP.[56] Rat peritoneal macrophages express low levels of SP and NK-1R mRNAs which can be substantially increased after LPS exposure.[57] Evidence also indicate that expression of NK-1R expression by macrophages can be increased by IL-4 and IFN-γ, suggesting a T cell macrophage communication that might involve SP and NK-1R.[58] SP-NK-1R interactions at the intestinal macrophage level might also modulate intestinal inflammation. Castagliuolo *et al.* indicate that LPMs isolated from toxin A-injected loops release large amounts of TNF-α and SP, compared to control LPMs. Moreover, pretreatment of rats with a NK-1R antagonist inhibited toxin A–mediated TNF-α release from isolated LPMs, while LPMs obtained from toxin A–exposed intestine incubated *in vitro* with SP showed enhanced TNF-α secretion compared to control LPMs, which did not respond to SP.[34] In addition, incubation of activated LPMs with the NK-1R antagonist CP-96345 showed diminished TNF-α release.[34] Thus, *in vivo* activated LPMs secrete SP during an intestinal inflammatory response, which leads to increased cytokine production, pointing to an autocrine/paracrine regulation of cytokine secretion by SP during intestinal inflammation.

ROLE OF SP AND NK-1R IN IMMUNE RESPONSES DURING *SALMONELLA* INFECTION

Salmonella gastroenteritis is an important foodborne infection associated with significant morbidity around the world. Studies in animal models indicate that SP participates in the pathophysiology of *Salmonella* infection. Thus, SP exposure to a strain of *Salmonella* inhibited binding to lymphocytes, with a more pronounced effect on the T-suppressor/cytotoxic T-cell subset.[59] Oral intake of *Salmonella* in mice promptly results in substantial NK-1R upregulation in the Peyer's patches and mesenteric lymph nodes.[60] In murine salmonellosis, administration of a NK-1R antagonist prior to *Salmonella* resulted in an earlier onset of infection, increased mortality, and reduced mucosal IL-12 and IFN-γ mRNA levels in infected mice.[60] Moreover, IL-12 protects mice from *Salmonella* infection,[61] and SP via its NK-1 receptor stimulates IL-12 release from macrophages.[62] Thus, on the basis of this evidence, SP and NK-1R might play an important role in protecting immune responses in *Salmonella* gastroenteritis, via macrophage-dependent responses. A recent study by Walters and colleagues using NK-1R-deficient mice, however, projects a different view. These studies showed that oral immunization of NK1R KO mice with a *Salmonella*-CFA/I vaccine resulted in elevated mucosal and systemic IgA responses to CFA/I fimbriae associated with increased IL-5- and IL-6-producing CD4$^+$ Th2 cell populations.[63] Moreover, there were no differences in the ability of these vaccines to protect mice between NK-1R KO and wild-type mice. However, innate resistance to wild-type *Salmonella* was significantly enhanced in NK-1R-deficient mice, suggesting diminished proinflammatory responses in the absence of SP/NK-1R system.[63] Despite the different results, however, it is clearly evident that SP and its NK-1R contributes to intestinal immunity during *Salmonella* infection.

SP-DEPENDENT NEUROIMMUNE INTERACTIONS IN PARASITIC INFECTIONS

Trichinella spiralis

Trichinella spiralis is a helminthic parasite affecting both animals and humans, whose pathophysiology involves extensive neuroimmune interactions. Mast cells and Th2 cells play an important role in the development of *T. spiralis* infection and several of its intestinal responses.[64,65] For example, increased levels of substance P are evident in the myenteric plexus of *T. spiralis*-infected rats,[66] although in the guinea pig and ferret intestine lower intestinal levels were noted.[66,67] Pretreatment with either a SP antibody or the NK-1R antagonist CP 96345 effectively diminished inflammatory responses in the jejunum of *T. spiralis*–infected mice.[68,69] Moreover, in the inflamed intestine of rats infected with *T. spiralis*, activity of the SP-limiting enzyme NEP is significantly downregulated, leading to reduced SP degradation.[70] Together, these results indicate that SP-NK-1R-dependent mechanisms might regulate intestinal inflammatory responses during this parasitic infection.

Nippostrongylus brasiliensis

Animal models of *N. brasiliensis* infection have been extensively used to study intestinal pathophysiology, including inflammation and permeability-related responses, where neuronal mast cell interactions appear to play an important role. In a rat *N. brasiliensis* model, the majority of intestinal mucosal mast cells were in contact with nerves in the small intestinal submucosa, including SP-containing nerves,[49,71] providing anatomical evidence for cross-talk between the immune and nervous systems in the gut. Ablation of extrinsic sensory neurons with capsaicin worsened intestinal inflammation in *N. brasiliensis*–infected rats, without affecting the duration of the infection.[72] Moreover, tissue from *N. brasiliensis*–infected rats contained increased amounts of immunoreactive SP immunoreactivity, primarily on nerve fibers.[73] Thus, SP-containing sensory neurons may play a protective role in the development of *N. brasiliensis* infection and SP–mast cell interactions might participate in this response.

Schistosoma mansoni

Schistostoma mansoni infections represent an important clinical condition affecting the intestine, the liver, and the spleen, characterized by formation of granulomas containing several immune cells.[74] Several pieces of evidence demonstrate extensive cross-talk between neuropeptides, including SP and NK-1R, and immune cells affecting the pathophysiology of schistosomiasis.[74] Thus, eosinophils from schistosoma granulomas express SP at the protein and mRNA level,[75] and NK-1R is evident in T lymphocytes from these ganulomas.[76] SP modulates immunoglobulin secretion in granuloma cells isolated from infected mice,[77] and stimulates IFN-γ secretion from primed granuloma cells.[78] SP mRNA is also detectable in lamina propria and spleen macrophages isolated from schistosome granulomas.[79] Moreover, granuloma macrophages from STAT6-deficient mice had several-fold higher SP mRNA expression, while, in contrast, STAT4 knockout mice had diminished SP mRNA expression in the same cell population.[79] Along these lines, IL-12, which signals via STAT4 to induce Th1-type inflammation, induced SP mRNA expression in macrophages from *Schistosoma*-infected mice and lamina propria mononuclear cells.[79] Thus, SP mRNA, expressed in macrophages during inflammatory responses, is regulated by IL-12 and STAT4-dependent signaling. The importance of SP and its receptor in the development of schistosomiasis granulomas is underscored by studies using NK-1R antagonists and mice deficient in NK-1R 1 receptor.[78,80] Preprotachykinin C mRNA and HK were also found in schistosoma granuloma T cells and macrophages and both SP and HK stimulated IFN-γ production, while a NK-1R antagonist inhibited this response.[81] Thus, it is quite evident that HK and SP are expressed at sites of chronic inflammation, and their expression is regulated during an inflammatory response during this helminthic infection. Moreover, SP and NK-1R immunomodulation and proinflammatory responses are also subject to regulation by another peptide, somatostatin, acting via its type 2 (SSR2) receptor.[82]

Inflammatory Bowel Disease

Inflammatory bowel disease (IBD), which includes Crohn's disease (CD) and ulcerative colitis (UC), is a group of chronic debilitating diseases with substantial morbidity and mortality affecting millions of patients worldwide. Although the etiology of IBD remains under investigation, several studies point to an important role for SP and its receptors in the pathophysiology of this disease. Early studies indicated increased expression of SP receptor binding sites in IBD patients expressed in the submucosa, muscularis mucosa and external circular, and longitudinal muscle.[10] Patients with CD showed increased NK-1R receptors in lymphoid aggregates, small blood vessels, and enteric neurons, while in UC patients, these receptors were only evident in lymphoid aggregates and small blood vessels, but not in enteric nerves.[83,84] Later studies confirmed increased NK-1R expression in the intestine of these patients and indicated that lamina propria mononuclear cells, as well as epithelial cells also express NK-1R.[12,14] Raithel *et al.* also indicated that colonic mucosal explants from IBD patients showed enhanced mucosal mast cell mediator secretion in response to SP,[85] suggesting a functional role for these receptors in IBD. While some studies found increased SP expression in IBD tissues,[86–88] other studies failed to demonstrate such a response.[89,90]

Diarrhea represents one of the predominant symptoms in IBD, and SP–NK-1R interaction appears to participate in this response. Electrophysiologic studies with animal small intestine and colon indicate the ability of SP to mediate intestinal secretion in normal intestine.[91–94,95] These studies also demonstrated that enteric nerves and mast cells might participate in these SP-mediated responses. Experiments with human colonic strips mounted in Ussing chambers indicate that SP, via NK-1R, is able to stimulate chloride secretion in human intestine via mast cell and nerve-dependent mechanisms.[13] These results suggest extensive neuroimmune modulation of NK-1R-mediated secretion in human colon. Moreover, Riegler *et al.* also showed that SP caused histamine and prostaglandin release from human colonic mucosa, while histamine and prostaglandin inhibitors reduced the secretory response to SP.[13] The pathophysiologic importance of the NK-1R diarrheal response was confirmed by Turvill *et al.*, demonstrating that the cholera toxin–mediated intestinal secretion involves NK-1 and NK-2 receptors.[96]

SP AND ANIMAL MODELS OF INFLAMMATORY BOWEL DISEASE

Apart from indirect evidence from human studies, results from animal models of IBD strongly suggest a functional role for SP receptors in the pathophysiology of this disease. For example, administration of a NK-1 receptor antagonist to rats reduced the severity of colitis and alterations of contractility 14 days after intracolonic administration of trinitrobenzene sulfonic acid (TNBS), an animal model resembling CD.[97] Genetically engineered NK-1R-deficient mice were also protected from acute colitis 2 days after intracolonic TNBS administration.[98] Moreover, injection of an NK-1R antagonist to rats also reduces colonic inflammation and oxidative stress in dextran sulfate–induced colitis, a model resembling UC.[99] Ileal pouch–anal anastomosis (IPAA) is a frequent surgical option for patients operated on for chronic UC requiring colectomy. However, this anastomosis is often associated with ileal pouch inflammation and this effect can be recapitulated in rats with experimental IPAA. Interestingly, administration of an NK-1R antagonist to rats with IPAA was effective in reducing inflammatory responses in the ileal pouch,[100] indicating that SP receptor antagonism might be a therapeutic option in clinical pouchitis. IL-10-deficient mice develop spontaneous colitis characterized by a Th1-driven response and have been used as model to study IBD. Administration of non-steroidal anti-inflammatory compounds (NSAIDs) to young IL-10 mice results promptly in dramatic ileitis and colitis,[101] characterized by the appearance of NK-1R in mucosal T cells regulated by an interplay between IL-12 and IL-10.[35] Moreover, NK-1R antagonism in these mice alters intestinal inflammation, confirming the importance of SP and its receptor in the development of intestinal inflammation.[35]

As discussed above, NEP is a SP-degrading enzyme that limits availability of this peptide during an inflammatory response. NEP knockout mice have substantially elevated SP colonic levels and increased colonic permeability under basal conditions than wild-type mice.[102] The severity of TNBS-induced colitis in NEP knockout mice was also substantially worsened compared to the wild-type, while this effect was prevented by recombinant NEP and NK-1R antagonism.[102] Thus, increased bioavailability of SP due to lack of the SP degrading enzyme NEP leads to increased colonic inflammation.

Mechanisms of the Proinflammatory Effects of SP

Many of the studies outlined above clearly indicate that SP, acting via NK-1R, plays an important role in the pathogenesis of intestinal inflammation. The mechanism of SP–NK-1R participation in intestinal inflammation involves release of inflammatory mediators because SP directly stimulates cytokine production such as IL-1β, IL-6, IL-8, and TNF-α from several diverse cell types.[34,55,103–105] Transcription of proinflammatory genes by SP–NK-1R interactions involves NK-1R-dependent activation of the inflammatory transcription factor NF-κB in target cells.[15,106,107] SP-induced NF-κB activation and cytokine gene transcription also involve the Rho family of small molecular weight GTPases, RhoA, Rac1, and cdc42,[15] and can be dependent[15,107] or independent of MAP kinase activation. Recent evidence also indicates that SP induces phosphorylation of protein kinase C, including the delta, theta, and epsilon isoforms[108] in human colonocytes. These studies also showed that SP-induced PKC delta activation is functionally involved in NK-1R-mediated NF-κB activation and IL-8 secretion in response to SP.[108]

As discussed above, NK-1R expression is increased in several models of intestinal inflammation. Because cytokine levels are also increased during colitis, cytokines can, in turn, affect expression of NK-1R. Consistent with this hypothesis, Simeonidis *et al.* demonstrated that exposure of human mono-cytic THP-1 cells expressing authentic NK-1R to IL-1β and TNF-α stimulated increased NK-1R gene expression at the mRNA and protein levels.[109] More-over, NK-1R expression in response to cytokine stimulation was diminished by transfection of THP-1 cells with the NF-κB inhibitor IκBα, indicating that this transcription factor is tightly involved in regulation of NK-1R gene expression during an inflammatory response. Along these lines, IL-12 and IL-18 induce T cells to express NK-1R through NF-κB activation, while IL-10 inhibits this response.[110] Similar NF-κB-dependent regulation of NK-1R expression has also been reported in astrocytes,[111] and human alveolar macrophages,[112] while Reed *et al.*[113] demonstrated that NF-κB activation precedes NK-1R expression in experimental colitis, providing a functional correlate to this response. Taken together, these results indicate that the proinflammatory factor NF-κB is involved in both SP proinflammatory signaling and regulation of the SP receptor NK-1 during colitis.

SP MEDIATES TISSUE RECOVERY VIA EPIDERMAL GROWTH FACTOR RECEPTOR ACTIVATION

Besides acting as a pro-inflammatory mediator, SP can also induce cell pro-liferation in several cell types such as T lymphocytes,[29] skin fibroblasts,[114] and smooth muscle cells.[114] Castagliuolo *et al.*[98] reported that mice lacking NK-1R had significantly worsened colitis in the chronic phase of both the DSS and TNBS colitis models, indicating that SP can also promote mucosal healing during an inflammatory response. Further experiments indicated that this effect is likely mediated by SP-induced cell proliferation via a communi-cation between the NK-1R and the epidermal growth factor receptor (EGFR) as shown in colonic fibroblasts *in vivo*, human astrocytoma cells, as well as hu-man colonic epithelial cells.[98,115,116] SP-induced transactivation and tyrosine phosphorylation of EGFR, leading to cell proliferation, involves the formation of activated EGFR complex with adapter proteins SHC and Grb2.[115] Moreover, in human colonocytes, NK-1R-induced EGFR and MAPK activation and cell proliferation involves release of matrix metalloproteinases (most likely TACE) and secretion of transforming growth factor (TGF-α), signaling mechanisms likely to be involved in the protective effects of NK-1R in chronic colitis.

SUMMARY AND THERAPEUTIC IMPLICATIONS

As we discussed in this review, substantial evidence from *in vitro* and *in vivo* approaches, as well as evaluation of responses in human colon with IBD, suggest that SP is an important mediator of the neuroimmune response related to several disease states. These interactions are important in the initiation and progress of inflammatory processes as well as in several symptoms related to inflammatory diarrhea of diverse etiologies. The ability of proinflammatory cytokines to modulate expression of SP receptors on neuronal, immune, and epithelial cells, together with increased expression of SP itself in intestinal inflammation, suggests that these molecules may represent a potential therapeutic target for treatment of several intestinal inflammatory states. The development of highly specific neurokinin-1 receptor antagonists by several major pharmaceutical companies and their current use in different clinical conditions, such as depression and anxiety, rheumatoid arthritis, chemotherapy- or radiotherapy-induced emesis, among others, opens up the possibility for their use in intestinal inflammation and IBD. Clinical trials in humans assessing the utility of NK-1R antagonists for the treatment of IBD are limited, and the results of a pilot study have not been reported.

REFERENCES

1. CHANG, M.M. & S.E. LEEMAN. 1970. Isolation of a sialogogic peptide from bovine hypothalamic tissue and its characterization as substance P. J. Biol. Chem. **245:** 4784–4790.
2. KIMURA, S. *et al.* 1984. Pharmacological characterization of novel mammalian tachykinins, neurokinin alpha and neurokinin beta. Neurosci. Res. **2:** 97–104.
3. HARRISON, S. & P. GEPPETTI. 2001. Substance P. Int. J. Biochem. Cell Biol. **33:** 555–576.
4. SEVERINI, C. *et al.* 2002. The tachykinin peptide family. Pharmacol. Rev. **54:** 285–322.
5. HOLZER, P. & U. HOLZER-PETSCHE. 1997. Tachykinins in the gut. Part I. Expression, release and motor function. Pharmacol. Ther. **73:** 173–217.
6. HOLZER, P. & U. HOLZER-PETSCHE. 1997. Tachykinins in the gut. Part II. Roles in neural excitation, secretion and inflammation. Pharmacol. Ther. **73:** 219–263.
7. ZHANG, Y. *et al.* 2000. Hemokinin is a hematopoietic-specific tachykinin that regulates B lymphopoiesis. Nat. Immunol. **1:** 392–397.
8. BELLUCCI, F. *et al.* 2002. Pharmacological profile of the novel mammalian tachykinin, hemokinin 1. Br. J. Pharmacol. **135:** 266–274.
9. MORTEAU, O. *et al.* 2001. Hemokinin 1 is a full agonist at the substance P receptor. Nat. Immunol. **2:** 1088.
10. MANTYH, C.R. *et al.* 1988. Receptor binding sites for substance P, but not substance K or neuromedin K, are expressed in high concentrations by arterioles, venules, and lymph nodules in surgical specimens obtained from patients with ulcerative colitis and Crohn's disease. Proc. Natl. Acad. Sci. USA **85:** 3235–3239.

11. POTHOULAKIS, C. *et al*. 1998. Substance P receptor expression in intestinal epithelium in *Clostridium difficile* toxin A enteritis in rats. Am. J. Physiol. **275:** G68–G75.

12. GOODE, T. *et al*. 2000. Neurokinin-1 receptor expression in inflammatory bowel disease: molecular quantitation and localisation. Gut **47:** 387–396.

13. RIEGLER, M. *et al*. 1999. Effects of substance P on human colonic mucosa *in vitro*. Am. J. Physiol. **276:** G1473–G1483.

14. RENZI, D. *et al*. 2000. Substance P (neurokinin-1) and neurokinin A (neurokinin-2) receptor gene and protein expression in the healthy and inflamed human intestine. Am. J. Pathol. **157:** 1511–1522.

15. ZHAO, D. *et al*. 2002. Substance P-stimulated interleukin-8 expression in human colonic epithelial cells involves Rho family small GTPases. Biochem. J. **368:** 665–672.

16. LIU, L. *et al*. 2002. Roles of substance P receptors in human colon circular muscle: alterations in diverticular disease. J. Pharmacol. Exp. Ther. **302:** 627–635.

17. CAO, W. *et al*. 2000. Gq-linked NK(2) receptors mediate neurally induced contraction of human sigmoid circular smooth muscle. Gastroenterology **119:** 51–61.

18. WARNER, F.J. *et al*. 2000. Circular muscle contraction, messenger signalling and localization of binding sites for neurokinin A in human sigmoid colon. Clin. Exp. Pharmacol. Physiol. **27:** 928–933.

19. MAGGI, C.A. *et al*. 1997. Tachykinin receptors and intestinal motility. Can. J. Physiol. Pharmacol. **75:** 696–703.

20. MANN, P.T. *et al*. 1997. Localisation of neurokinin 3 (NK3) receptor immunoreactivity in the rat gastrointestinal tract. Cell Tissue Res. **289:** 1–9.

21. WANG, H. *et al*. 2002. Localization of neurokinin B receptor in mouse gastrointestinal tract. World J. Gastroenterol. **8:** 172–175.

22. MANNING, B.P. & G.M. MAWE. 2001. Tachykinins mediate slow excitatory postsynaptic transmission in guinea pig sphincter of Oddi ganglia. Am. J. Physiol. Gastrointest. Liver Physiol. **281:** G357–G364.

23. LAMBRECHT, B.N. *et al*. 1999. Endogenously produced substance P contributes to lymphocyte proliferation induced by dendritic cells and direct TCR ligation. Eur. J. Immunol. **29:** 3815–3825.

24. MARRIOTT, I. & K.L. BOST. 2001. Substance P receptor mediated macrophage responses. Adv. Exp. Med. Biol. **493:** 247–254.

25. LAI, J.P. *et al*. 2000. Detection of substance P and its receptor in human fetal microglia. Neuroscience **101:** 1137–1144.

26. HO, W.Z. *et al*. 1997. Human monocytes and macrophages express substance P and neurokinin-1 receptor. J. Immunol. **159:** 5654–5660.

27. LAI, J.P. *et al*. 1998. Identification of a delta isoform of preprotachykinin mRNA in human mononuclear phagocytes and lymphocytes. J. Neuroimmunol. **91:** 121–128.

28. LAI, J.P., S.D. DOUGLAS & W.Z. HO. 1998. Human lymphocytes express substance P and its receptor. J. Neuroimmunol. **86:** 80–86.

29. PAYAN, D.G., D.R. BREWSTER & E.J. GOETZL. 1983. Specific stimulation of human T lymphocytes by substance P. J. Immunol. **131:** 1613–1615.

30. STANISZ, A.M. *et al*. 1987. Distribution of substance P receptors on murine spleen and Peyer's patch T and B cells. J. Immunol. **139:** 749–754.

31. WOZNIAK, A. *et al*. 1989. Activation of human neutrophils by substance P: effect on FMLP-stimulated oxidative and arachidonic acid metabolism and on antibody-dependent cell-mediated cytotoxicity. Immunology **68:** 359–364.

32. SHANAHAN, F. *et al*. 1985. Mast cell heterogeneity: effects of neuroenteric peptides on histamine release. J. Immunol. **135:** 1331–1337.
33. FEISTRITZER, C. *et al*. 2003. Natural killer cell functions mediated by the neuropeptide substance P. Regul. Pept. **116:** 119–126.
34. CASTAGLIUOLO, I. *et al*. 1997. Increased substance P responses in dorsal root ganglia and intestinal macrophages during *Clostridium difficile* toxin A enteritis in rats. Proc. Natl. Acad. Sci. USA **94:** 4788–4793.
35. WEINSTOCK, J.V. *et al*. 2003. Substance P regulates Th1-type colitis in IL-10 knockout mice. J. Immunol. **171:** 3762–3767.
36. KELLY, C.P., C. POTHOULAKIS & J.T. LAMONT. 1994. *Clostridium difficile* colitis. N. Engl. J. Med. **330:** 257–262.
37. POTHOULAKIS, C. & J.T. LAMONT. 2001. Microbes and microbial toxins: paradigms for microbial-mucosal interactions II. The integrated response of the intestine to *Clostridium difficile* toxins. Am. J. Physiol. Gastrointest. Liver Physiol. **280:** G178–G183.
38. CASTAGLIUOLO, I. *et al*. 1994. Neuronal involvement in the intestinal effects of *Clostridium difficile* toxin A and *Vibrio cholerae* enterotoxin in rat ileum. Gastroenterology **107:** 657–665.
39. MANTYH, C.R. *et al*. 1996. Substance P activation of enteric neurons in response to intraluminal *Clostridium difficile* toxin A in the rat ileum. Gastroenterology **111:** 1272–1280.
40. MANTYH, C.R., D.C. MCVEY & S.R. VIGNA. 2000. Extrinsic surgical denervation inhibits *Clostridium difficile* toxin A-induced enteritis in rats. Neurosci. Lett. **292:** 95–98.
41. MCVEY, D.C. & S.R. VIGNA. 2001. The capsaicin VR1 receptor mediates substance P release in toxin A-induced enteritis in rats. Peptides **22:** 1439–1446.
42. POTHOULAKIS, C. *et al*. 1994. CP-96,345, a substance P antagonist, inhibits rat intestinal responses to *Clostridium difficile* toxin A but not cholera toxin. Proc. Natl. Acad. Sci. USA **91:** 947–951.
43. MANTYH, C.R. *et al*. 1996. Increased substance P receptor expression by blood vessels and lymphoid aggregates in *Clostridium difficile*-induced pseudomembranous colitis. Dig. Dis. Sci. **41:** 614–620.
44. CASTAGLIUOLO, I. *et al*. 1998. Neurokinin-1 (NK-1) receptor is required in *Clostridium difficile*-induced enteritis. J. Clin. Invest. **101:** 1547–1550.
45. CASTAGLIUOLO, I. *et al*. 1999. Neurotensin is a proinflammatory neuropeptide in colonic inflammation. J. Clin. Invest. **103:** 843–849.
46. ANTON, P.M. *et al*. 2004. Corticotropin-releasing hormone (CRH) requirement in *Clostridium difficile* toxin A-mediated intestinal inflammation. Proc. Natl. Acad. Sci. USA **101:** 8503–8508.
47. OKAMOTO, A. *et al*. 1994. Interactions between neutral endopeptidase (EC 3.4.24.11) and the substance P (NK1) receptor expressed in mammalian cells. Biochem. J. **299**(Pt 3): 683–693.
48. KIRKWOOD, K.S. *et al*. 2001. Deletion of neutral endopeptidase exacerbates intestinal inflammation induced by *Clostridium difficile* toxin A. Am. J. Physiol. Gastrointest. Liver Physiol. **281:** G544–G551.
49. BIENENSTOCK, J. *et al*. 1987. The role of mast cells in inflammatory processes: evidence for nerve/mast cell interactions. Int. Arch. Allergy Appl. Immunol. **82:** 238–243.
50. MORIARTY, D. *et al*. 2001. Potent NK1 antagonism by SR-140333 reduces rat colonic secretory response to immunocyte activation. Am. J. Physiol. Cell Physiol. **280:** C852–C858.

51. POTHOULAKIS, C. *et al.* 1993. Ketotifen inhibits *Clostridium difficile* toxin A-induced enteritis in rat ileum. Gastroenterology **105:** 701–707.
52. WERSHIL, B.K., I. CASTAGLIUOLO & C. POTHOULAKIS. 1998. Direct evidence of mast cell involvement in *Clostridium difficile* toxin A-induced enteritis in mice. Gastroenterology **114:** 956–964.
53. BISCHOFF, S.C. *et al.* 2004. Substance P and other neuropeptides do not induce mediator release in isolated human intestinal mast cells. Neurogastroenterol. Motil. **16:** 185–193.
54. LIGUMSKY, M. *et al.* 1990. Role of interleukin 1 in inflammatory bowel disease—enhanced production during active disease. Gut 31: 686–689.
55. LAURENZI, M.A. *et al.* 1990. The neuropeptide substance P stimulates production of interleukin 1 in human blood monocytes: activated cells are preferentially influenced by the neuropeptide. Scand. J. Immunol. **31:** 529–533.
56. LOTZ, M., J.H. VAUGHAN & D.A. CARSON. 1988. Effect of neuropeptides on production of inflammatory cytokines by human monocytes. Science **241:** 1218–1221.
57. BOST, K.L., S.A. BREEDING & D.W. PASCUAL. 1992. Modulation of the mRNAs encoding substance P and its receptor in rat macrophages by LPS. Reg. Immunol. **4:** 105–112.
58. MARRIOTT, I. & K.L. BOST. 2000. IL-4 and IFN-γ up-regulate substance P receptor expression in murine peritoneal macrophages. J. Immunol. **165:** 182–191.
59. DE SIMONE, C. *et al.* 1989. Effects of substance P on the spontaneous binding of *Salmonella minnesota* R345 (Rb) to human peripheral blood lymphocytes. J. Clin. Lab. Anal. **3:** 345–349.
60. KINCY-CAIN, T. & K.L. BOST. 1996. Increased susceptibility of mice to *Salmonella* infection following *in vivo* treatment with the substance P antagonist, spantide II. J. Immunol. **157:** 255–264.
61. KINCY-CAIN, T., J.D. CLEMENTS & K.L. BOST. 1996. Endogenous and exogenous interleukin-12 augment the protective immune response in mice orally challenged with *Salmonella dublin*. Infect. Immun. **64:** 1437–1440.
62. KINCY-CAIN, T. & K.L. BOST. 1997. Substance P-induced IL-12 production by murine macrophages. J. Immunol. **158:** 2334–2339.
63. WALTERS, N. *et al.* 2005. Enhanced immunoglobulin A response and protection against *Salmonella enterica* serovar typhimurium in the absence of the substance P receptor. Infect. Immun. **73:** 317–324.
64. WOODBURY, R.G. *et al.* 1984. Mucosal mast cells are functionally active during spontaneous expulsion of intestinal nematode infections in rat. Nature **312:** 450–452.
65. KHAN, W.I. & S.M. COLLINS. 2004. Immune-mediated alteration in gut physiology and its role in host defence in nematode infection. Parasite Immunol. **26:** 319–326.
66. SWAIN, M.G. *et al.* 1992. Increased levels of substance P in the myenteric plexus of *Trichinella*-infected rats. Gastroenterology **102:** 1913–1919.
67. GREENWOOD, B. & J.M. PALMER. 1996. Neural integration of jejunal motility and ion transport in nematode-infected ferrets. Am. J. Physiol. **271:** G48–G55.
68. AGRO, A. & A.M. STANISZ. 1993. Inhibition of murine intestinal inflammation by anti-substance P antibody. Reg. Immunol. **5:** 120–126.
69. KATAEVA, G., A. AGRO & A.M. STANISZ. 1994. Substance-P-mediated intestinal inflammation: inhibitory effects of CP 96345 and SMS 201-995. Neuroimmunomodulation **1:** 350–356.

70. HWANG, L. *et al*. 1993. Downregulation of neutral endopeptidase (EC 3.4.24.11) in the inflamed rat intestine. Am. J. Physiol. **264:** G735–G743.
71. STEAD, R.H. *et al*. 1987. Intestinal mucosal mast cells in normal and nematode-infected rat intestines are in intimate contact with peptidergic nerves. Proc. Natl. Acad. Sci. USA **84:** 2975–2979.
72. GAY, J. *et al*. 2000. Development and sequels of intestinal inflammation in nematode-infected rats: role of mast cells and capsaicin-sensitive afferents. Neuroimmunomodulation **8:** 171–178.
73. MASSON, S.D. *et al*. 1996. *Nippostrongylus brasiliensis* infection evokes neuronal abnormalities and alterations in neurally regulated electrolyte transport in rat jejunum. Parasitology **113**(Pt 2): 173–182.
74. WEINSTOCK, J.V. 2004. The role of substance P, hemokinin and their receptor in governing mucosal inflammation and granulomatous responses. Front. Biosci. **9:** 1936–1943.
75. WEINSTOCK, J.V. *et al*. 1988. Eosinophils from granulomas in murine schistosomiasis mansoni produce substance P. J. Immunol. **141:** 961–966.
76. COOK, G.A. *et al*. 1994. Molecular evidence that granuloma T lymphocytes in murine schistosomiasis mansoni express an authentic substance P (NK-1) receptor. J. Immunol. **152:** 1830–1835.
77. NEIL, G.A., A. BLUM & J.V. WEINSTOCK. 1991. Substance P but not vasoactive intestinal peptide modulates immunoglobulin secretion in murine schistosomiasis. Cell Immunol. **135:** 394–401.
78. BLUM, A.M. *et al*. 1993. Substance P modulates antigen-induced, IFN-γ production in murine Schistosomiasis mansoni. J. Immunol. **151:** 225–233.
79. ARSENESCU, R. *et al*. 2005. IL-12 induction of mRNA encoding substance P in murine macrophages from the spleen and sites of inflammation. J. Immunol. **174:** 3906–3911.
80. BLUM, A.M. *et al*. 1999. The substance P receptor is necessary for a normal granulomatous response in murine schistosomiasis mansoni. J. Immunol. **162:** 6080–6085.
81. METWALI, A. *et al*. 2004. Cutting edge: hemokinin has substance P-like function and expression in inflammation. J. Immunol. **172:** 6528–6532.
82. WEINSTOCK, J.V. & D. ELLIOTT. 2000. The somatostatin immunoregulatory circuit present at sites of chronic inflammation. Eur. J. Endocrinol. **143**(Suppl 1): S15–S19.
83. MANTYH, C.R. *et al*. 1995. Differential expression of substance P receptors in patients with Crohn's disease and ulcerative colitis. Gastroenterology **109:** 850–860.
84. MANTYH, C.R. *et al*. 1994. Substance P binding sites on intestinal lymphoid aggregates and blood vessels in inflammatory bowel disease correspond to authentic NK-1 receptors. Neurosci. Lett. **178:** 255–259.
85. RAITHEL, M., H.T. SCHNEIDER & E.G. HAHN. 1999. Effect of substance P on histamine secretion from gut mucosa in inflammatory bowel disease. Scand. J. Gastroenterol. **34:** 496–503.
86. GOLDIN, E. *et al*. 1989. Colonic substance P levels are increased in ulcerative colitis and decreased in chronic severe constipation. Dig. Dis. Sci. **34:** 754–757.
87. MAZUMDAR, S. & K.M. DAS. 1992. Immunocytochemical localization of vasoactive intestinal peptide and substance P in the colon from normal subjects and patients with inflammatory bowel disease. Am. J. Gastroenterol. **87:** 176–181.

88. BERNSTEIN, C.N., M.E. ROBERT & V.E. EYSSELEIN. 1993. Rectal substance P concentrations are increased in ulcerative colitis but not in Crohn's disease. Am. J. Gastroenterol. **88:** 908–913.
89. YAMAMOTO, H. *et al.* 1996. Abnormal neuropeptide concentration in rectal mucosa of patients with inflammatory bowel disease. J. Gastroenterol. **31:** 525–532.
90. RENZI, D. *et al.* 1998. Substance P and vasoactive intestinal polypeptide but not calcitonin gene-related peptide concentrations are reduced in patients with moderate and severe ulcerative colitis. Ital. J. Gastroenterol. Hepatol. **30:** 62–70.
91. BROWN, D.R., A.M. PARSONS & S.M. O'GRADY. 1992. Substance P produces sodium and bicarbonate secretion in porcine jejunal mucosa through an action on enteric neurons. J. Pharmacol. Exp. Ther. **261:** 1206–1212.
92. PARSONS, A.M. *et al.* 1992. Neurokinin receptors and mucosal ion transport in porcine jejunum. J. Pharmacol. Exp. Ther. **261:** 1213–1221.
93. WANG, L. *et al.* 1995. Substance P induces ion secretion in mouse small intestine through effects on enteric nerves and mast cells. Am. J. Physiol. **269:** G85–G92.
94. KUWAHARA, A. & H.J. COOKE. 1990. Tachykinin-induced anion secretion in guinea pig distal colon: role of neural and inflammatory mediators. J. Pharmacol. Exp. Ther. **252:** 1–7.
95. RIEGLER, M. *et al.* 1999. Substance P causes a chloride-dependent short-circuit current response in rabbit colonic mucosa *in vitro.* Scand. J. Gastroenterol. **34:** 1203–1211.
96. TURVILL, J.L., P. CONNOR & M.J. FARTHING. 2000. Neurokinin 1 and 2 receptors mediate cholera toxin secretion in rat jejunum. Gastroenterology **119:** 1037–1044.
97. DI SEBASTIANO, P. *et al.* 1999. SR140333, a substance P receptor antagonist, influences morphological and motor changes in rat experimental colitis. Dig. Dis. Sci. **44:** 439–444.
98. CASTAGLIUOLO, I. *et al.* 2002. Protective effects of neurokinin-1 receptor during colitis in mice: role of the epidermal growth factor receptor. Br. J. Pharmacol. **136:** 271–279.
99. STUCCHI, A.F. *et al.* 2000. NK-1 antagonist reduces colonic inflammation and oxidative stress in dextran sulfate-induced colitis in rats. Am. J. Physiol. Gastrointest. Liver Physiol. **279:** G1298–G1306.
100. STUCCHI, A.F. *et al.* 2003. A neurokinin 1 receptor antagonist reduces an ongoing ileal pouch inflammation and the response to a subsequent inflammatory stimulus. Am. J. Physiol. Gastrointest. Liver Physiol. **285:** G1259–G1267.
101. BERG, D.J. *et al.* 2002. Rapid development of colitis in NSAID-treated IL-10-deficient mice. Gastroenterology **123:** 1527–1542.
102. STURIALE, S. *et al.* 1999. Neutral endopeptidase (EC 3.4.24.11) terminates colitis by degrading substance P. Proc. Natl. Acad. Sci. USA **96:** 11653–11658.
103. LIEB, K. *et al.* 1996. Effects of substance P and selected other neuropeptides on the synthesis of interleukin-1 beta and interleukin-6 in human monocytes: a re-examination. J. Neuroimmunol. **67:** 77–81.
104. FIEBICH, B.L. *et al.* 2000. The neuropeptide substance P activates p38 mitogen-activated protein kinase resulting in IL-6 expression independently from NF-kappa B. J. Immunol. **165:** 5606–5611.
105. DEROCQ, J.M. *et al.* 1996. Effect of substance P on cytokine production by human astrocytic cells and blood mononuclear cells: characterization of novel tachykinin receptor antagonists. FEBS Lett. **399:** 321–325.

106. LIEB, K. *et al.* 1997. The neuropeptide substance P activates transcription factor NF-kappa B and kappa B-dependent gene expression in human astrocytoma cells. J. Immunol. **159:** 4952–4958.
107. AZZOLINA, A., A. BONGIOVANNI & N. LAMPIASI. 2003. Substance P induces TNF-alpha and IL-6 production through NF kappa B in peritoneal mast cells. Biochem. Biophys. Acta. **1643:** 75–83.
108. KOON, H.W. *et al.* 2005. Substance P-stimulated interleukin-8 expression in human colonic epithelial cells involves PKC{delta} activation. J. Pharmacol. Exp. Ther **314:** 1393–1400.
109. SIMEONIDIS, S. *et al.* 2003. Regulation of the NK-1 receptor gene expression in human macrophage cells via an NF-kappa B site on its promoter. Proc. Natl. Acad. Sci. USA **100:** 2957–2962.
110. WEINSTOCK, J.V. *et al.* 2003. IL-18 and IL-12 signal through the NF-kappa B pathway to induce NK-1R expression on T cells. J. Immunol. **170:** 5003–5007.
111. GUO, C.J. *et al.* 2004. Interleukin-1beta upregulates functional expression of neurokinin-1 receptor (NK-1R) via NF-kappaB in astrocytes. Glia **48:** 259–266.
112. BARDELLI, C. *et al.* 2005. Expression of functional NK1 receptors in human alveolar macrophages: superoxide anion production, cytokine release and involvement of NF-kappaB pathway. Br. J. Pharmacol. **145:** 385–396.
113. REED, K.L. *et al.* 2005. NF-kappaB activation precedes increases in mRNA encoding neurokinin-1 receptor, proinflammatory cytokines, and adhesion molecules in dextran sulfate sodium-induced colitis in rats. Dig. Dis. Sci. **50:** 2366–2378.
114. NILSSON, J., A.M. VON EULER & C.J. DALSGAARD. 1985. Stimulation of connective tissue cell growth by substance P and substance K. Nature **315:** 61–63.
115. CASTAGLIUOLO, I. *et al.* 2000. Epidermal growth factor receptor transactivation mediates substance P-induced mitogenic responses in U-373 MG cells. J. Biol. Chem. **275:** 26545–26550.
116. KOON, H.W. *et al.* 2004. Metalloproteinases and transforming growth factor-alpha mediate substance P-induced mitogen-activated protein kinase activation and proliferation in human colonocytes. J. Biol. Chem. **279:** 45519–45527.

Hypothalamic-Pituitary-Adrenal Axis Function in Sjögren's Syndrome

Mechanisms of Neuroendocrine and Immune System Homeostasis

ELIZABETH O. JOHNSON,[a] MARIA KOSTANDI,[b]
AND HARALAMPOS M. MOUTSOPOULOS[c]

[a]Department of Anatomy-Histology-Embryology, School of Medicine, University of Ioannina, Ioannina 45-110, Greece

[b]Department of Pharmacology, School of Medicine, University of Ioannina, Ioannina 45-110, Greece

[c]Department of Pathophysiology, School of Medicine, University of Athens, Athens, Greece

ABSTRACT: To date, evidence suggests that rheumatic diseases are associated with hypofunctioning of the hypothalamic-pituitary-adrenal (HPA) axis. Sjögren's syndrome (SS), the second most common autoimmune disorder, is characterized by diminished lacrimal and salivary gland secretion. To examine HPA axis activity in SS patients, the adrenocorticotropin (ACTH) response to ovine corticotropin-releasing factor (oCRH) was used as a direct measure of corticotrophic function, and the plasma cortisol response to the ACTH released during oCRH stimulation as an indirect measure of adrenal function. Significantly lower basal ACTH and cortisol levels were found in patients with SS and were associated with a blunted pituitary and adrenal response to oCRH compared to normal controls. Fibromyalgia (FM) patients demonstrated elevated evening basal ACTH and cortisol levels and a somewhat exaggerated peak, delta, and net integrated ACTH response to oCRH. A subgroup of SS patients also met the diagnostic criteria for FM and demonstrated a pituitary-adrenal response that was intermediate to SS and FM. These findings suggest not only adrenal axis hypoactivity in SS and FM patients, but also that varying patterns of adrenal and thyroid axes dysfunction may exist in patients with different rheumatic diseases.

KEYWORDS: HPA axis; CRH; ACTH; Sjögren's syndrome; fibromyalgia; hypothalamus

Address for correspondence: Elizabeth O. Johnson, Ph.D., Department of Anatomy-Histology-Embryology, University of Ioannina, School of Medicine, Ioannina 45-110, Greece. Voice: +30-26510-97584; fax: +30-26510-97861.
e-mail: ejohnson@cc.uoi.gr

Ann. N.Y. Acad. Sci. 1088: 41–51 (2006). © 2006 New York Academy of Sciences.
doi: 10.1196/annals.1366.018

INTRODUCTION

Over the last decade, novel and truly exciting developments have emerged in several areas of neuroimmunology. There is now a growing emphasis on an integrative approach that attempts to explore possible common pathophysiological and genetic mechanisms in inflammatory and stress-related disorders. These studies explore the interface between immunologic, neurobiologic, endocrinologic, and metabolic factors. As a result, substantial strides have been made in our understanding of the biochemical, molecular, and behavioral mechanisms of action for the chemical mediators responsible for the communication and integration of the immune and nervous systems over a wide range of biomedical phenomena.[1–3]

The study of the neuroimmunological aspects in immune diseases has emerged from a tradition of mechanistic descriptions of cell-to-cell communication in the immune system, a growing awareness of the psychiatric and neurologic manifestations in several inflammatory disorders, and a series of investigations assessing the role of the neuroendocrine system in maintaining physiological homeostasis.[1–3] Recent advances in cellular and molecular biological techniques have facilitated our understanding of major and rapid alterations in traditional concepts of the regulation of immune and neuroendocrine systems. Today, it is generally accepted that the immune and inflammatory processes bidirectionally communicate with the central nervous system (CNS), which in turn, plays a role in modulating the inflammatory response.[1,4] This communicatory link involves hormonal and neuronal mechanisms through which the brain can regulate immune system function, and conversely immune factors, such as cytokines, that can influence CNS function.

Several neurohormonal systems and immunologic factors appear to play a fundamental role in these communicatory links which enable the peripheral immunologic apparatus to signal and interact with the brain and participate in maintaining immunologic homeostasis.[5–7] This is facilitated by an extensive coexpression of receptors and overlap of synthesis of a multitude of hormone-like molecules that regulate cell function. In this regard, interleukin-1 (IL-1), a major product of activated macrophages, has extensively been studied. IL-1 receptors are expressed not only on peripheral T lymphocytes, but also in the brain.[8,9] In addition to regulating a wide range of neural functions that are under direct CNS control including arousal, body temperature, sleep, food intake, reproductive behavior and mood, some of the actions of IL-1 on peripheral immune function also appear to be mediated by IL-1 in the CNS.[10] However, the relation of CNS IL-1 to peripheral immune system–derived IL-1 remains to be elucidated. IL-1 is also a potent stimulator of the hypothalamic-pituitary-adrenal (HPA) axis, resulting in the release of corticosteroids. Corticosteroids, in turn, feed back to inhibit macrophage release of IL-1.[11] Other examples of this intricate communication between the immune and nervous system are increasingly being characterized.

TABLE 1. HPA axis function parameters in SS patients [2,3,23]

Locus	Hormone	Conditions	pSS	sSS	Normal
Pituitary	Basal ACTH	Evening	$5.1 \pm 0.5*$	11.8 ± 6.3	11.4 ± 1.5
	Peak ACTH	oCRH Stimulus	$46.2 \pm 5.4*$	56.9 ± 15.9	61.5 ± 3.8
Adrenal	Basal Cortisol	Evening	$2.4 \pm 0.6*$	6.8 ± 2.5	5.9 ± 1.2
	Peak Cortisol	oCRH Stimulus	$15.7 \pm 1.6*$	6.8 ± 4.4	19.6 ± 0.7

ACTH levels in pg/mL.
Cortisol levels in μg/mL.
*$P \leq 0.05$ ANOVA followed by Fisher protected least significant difference (PSLD) (pSS compared to normal controls).

Recent evidence suggests that there are two major pathways by which the CNS can regulate the immune system. The first pathway is through neuro-hormonal systems, particularly the HPA or stress axis. Other neurohormonal systems that appear to also play important roles include the hypothalamic-pituitary-gonadal (HPG) axis, the hypothalamic-pituitary-thyroid (HPT) axis, and the hypothalamic-growth hormone axis. The second major pathway is the autonomic nervous system and the release of norepinephrine and acetyl-choline. Glucocorticoids inhibit the functions of virtually all inflammatory cells via the alteration of transcription of cytokine genes (tumor necrosis factor [TNF], IL-1, IL-6) and inhibiting the production of arachidonic-acid-derived proinflammatory substances, such as leukotrienes and prostragladins.

Conversely, the immune system modulates CNS function through various factors, particularly cytokines that can act independently or synergistically. The CNS contains IL-1 receptors in areas that control the acute-phase response.[12] In addition, IL-1 stimulates the production of endothelia cell prostaglandins that, in turn, induce corticotropin-releasing factor (CRH) release from the median eminence.[13] In contrast, IL-6 acts as a potent stimulator of adrenocorticotropin (ACTH) and cortisol release.[14]

In healthy individuals, this bidirectional regulatory system forms a negative feedback loop, which keeps the CNS and immune system in balance. Perturbations of these regulatory systems could potentially lead to either overactivation or oversuppression of the immune responses. One working hypothesis is that disruptions of the communication links between the immune system and the CNS may be associated with susceptibility or severity of autoimmune/inflammatory disease.

THE HPA AXIS

The stress system consists of three central and two peripheral components. The central components of the stress system comprise the locus ceruleus in the reticular formation, which regulates arousal, the brainstem centers of the autonomic system, which regulate sympathetic/adrenomedullary function, and the hypothalamic paraventricular nucleus (PVN), which regulates adrenocortical function. The peripheral components consist of the sympa-thetic/adrenomedullary system and the pituitary-adrenal axis. The interactions between the various components of the stress system are numerous and com-plex.[4] CRH-secreting neurons of the lateral PVN project toward the arousal and sympathetic system in the hindbrain, and, conversely, catecholaminergic fibers from the locus ceruleus and central sympathetic system project via the ascending noradrenergic bundle to the PVN in the hypothalamus. Activation of the CRH neurons in the PVN results in the release of CRH into the hypophy-seal portal system, and stimulation of the arousal and sympathetic centers in the brainstem, in a positive, reverberating feedback loop.

Both endrophin and ACTH secreted by the proopiomelano cortin (POMC) neurons of the arcuate nucleus exert inhibitory effects on CRH secretion. As POMC neurons are stimulated by CRH, they provide another negative feedback control loop on the HPA axis. ACTH stimulates the release of cortisol from the adrenal cortex, the latter which feeds back in a negative fashion, both at the level of the pituitary and the hypothalamus.[4] Activation of the stress system has direct consequences on the function of other major systems, particularly those responsible for reproduction, growth, and immunity.[4]

HPA AXIS AND IMMUNE SYSTEM DYSFUNCTION

Psychological stress has long been thought to be associated with the onset and exacerbations of autoimmune/inflammatory disease, with recent devel-opments indicating that a relationship between stress-related disorders and autoimmunity may be rooted in a common neuroendocrine defect. Physical, behavioral, and inflammatory stresses, through stimulation of the CRH neu-ron, activate a final common neuroendocrine pathway: the HPA axis. This suggests that an association between stress and development of inflammatory disease may be related to alterations of this common pathway, or to defects in the intricate feedback loops that exist between the immune system and the central components of the nervous system.

Corticosteroids represent one of the most potent endogenous anti-inflammatory agents known. They have the capacity to inhibit and suppress virtually all critical inflammatory and immune cell functions, even at physi-ological concentrations, and particularly during the early development of the immune/inflammatory response.[15] At the molecular level, they inhibit the pro-duction of most inflammatory mediators including IL-1, TNF, phospholipase A2, and prostaglandins. Hence, stress-induced enhanced production and se-cretion of glucocorticoids appears to counter-regulate and suppress excessive immune/inflammatory cell activation and mediator production that could oth-erwise result in self-induced tissue injury. This suggests a critical role for corticosteroids in maintaining physiological homeostasis during the adaptive response to noxious stressors.

Based on this counter-regulatory effect of corticosteroids in monitoring the immune system, several possible mechanisms by which clinical hyperimmune or autoimmune states may arise have been hypothesized.[16] For example, a predisposition to autoimmune disease could develop with abnormally rapid or altered catabolism of corticosteroids, which would result in functionally inappropriate levels of anti-inflammatory glucocorticoids. Patients with systemic lupus erythematosus (SLE) appear to have functionally deficient concentrations of glucocorticoids as a consequence of lymphocytes that catabolize cortisol more rapidly than normal.[17] Glucocorticoid resistance at the cellular level could also predispose an organism to develop a hyperimmune or autoimmune condition. For example, rheumatoid arthritis (RA) patients demonstrate deficient glucocorticoid-induced protein induction in polymorphonuclear leukocytes.[18] A common observation is that female patients with RA frequently go into remission during pregnancy and into a state of severe exacerbation in the postpartum period.[19]

Finally, another mechanism by which a hyperimmune state and autoimmune disease might develop would be when an individual is incapable of mounting an appropriate corticosteroid response during an invasive challenge and engagement of the inflammatory/immune system. In an animal model of autoimmune inflammatory disease, the Lewis (LEW/N) rat, a hypofunctional CRH neuron appears to allow development of RA and other autoimmune inflammatory diseases. This is related to an apparent interruption in the inflammatory mediator–CRH negative loop that leads to adequate counter-regulation of the inflammatory response via glucocorticoids.[20,21] The defect of the CRH neuron in this animal is generalized so that the CRH gene is hyporesponsive not only to any of the physiological stimuli, but to neurochemical and environmental stimuli as well. Hence, the Lewis rat shows not only evidence of defective immune counter-regulation, as a consequence of the deficient CRH neuron responsiveness, but also evidence of behavioral alterations compatible with decreased CRH synthesis and release in the CNS.

SJÖGREN'S SYNDROME

Sjögren's syndrome (SS) is a chronic, slowly progressing inflammatory-autoimmune exocrinopathy of unknown etiology. The typical clinical presentation of Sjögren's syndrome includes keratoconjunctivitis sicca and xerostomia, due to diminished lacrimal and salivary gland secretion. This autoimmune disease expands from an organ-specific (exocrine glands) to a systemic (extraglandular) disorder affecting lungs, kidneys, blood vessels, and muscles, as well as a B cell lymphoproliferative disorder. These features are believed to be the consequence of overt immune system activation, expressed by various autoantibodies, and lymphocytic invasion of the exocrine glands and the other affected organs.[22]

When not associated with other connective tissue diseases, the syndrome is classified as primary SS (pSS). Secondary SS (sSS) defines the disease complex in the presence of other autoimmune disorders, such as RA and SLE.[22] About half of the patients have an associated autoimmune disease, and patients often express fatigue, arthralgias, and myalgias, among other, symptoms which typically characterizes fibromyalgia (FM). FM is a nonarticular rheumatic syndrome that can occur as a feature of SS. SS is the second most common autoimmune rheumatic disorder after RA. It progresses very slowly, with 8–10 years elapsing from the initial symptoms to the full-blown development of the syndrome. It has a strong predilection for women in the fourth or fifth decade of life. The presence of focal lymphoid infiltrate lesions and marked autoantibody responses against the Ro SSA antigen (SSA) and La SSB antigen (SSB) ribonucleoproteins ranks SS exocrinopathy as an autoimmune disorder.[22]

THE HPA AXIS IN SJÖGREN'S SYNDROME

SS is associated with a low basal activity of the HPA axis, as indicated by low basal plasma ACTH levels and cortisol levels in the evening. As the HPA axis is normally at its nadir in the evening, this reduction in the mean evening basal ACTH and cortisol concentrations in SS patients is noteworthy. Although these evening measures provide some information about basal HPA axis function in this patient population, precise basal evaluation is not possible on account of the pulsatile, episodic nature of HPA axis function and its distinct circadian variation. Interestingly, patients with both SS and fibromyalgia (FMS, previously defined as FM) had evening basal ACTH and cortisol levels that were not significantly different from controls, and intermediate to those measured in patients with either FMS or SS alone.[23]

The functional integrity of the HPA was assessed using the ovine (o)CRH stimulation test in the evening in medication-free, female patients with SS during the prefollicular phase.[23] In this study, ACTH response to oCRH was used as a direct measure of corticotrophic function and the plasma cortisol response to ACTH released during oCRH stimulation was an indirect measure of adrenal function. Although patients with SS responded to the oCRH stimulation with a time-dependent increase in ACTH and cortisol levels, the low basal activity was associated with both pituitary and adrenal hyporesponsiveness, as seen with attenuation of the ACTH and cortisol responses (TABLE 1).

The blunted rather than exaggerated ACTH response to oCRH, despite basal hypocortisolism, suggests insufficient priming of the pituitary corticotrophs by endogenous CRH. If either the pituitary or hypothalamus were normal, the ACTH response to CRH would be expected to be exaggerated in the context of a relative lack of glucocorticoid negative feedback due to the low levels of cortisol.

The relative hyporesponsiveness of the adrenal glands to the endogenous ACTH released during the course of stimulation by oCRH could occur in two contexts. First, SS patients could express a primary adrenal insufficiency in which the adrenals are themselves intrinsically hypoactive. Secondly, it could occur in the context of insufficient stimulation of the adrenal cortex by ACTH, owing either to a pituitary or hypothalamic defect. The blunted cortisol response in SS patients compared to controls indicates a relative hyporesponsiveness of the adrenal glands to the endogenous ACTH released during the course of stimulation by oCRH. Because the ACTH response was also blunted in SS, this suggests that the adrenal has become hypofunctional, due to chronic understimulation by ACTH or to a process related to the disease itself.

Similar to our findings in SS, studies in RA patients reported normal or low normal cortisol secretion rates and basal levels.[23,25] We have shown that despite significant reduction in evening basal cortisol levels, patients with SS have attenuated, but clear ACTH responses to oCRH. We surmise that as in postoperative patients with Cushing's disease, chronic fatigue syndrome, seasonal affective disorder (SAD), atypical depression, and hypothyroidism, this attenuated ACTH response to CRH in the context of hypocortisolism reflects pituitary corticotrophs that are insufficiently primed by endogenous CRH. This suggests a subtle central adrenal insufficiency where CRH-activation of the pituitary-adrenal axis does not develop normally. In turn, a deficient HPA counter-regulatory response may allow the development of unchecked and, as a result, enhanced, inflammatory/immune cell activation. This apparent secondary or central adrenal insufficiency in SS patients is particularly intriguing in light of the Lewis (LEW/N) rat model. The Lewis rat, which develops severe arthritis to streptococcal cell wall, demonstrates a premorbid HPA axis hyporesponsiveness.[15,26]

Interleukin-1 (IL-1) is now viewed as a mediator of the stress response to noxious stimuli, including stimulation of the HPA axis in addition to the regulation of various related neural functions, such as arousal, body temperature, sleep, food intake, reproductive behavior, and mood.[27] Thus, in addition to its effects on immune cells, IL-1 directly stimulates the HPA axis to release corticosteroids, which, in turn, feed back to inhibit macrophage release of IL-1. Additional evidence that the neuroimmune axis is impaired in SS patients is the significantly higher levels of plasma IL-1 in these patients in the context of significant basal hypocortisolism and HPA axis hyporesponsiveness.[1–3] IL-6 is also significantly elevated in both serum and saliva of SS patients.[28] TNF plasma levels tend to be only slightly elevated in pSS patients compared to normal controls.

Similar to our findings in SS, studies in RA patients report normal or low-normal basal cortisol levels and secretion rates in association with increased levels of IL-6.[29] Although recombinant IL-6 activates the HPA axis, the ACTH and cortisol levels in patients with RA were found comparable to those of controls, despite increased IL-6 production in these patients. These findings underscore the insufficient HPA axis response to stimuli such as IL-6 or oCRH.

PSYCHIATRIC PROFILE IN SS

After an initial case report of "neurotic behavior" in a female with pSS,[30] several studies have provided ample evidence of psychiatric disturbances in SS patients.[23,31,32] In a detailed study of psychiatric dysfunction in pSS, the authors noted that the most common psychiatric abnormality entailed affective disturbances.[32] The authors noted that the behavioral symptoms closely fulfilled the criteria of the American Psychiatric Association's diagnostic and statistical manual for atypical depression rather than those of a major depressive episode. We have found that the majority of women with SS experienced a stressful life event 6 months to 2 years before the onset of their symptoms and expressed anxiety, fatigue, irritability, and impaired sleep quality as assessed by structured interviews.[23] The behavioral traits expressed by SS patients were found similar in nature to those characterizing atypical depression and chronic fatigue syndrome, among others. It is noteworthy that an unusually large cohort (16%) of chronic fatigue syndrome patients with complaints of severe, dominating, chronic fatigue, have been detected as also having SS.[33]

Perturbations in the CRH system in humans have been clearly associated with depressive symptoms.[4] In contrast to the enhanced arousal seen in melancholic depression, atypical depression represents an excessive counter-regulation of the generalized stress response, featuring lethargy, apathy, and passivity. Such a depressive syndrome also occurs during the course of various diseases including Cushing's disease, hypothyroidism, chronic fatigue syndrome, and RA.[13]

In a recent study by Stevenson, pSS was found to be associated with an increased risk for depression.[34] Although peripheral nervous system disease is a well-established complication in pSS,[35] until relatively recently little attention has been focused on CNS complications of this disorder. To date, CNS involvement in pSS is controversial with regard to frequency, significance, and etiology. MRI studies suggest increased discrete cerebral tissue damage in pSS patients.[36] Similarly, Escudero and colleagues detected hypertensive small subcortical lesions in 51% of the SS patients examined with cranial MRI.[37]

Similar to our findings in SS patients, studies which examined the activity of the HPA axis in patients with SAD reported a delayed and significantly blunted ACTH response to exogenous CRH in the setting of low-normal cortisol levels, suggesting that either the pituitary or hypothalamus was hyporesponsive.[38] Centrally mediated adrenal axis insufficiency has been documented in atypical depression,[39] postoperative Cushing's syndrome,[39] chronic fatigue syndrome,[40] and hypothyroidism.[41]

Taken together, the clinical relevance of the available data is not yet clear, although the findings suggest that patients with SS often show signs of the atypical form of major depression. Whether the clinical picture of SS and possible other forms of autoimmune disease in humans represents a confluence of immunological and behavioral deficits related to a deficiency in CRH responsiveness remains to be determined.

REFERENCES

1. JOHNSON, E.O. & H.M. MOUTSOPOULOS. 1992. Neuroimmunological axis and rheumatic diseases [editorial]. Eur. J. Clin. Invest. **22**(Suppl.1): 2–5.
2. JOHNSON, E.O. & H.M. MOUTSOPOULOS. 2000. Neuroendocrine manifestations in Sjögren's syndrome. Relation to neurobiology of stress. Ann. N. Y. Acad. Sci. **917:** 797–808.
3. JOHNSON, E.O., F. SKOPOULI & H.M. MOUTSOPOULOS. 2000. Neuroendocrine alterations in Sjögren's syndrome. *In* Rheumatic Disease Clinics of North America.Vol 26. A.T. Masi, Ed.: 927–949. W.B. Saunders, Philadelphia, PA
4. JOHNSON, E.O., T.C. KAMILARIS, G.P. CHROUSOS & P.W. GOLD. 1992. Mechanisms of stress: a dynamic overview of hormonal and behavioral homeostasis. Neurosci. Biobehav. Rev. **16:** 115–130.
5. BATEMAN, A., A. SINGH, K. THOMAS & S. SOLOMON. 1989. The immune-hypothalamic-pituitary-adrenal axis. Endocr. Rev. **10:** 92–112.
6. SMITH, E.M. & J.E. BLALOCK. 1989. A molecular basis for interaction between the immune and neuroendocrine systems. Intern. J. Neurosci. **38:** 455–465.
7. WILDER, R.L. & E.M. STERNBERG. 1990. Neuroendocrine hormonal factors in rheumatoid arthritis and related conditions. Curr. Opin. Rheumatol. **2:** 436–440.
8. FARRAR, W.L, P.L. KILIAN, M.R. RUFF *et al.* 1987. Visualization and characterization of interleukin-1 receptors in brain. J. Immunol. **139:** 459–465.
9. FONTANA, A., E. WEBER & J.M. DAYER. 1984. Synthesis of interleukin-1/endogenous pyrogen in the brain of endotoxin-treated mice: a step in fever induction? J. Immunol. **133:** 1696–1698.
10. ROTHWELL, N.J. 1991. Functions and mechanisms of interleukin 1 in the brain. Trends Pharm. Sci. **12:** 430–436.
11. MUNCK, A., P.M. GUYRE & N.J. HOLBROOK. 1984. Physiological functions of glucocorticoids in stress and their relation to pharmacological actions. Endocr. Rev. **5:** 25–44.
12. ERICSSON, A., C. LIU, R.P. HART & P.E. SAWCHENKO. 1995. Type 1 interleukin-1 receptor in the rat brain: distribution, regulation and relationship to sites of IL-1 induced cellular activation. J. Comp. Neurol. **361:** 681–698.
13. STERNBERG, E.M., G.P. CHROUSOS, R.L. WILDER & P.W. GOLD. 1992. The stress response and the regulation of inflammatory disease. Ann. Intern. Med. **117:** 854–866.
14. MASTORAKOS, G., G.P. CHROUSOS & J.S. WEBER. 1993. Recombinant interleukin-6 activates the hypothalamic-pituitary-adrenal axis in humans. J. Clin. Endocrinol. Metab. **77:** 1690–1694.
15. STERNBERG, E.M. & C.W. PARKER. 1988. Pharmacologic aspects of lymphocyte regulation. *In* The Lymphocyte, Structure and Function, 2nd edition. J.J. Marchalonis, Ed.: 1–54. Marcel Dekker. New York.

16. WILDER, R.L. & E.M. STERNBERG. 1990. Neuroendocrine hormonal factors in rheumatoid arthritis and related conditions. Curr. Opin. Rheumatol. **2:** 436–440.
17. KLEIN, A., D. BUSKILA, D. GLADMAN, et al. 1990. Cortisol catabolism by lymphocytes of patients with systemic lupus erythematosus and rheumatoid arthritis. J. Rheumatol. **17:** 30–33.
18. BLOWERS, L.E., M.I. JAYSON & M. JASANI. 1988. Dexamethasone modulated protein synthesis in polymorphonuclear leukocytes: response in rheumatoid arthritis. J. Rheumatol. **15:** 785–791.
19. LAHITA, R.G. 1987. Sex and age in systemic lupus erythematosus. *In* Systemic Lupus Erythematosus. R.G. Lahita, Ed.: 523–539. John Wiley & Sons. New York.
20. STERNBERG, E.M., J.M. HILL, G.P. CHROUSOS, *et al.* 1989. Inflammatory mediator-induced hypothalmic-pituitary-adrenal axis activation is defective in streptococcal cell wall arthritis-susceptible Lewis rats. Proc. Natl. Acad. Sci. USA **86:** 2374–2378.
21. STERNBERG, E.M. & R.L. WILDER. 1989. The role of the hypothalamic-pituitary-adrenal axis in an experimental model of arthritis. Prog. Neuroendocrinimmun **2:** 102–108.
22. MOUTSOPOULOS, H.M. & P. YOUINOU. 1991. New developments in Sjögren's syndrome. Curr. Opin. Rheumatol. **3:** 815–822.
23. JOHNSON, E.O., P. VLACHOYIANNOPOULOS, F.N. SKOPOULI, *et al.* 1998. Hypofunction of the stress axis in Sjogren's syndrome. J. Rheumatol. **25:** 1508–1514.
24. HILL, S.R., A. ULLAO, W.R. STARNESS & A.L. HOLLWY. 1963. Corticosteroids in rheumatoid arthritis. Arch. Intern. Med. **112:** 603.
25. PAL, S.B. 1970. The secretion rate of cortisol in patients with rheumatoid arthritis. Clin. Chim. Acta. **29:** 129.
26. STERNBERG, E.M., R.L. WILDER, G.P. CHROUSOS & P.W. GOLD. 1991. Stress responses and the pathogenesis of arthritis. *In* Stress, Neuropeptides, and Systemic Disease. McCubbin, Ed.: 287–300. Academic Press. New York.
27. STERNBERG, E.M. 1997. Emotions and disease. From balance of humors to balance of molecules. Nat. Med. **3:** 264–267.
28. GRISIUS, M.M., D.K. BERMUDEZ & P.C. FOX. 1997. Salivary and serum interleukin 6 in primary Sjogren's syndrome. J. Rheumatol. **24:** 1291–1295.
29. AL-JANADI, M., S. AL-BALLA, A. AL-DALAAN & S. RAZIUDDIN. 1993. Cytokine profile in systemic lupus erythematosus, rheumatoid arthritis and other rheumatic diseases. J. Clin. Immunol. **13:** 58.
30. SHELDON, J.H. 1938. Sjogren's syndrome associated with pigmentation and scleroderma of the legs. Proc. R. Soc. Med. **32:** 255.
31. DROSOS, A.A., A.P. ANDONOPOULOS, G. LAGOS, *et al.* 1989. Neuropsychiatric abnormalities in primary Sjogren's syndrome. Clin. Exp. Rheumatol. **7:** 207.
32. MALINOW, K.L., R. MOLINA B. GORDON, *et al.* 1985. Neuropsychiatric dysfunction in primary Sjogren's syndrome. Ann. Intern. Med. **103:** 344–349.
33. CALABRESE, L.H., M.E. DAVIS & W.S. WILKE. 1994. Chronic fatigue syndrome and a disorder resembling Sjögren's syndrome: preliminary report. Clin. Infect. Dis. **18**(Suppl. 1): S28–S31.
34. STEVENSON, H.A., M.E. JONES, J.L. ROSTRON, *et al.* 2004. UK patients with priamry Sjogren's syndrome are at increased risk from clinical depresion. Gerodontology **21:** 141–145.
35. VALTYSDOTTIR, S.T., B. GUDBJORNSSON U. LINDQVIST, *et al.* 1989. Anxiety and depression in patients with primary Sjogren's syndrome. Scand. J. Rheumatol. **18:** 21–27.

36. COATES, T., J.P. SLAVOTINEK, M. RISCHMUELLER, *et al.* 2000. Cerebral white matter lesions in primary Sjogren's syndrome: a controlled study. J. Neurol. Neurosurg. Psychiatry **68:** 170–177.

37. ESCUDER, D., P. LATORE, M. CODINA, *et al.* 1999. Central nervous system disease in Sjogren's syndrome. Clin. Rheumatol. **18:** 299–303.

38. VANDERPOOL, J., N. ROSENTHAL G.P. CHROUSOS, *et al.* 1991. Evidence for hypothalamic CRH deficiency in patients with seasonal affective disorder. J. Clin. Endocrinol. Metab. **72:** 1382–1387.

39. GOLD, P.W., F.K. GOODWIN & G.P. CHROUSOS. 1988. Clinical and biochemical manifestations of depression: relation to the neurobiology of stress. N. Engl. J. Med. **319:** 384–393.

40. DEMITRACK, M.A., J.K. DALE S.E. STRAUS, *et al.* 1991. Evidence for impaired activation of the hypothalamic-pituitary-adrenal axis in patients with chronic fatigue syndrome. J. Clin. Endocrinol. Metab. **73:** 1224–1234.

41. KAMILARIS, T.C., C.R. DEBOLD E.O. JOHNSON, *et al.* 1991. Effects of short and long duration hypothyroidism and hyperthroidism on the plasma adrenocorticotropin and corticosterone responses to ovine corticotropin-releasing hormone in rats. Endocrinology **128:** 2567–2576.

The Role of Chaperone Proteins in Autoimmunity

JOHN G. ROUTSIAS AND ATHANASIOS G. TZIOUFAS

Department of Pathophysiology, School of Medicine, University of Athens, 11527 Athens, Greece

ABSTRACT: Heat-shock or stress proteins (HSPs) are intracellular molecules that are expressed under cellular stress and have housekeeping and cytoprotective functions. Many of them act also as molecular chaperones, assisting the correct folding, stabilization, and translocation of proteins. In pathological situations, such as necrotic cell death, they can be released into the extracellular environment complexed with intact or fragmented cellular proteins. Evidence is now accumulating to indicate that, under certain circumstances, these complexes can contribute to induction of autoimmunity by receptor-mediated activation of the innate immune response (signaling the "danger") and by participation in the presentation of autoantigens for the adaptive immune response (acting as natural adjuvants). In addition, the conservation of HSPs through prokaryotes and eukaryotes, together with the increased production of host and microbial HSPs at the site of infection, has led to the proposition that these proteins may provide a link between infection and autoimmunity. This review outlines the mechanisms for the potential involvement of chaperones in the induction of autoimmune disease.

KEYWORDS: autoimmunity; chaperones; heat shock stress proteins; epitopes; calreticulin; HSP70; HSP60; Bip

HEAT-SHOCK / STRESS PROTEINS AND MOLECULAR CHAPERONES

Cell stressors including heat, irradiation, reactive oxygen species, hypoxia, pH shift, infection, inflammation, nutritional deficiency, and exposure to chemical agents cause modifications of the intracellular milieu. They include downregulation of many housekeeping genes and activation of stress genes that are usually transcribed at low levels in the absence of stress.[1,2] The products of these genes are called heat-shock stress proteins (HSPs) and have the capacity

Address of correspondence: Athanasios G. Tzioufas, M.D., Department of Pathophysiology, School of Medicine, University of Athens, 75, M. Asias St., 11527 Athens, Greece. Voice: +30-210-7462670; fax: +30-210-7462664.

e-mail: agtzi@med.uoa.gr

Ann. N.Y. Acad. Sci. 1088: 52–64 (2006). © 2006 New York Academy of Sciences.
doi: 10.1196/annals.1366.029

to stabilize and refold the partially denatured proteins or mediate the degradation of nonreversibly damaged proteins under stress conditions. Under physiological conditions, some of these proteins function as molecular chaperones. They assist a nascent polypeptide chain to attain a functional conformation and then bring the protein to the cellular site where it carries out its functions.[3] The term "heat shock proteins" is somewhat of a misnomer, as they are not induced solely by heat shock. However, for historical reasons, the term "HSP" is used even if the parent gene is induced by other than heat-shock stressors. We should also note that many HSPs are not chaperones and, conversely, only a fraction of chaperones are encoded in genes that are inducible by stressors and thus belong to the stress proteins. Therefore, the terms "HSPs" and "chaperones" have to be used carefully to avoid misunderstanding (e.g., a HSP is not necessarily induced by heat shock and a chaperone is not necessarily a HSP).

Chaperones and HSPs are classified into groups according their localization and molecular mass in kilodaltons (kDa). The best-understood HSPs are those with a molecular weight of 110, 90, 70, and 60 kDa, respectively, called also major HSPs. They are constitutively expressed primarily in the cytosol and mitochondria in the absence of heat stress and their expression can be upregulated by various stressors. The second group comprises the "minor" HSPs, which are located primary in the rough endoplasmic reticulum (ER) and are induced by glucose deprivation. This group includes glucose-regulated proteins (grp) with molecular weights of 34, 47, 56, 75, 78, 94, and 174 kDa. A third group consists of low (about 20 kDa) molecular mass HSPs.

HSP60 and HSP70 families are the major chaperones of the cytosol. HSP70s are highly conserved and demonstrate a 60–78% base identity among eukaryotic cells and a 40–60% identity between eukaryotic HSP70 and *Escherichia coli* DNAK.[4,5] HSP70 family members are equipped with two major functional domains, including a C-terminal region that binds peptides and denatured proteins, and an N-terminal ATPase domain that controls the opening and closing of the peptide-binding domain.[6] The HSP60 family comprises HSP60 in mammals, mycobacterial homologue mHSP65, chlamydial HSP60, and the *E. coli* homologue GroEL.[7] HSP60 family members bind to partially folded polypeptides and assist in their correct folding as well as in their assembly in multimeric complexes.[6]

In the ER the major chaperones include Grp78, Grp58, calnexin, and calreticulin. Grp78 (also referred to as BiP, the immunoglobulin binding protein)[8] interacts with many secretory and membrane proteins within the ER during the course of their maturation. Grp58 belongs to the family of disulfide isomerases, the folding enzymes of the ER, which catalyze the formation of disulfide bonds.[9] Calnexin and calreticulin are thought to function as chaperones monitoring the folding and assembly of glycoproteins.[10] Calreticulin is also considered to recognize specific oligosaccharides in the carbohydrate portion of glycoproteins, acting like a lectin.[11]

CHAPERONES AND THE IMMUNE SYSTEM

The most appropriate stimulus for innate immunity is the exposure to a foreign molecule in a "dangerous" milieu. In this context, "danger" is signaled by certain conserved molecules of invading pathogens (pathogen-associated molecular pattern, PAMP). The essential decision for responding to or ignoring a particular antigen is made by innate immune recognition receptors upon activation by PAMP molecules, such as lipopolysaccharide (LPS) or bacterial CpG DNA.[12] Receptors of this type, called pattern recognition receptors (PRRs) have been identified in large numbers. Many recently cloned PRRs belong to the expanding family of toll-like receptors (TLRs). An alternative pathway for the activation of innate immunity was proposed by Matzinger. The so-called "danger theory" states that, in addition, innate immunity can be activated by endogenous substances released by damaged or stressed tissue.[13] Thus, stressed mammalian cells can messenger stress to other (immune or nonimmune) cells. Potential candidates for signaling tissue damage or cellular stress are heat-shock proteins. In this regard, HSP60 and HSP70 have been found capable of signaling through CD14, TLR-2, and TLR-4.[14–16]

In addition to having a function as stimulators of the innate immune system, HSPs have been also shown to play a role in generating antigen-specific T cell responses.[17,18] The proposed mechanism is that peptides, complexed with the HSPs—including HSP70, Gp96, and calreticulin—are delivered to antigen-presenting cells (APCs) by receptor-mediated internalization of the HSPs, making them available for processing and presentation on major histocompatibility complex (MHC) molecules. Specific receptor-mediated mechanisms exist for the capture and internalization of HSPs,[19] suggesting that cross-presentation of HSP-derived antigenic determinants is a legitimate mechanism for cross-priming by professional APCs.

Moreover, HSPs can be overexpressed in different pathologic conditions and serve as specific targets of the adaptive immune response. All these discrete immunological functions of HSPs are discussed in detail in the following paragraphs.

HSPs as Targets of the Immune Response

Infection is a stressful process—for both the pathogen and the host—and therefore inevitably results in increased production of molecular chaperones by the pathogen as well as by the host. The conservation of HSPs through prokaryotes and eukaryotes, together with the increased production of host and microbial HSPs at the site of infection, has led to suggestions that cross-reactivity between host and pathogen HSPs might be responsible for a variety of autoreactive disorders that are associated with high frequency recognition of HSPs.[7,20] In this context, the possible involvement of mycobacterial HSP70 in the autoantibody production in systemic lupus erythematosus (SLE) has been indicated in one study.[21]

Regardless of the participation of HSPs in the pathogenesis of autoimmunity via antigenic cross-reactivity, HSPs are capable of eliciting immune responses.[22] Autoantibodies and cells reactive to HSP have been detected in patients with rheumatoid arthritis,[23] SLE,[24] inflammatory bowel disease,[25] multiple sclerosis,[26,27] Bechet's disease,[28] ocular inflammation,[29] and development of vascular lesions.[30] The role of this autoimmune response to HSPs in various diseases has not been yet identified. In one case autoantibodies to HSP90 have been correlated with elevated levels of IL-6 in SLE.[31] In another study, a cross-recognition between the HSP60 and the Ro60 autoantigen, has been demonstrated.[32,33]

Besides molecular mimicry, a process known as intermolecular spreading of humoral autoimmunity has been implicated for the induction of autoantibodies against HSPs. As a model for epitope spreading, the Ro/La ribonucleoprotein complex (RNP) was used. This autoantigenic complex is formed by the noncovalent association of the Ro52, La, and Ro60 autoantigens with a small cytoplasmic RNA (hYRNA).[34] The chaperone calreticulin has been also identified as an additional component of the complex.[35] Immunization experiments showed spreading of the immune response from Ro52 and Ro60—but not La—to calreticulin in murine experimental autoimmunity, consistent with the notion that calreticulin may associate with the subpopulation of Ro particles from which La has already dissociated.[36] Subsequent work from the same group demonstrated additional spreading of autoimmunity to the Bip and HSP70 chaperones after immunization with Ro52 and Ro60 autoantigens, suggesting that these components may co-localize and physically associate under certain conditions. The potential importance of the ER-resident chaperones, Bip and calreticulin, in autoimmune response against Ro/La RNP is further supported by their co-localization with Ro in small apoptotic membrane blebs[37] and the finding that Bip interacts with the Ro52 autoantigen.[38]

HSPs as Pro-inflammatory Mediators

The "danger theory" asserts that—in addition to infectious non-self-agents—professional APCs can be activated by endogenous substances released by damaged, infected, stressed, or transformed cells.[13,39] The first piece of evidence demonstrating that HSP60 and HSP70 stimulate human monocytes to release proinflammatory cytokines was presented in 1993.[40–42] Later, many authors provided further evidence for signaling and activation of different cells by HSP60 and HSP70.[43] However, it was found that LPS contamination has biased the results of these early experiments. The remarkable findings of Bausinger et al. call more attention to the interpretation of the results obtained before 2002.[44] These authors reported that endotoxin-free recombinant HSP70 fails to activate dendritic cells. In line with these observations, Gao et al. published two papers on the meticulous investigation of HSP-induced cytokine production by murine macrophages. HSP70 or HSP60 preparations with very low endotoxin contamination had no stimulatory effect on murine macrophages.[45,46] For this reason, researchers introduced more appropriate controls to rule out the potential LPS contamination present in recombinant preparations used for cell stimulation. In recent years, convincing evidence from well-documented studies indicate that the recognition of HSPs by different cells and the activation of targeted cells is a receptor-mediated process. Extracellular HSP60 from both bacteria and humans can stimulate a proinflammatory phenotype in various cells including monocytes/macrophages, dendritic cells, and vascular endothelial cells. These cells present increased expression of cell-surface adhesion molecules and release proinflammatory cytokines. The receptor(s) for human HSP60 is CD14 and/or TLR2 and/or TLR4.[47] Exogenous human and bacterial HSP70 proteins also stimulate monocytes/macrophages and dendritic cells via a plethora of receptors including CD14,[48] TLR2, TLR4,[49] CD40,[50,51] CD91,[52] and LOX-1.[53] The stimulation of proinflammatory behavior in various cells can also trigger the generation of adaptive immune response. Thus, both HSP60 and HSP70 seem to initiate the MyD88-dependent, Th1-type response–inducing pathway.[54]

HSPs as Potent Antigen Carriers

HSPs such as HSP70, HSP90, gp96, HSP110, grp170, and calreticulin (CRT) associate with a broad array of peptides generated within the cells.[55,56] These peptides include normal self-peptides as well as antigenic peptides derived from tumor,[57] bacterial antigens,[58] or viral antigens.[59] The cross-presentation hypothesis suggests that the complexes of HSP-chaperoned peptides released from the cells, after stress or cell death, are taken up by the APCs, resulting in representation (cross-presentation) of the peptides by MHC molecules of the APCs[56] A large body of evidence suggests that HSP–peptide complexes, which are generated within cells, can be used to immunize mice and elicit antigen-specific CD8$^+$ T cell responses. Immunization with femtomolar quantities of antigenic peptides chaperoned by HSPs (but not other proteins) is effective in eliciting such T cell responses.[60] On theoretical grounds, immunization with such a small quantity can be effective only after receptor-mediated endocytosis of the HSP-chaperoned peptides.[61] In attempting to identify the HSP receptor, Binder et al.[62] applied solubilized membranes of APCs to gp96 affinity columns and eluted and sequenced a gp96-binding protein. This turned out to be the previously known receptor of α2-macroglobulin, CD91. The CD91 molecule appears to function as the receptor not only for gp96, but also for

HSP90, HSP70, and calreticulin–peptide complexes,[52] although other receptors have also been proposed, including CD40[50] and LOX-1.[53]

It is now well accepted that HSPs act to chaperone peptides present in the cytosol for presentation and processing via the MHC class I molecule-loading pathway.[61,63] It has also been shown that gp96-associated peptides, besides MHC class I molecule-loading pathway, can enter an acidic compartment and load onto MHC class II molecules, implicating gp96 in MHC class II presentation.[64] Previous studies showed that exogenous bacterial HSPs enhance the class II MHC antigen processing and presentation of chaperoned peptides to CD4[+] T cells. Roth *et al.* demonstrated an enhancing effect of bacterial DNAK, the *E. coli* analogue of HSP70, in the MHC class II-dependent presentation of recombinant human acetylcholine receptor alpha-subunit Ag.[65] Similarly, Tobian *et al.* showed that exogenous bacterial HSPs (*E. coli* DNAK and *Mycobacterium tuberculosis* HSP70) delivered an extended OVA peptide for processing and MHC-II presentation, as detected by hybridoma T cells. These HSPs enhanced MHC-II presentation only if the peptide was chaperoned by the HSP. This process was found to be independent of TLR-induced induction of accessory molecules since it was intact in MyD88 knockout cells, which lack most TLR signaling.[66]

Recently, evidence that endogenous HSPs are involved in MHC class II antigen presentation has been provided. Mycko *et al.*, using MHC class II APCs, overexpressing HSP70 and an MBP-specific TCR hybridoma as well as T cell lines, demonstrated that HSP70 binds MBP peptides in an ATP/ADP-dependent manner and is actively involved in MHC class II-dependent autoantigen processing by the APCs.[67] Doody *et al.* compared the ability of the ER-resident HSP gp96 to prime CD4 and CD8 cells using TCR transgenic adoptive transfer systems and soluble gp96–peptide complexes. It was found that gp96 facilitated the *in vivo* cross-presentation of both class-I and class-II restricted peptides to CD8 and CD4 T cells, respectively. However, gp96 preferentially primed CD8—but not CD4—cell effector function.[68] In another study, using a soluble heat-shock fusion protein (Hsfp) having peptide sequences capable of inducing both CD4[+] and CD8[+] cells, it was found that many more class-II MHC peptide than class-I MHC peptide complexes are displayed on dendritic cells. In this study, the CD4 cells were found to respond far more vigorously than the CD8 cells.[69] In a similar way, taking advantage of an identified region in HIV Gag p24 that contains overlapping CTL and Th epitopes, Sen *et al.* studied the simultaneous presentation of these epitopes from a single precursor peptide complexed to HSP gp96. They demonstrated an efficient HSP-mediated presentation of at least eight different CTL and Th epitopes from the same precursor peptide sequence and induction of both CD8[+] and CD4[+]T-cell responses, respectively.[70]

Taken together, internalized HSP–peptide complexes can enter the MHC class I- and class II-enriched compartments by a receptor-mediated uptake and be presented to CD8 and CD4 T cells, eliciting a peptide-specific response.

HSPs as Natural Adjuvants

HSPs chaperone peptides, enchancing their antigenicity. One of the best-studied examples is the ER-resident chaperone calreticulin. Calreticulin is upregulated in response to various types of ER stress and has the ability to bind to glycoproteins containing monoglucosylated core glycans as well as to several nonglycosylated peptides. The ability of calreticulin to interact with nonglycosylated polypeptide substrates *in vitro* is highly influenced by environmental parameters, including the temperature and the presence of ATP and divalent cations. It has been suggested that exposure at high temperatures permits the exchange of naturally bound peptides to calreticulin with those added exogenously.[71,72] ATP binding to calreticulin increases its hydrophobicity, resulting in significant conformational alterations of the molecule.[73] Similarly, divalent cations appear to play a regulatory role on its activity as chaperone, most probably by neutralizing its negative charges, thereby inducing specific conformational changes.[74] A recent study demonstrated that the polypeptide-binding conformation of calreticulin is induced by heat shock, calcium depletion, or by deletion of the C-terminal acidic region.[75] Thus, cell stress conditions that generate nonnative substrates of calreticulin also affect the conformational properties of calreticulin itself, and enhance its binding to substrates, independent of substrate glucosylation.

We observed previously that calreticulin can be complexed with specific epitopes, inducing conformation-dependent recognition by autoantibodies from autoimmune human sera.[76] In our study calreticulin was isolated from human spleen, using a multistep purification method, and allowed to interact with seven biotinylated epitopes of Ro60, La, and Sm autoantigens. Among the synthetic peptides tested, only the two epitopes of Ro60 kDa autoantigen, spanning the sequences 175–184aa and 216–232aa, exhibited a substantial binding to calreticulin. Our results indicated that calreticulin–Ro60 kD peptide interaction was favored by heating at 40°C, the presence of ATP, and optimum concentrations of divalent ions. These conditions not only increased the interaction of calreticulin with Ro60 kDa epitopes, but also the antigenicity of the complex that exhibited a much more stronger anti-Ro60 kDa reactivity compared to that observed when calreticulin and peptides were tested individually. In fact, all anti-Ro60 kDa–positive sera of patients with autoimmune rheumatic diseases recognized the complex calreticulin–peptide, while the same sera displayed very low reactivity when tested individually with calreticulin or the Ro epitopes alone (TABLE 1). It was therefore proposed that calreticulin may play a more active role for the generation of autoimmune response against Ro60 kDa. According to our hypothesis, calreticulin can be released into the extracellular space, together with Ro fragments, after necrosis or cell lysis by cytotoxic T cells.[77,78] Under certain physicochemical conditions favored by the microenviromental milieu, calreticulin can bind Ro peptides, eventually increasing their antigenicity. The complex is then transported to professional APCs and the peptides are

TABLE 1. Reactivity of autoimmune sera against calreticulin (Crtc), Ro60 epitopes (10p and 17p), and calreticulin peptide complexes (Crtc-17p and Crtc-10p)

	Crtc-17p (%)	Crtc-10p (%)	Crtc (%)	17p (%)	10p
anti-Ro (+)	100	95	8	29	11%
anti-Ro (−)	8	4	4	0	4%

presented to autoreactive Th cells. In this regard calreticulin is used as a vehicle to deliver peptides in the immune system, augmenting the specific autoimmune response.

Recently, evidence for a similar mechanism has been provided for HSP70.[79] The heat-shock protein HSP70 was found to enhance antigen-specific proliferation of human CD4[+] memory T cells and to increase the immunogenicity of presented peptides. At low doses of antigen, stimulation with HSP70–peptide complexes was found to be far superior to stimulation with peptide alone. The complex formation of the antigenic peptide with HSP70 was found to be absolutely required in order to elicit an antigen-specific amplification. In this scenario, the induction of HSP70 decreases the threshold of activation of human CD4[+] T cells by the antigenic peptide. The increased reactivity of T cells against a peptide chaperoned by HSP indicates a putative involvement of HSP in the pathogenesis of autoimmune diseases. Thus, the induction of HSP by certain stress factors, such as infection, would facilitate an immune response

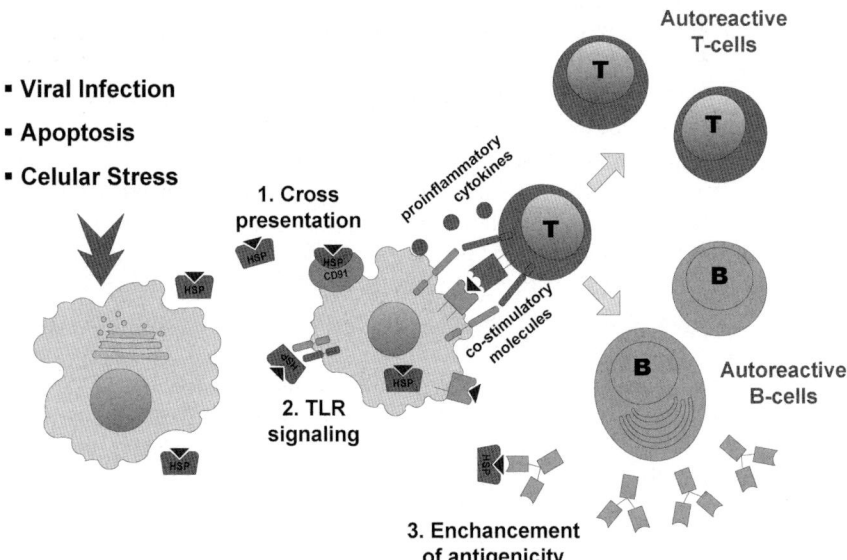

FIGURE 1. Proposed mechanism for the role of chaperones in the pathogenesis of autoimmunity.

to a given peptide of the self that would not be immunogenic under conditions where HSP is not available.

CHAPERONES AND AUTOIMMUNITY

HSPs seem to be directly involved in the pathogenesis of autoimmunity. They can also be directly implicated for the induction of autoimmunity if we summarize the functions of HSPs and consider the following series of events: Under specific conditions HSPs can meet self proteins, which are normally resident in different compartments of the cell. For example after induction of apoptosis or after a viral infection, which is accompanied by ER remodeling, the ER-resident chaperones can interact with intact or fragmented cytoplasmic autoantigens, thus enchancing their antigenicity.[76,38] Following subsequent secondary necrosis, extracellular HSPs may be released that can act as both proinflammatory mediators (signaling the "danger") and antigen carriers, facilitating cross-presentation of their "antigenic cargo" to sensitized Th and CTL cells. The activation of autoreactive T cells in the "proinflammatory milieu" of their microenvironment seems to be sufficient for the induction of humoral and cellular autoimmunity (FIG. 1).

REFERENCES

1. VERBEKE, P. *et al.* 2001. Heat shock response and ageing: mechanisms and applications. Cell Biol. Int. **25:** 845–857.
2. GAO, H. *et al.* 2004. Global transcriptome analysis of the heat shock response of *Shewanella oneidensis.* J. Bacteriol. **186:** 7796–7803.
3. KLEIZEN, B. & I. BRAAKMAN. 2004. Protein folding and quality control in the endoplasmic reticulum. Curr. Opin. Cell Biol. **16:** 343–349.
4. LINDQUIST, S. 1986. The heat-shock response. Annu. Rev. Biochem. **55:** 1151–1191.
5. CAPLAN, A.J., D.M. CYR & M.G. DOUGLAS. 1993. Eukaryotic homologues of *Escherichia coli* dnaj: a diverse protein family that functions with HSP70 stress proteins. Mol. Biol. Cell. **4:** 555–563.
6. BUKAU, B. & A.L. HORWICH. 1998. The HSP70 and HSP60 chaperone machines. Cell **92:** 351–366.
7. YOUNG, R.A. & T.J. ELLIOTT. 1989. Stress proteins, infection, and immune surveillance. Cell **59:** 5–8.
8. HAAS, I.G. 1991. BiP—a heat shock protein involved in immunoglobulin chain assembly. Curr. Top. Microbiol. Immunol. **167:** 71–82.
9. MAZZARELLA, R.A. *et al.* 1994. Erp61 is grp58, a stress-inducible luminal endoplasmic reticulum protein, but is devoid of phosphatidylinositide-specific phospholipase C activity. Arch. Biochem. Biophys. **308:** 454–460.
10. MICHALAK, M. *et al.* 1992. Calreticulin. Biochem. J. **285:** 681–692.
11. HELENIUS, A. 1994. How N-linked oligosaccharides affect glycoprotein folding in the endoplasmic reticulum. Mol. Biol. Cell. **5:** 253–265.

12. JANEWAY, C.A. Jr. & R. MEDZHITOV. 2002. Innate immune recognition. Annu. Rev. Immunol. **20:** 197–216.
13. MATZINGER, P. 1998. An innate sense of danger. Semin. Immunol. **10:** 399–415.
14. ASEA, A. 2003. Chaperokine-induced signal transduction pathways. Exerc. Immunol. Rev. **9:** 25–33.
15. OHASHI, K. *et al.* 2000. Cutting edge: heat shock protein 60 is a putative endogenous ligand of the toll-like receptor-4 complex. J. Immunol. **164:** 558–561.
16. VABULAS, R.M. *et al.* 2001. Endocytosed HSP60s use toll-like receptor 2 (TLR2) and TLR4 to activate the toll/interleukin-1 receptor signaling pathway in innate immune cells. J. Biol. Chem. **276:** 31332–31339.
17. SRIVASTAVA, P. 2002. Roles of heat-shock proteins in innate and adaptive immunity. Nat. Rev. Immunol. **2:** 185–194.
18. POCKLEY, A.G. 2003. Heat shock proteins as regulators of the immune response. Lancet **362:** 469–476.
19. ARNOLD-SCHILD, D. *et al.* 1999. Cutting edge: receptor-mediated endocytosis of heat shock proteins by professional antigen-presenting cells. J. Immunol. **162:** 3757–3760.
20. ZUGEL, U. & S.H. KAUFMANN. 1999. Role of heat shock proteins in protection from and pathogenesis of infectious diseases. Clin. Microbiol Rev. **12:** 19–39.
21. TASNEEM, S., N. ISLAM & R. ALI. 2001. Crossreactivity of SLE autoantibodies with 70 kDa heat shock proteins of *Mycobacterium tuberculosis*. Microbiol. Immunol. **45:** 841–846.
22. WINFIELD, J.B. & W.N. JARJOUR. 1991. Stress proteins, autoimmunity, and autoimmune disease. Curr. Top. Microbiol. Immunol. **167:** 161–189.
23. PANCHAPAKESAN, J., M. DAGLIS & P. GATENBY. 1992. Antibodies to 65 kDa and 70 kDa heat shock proteins in rheumatoid arthritis and systemic lupus erythematosus. Immunol. Cell Biol. **70:** 295–300.
24. JARJOUR, W.N. *et al.* 1991. Autoantibodies to human stress proteins. A survey of various rheumatic and other inflammatory diseases. Arthritis Rheum. **34:** 1133–1138.
25. STEVENS, T.R. *et al.* 1992. Circulating antibodies to heat-shock protein 60 in Crohn's disease and ulcerative colitis. Clin. Exp. Immunol. **90:** 271–274.
26. SALVETTI, M. *et al.* 1992. T-lymphocyte reactivity to the recombinant mycobacterial 65- and 70-kDa heat shock proteins in multiple sclerosis. J. Autoimmun. **5:** 691–702.
27. GEORGOPOULOS, C. & H. MCFARLAND. 1993. Heat shock proteins in multiple sclerosis and other autoimmune diseases. Immunol. Today **14:** 373–375.
28. STANFORD, M.R. *et al.* 1994. Heat shock protein peptides reactive in patients with Behcet's disease are uveitogenic in Lewis rats. Clin. Exp. Immunol. **97:** 226–231.
29. DE SMET, M.D. & A. RAMADAN. 2001. Circulating antibodies to inducible heat shock protein 70 in patients with uveitis. Ocul. Immunol Inflamm. **9:** 85–92.
30. GROMADZKA, G. *et al.* 2001. Elevated levels of anti-heat shock protein antibodies in patients with cerebral ischemia. Cerebrovasc. Dis. **12:** 235–239.
31. RIPLEY, B.J., D.A. ISENBERG & D.S. LATCHMAN. 2001. Elevated levels of the 90 kDa heat shock protein (HSP90) in SLE correlate with levels of IL-6 and autoantibodies to HSP90. J. Autoimmun. **17:** 341–346.
32. TEZEL, G., J. YANG & M.B. WAX. 2004. Heat shock proteins, immunity and glaucoma. Brain Res. Bull. **62:** 473–480.
33. WAX, M.B. *et al.* 1998. Anti-Ro/SS-A positivity and heat shock protein antibodies in patients with normal-pressure glaucoma. Am. J. Ophthalmol. **125:** 145–157.

34. SLOBBE, R.L. *et al.* 1992. Ro ribonucleoprotein assembly in vitro. Identification of RNA-protein and protein-protein interactions. J. Mol. Biol. **227:** 361–366.
35. CHENG, S.T. *et al.* 1996. Calreticulin binds hYRNA and the 52-kDa polypeptide component of the Ro/SS-A ribonucleoprotein autoantigen. J. Immunol. **156:** 4484–4491.
36. KINOSHITA, G. *et al.* 1998. Spreading of the immune response from 52 kDaRo and 60 kDaRo to calreticulin in experimental autoimmunity. Lupus **7:** 7–11.
37. CASCIOLA-ROSEN, L.A., G. ANHALT & A. ROSEN. 1994. Autoantigens targeted in systemic lupus erythematosus are clustered in two populations of surface structures on apoptotic keratinocytes. J. Exp. Med. **179:** 1317–1330.
38. PURCELL, A.W. *et al.* 2003. Association of stress proteins with autoantigens: a possible mechanism for triggering autoimmunity? Clin. Exp. Immunol. **132:** 193–200.
39. GALLUCCI, S. & P. MATZINGER. 2001. Danger signals: SOS to the immune system. Curr. Opin. Immunol. **13:** 114–119.
40. FRIEDLAND, J.S. *et al.* 1993. Mycobacterial 65-kD heat shock protein induces release of proinflammatory cytokines from human monocytic cells. Clin. Exp. Immunol. **91:** 58–62.
41. PEETERMANS, W.E. *et al.* 1993. Murine peritoneal macrophages activated by the mycobacterial 65-kilodalton heat shock protein express enhanced microbicidal activity in vitro. Infect. Immun. **61:** 868–875.
42. BEAGLEY, K.W. *et al.* 1993. The *Mycobacterium tuberculosis* 71-kDa heat-shock protein induces proliferation and cytokine secretion by murine gut intraepithelial lymphocytes. Eur. J. Immunol. **23:** 2049–2052.
43. RANFORD, J.C., A.R. COATES & B. HENDERSON. 2000. Chaperonins are cell-signalling proteins: the unfolding biology of molecular chaperones. Expert Rev. Mol. Med. **2000:** 1–17.
44. BAUSINGER, H. *et al.* 2002. Endotoxin-free heat-shock protein 70 fails to induce APC activation. Eur. J. Immunol. **32:** 3708–3713.
45. GAO, B. & M.F. TSAN. 2003. Recombinant human heat shock protein 60 does not induce the release of tumor necrosis factor alpha from murine macrophages. J. Biol. Chem. **278:** 22523–22529.
46. GAO, B. & M.F. TSAN. 2003. Endotoxin contamination in recombinant human heat shock protein 70 (HSP70) preparation is responsible for the induction of tumor necrosis factor alpha release by murine macrophages. J. Biol. Chem. **278:** 174–179.
47. TSAN, M.F. & B. GAO. 2004. Cytokine function of heat shock proteins. Am. J. Physiol Cell Physiol. **286:** C739-C744.
48. ASEA, A. *et al.* 2000. HSP70 stimulates cytokine production through a CD14-dependant pathway, demonstrating its dual role as a chaperone and cytokine. Nat. Med. **6:** 435–442.
49. ASEA, A. *et al.* 2002. Novel signal transduction pathway utilized by extracellular HSP70: role of toll-like receptor (TLR) 2 and TLR4. J. Biol. Chem. **277:** 15028–15034.
50. BECKER, T., F.U. HARTL & F. WIELAND. 2002. CD40, an extracellular receptor for binding and uptake of HSP70-peptide complexes. J. Cell Biol. **158:** 1277–1285.
51. WANG, Y. *et al.* 2001. CD40 is a cellular receptor mediating mycobacterial heat shock protein 70 stimulation of CC-chemokines. Immunity **15:** 971–983.
52. BASU, S. *et al.* 2001. CD91 is a common receptor for heat shock proteins gp96, hsp90, hsp70, and calreticulin. Immunity **14:** 303–313.

53. DELNESTE, Y. *et al*. 2002. Involvement of LOX-1 in dendritic cell-mediated antigen cross-presentation. Immunity. **17:** 353–362.
54. BULUT, Y. *et al*. 2002. Chlamydial heat shock protein 60 activates macrophages and endothelial cells through Toll-like receptor 4 and MD2 in a MyD88-dependent pathway. J. Immunol. **168:** 1435–1440.
55. SRIVASTAVA, P.K. *et al*. 1998. Heat shock proteins come of age: primitive functions acquire new roles in an adaptive world. Immunity **8:** 657–665.
56. LI, Z., A. MENORET & P. SRIVASTAVA. 2002. Roles of heat-shock proteins in antigen presentation and cross-presentation. Curr. Opin. Immunol. **14:** 45–51.
57. CASTELLI, C. *et al*. 2001. Human heat shock protein 70 peptide complexes specifically activate antimelanoma T cells. Cancer Res. **61:** 222–227.
58. ZUGEL, U. *et al*. 2001. gp96-peptide vaccination of mice against intracellular bacteria. Infect. Immun. **69:** 4164–4167.
59. NAVARATNAM, M. *et al*. 2001. Heat shock protein-peptide complexes elicit cytotoxic T-lymphocyte and antibody responses specific for bovine herpesvirus 1. Vaccine. **19:** 1425–1434.
60. BLACHERE, N.E. *et al*. 1997. Heat shock protein-peptide complexes, reconstituted in vitro, elicit peptide-specific cytotoxic T lymphocyte response and tumor immunity. J. Exp. Med. **186:** 1315–1322.
61. SINGH-JASUJA, H. *et al*. 2000. Cross-presentation of glycoprotein 96-associated antigens on major histocompatibility complex class I molecules requires receptor-mediated endocytosis. J. Exp. Med. **191:** 1965–1974.
62. BINDER, R.J., D.K. HAN & P.K. SRIVASTAVA. 2000. CD91: a receptor for heat shock protein gp96. Nat. Immunol. **1:** 151–155.
63. CASTELLINO, F. *et al*. 2000. Receptor-mediated uptake of antigen/heat shock protein complexes results in major histocompatibility complex class I antigen presentation via two distinct processing pathways. J. Exp. Med. **191:** 1957–1964.
64. MATSUTAKE, T. & P.K. SRIVASTAVA. 2000. CD91 is involved in MHC class II presentation of gp96 chaperoned peptides. *In* Second International Conference on Heat Shock Proteins in Immune Response. Cahperone, C.S., Ed.: pp 8–12. Vol. 378. Cell Stress Society International. Farmington, CT, USA.
65. ROTH, S. *et al*. 2002. Major differences in antigen-processing correlate with a single Arg71<−>Lys substitution in HLA-DR molecules predisposing to rheumatoid arthritis and with their selective interactions with 70-kDa heat shock protein chaperones. J. Immunol. **169:** 3015–3020.
66. TOBIAN, A.A., D.H. CANADAY & C.V. HARDING. 2004. Bacterial heat shock proteins enhance class II MHC antigen processing and presentation of chaperoned peptides to CD4+ T cells. J. Immunol. **173:** 5130–5137.
67. MYCKO, M.P. *et al*. 2004. Inducible heat shock protein 70 promotes myelin autoantigen presentation by the HLA class II. J. Immunol. **172:** 202–213.
68. DOODY, A.D. *et al*. 2004. Glycoprotein 96 can chaperone both MHC class I- and class II-restricted epitopes for in vivo presentation, but selectively primes CD8+ T cell effector function. J. Immunol. **172:** 6087–6092.
69. PALLISER, D. *et al*. 2005. Multiple intracellular routes in the cross-presentation of a soluble protein by murine dendritic cells. J. Immunol. **174:** 1879–1887.
70. SENGUPTA, D. *et al*. 2004. Heat shock protein-mediated cross-presentation of exogenous HIV antigen on HLA class I and class II. J. Immunol. **173:** 1987–1993.
71. BASU, S. & P.K. SRIVASTAVA. 1999. Calreticulin, a peptide-binding chaperone of the endoplasmic reticulum elicits tumor- and peptide-specific immunity. J. Exp. Med. **189:** 797–802.

72. JORGENSEN, C.S. *et al*. 2003. Dimerization and oligomerization of the chaperone calreticulin. Eur. J. Biochem. **270:** 4140–4148.
73. CORBETT, E.F. *et al*. 2000. The conformation of calreticulin is influenced by the endoplasmic reticulum luminal environment. J. Biol. Chem. **275:** 27177–27185.
74. SVAERKE, C. & G. HOUEN. 1998. Chaperone properties of calreticulin. Acta Chem. Scand. **52:** 942–949.
75. RIZVI, S.M. *et al*. 2004. A polypeptide binding conformation of calreticulin is induced by heat shock, calcium depletion, or by deletion of the C-terminal acidic region. Mol. Cell. **15:** 913–923.
76. STAIKOU, E.V. *et al*. 2003. Calreticulin binds preferentially with B cell linear epitopes of Ro60 kD autoantigen, enhancing recognition by anti-Ro60 kD autoantibodies. Clin. Exp. Immunol. **134:** 143–150.
77. BASU, S. *et al*. 2000. Necrotic but not apoptotic cell death releases heat shock proteins, which deliver a partial maturation signal to dendritic cells and activate the NF-kappa B pathway. Int. Immunol. **12:** 1539–1546.
78. DUPUIS, M. *et al*. 1993. The calcium-binding protein calreticulin is a major constituent of lytic granules in cytolytic T lymphocytes. J. Exp. Med. **177:** 1–7.
79. HAUG, M. *et al*. 2005. The heat shock protein HSP70 enhances antigen-specific proliferation of human CD4$^+$ memory T cells. Eur. J. Immunol. **35:** 3163–3172.

The Role of Stress in Asthma

Insight from Studies on the Effect of Acute and Chronic Stressors in Models of Airway Inflammation

RATTANJEET S. VIG,[a] PAUL FORSYTHE,[b]
AND HARISSIOS VLIAGOFTIS[a]

[a]Department of Medicine, University of Alberta, Edmonton, Alberta, Canada

[b]The Brain-Body Institute and McMaster University Department of Pathology, Hamilton, Ontario, Canada

ABSTRACT: Asthma, a chronic inflammatory disease of the airways, is greatly influenced by psychosocial factors and stress. This review looks at clinical studies that have shown strong associations between psychological stress and asthma to identify potential mechanisms for these interactions. Furthermore, we review animal studies involving stress and airway inflammation or airway hyperresponsiveness, and discuss possible mechanisms of stress action in asthma. In conclusion, further research, both in humans and in animal models, into the mechanisms of stress-induced changes in asthma exacerbation are required to help better understand the complex makeup of asthma and assist in the development of therapies directed at the interplay between the nervous system and airway inflammation.

KEYWORDS: asthma; atopy; psychological stress; neuroimmunomodulation; acute stress; chronic stress; animal models; inflammation; disease; clinical studies

INTRODUCTION

Asthma is a chronic inflammatory disease of the airways defined by persistent symptoms of wheezing, chest tightness, coughing, variable reversible airway obstruction, and airway hyperresponsiveness (AHR). Although asthma can be characterized as a syndrome because of its wide variety of pathogenesis and manifestations, the resulting symptoms are largely due to epithelial damage, infiltration of the bronchial mucosa with lymphocytes, eosinophils and

Address for correspondence: Harissios Vliagoftis, 550A HMRC Department of Medicine, University of Alberta, Edmonton, Alberta, Canada T6G 2S2. Voice: 780-492-9295; fax: 780-492-5329.
e-mail: hari@ualberta.ca

Ann. N.Y. Acad. Sci. 1088: 65–77 (2006). © 2006 New York Academy of Sciences.
doi: 10.1196/annals.1366.023

other inflammatory cells, increased mucus production, and edema that may lead to airway smooth muscle hyperplasia and airway remodeling.[1,2] Until the inflammatory basis of the disease was described in the second half of the 20th century, asthma was considered as purely or primarily psychogenic, and was commonly referred to as "asthma nervosa."

A number of observational studies indicate that psychological stress is closely related to asthma severity in both children and adults and may also be involved in the development of the disease. Between 20% and 35% of asthmatics experience exacerbations of their disorder during periods of stress.[3] The mental health of asthmatic children is an important predictor of asthma morbidity,[4] and has been linked to asthma mortality.[5,6] Psychological distress in children is associated with asthma that is more difficult to manage,[7] with more frequent and lengthier hospital admissions,[8] and functional disability.[9]

What is missing from these studies is a clear indication of the mechanism of the interactions between stress and asthma. A workshop by the National Heart, Lung and Blood Institute[10] suggested that the role of psychological stress in asthma should be an area of intense study. Since then, it has been increasingly recognized that psychosocial factors, as an environmental stressor, may have important roles in the severity of asthma symptoms and potentially in the induction of allergic diseases in general. However, to date there is little understanding of the mechanisms of the interaction between stress and the asthmatic response and further studies are needed to elucidate these important pathways.

STRESS

Stress, or the general adaptation syndrome, was first described by Hans Selye[11,12] as "the state manifested by a specific syndrome, which consists of all the nonspecifically induced changes within a biological system." Stress is considered the common denominator of all the adaptive reactions in the body, and, as such, stress cannot be directly detrimental for health. The concept that stress in certain cases may precipitate physiological changes leading to disease was first explored by Hans Selye,[11] who called that stress "distress." This stress response may be defined as the psychophysiologic reaction to noxious physical or psychological stimuli.

When the body is challenged physically or psychologically, short-term activation of the neuroendocrine and autonomic nervous systems promotes adaptation and survival during the period of challenge. This has been termed *allostasis* meaning literally "reestablishing stability through change."[13] During allostasis, physiological systems operate at a higher or lower level than during "normal" homeostasis; for example, emotional distress may lead to elevated heart rate and blood pressure as well as elevated glucocorticoid levels that in turn suppress the production of inflammatory cytokines. Providing allostatic responses are shut off when they are no longer needed, the body is able to adapt to and survive the immediate challenge without suffering long-term consequences. However, if the same response systems are activated over a longer period of time or remain active when no longer needed, these adaptive changes lead to other consequences, including receptor desensitization and tissue damage that may precipitate or exacerbate disease processes. This has been termed *allostatic load*, and it refers to the price the tissue or organ pays for an overactive or inefficiently managed allostatic response.

In humans, stress can manifest itself in various ways. Acute stress, often dubbed the flight-or-fight response or positive stress, is one where there is a perceived threat or challenge, which requires a small period of time for which to successfully adapt, like an immediate threat of an exam.[14] This stress leads to the immediate activation of the hypothalamic-pituitary-adrenal (HPA) axis. Release of the hypothalamic corticotrophin-releasing hormone (CRH or CRF) stimulates release of adrenocorticotropic hormone (ACTH) from the pituitary, which in turn promotes the release of corticosteroids from the adrenal cortex.[15] The HPA axis is one of the central mechanisms by which stress, detected by the brain, alters physiological function throughout the body. Acute stressors, via the stimulation of the sympathetic immune system, prepare the body for an immediate response and can lead to beneficial effects.[16] The overall effect of the HPA axis on immune/inflammatory responses is to prevent them from proceeding unchecked by suppressing the response as soon as they begin.

These effects are clinically opposite to chronic stressors, where the presence of a long-term stress maintains the output of stress molecules via the HPA axis and sympathetic stimulation, exhausting the body of its resources.[14] The reference to stress in clinical studies usually refers to chronic psychological stress. These types of stress include reduced social status, death of a friend or family member, loss of a job, long-term anxiety, and depression.

STRESS ON THE IMMUNE SYSTEM

Stress activates a number of biological pathways and has a number of biological effects that may be involved in asthma pathophysiology (FIG. 1). Whether stress activates or inhibits these pathways is often dependent on the duration and quality of the stress stimulus. In this review we will discuss primarily the effects of stress on airway inflammation.

Stress has been shown to have a variety of immunomodulatory effects both positive and negative. There is a substantial volume of literature demonstrating that psychological stress may influence inflammatory and immune cell trafficking, cell proliferation, and cell function including cytokine and inflammatory mediator production. Stress can modulate these responses through nerve pathways that connect the autonomic nervous and the immune systems as well as through the release of hormones and neuropeptides, which have the potential to interact with immune cells.

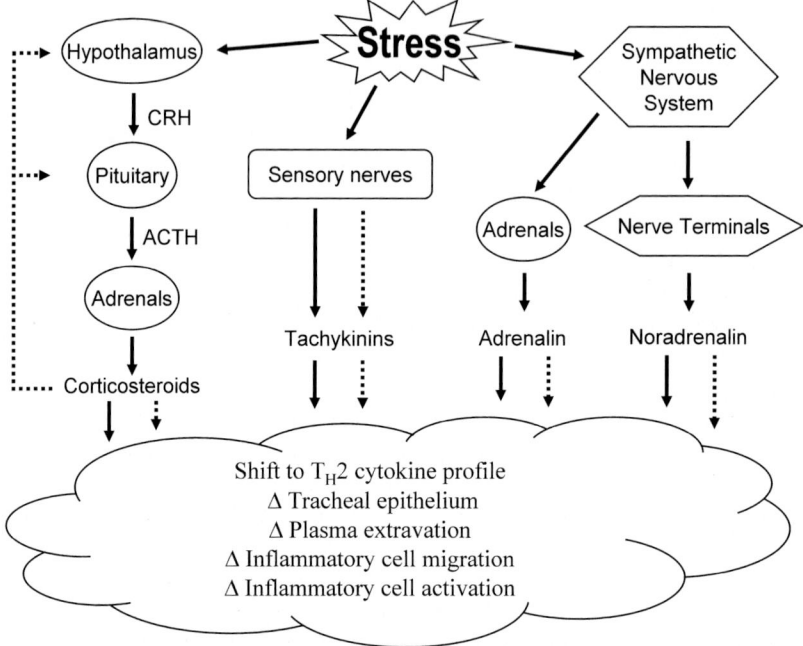

FIGURE 1. Mechanisms of action of the stress response (*solid arrows* indicate stimulation, *dashed arrows* indicate inhibition). The stress response via the brain activates the HPA axis, which produces corticosteroids as the final hormone, and also the sympathetic nervous system. Additionally, stress can induce or inhibit release of tachykinins from primary sensory nerves. The release of these molecules, depending on the duration and intensity of the stress, can exert numerous positive or negative effects on the body.

Acute stress induces an adrenal hormone-mediated redistribution of immune cells from the blood to other compartments of the immune system.[17] There is evidence that immune cells in these cases redistribute to the skin, where they may enhance skin immune function,[18,19] which is partly mediated by gamma interferon (IFN-γ).[20] In a similar fashion, exposure to laboratory stressor tasks for a few minutes has been shown to induce suppression of T cell mitogenesis and increase the number of circulating $CD8^+$ and natural killer cells.[21,22] These effects appear to be mediated by the autonomic nervous system[23] and are associated with alterations in the production of cytokines, such as interleukin (IL)-1-β, IL-2, and IFN-γ.[24,25]

Although acute stress augments certain immune responses, it has also been shown to inhibit other aspects of the immune response. In humans for example, stress induced by examinations can cause downregulation of T cell function and altered cytokine levels and ratios in human patients.[10] This is due to the shift of the immune response induced by stress from an antibacterial T_H1 response toward a humoral T_H2 response.[26]

In contrast to the effect of acute stress, which augments immune responses, chronic stress seems to depress the migration of immune cells from the blood,[27] an effect that correlates with the attenuation of responsiveness to corticosteroids. Although many of the factors released by the HPA axis remain the same between acute and chronic stresses, the temporal nature of the stress response induces opposite effects in chronic stress as compared to acute stress. These differences may be due to the differing mechanisms that take place with regard to acute and chronic stress states, as well as exhaustion of the body attempting to cope with repeated or chronic stressors.

It has been observed that not all individuals show the same response to stress-induced alterations in immune function. There is some evidence that patients with conditions believed to be affected by stress, such as atopic dermatitis, are more sensitive to stress-induced immune system dysfunction than normal individuals.[28]

In humans, chronic clinical stress has been shown to play an important role in disease, usually resulting in exacerbation of symptoms, primarily in inflammatory diseases. Mental stress, anxiety, and anger have been found to be positively correlated with cardiac ischemia,[29] periodontal disease,[30] inflammatory bowel disease,[31] as well as ulcerative colitis [32,33] and it is hypothesized to play major roles in autoimmune diseases, such as Graves' disease, multiple sclerosis, rheumatoid arthritis, and others.[34–37] Chronic stress also promotes lymphocyte apoptosis via a mechanism independent of the HPA axis.[38]

Working knowledge into the functions of the HPA axis, the primary mechanism whereby the effects of stress are carried throughout the body, has greatly increased only in the last few decades, and, combined with existing knowledge of the sympathetic nervous system, only recently has stress begun to be recognized as a fundamental physiological process that regularly influences well-being and disease states.

HUMAN STUDIES RELATING STRESS AND ASTHMA

Good clinical evidence regarding the effect of stress and asthma is relatively sparse apart from observational and some epidemiological studies. Many of the early studies examined the link between the nervous system and asthma using suggestion (hypnotic or conscious), and they described its effects on asthma symptoms. A review by Isenberg *et al.*[3] shows that studies in this field reveal that 35% to 40% of asthmatics develop bronchoconstriction following relevant suggestion or following other stressful stimuli. This effect is greater and more consistent in asthmatics, although even nonasthmatic individuals develop bronchoconstriction as a result of suggestion. Pastorello *et al.* used suggestion to indicate that a saline solution was a bronchodilator or bronchoconstrictor, but found no significant changes in respiratory measures.[39] In contrast, a study in elderly male patients, showed that the recollection of an asthma attack either consciously or through hypnotism, was sufficient to cause a significant rise in minute ventilation.[40] In some of these studies the effect of suggestion in normal controls was not studied. Despite this important criticism, a number of studies show an increase in airway resistance and reduction in forced expiratory volume following hypnotism and suggestion of anger, fear, and recollection of asthma in adults[41,42] and children.[43]

Other prolonged clinical studies in asthmatic patients tend to show similar stress-induced effects. In one set of studies,[44,45] Sandberg et al. followed a large cohort of chronic asthmatic children over an 18-month time course, using a diary system to record positive and negative events, and showed a significant correlation between stressors and the induction of asthma exacerbations. The first study concluded that severe events without the presence of a chronic stress increased the risk of an asthma attack significantly between 2–6 weeks after the event. However, in children with chronic stress, a severe event could precipitate an increased risk of asthma attack within the first 2 weeks. Another study conducted by Smyth et al. [46] also found an association between variable mood states or the presence of stressors with lower peak expiratory volumes in asthmatic patients. Other studies have associated psychological distress in children with asthma that is more difficult to manage,[7] with more frequent and lengthier admissions to the hospital,[8] and functional disability.[9] One of these studies was also able to correlate the length and number of hospitalizations with anxiety, stigma of being asthmatic, neuroticism, and hostility.[8] Similar findings linking psychological morbidity to asthma mortality in children have been conducted in Australia,[6] the United States,[5] and in adults in England.[47] All of these studies show that stress plays a very strong role in the development of chronic asthma and on the probability, number, and severity of asthma exacerbations. In addition, asthma induces stress and negative emotional responses, which some studies above could correlate with a further deterioration of asthma.[48]

So, is the correlation between stress and asthma a result of asthma inducing negative stress or does stress in fact worsen asthma symptoms? A third form of human studies in this area involves inducing a short-term stress on an individual in an attempt to answer that very question. Asthmatics that are stressed with a method of forced oscillation have significantly higher airway impedance as compared to controls.[49] Other methods of inducing stress, via an examination or computer puzzle test, have also been used. Adolescent asthmatics undertaking a stressful computer puzzle test have increased breathlessness.[16] Asthmatic students respond to allergen challenge with increased airway inflammation during stressful examination periods compared to low-stress periods.[50] Other studies are not as conclusive. One paper found no significant relationship between daily life stress ands serum IgE levels or bronchial hyperresponsiveness.[51] Studies have shown that stress-induced changes in physiological parameters of breathing may be similar in asthmatic and nonasthmatic children but these changes may have higher clinical significance in asthmatics due to their higher baseline airway resistance.[52] Such changes may be the result of differences in coping behavior, as passive stressful tasks like watching bloody surgeries or other stress-inducing videos cause increased airway resistance in asthmatics in comparison to active stressful tasks like arithmetic.[41] Similarly, relieving stress by writing about stressful experiences, a task that helps to improve coping, improves a number of physiological parameters of asthma for long periods.[53]

Explanations for the purported enhancement of asthmatic symptoms by stress which do not involve directly alteration of airway physiology or inflammation have also been suggested. Stress can change an asthmatic's perception of breathlessness and lead him or her to believe that his condition is deteriorating despite an absence of changes in physiologic parameters of breathing.[16] Additionally, stress might affect self-management strategies and adherence to treatment plans and therefore can lead to deterioration of asthma control during periods of stress. It is also commonly believed that asthma can induce stress in patients, although one study demonstrated that in most patients, asthma exacerbations do not provoke a physiological stressor response.[54] This is a possible explanation for the observation of Rimington *et al.* [55] that increases in Hospital Anxiety and Depression scale scores lead to symptom scores above what is expected by lung function and other objective measurements. Finally, psychological stress correlates with an increased risk of acute respiratory infections,[56,57] which are an important trigger of asthma exacerbation. Although the foregoing explanations are possible, we believe that there is an abundance of epidemiological data to suggest that the regulatory mechanisms affected by stress are more complicated than previously supposed, and directly affect the pathophysiology of the asthmatic response.

Overall, the consensus has emerged that stressful situations and events are affecting the severity of asthma. What is not clear is whether this increased severity of asthma is the direct result of increased inflammation during high stress states or results from other effects of the nervous or endocrine systems directly on pulmonary physiology. The study of Liu *et al.* [50] shows that stressed individuals have the potential to develop higher degrees of inflammation but did not show any baseline differences between high and low stress states. Several other important questions also remain. Many of the studies above seem to identify only a subpopulation that is more greatly affected by stressors than others. Is this a result of the cumulative effect of stress, or do genetic aspects of the individual make certain individuals more prone to the effects of stress? Does stress only exacerbate existing symptoms, or is it also responsible for the development of atopy in the individual initially? Our ability to answer these questions and determine the mechanisms of stress in human patients is limited beyond the studies that have already been described. In order to see the effect of stress on asthma and be able to discern the mechanisms behind such outcomes, it becomes vital to use animal models.

THE USE OF ANIMAL MODELS TO STUDY THE
RELATIONSHIP BETWEEN STRESS AND ASTHMA

Human studies have established the association between stress and immune function. More recent cohort studies are further looking into these effects by collecting more data on these associations. Since human studies are not often suitable to identify the mechanism of these interactions, much of the evidence regarding the pathways of the effects of stress on asthma comes from animal models. Using animal models, the level and type of stress can be controlled and quantified and other interventions can be used to define the desired pathways. Just as in some of the human studies, the animal models of stress can use short-term stressors and chronic or repeated stressors that may have different effects on allergic inflammation.

Short-Term Stress

The literature has provided much insight into the effects of acute stress on allergic inflammation models. Our group, using a Balb/c mouse model of allergic airway inflammation and restraint stress for 1 h per day for three consecutive days, showed a significant reduction in accumulation of inflammatory cells in the BAL, but increased levels of BAL IL-6, IL-9, IL-13, and no change in IL-10 and IFN-γ levels.[58] The use of a specific corticosteroid inhibitor, RU486, reversed these BAL changes.[58] It is thus apparent that in this short-term stress model, the elevated levels of corticosteroids in stressed animals (unpublished data) may result in a reduction of inflammatory cell infiltration in the airways and may alter BAL cytokine levels. This observation is supported by the fact that CRH-deficient mice develop increased airway inflammation and elevated IL-4, 5, 13, RANTES, IFN-γ, and Eotaxin BAL levels after OVA sensitization and challenge compared to normal controls.[59] This effect is believed to be the result of near-absent corticosteroid and catecholamine production from the adrenal gland because of the absence of the stimulus for their release.

Similar to our study, an elevation in corticosteroids is also seen in a rat model of water-avoidance stress, which also results in increased tracheal epithelial short-circuit activity and elevated response to CRH.[60] This confirms that stress may induce not only inflammatory changes that may affect asthma, but also physiological changes in the airways, which may contribute to it. Another physiological change can be seen in guinea pigs, where injection of CRH, which not only is a stress hormone itself but also an indirect stimulator of corticosteroid release, reduces OVA-induced plasma extravation in guinea pig airways via the inhibition of tachykinin release from primary sensory nerves.[61] These studies, despite using different animal models, together show that short-term stress results in the activation of CRH and corticosteroid release, which reduces inflammation and plasma extravation, and that this mechanism may involve the inhibition of tachykinin release and physiological changes in the tracheal epithelium. This correlates with the current asthma research into the important role that neuronal and nonneuronal tachykinins play in airway inflammation, mast cell activation, cytokine secretion, bronchial hyperresponsiveness, and mucoid secretion.[62–64]

Long-Term Stress

In contrast to short-term stress, chronic or repeated stress induces the reverse phenotype with regard to inflammation in animal models of asthma. Extending the 1-h daily restraint stress to a week in the mouse model we described above, we have shown a significant increase in BAL accumulation of all inflammatory cell types, but with no significant change in the cytokines tested.[58] A similar result was seen using unavoidable repeated sound stress for 24 h with increased BAL leukocytes (especially eosinophils) and increased airway hyperresponsiveness of tracheal smooth muscle.[65] However, in contrast to our studies, Joachim *et al.* identified increased AHR in addition to airway inflammation in stressed versus nonstressed controls. The two studies have a number of differences that may explain this discrepancy. Joachim *et al.* evaluated AHR using a different technique, an event that may or may not be involved in the described differences. More importantly, the latter paper used a different background of mice (CBA/J instead of Balb/c). This would indicate that genetic differences may be important for the manifestation of stress-induced or exacerbated asthma and may explain the fact that only a subgroup of patients with asthma experiences increased severity during episodes of stress.[3] Also, the stressor in the latter study was of much longer duration compared to the stress in our study. This could indicate that different mediators of stress or different adaptation mechanisms employed, depending on the stressor, may have diverse effects on asthma symptoms.

The effects of long-term stress on airway inflammation have also been replicated in a rat [66] and a guinea pig model.[67] The rat model also showed an increase in allergen-induced plasma extravasation in the paw of stressed animals[66]; however, another study of plasma extravasation in the synovium showed that repeated stress induces the opposite response.[68] This discrepancy may indicate tissue-specific responses to stress or possibly the result of different stress protocols.

These studies have confirmed the predictions from the observational human studies on the effects of stress on asthma. However, the main focus of future studies should be the identification of the pathways mediating these effects. The different response of airway inflammation in long-term stress as opposed to short-term stress models indicates that different mechanisms are at play. Our group has shown that corticosteroids are not involved in the effects of long-term stress on airway inflammation the way they are involved in the effects of short-term stress.[58] Joachim *et al.* have shown that the long-term stress mechanism likely involves the role of the neurokinin-1 (NK-1) receptor, which is present in the human lung and submucosal glands, in addition to on mast cells, lymphocytes, and macrophages in rodents.[67] Substance P is the primary tachykinin that acts on the NK-1 receptor, whose inhibition in a sound stress guinea pig model with a highly specific inhibitor results in ablation of long-term stress-induced effects in the lung.[67]

CONCLUSIONS

Stress is more than a mental construct; it is a physiologically relevant effector that has the capacity to significantly alter the human immune system and possibly airway physiology, and therefore has the potential to affect the development and manifestations of asthma. Studies in humans show the significant role that stress plays in stimulating asthma exacerbations, including negative correlations with important physiological markers of airway function. Discovering that stress does play a significant role in the quality of life of asthmatics is important, as will be discovering the mechanisms behind the negative impact of stress.

It is likely that a wide variety of factors may play a role, including psychological changes in perception of breathlessness [16] and changes in coping behavior in combination with physiological changes, which may include alterations in airway structure or function, immune deregulation, and even possibly changes in smooth muscle reactivity. With many unanswered questions, more research is required to ascertain the exact effect of stress and the mechanisms in play. For example, much of the current research on the topic deals with the importance of stress on those currently diagnosed with asthma. However, stress affects those of all ages, including neonates, children, and even fetuses *in utero*. Stress may have a more profound and permanent impact on lung function and asthma phenotype in these cases. Additionally, while stress influences those with asthma, it is still to be seen whether it plays an important role in the sensitization to allergens or the development of asthma.

Regardless, to discover how stress affects immunity will undoubtedly provide further insights into the crosstalk between the nervous, immune, and endocrine systems and give us a better understanding of the root causes of asthma, and even possibly superior tools with which we can deal with, and hopefully prevent, this costly ailment.

REFERENCES

1. KAY, A.B. 2001. Allergy and allergic diseases. Second of two parts. N. Engl. J. Med. **344:** 109–113.
2. DJUKANOVIC, R. 2000. Asthma: a disease of inflammation and repair. J. Allergy Clin. Immunol. **105:** S522–S526.
3. ISENBERG, S.A., P.M. LEHRER & S. HOCHRON. 1992. The effects of suggestion and emotional arousal on pulmonary function in asthma: a review and a hypothesis regarding vagal mediation. Psychosom. Med. **54:** 192–216.

4. WEIL, C.M. *et al.* 1999. The relationship between psychosocial factors and asthma morbidity in inner-city children with asthma. Pediatrics **104:** 1274–1280.
5. STRUNK, R.C. *et al.* 1985. Physiologic and psychological characteristics associated with deaths due to asthma in childhood. A case-controlled study. JAMA **254:** 1193–1198.
6. SEARS, M.R. *et al.* 1986. Deaths from asthma in New Zealand. Arch. Dis. Child. **61:** 6–10.
7. FRITZ, G.K. & J.C. OVERHOLSER. 1989. Patterns of response to childhood asthma. Psychosom. Med. **51:** 347–355.
8. KAPTEIN, A.A. 1982. Psychological correlates of length of hospitalization and rehospitalization in patients with acute, severe asthma. Soc. Sci. Med. **16:** 725–729.
9. GUTSTADT, L.B. *et al.* 1989. Determinants of school performance in children with chronic asthma. Am. J. Dis. Child. **143:** 471–475.
10. BUSSE, W.W. *et al.* 1995. NHLBI Workshop summary. Stress and asthma. Am. J. Respir. Crit. Care Med. **151:** 249–252.
11. SELYE, H. 1934. On the nervous control of lactation. Am. J. Physiol. **107:** 535–538.
12. SELYE, H. 1970. The evolution of the stress concept. Stress and cardiovascular disease. Am. J. Cardiol. **26:** 289–299.
13. STERLING, P. & J. EYER 1988. Allostasis: A New Paradigm to Explain Arousal Pathology. John Wiley & Sons. New York.
14. MCEWEN, B.S. 1998. Protective and damaging effects of stress mediators. N. Engl. J. Med. **338:** 171–179.
15. TSIGOS, C. & G.P. CHROUSOS. 2002. Hypothalamic-pituitary-adrenal axis, neuroendocrine factors and stress. J. Psychosom. Res. **53:** 865–871.
16. RIETVELD, S., I. VAN BEEST & W. EVERAERD. 1999. Stress-induced breathlessness in asthma. Psychol. Med. **29:** 1359–1366.
17. DHABHAR, F.S. *et al.* 1995. Effects of stress on immune cell distribution. Dynamics and hormonal mechanisms. J. Immunol. **154:** 5511–5527.
18. DHABHAR, F.S. 2000. Acute stress enhances while chronic stress suppresses skin immunity. The role of stress hormones and leukocyte trafficking. Ann. N. Y. Acad. Sci. **917:** 876–893.
19. DHABHAR, F.S. & B.S. MCEWEN. 1996. Stress-induced enhancement of antigen-specific cell-mediated immunity. J. Immunol. **156:** 2608–2615.
20. DHABHAR, F.S. *et al.* 2000. Stress-induced enhancement of skin immune function: A role for gamma interferon. Proc. Natl. Acad. Sci. USA **97:** 2846–2851.
21. KIECOLT-GLASER, J.K. *et al.* 1992. Acute psychological stressors and short-term immune changes: what, why, for whom, and to what extent? Psychosom. Med. **54:** 680–685.
22. SCHMID-OTT, G. *et al.* 2001. Levels of circulating CD8(+) T lymphocytes, natural killer cells, and eosinophils increase upon acute psychosocial stress in patients with atopic dermatitis. J. Allergy Clin. Immunol. **107:** 171–177.
23. HERBERT, T.B. *et al.* 1994. Cardiovascular reactivity and the course of immune response to an acute psychological stressor. Psychosom. Med. **56:** 337–344.
24. DOBBIN, J.P. *et al.* 1991. Cytokine production and lymphocyte transformation during stress. Brain Behav. Immun. **5:** 339–348.
25. GLASER, R. *et al.* 1990. Psychological stress-induced modulation of interleukin 2 receptor gene expression and interleukin 2 production in peripheral blood leukocytes. Arch. Gen. Psychiatry **47:** 707–712.

26. ELENKOV, I.J. & G.P. CHROUSOS. 1999. Stress hormones, Th1/Th2 patterns, pro/anti-inflammatory cytokines and susceptibility to disease. Trends Endocrinol. Metab. **10:** 359–368.
27. DHABHAR, F.S. & B.S. MCEWEN. 1997. Acute stress enhances while chronic stress suppresses cell-mediated immunity *in vivo*: a potential role for leukocyte trafficking. Brain Behav. Immun. **11:** 286–306.
28. SCHMID-OTT, G. *et al.* 2001. Different expression of cytokine and membrane molecules by circulating lymphocytes on acute mental stress in patients with atopic dermatitis in comparison with healthy controls. J. Allergy Clin. Immunol. **108:** 455–462.
29. KRANTZ, D.S. *et al.* 2000. Effects of mental stress in patients with coronary artery disease: evidence and clinical implications. JAMA **283:** 1800–1802.
30. VETTORE, M.V. *et al.* 2003. The relationship of stress and anxiety with chronic periodontitis. J. Clin. Periodontol. **30:** 394–402.
31. MAWDSLEY, J.E. & D.S. RAMPTON. 2005. Psychological stress in IBD: new insights into pathogenic and therapeutic implications. Gut **54:** 1481–1491.
32. LEVENSTEIN, S. *et al.* 2000. Stress and exacerbation in ulcerative colitis: a prospective study of patients enrolled in remission. Am. J. Gastroenterol. **95:** 1213–1220.
33. LEVENSTEIN, S. *et al.* 1994. Psychological stress and disease activity in ulcerative colitis: a multidimensional cross-sectional study. Am. J. Gastroenterol. **89:** 1219–1225.
34. MARTINELLI, V. 2000. Trauma, stress and multiple sclerosis. Neurol. Sci. **21:** S849–S852.
35. MIZOKAMI, T. *et al.* 2004. Stress and thyroid autoimmunity. Thyroid **14:** 1047–1055.
36. POTTER, P.T. & A.J. ZAUTRA. 1997. Stressful life events' effects on rheumatoid arthritis disease activity. J. Consult. Clin. Psychol. **65:** 319–323.
37. ZAUTRA, A.J. *et al.* 1994. Interpersonal stress, depression, and disease activity in rheumatoid arthritis and osteoarthritis patients. Health Psychol. **13:** 139–148.
38. YIN, D. *et al.* 2000. Chronic restraint stress promotes lymphocyte apoptosis by modulating CD95 expression. J. Exp. Med. **191:** 1423–1428.
39. PASTORELLO, E.A. *et al.* 1987. The role of suggestion in asthma. I. Effects of inactive solution on bronchial reactivity under bronchoconstrictor or bronchodilator suggestion. Ann. Allergy **59:** 336–338.
40. CLARKE, P.S. & J.R. GIBSON. 1980. Asthma hyperventilation and emotion. Aust. Fam. Physician **9:** 715–719.
41. LEHRER, P.M. *et al.* 1996. Behavioral task-induced bronchodilation in asthma during active and passive tasks: a possible cholinergic link to psychologically induced airway changes. Psychosom. Med. **58:** 413–422.
42. RITZ, T. *et al.* 2000. Emotions and stress increase respiratory resistance in asthma. Psychosom. Med. **62:** 401–412.
43. TAL, A. & D.R. MIKLICH. 1976. Emotionally induced decreases in pulmonary flow rates in asthmatic children. Psychosom. Med. **38:** 190–200.
44. SANDBERG, S. *et al.* 2004. Asthma exacerbations in children immediately following stressful life events: a Cox's hierarchical regression. Thorax **59:** 1046–1051.
45. SANDBERG, S. *et al.* 2000. The role of acute and chronic stress in asthma attacks in children. Lancet **356:** 982–987.
46. SMYTH, J.M. *et al.* 1999. Daily psychosocial factors predict levels and diurnal cycles of asthma symptomatology and peak flow. J. Behav. Med. **22:** 179–193.
47. INNES, N.J. *et al.* 1998. Psychosocial risk factors in near-fatal asthma and in asthma deaths. J. R. Coll. Physicians Lond. **32:** 430–434.

48. WRIGHT, R.J., M. RODRIGUEZ & S. COHEN. 1998. Review of psychosocial stress and asthma: an integrated biopsychosocial approach. Thorax **53:** 1066–1074.
49. CARR, R.E. *et al.* 1996. Effect of psychological stress on airway impedance in individuals with asthma and panic disorder. J. Abnorm. Psychol. **105:** 137–141.
50. LIU, L.Y. *et al.* 2002. School examinations enhance airway inflammation to antigen challenge. Am. J. Respir. Crit. Care Med. **165:** 1062–1067.
51. KOH, K.B. & C.S. HONG. 1993. The relationship of stress with serum IgE level in patients with bronchial asthma. Yonsei Med. J. **34:** 166–174.
52. MCQUAID, E.L. *et al.* 2000. Stress and airway resistance in children with asthma. J. Psychosom. Res. **49:** 239–245.
53. SMYTH, J.M. *et al.* 1999. Effects of writing about stressful experiences on symptom reduction in patients with asthma or rheumatoid arthritis: a randomized trial. JAMA **281:** 1304–1309.
54. CYDULKA, R.K. & C.L. EMERMAN. 1998. Adrenal function and physiologic stress during acute asthma exacerbation. Ann. Emerg. Med. **31:** 558–561.
55. RIMINGTON, L.D. *et al.* 2001. Relationship between anxiety, depression, and morbidity in adult asthma patients. Thorax **56:** 266–271.
56. COHEN, S., D.A. TYRRELL & A.P. SMITH. 1991. Psychological stress and susceptibility to the common cold. N. Engl. J. Med. **325:** 606–612.
57. COHEN, S., D.A. TYRRELL & A.P. SMITH. 1993. Negative life events, perceived stress, negative affect, and susceptibility to the common cold. J. Pers. Soc. Psychol. **64:** 131–140.
58. FORSYTHE, P. *et al.* 2004. Opposing effects of short- and long-term stress on airway inflammation. Am. J. Respir. Crit. Care Med. **169:** 220–226.
59. SILVERMAN, E.S. *et al.* 2004. Corticotropin-releasing hormone deficiency increases allergen-induced airway inflammation in a mouse model of asthma. J. Allergy Clin. Immunol. **114:** 747–754.
60. AKIYAMA, H., H. AMANO & J. BIENENSTOCK. 2005. Rat tracheal epithelial responses to water avoidance stress. J. Allergy Clin. Immunol. **116:** 318–324.
61. YOSHIHARA, S. *et al.* 1995. Corticotropin-releasing factor inhibits antigen-induced plasma extravasation in airways. Eur. J. Pharmacol. **280:** 113–118.
62. JESSOP, D.S., M.S. HARBUZ & S.L. LIGHTMAN. 2001. CRH in chronic inflammatory stress. Peptides **22:** 803–807.
63. JOOS, G.F., K.O. DE SWERT & R.A. PAUWELS. 2001. Airway inflammation and tachykinins: prospects for the development of tachykinin receptor antagonists. Eur J Pharmacol. **429:** 239–250.
64. MANTYH, P.W. 2002. Neurobiology of substance P and the NK1 receptor. J. Clin. Psychiatry **63(Suppl 11):** 6–10.
65. JOACHIM, R.A. *et al.* 2003. Stress enhances airway reactivity and airway inflammation in an animal model of allergic bronchial asthma. Psychosom. Med. **65:** 811–815.
66. DATTI, F. *et al.* 2002. Influence of chronic unpredictable stress on the allergic responses in rats. Physiol. Behav. **77:** 79–83.
67. JOACHIM, R.A. *et al.* 2004. Neurokinin-1 receptor mediates stress-exacerbated allergic airway inflammation and airway hyperresponsiveness in mice. Psychosom. Med. **66:** 564–571.
68. STRAUSBAUGH, H.J., M.F. DALLMAN & J.D. LEVINE. 1999. Repeated, but not acute, stress suppresses inflammatory plasma extravasation. Proc. Natl. Acad. Sci. USA **96:** 14629–14634.

The Critical Role of Mast Cells in Allergy and Inflammation

THEOHARIS C. THEOHARIDES,[a,b,c]
AND DIMITRIOS KALOGEROMITROS[d]

[a]*Department of Pharmacology and Experimental Therapeutics, Tufts University School of Medicine, Tufts–New England Medical Center, Boston, Massachusetts 02111, USA*

[b]*Department of Biochemistry, Tufts University School of Medicine, Tufts–New England Medical Center, Boston, Massachusetts 02111, USA*

[c]*Department of Internal Medicine, Tufts University School of Medicine, Tufts–New England Medical Center, Boston, Massachusetts 02111, USA*

[d]*Allergy Division, Attikon Hospital, Athens University Medical School, Athens, Greece*

ABSTRACT: Mast cells are well known for their involvement in allergic and anaphylactic reactions, but recent findings implicate them in a variety of inflammatory diseases affecting different organs, including the heart, joints, lungs, and skin. In these cases, mast cells appear to be activated by triggers other than aggregation of their IgE receptors (FcεRI), such as anaphylatoxins, immunoglobulin-free light chains, superantigens, neuropeptides, and cytokines leading to selective release of mediators without degranulation. These findings could explain inflammatory diseases, such as asthma, atopic dermatitis, coronary inflammation, and inflammatory arthritis, all of which worsen by stress. It is proposed that the pathogenesis of these diseases involve mast cell activation by local release of corticotropin-releasing hormone (CRH) or related peptides. Combination of CRH receptor antagonists and mast cell inhibitors may present novel therapeutic interventions.

KEYWORDS: asthma; coronary artery disease; inflammation; dermatoses; mast cells; skin; stress; vascular permeability

SELECTIVE RELEASE OF MAST CELL MEDIATORS

Mast cells are necessary for the development of allergic reactions, through cross-linking of their surface receptors for IgE (FcεRI),[1,2] leading to degranulation and the release of vasoactive, proinflammatory, and nociceptive

Address for correspondence: T.C. Theoharides, Ph.D., M.D., Department of Pharmacology and Experimental Therapeutics, Tufts University School of Medicine, 136 Harrison Avenue, Boston, MA 02111, USA. Voice: 617-636-6866; fax: 617-636-2456.
  e-mail: theoharis.theoharides@tufts.edu

Ann. N.Y. Acad. Sci. 1088: 78–99 (2006). © 2006 New York Academy of Sciences.
doi: 10.1196/annals.1366.025

mediators that include histamine, IL-6, IL-8, PGD$_2$, tryptase, and vascular endothelial growth factor (VEGF).[3–5] Mast cells derive from a distinct precursor in the bone marrow[6,7] and mature under local tissue microenvironmental factors.[5] In addition to stem cell factor (SCF), mast cell chemoattractants include nerve growth factor (NGF),[8] RANTES, and monocyte chemoattractor protein 1 (MCP-1).[9] They can secrete a multitude of biologically potent mediators (TABLE 1), giving rise to speculations about their possible role in innate or acquired immunity.[5,10,11] In addition to allergic triggers, mast cells can be activated by anaphylatoxins, antibody light chains, bacterial and viral antigens, cytokines, and neuropeptides.[12] Immunoglobulin-free light chains appear to elicit immediate hypersensitivity-like responses[13,14] through mast cell activation and subsequent induction of T-cell-mediated immune responses[15] (TABLE 2). Increasing evidence also indicates that mast cells are critical for the development of inflammatory diseases, especially in the pathogenesis of diseases such as arthritis, asthma, chronic dermatitis, and coronary artery disease (CAD) (TABLE 3).[12] However, unlike the case in allergic reactions, mast cells are rarely seen to degranulate during autoimmune[16] or inflammatory processes.[17] The only way to explain mast cell involvement in nonallergic processes would be through "differential" or "selective" secretion of mediators[18] without degranulation.[19] In fact, this may be the only way this ubiquitous and versatile cell may regulate immune responses without causing anaphylactic shock.

Instead, mast cells can undergo ultrastructural alterations of their electron-dense granular core, indicative of secretion, but without degranulation, a process that has been termed "activation,"[20–22] "intragranular activation,"[23] or "piecemeal" degranulation.[24] During such processes, mast cells can release many mediators *selectively* (TABLE 4)[25–27] as shown for serotonin[18] and eicosanoids.[28–30] Triggers include innate molecules, such as stem cell factor (SCF), which releases IL-6.[31–34] IL-1 can also stimulate human mast cells to release IL-6 selectively through 40–80-nm vesicles unrelated to the secretory granules (800–1000 nm).[35] Corticotropin-releasing hormone (CRH) can stimulate selective release of VEGF without degranulation.[36]

SKIN INFLAMMATION

Mast cells are well known for their role in skin hypersensitivity reactions.[37–41] Skin mast cells are located close to sensory nerve endings[42] and can be triggered by neuropeptides,[43–46] such as neurotensin (NT),[47] nerve growth factor (NGF),[48] substance P (SP),[49] and pituitary adenylate cyclase activating polypeptide (PACAP), all of which can be released from dermal neurons.[50] In fact, skin mast cells contain SP,[51] while cultured mouse and human mast cells were shown to contain and secrete NGF.[52]

Skin appears to have its own equivalent of the hypothalamic–pituitary–adrenal (HPA) axis,[53,54] the main regulator of which, CRH and its receptors,

TABLE 1. Mast cell mediators

Mediators	Main pathophysiologic effects
Prestored	
Biogenic amines	
Histamine	Vasodilation, angiogenesis, mitogenesis, pain
5-Hydroxytryptamine (5-HT, serotonin)	Vasoconstriction, pain
Chemokines	
IL-8, MCP-1, MCP-3, MCP-4, RANTES	Chemoattraction and tissue infiltration of leukocytes
Enzymes	
Arylsulfatases	Lipid/proteoglycan hydrolysis
Carboxypeptidase A	Peptide processing
Chymase	Tissue damage, pain, angiotensin II synthesis
Kinogenases	Synthesis of vasodilatory kinins, pain
Phospholipases	Arachidonic acid generation
Tryptase	Tissue damage, activation of PAR, inflammation, pain
Peptides	
Corticotropin-releasing hormone (CRH)	Inflammation, vasodilation
Endorphins	Analgesia
Endothelin	Sepsis
Kinins (bradykinin)	Inflammation, pain, vasodilation
Somatostatin (SRIF)	Anti-inflammatory action
Substance P (SP)	Inflammation, pain
Vasoactive intestinal peptide (VIP)	Vasodilation
Urocortin	Inflammation, vasodilation
Vascular endothelial growth factor (VEGF)	Neovascularization, vasodilation
Proteoglycans	
Chondroitin sulfate	Cartilage synthesis, anti-inflammatory action
Heparin	Angiogenesis, nerve growth factor stabilization
Hyaluronic acid	Connective tissue, nerve growth factor stabilization
De novo synthesized	
Cytokines	
Interleukins (IL)-1,2,3,4,5,6,9,10,13,16	Inflammation, leukocyte migration, pain
INF-γ; MIF; TNF-α	Inflammation, leukocyte proliferation/activation
Growth factors	
CSF, GM-CSF, b-FGF, NGF, VEGF	Growth of a variety of cells
Phospholipid metabolites	
Leukotriene B$_4$ (LTB$_4$)	Leukocyte chemotaxis
Leukotriene C$_4$ (LTC$_4$)	Vasoconstriction, pain
Platelet-activating factor (PAF)	Platelet activation, vasodilation
Prostaglandin D$_2$ (PGD$_2$)	Bronchonstriction, pain
Nitric oxide (NO)	Vasodilation

ABBREVIATIONS: TNF-α: tumor necrosis factor-α; INFγ: Interferon-γ; MIF: macrophage inflammatory factor; GM-CSF: granulocyte monocyte-colony stimulating factor; b-FGF: fibroblast growth factor; NGF: nerve growth factor; SCF: stem cell factor; VEGF: vascular endothelial growth factor.

TABLE 2. Mast cell triggers

Antigen + IgE
Anaphylatoxins
CRH
IL-1
Immunoglobulin-free light chains
LPS
NGF
NT
SCF
SP
Superantigens
Ucn
VIP
Viral DNA sequences

ABBREVIATIONS: CRH: corticotropin-releasing hormone; IL: interleukin; LPS: lipopolysaccharide; NGF: nerve growth factor; NT: neurotensin; SCF: stem cell factor; SP: substance P; Ucn: urocortin; VIP: vasoactive intestinal peptide.

are present in the skin.[55] Acute stress releases CRH in the skin,[56] inducing a local response.[54] Acute stress also induces redistribution of leukocytes from the systemic circulation to the skin[57]; it also exacerbates skin delayed hypersensitivity reactions[58] and chronic contact dermatitis in rats, an effect that depends on mast cells and CRH-1 receptors (CRHR-1).[59]

Computer-induced stress enhanced allergen-specific responses with concomitant increase in plasma SP levels in patients with atopic dermatitis.[60] Similar findings with increased plasma levels of SP, VIP, and NGF, along with a switch to a TH2 cytokine pattern, were reported in patients with atopic dermatitis playing video games.[61] Exercise was also shown to increase the

TABLE 3. Inflammatory diseases involving mast cells

Disease	Pathophysiologic effects
Asthma	Bronchonstriction, pulmonary inflammation
Atopic dermatitis	Skin vasodilation, T-cell recruitment, inflammation, itching
Coronary artery disease	Coronary inflammation, myocardial ischemia
Chronic prostatitis	Prostate inflammation
Chronic rhinitis	Nasal inflammation
Fibromyalgia	Muscle inflammation, pain
Interstitial cystitis	Bladder mucosal damage, inflammation, pain
Migraine	Meningeal vasodilation, inflammation, pain
Multiple sclerosis	Increased blood–brain barrier permeability, brain inflammation, Demyelination
Neurofibromatosis	Skin nerve growth, fibrosis
Osteoarthritis	Articular erosion, inflammation, pain
Rheumatoid arthritis	Joint inflammation, cartilage erosion

TABLE 4. Selective release of mast cell mediators

Stimuli	MC type	Mediators released	Mediators not released	Physiological importance	References
Endogenous					
IL-1β	RPMC	NO	PAF, H	Inflammation	194
PGE$_2$	RPMC	IL-6	H, TNF-α	Cytoprotection	195
SCF	BMMC	IL-6	H, LTC$_4$, TNF-α	MC development	33
IL-12	RPMC	INF-γ	H	Th1 immunity	196
CD8 ligands	RPMC	TNF-α, NO	H	T cell interaction	197
Thrombin	BMMC	IL-6	5HT, TNF-α	Anticlotting	198
SCF	hCBMC	IL-8	H, GM-CSF, INF-γ, IL-1β	Endothelial transmigration	199
Monomeric IgE	BMMC	IL-6	H, LTC$_4$	MC survival	200
Endothelin-1-3	RMMC	TNF-α, IL-12↑	IL-4, IL-10, IL-13↓*	Th1 immunity	201
LTC$_4$/LTD$_4$	IL-4-primed hCBMC	TNF-α, MIP-1α, IL-5	H	Non-IgE mediated inflammation	202
IL-1	hCBMC	IL-6, IL-8, TNF	H, tryptase	Inflammation	35
CRHR-1	hCBMC	VEGF	H, tryptase, IL-8	Inflammation	77
CRHR-2	hCBMC	IL-6	H, tryptase, IL-8, VEGF	Inflammation	203
Exogenous/ Pharmacological					
Amitriptyline	RPMC	Serotonin	H	Headaches	18
LPS	RPMC	IL-6	H	Bacterial infection	31
CpG DNA	BMMC	TNF-α, IL-6	HA, IL-4, IL-12, GM-CSF, INF-γ	Host response to bacteria	204
Cholera Toxin	RPMC	IL-6	H, TNF-α	Inflammation	205
PMA	BMMC	VPF/VEGF	5HT	Angiogenesis	4
Clostridium difficile toxin A	RPMC	TNF-α	H	GI tract inflammation	206
H. pylori VacA toxin	BMMC	IL-6, IL-8, TNF-α	H	Gastric injury	150
Suboptimal FcεRI stimulation	BMMC	MCP-1	IL-10, H	Chemokines ≫cytokines /H	207
S.a. peptidoglycan or zymosan	hCBMC	GM-CSF, IL-1β, RANTES, LTC$_4$	β-hexosaminidase, IL-6	Exacerbation of asthma by bacterial infection	141

ABBREVIATIONS: BMMC: bone marrow mast cells; CRHR: corticotropin-releasing hormone; H: histamine; hCBMC: human cord blood mast cells; LPS: lipopolysaccharide; LTC$_4$: leukotriene C$_4$; PMA: phorbol myristate acetate; TNF-α: tumor necrosis factor-α; NO: nitric oxide; MIP: macrophage inhibitory protein; GM-CSF: granulocyte monocyte-colony stimulating factor; 5HT: 5-hydroxytryptamine; INF-γ: interferon-γ; MCP-1: monocyte chemoattractant protein-1; RMMC: rat mucosal mast cells; RPMC: rat peritoneal mast cells; VPF: vascular proliferating factor; MC: mast cells; IgE: immunoglobulin E; SCF: stem cell factor; GI: gastrointestinal.

responsiveness of skin mast cells to morphine only in patients with exercise-induced asthma.[62]

CRH[63] and its structurally related peptide, urocortin (Ucn),[64] can activate skin mast cells and induce mast-cell-dependent vascular permeability in rodents. CRH also increases vascular permeability in human skin,[65] a process dependent on mast cells. CRH-R2 receptor expression was shown to be up-regulated in stress-induced alopecia in humans,[66] CRH-R2 expression was increased in chronic urticaria.[67] Acute restraint stress induces rat skin vascular permeability,[68] an effect inhibited by a CRH receptor antagonist and absent in mast-cell-deficient mice.[63,64]

Proteases released from mast cells could act on plasma albumin to generate histamine-releasing peptides,[69,70] which would further propagate mast cell activation and inflammation. Proteases could also stimulate protease-activated receptors (PARs), inducing microleakage and widespread inflammation.[71,72] Many dermatoses, such as atopic dermatitis (AD), chronic urticaria, and psoriasis, are triggered or exacerbated by stress,[73] which also worsens eczema[74] and acne vulgaris.[75]

Mast cells are localized close to CRH-positive neurons in the median eminence[76] and express functional CRH receptors.[77] The median eminence is rich in mast cells[78,79] and contains most of the histamine in the brain.[80] Hypothalamic mast cell activation can stimulate the HPA axis.[81–83] Histamine is considered a major regulator of hypothalamus[84] and can increase CRH mRNA expression there.[85] Moreover, human mast cells can synthesize and secrete large amounts of CRH[86] as well as IL-1 and IL-6, which are independent activators of the HPA axis.[87] The immunoendocrine responses to stress in chronic skin inflammatory diseases have been reviewed,[12,88] and it was proposed that mast cells constitute the "sensor" of a "brain–skin" connection.[89]

INFLAMMATORY ARTHRITIS

The presence of mast cells in joints has been known for many years.[17,90–96] Moreover, fluid aspirated from joints of patients with arthrosynovitis contains RANTES and MCP-1,[97] both of which are potent mast cell chemoattractants.[9] Mast cells are required for autoimmune arthritis[98] and inflammatory arthritis,[99] as knee involvement was absent in the joints of W/W^v mast cell–deficient mice as compared to their +/+ controls. Inflammatory arthritis was also significantly reduced in CRH knockout mice[99] and in mice treated with the CRH receptor-1 antagonist, Antalarmin.[100]

Mast cells in the joints of rheumatoid arthritis (RA) patients express CRH receptors.[101] Moreover, CRH,[101,102] Ucn,[103,104] and CRH receptors are increased in the joints of inflammatory and RA patients, the symptoms of whom worsen by stress.[105,106]

ASTHMA

Asthma is one of the most common chronic illnesses, affecting roughly 300 million people worldwide.[107,108] The morbidity and mortality due to asthma continues to increase despite advances in both our scientific knowledge, as well as in hygiene and drugs for this disease.[108] The World Health Organization has estimated that 1 of 250 deaths worldwide is due to asthma. These facts highlight the need for an improved understanding of the cellular and molecular mechanisms that contribute to the pathogenesis of asthma.

Recent reports indicate that stress can exacerbate asthma.[109–114] One study indicated that maternal stress may be responsible for the subsequent cellular response in childhood asthma.[115] It has been postulated that stress associated with urban living may contribute to poor asthma control.[116] Stress has long been postulated to have a negative impact on asthma, but the mechanisms by which this occurs remain poorly defined.[109,111,112,114,117,118] One study showed that adolescents with asthma in a low socioeconomic group, who reported more stressful and acute life events, had more asthma exacerbation and higher serum Th-2 cytokines than those in higher socioeconomic status.[119] The Inner City Asthma Study showed a correlation between community violence and asthma morbidity.[120] Post-traumatic psychological stress following the 9/11 attacks on the World Trade Center correlated with increased symptom severity in subjects with moderate-to-severe asthma and with utilization of urgent care in New York City.[121,122] In an epidemiological study carried out among 10,667 Finnish first-year university students (18–25 years old), it was shown that an excess of stressful events, such as concomitant severe disease or death of immediate family members or family conflicts, were associated with exacerbation of asthma.[111]

Stress associated with final examinations, as compared to mid semester, of college students with mild asthma increased sputum eosinophil counts, as well as eosinophil-derived neurotoxin and IL-5 once the eosinophils were cultured for up to 24 h.[117] It was suggested that a shift in cytokine generation to that of a Th2 type may be the defining parameter.[113] In one longitudinal study of 92 adults with asthma, it was determined that subjects who reported more negative life events and had low levels of social support had more episodes of asthma exacerbation induced by upper respiratory tract infections.[123] A large prospective long-term follow-up community-based cohort study of young adults showed a dose–response relationship between panic and asthma.[124] In fact, one study indicated that maternal stress may be responsible for the cellular response in childhood asthma,[115] while another showed that greater levels of caregiver-perceived stress at 2–3 months was associated with increased risk of subsequent repeated wheezing among children during the first 14 months of life.[125] Such findings cannot be easily explained as the HPA axis apparently functions normally in asthmatic adult patients, producing appropriate plasma cortisol increases in response to stress[126] which might be expected to reduce rather than exacerbate asthma symptoms. One publication showed a significantly blunted cortisol response to stress only in asthmatic children,[127] suggesting there may be differences due to age.

While no animal model exactly replicates human asthma, the use of animals has provided helpful information about the mechanisms of airway inflammation and hyperreactivity seen in asthma.[128,129] Chronic exposure to aerosolized ovalbumin has been shown to be a useful murine model of asthma leading to airway inflammation, airway hyperresponsiveness (AHR),[130] as well as microvascular leakage in the airways.[130–132] Microvascular leakage in the airway wall may also be important for the airway wall remodeling that is found in most asthmatics.[133,134] More recently, the house dust mite allergen model has been shown to effectively induce chronic airway inflammation and AHR.[133,135] Stress has been shown to increase AHR[114] and inflammation[114,136] in response to ovalbumin challenge in murine models of asthma. In one case, exposure to an ultrasonic stressor, coinciding with the first aerosol challenge, significantly increased allergen-induced pulmonary reactivity and bronchial inflammation. Short-term (3 days) stress before allergen challenge decreased the number of inflammatory cells, but increased IL-6, while long-term (7 days) stress evidently increased the number of inflammatory cells but did not alter IL-6 levels.[136]

The role of mast cells in asthma is undisputed.[137–139] Rodent mast cells express bacterial Toll-like receptors (TLRs) 2 and 4.[140,141] However, the pattern of response may be species- and tissue-specific, making generalizations difficult. TLRs were initially discovered in *Drosophila* as the receptors responsible for dorso-ventral patterning in the developing embryo; however, soon after they were shown to be important in the development of innate immunity to invading pathogens.[142] Subsequently, human homologues for TLRs were identified beginning with TLR-4, which was shown to bind lipopolysaccharide (LPS). Ten human TLRs have been identified so far.[143–145] Evidence is building that TLRs play an important role in recognition of ligands associated with bacterial or viral infections, and play a key role in the development of adaptive immune responses,[144] especially in asthma.[146] LPS induced release of TNF-α through TLR-4, while peptidoglycan induced histamine release through TLR-2 from rodent mast cells. Fetal rat skin-derived mast cells expressed TLR-3, 7, and 9 and activation by CPG oligodeoxynucleotide induced release of TNF and IL-6, as well as RANTES and MIP, but without degranulation.[147,148] In another paper, LPS could not induce release of GM-CSF, IL-1, or LTC$_4$.[141] However, LPS did induce secretion of TH2 cytokines IL-5, IL-10, and IL-13 and increased their production by FcϵRI cross-linking.[149] Elsewhere, it was shown that TLR-2 activation produced IL-4, IL-6, and IL-13, but not IL-1,[150] while LPS produced TNF, IL-1, IL-6, and IL-13, but not IL-4 or IL-5, without degranulation.[150] Activation of these receptors even in human cultured mast cells leads to distinct biological effects: Human mast cells express viral TLR-9,[151] activation of which produced the proinflammatory cytokine IL-6,[151] while they produced IFN in response to double-stranded RNA through TLR-3.[152] These findings may explain how viral infections worsen asthma.

Viral infections have been shown to exacerbate asthma and contribute to as many as 50% of asthma-associated deaths; moreover, more than 80% of childhood asthma exacerbations are associated with viral airway infections.[153] A number of studies have shown that viral infections increase airway hyperresponsiveness and antigen sensitization,[154] as well as recruitment of inflammatory cells.[155] Synoptical virus, metapneumovirus, rhinovirus, adenovirus,[156] as well as influenza and parainfluenza virus have been implicated in the pathogenesis of asthma.[157–159] In fact, rhinovirus infections during infancy appear to predict childhood wheezing,[160] while respiratory syncytial virus during the first 3 months of life was shown to promote a TH2 response, especially significantly high levels of IL-4.[161] Such early-infancy viral respiratory infections may also induce metalloproteinases, which are involved in airway remodeling in asthma.[162] However, this field is quite confusing because current discussions focus on viral nucleic acid inoculation.[163]

CORONARY INFLAMMATION

Increasing evidence implicates acute psychological stress and cardiac mast cells in coronary artery disease (CAD), especially when it occurs without angina, which appears to involve a sizable portion of myocardial infections (MI).[164–167] Cardiac mast cells can participate in the development of atherosclerosis, coronary inflammation, and cardiac ischemia.[168] Mast cells are particularly prominent in coronary arteries during spasm[169] and accumulate in the shoulder region of human coronary plaque rupture.[170–172] The human mast cell proteolytic enzyme chymase is the main cardiac source of converting enzyme that generates the coronary constrictor angiotensin II;[173] the chymase can also induce the removal of cholesterol from HDL particles and uptake by macrophages that become "foam" cells, major components of coronary atheromas.[174–177] Cardiac mast-cell-derived histamine[178] can constrict the coronary arteries[179] and can sensitize nerve endings;[180] this is particularly important because mast cells are localized close to nerve endings in atherosclerotic coronary arteries.[181]

Acute stress induces rat cardiac mast cell activation, an effect blocked by the "mast cell stabilizer" disodium cromoglycate (cromolyn).[182] Acute stress can also induce histamine release from mouse heart,[183] as well as increase serum histamine and IL-6.[183,184] These effects are dependent on mast cells and are greater in apolipoprotein E (ApoE) knockout mice that develop atherosclerosis.[183,184] Serum IL-6 elevations in patients with acute CAD were documented to derive primarily from the coronary sinus.[185] Both histamine[186] and

IL-6[187] are significant independent factors of CAD morbidity and mortality. There are also reports of anaphylactic CAD that has been termed the "Kounis" syndrome.[188,189]

CONCLUSION

Mast cells have emerged as unique immune cells that can be activated by many immune and nonimmune triggers, including acute stress through CRH; it is, therefore, proposed that CRH be renamed SRH (**Stress Response Hormone**) to reflect its versatile role in stress. Mast cells are critical in the development of inflammatory diseases, especially dermatoses, asthma, arthritis, and CAD. Inhibition of mast cell activation by CRH,[190] therefore, is a novel target for the development of new treatments for inflammatory and autoimmune disorders. Certain dietary supplements have recently been shown to be effective in this regard[191] because they combine the proteoglycan chondroitin sulfate[192] and the flavonoid quercetin,[193] both of which have mast cell inhibitory and anti-inflammatory actions.

ACKNOWLEDGMENTS

Aspects of the work discussed were supported in part by NIH Grant No. AR47652, and by a grant from Theta Biomedical Consulting and Development Co., Inc. (Brookline, MA) to T.C.T. who has been awarded U.S. patents #5250529; #6020305; #5648350; #5855884; #5821259; #5994357; #6624148 and #6984667 covering the use of CRH and mast cell blockers in the diseases described above. We thank Ms. Jessica Christian for her patience and word processing skills.

REFERENCES

1. BLANK, U. & J. RIVERA. 2004. The ins and outs of IgE-dependent mast-cell exocytosis. Trends Immunol. **25:** 266–273.
2. KRAFT, S., S. RANA, M.H. JOUVIN, et al. 2004. The role of the FcεRI beta-chain in allergic diseases. Int. Arch. Allergy Immunol. **135:** 62–72.
3. GRUTZKAU, A., S. KRUGER-KRASAGAKES, H. BAUMEISTER, et al. 1998. Synthesis, storage and release of vascular endothelial growth factor/vascular permeability factor (VEGF/VPF) by human mast cells: implications for the biological significance of VEGF$_{206}$. Mol. Biol. Cell **9:** 875–884.
4. BOESIGER, J., M. TSAI, M. MAURER, et al. 1998. Mast cells can secrete vascular permeability factor/vascular endothelial cell growth factor and exhibit enhanced release after immunoglobulin E-dependent upregulation of Fce receptor I expression. J. Exp. Med. **188:** 1135–1145.

5. GALLI, S.J., S. NAKAE & M. TSAI. 2005. Mast cells in the development of adaptive immune responses. Nat. Immunol. **6:** 135–142.
6. RODEWALD, H.R., M. DESSING, A.M. DVORAK, *et al.* 1996. Identification of a committed precursor for the mast cell lineage. Science **271:** 818–822.
7. CHEN, C.C., M.A. GRIMBALDESTON, M. TSAI, *et al.* 2005. Identification of mast cell progenitors in adult mice. Proc. Natl. Acad. Sci. USA **102:** 11408–11413.
8. ALOE, L. & R. LEVI-MONTALCINI. 1977. Mast cells increase in tissues of neonatal rats injected with the nerve growth factor. Brain Res. **133:** 358–366.
9. CONTI, P., X. PANG, W. BOUCHER, *et al.* 1997. Impact of RANTES and MCP-1 chemokines on *in vivo* basophilic mast cell recruitment in rat skin injection model and their role in modifying the protein and mRNA levels for histidine decarboxylase. Blood **89:** 4120–4127.
10. ROTTEM, M. & Y.A. MEKORI. 2005. Mast cells and autoimmunity. Autoimmun. Rev. **4:** 21–27.
11. GALLI, S.J., J. KALESNIKOFF, M.A. GRIMBALDESTON, *et al.* 2005. Mast cells as "tunable" effector and immunoregulatory cells: recent advances. Annu. Rev. Immunol. **23:** 749–786.
12. THEOHARIDES, T.C. & D.E. COCHRANE. 2004. Critical role of mast cells in inflammatory diseases and the effect of acute stress. J. Neuroimmunol. **146:** 1–12.
13. KRANEVELD, A.D., M. KOOL, A.H. VAN HOUWELINGEN, *et al.* 2005. Elicitation of allergic asthma by immunoglobulin free light chains. Proc. Natl. Acad. Sci. USA **102:** 1578–1583.
14. REDEGELD, F.A., M.W. VAN DER HEIJDEN, M. KOOL, *et al.* 2002. Immunoglobulin-free light chains elicit immediate hypersensitivity-like responses. Nat. Med. **8:** 694–701.
15. REDEGELD, F.A. & F.P. NIJKAMP. 2003. Immunoglobulin free light chains and mast cells: pivotal role in T-cell-mediated immune reactions? Trends Immunol. **24:** 181–185.
16. BENOIST, C. & D. MATHIS. 2002. Mast cells in autoimmune disease. Nature **420:** 875–878.
17. WOOLLEY, D.E. 2003. The mast cell in inflammatory arthritis. N. Engl. J. Med. **348:** 1709–1711.
18. THEOHARIDES, T.C., P.K. BONDY, N.D. TSAKALOS, *et al.* 1982. Differential release of serotonin and histamine from mast cells. Nature **297:** 229–231.
19. THEOHARIDES, T.C. & W.W. DOUGLAS. 1978. Somatostatin induces histamine secretion from rat peritoneal mast cells. Endocrinology **102:** 1637–1640.
20. DIMITRIADOU, V., M. LAMBRACHT-HALL, J. REICHLER, *et al.* 1990. Histochemical and ultrastructural characteristics of rat brain perivascular mast cells stimulated with compound 48/80 and carbachol. Neuroscience **39:** 209–224.
21. DIMITRIADOU, V., M.G. BUZZI, M.A. MOSKOWITZ, *et al.* 1991. Trigeminal sensory fiber stimulation induces morphologic changes reflecting secretion in rat dura mast cells. Neuroscience **44:** 97–112.
22. THEOHARIDES, T.C., G.R. SANT, M. EL-MANSOURY, *et al.* 1995. Activation of bladder mast cells in interstitial cystitis: a light and electron microscopic study. J. Urol. **153:** 629–636.
23. LETOURNEAU, R., X. PANG, G.R. SANT, *et al.* 1996. Intragranular activation of bladder mast cells and their association with nerve processes in interstitial cystitis. Br. J. Urol. **77:** 41–54.

24. DVORAK, A.M., R.S. MCLEOD, A. ONDERDONK, *et al.* 1992. Ultrastructural evidence for piecemeal and anaphylactic degranulation of human gut mucosal mast cells *in vivo*. Int. Arch. Allergy Immunol. **99:** 74–83.

25. KOPS, S.K., H. VAN LOVEREN, R.W. ROSENSTEIN, *et al.* 1984. Mast cell activation and vascular alterations in immediate hypersensitivity-like reactions induced by a T cell derived antigen-binding factor. Lab. Invest. **50:** 421–434.

26. VAN LOVEREN, H., S.K. KOPS & P.W. ASKENASE. 1984. Different mechanisms of release of vasoactive amines by mast cells occur in T cell-dependent compared to IgE-dependent cutaneous hypersensitivity responses. Eur. J. Immunol. **14:** 40–47.

27. KOPS, S.K., T.C. THEOHARIDES, C.T. CRONIN, *et al.* 1990. Ultrastructural characteristics of rat peritoneal mast cells undergoing differential release of serotonin without histamine and without degranulation. Cell Tissue Res. **262:** 415–424.

28. BENYON, R., C. ROBINSON & M.K. CHURCH. 1989. Differential release of histamine and eicosanoids from human skin mast cells activated by IgE-dependent and non-immunological stimuli. Br. J. Pharmacol. **97:** 898–904.

29. LEVI-SCHAFFER, F. & M. SHALIT. 1989. Differential release of histamine and prostaglandin D_2 in rat peritoneal mast cells activated with peptides. Int. Arch. Allergy Appl. Immunol. **90:** 352–357.

30. VAN HAASTER, C.M., W. ENGELS, P.J.M.R. LEMMENS, *et al.* 1995. Differential release of histamine and prostaglandin D_2 in rat peritoneal mast cells: roles of cytosolic calcium and protein tyrosine kinases. Biochim. Biophys. Acta **1265:** 79–88.

31. LEAL-BERUMEN, I., P. CONLON & J.S. MARSHALL. 1994. IL-6 production by rat peritoneal mast cells is not necessarily preceded by histamine release and can be induced by bacterial lipopolysaccharide. J. Immunol. **152:** 5468–5476.

32. MARQUARDT, D.L., J.L. ALONGI & L.L. WALKER. 1996. The phosphatidylinositol 3-kinase inhibitor wortmannin blocks mast cell exocytosis but not IL-6 production. J. Immunol. **156:** 1942–1945.

33. GAGARI, E., M. TSAI, C.S. LANTZ, *et al.* 1997. Differential release of mast cell interleukin-6 via c-kit. Blood **89:** 2654–2663.

34. HOJO, H., R. SUN, Y. ONO, *et al.* 1996. Differential production of interleukin-6 and its close relation to liver metastasis in clones from murine P815 mastocytoma. Cancer Lett. **108:** 55–59.

35. KANDERE-GRZYBOWSKA, K., R. LETOURNEAU, W. BOUCHER, *et al.* 2003. IL-1 induces vesicular secretion of IL-6 without degranulation from human mast cells. J. Immunol. **171:** 4830–4836.

36. CAO, J., C.L. CURTIS & T.C. THEOHARIDES. 2006. Corticotropin-releasing hormone (CRH) induces vascular endothelial growth factor (VEGF) release from human mast cells via the cAMP/protein kinase A/p38 MAPK pathway Mol. Pharmacol. **69:** 998–1006.

37. LEUNG, D.Y., L.A. DIAZ, V. DELEO, *et al.* 1997. Allergic and immunologic skin disorders. JAMA **278:** 1914–1923.

38. CHARLESWORTH, E.N. 1995. Role of basophils and mast cells in acute and late reactions in the skin. Chem. Immunol. **62:** 84–107.

39. CHURCH, M.K. & G.F. CLOUGH. 1999. Human skin mast cells: *in vitro* and *in vivo* studies. Ann. Allergy Asthma Immunol. **83:** 471–475.

40. NOLI, C. & A. MIOLO. 2001. The mast cell in wound healing. Vet. Dermatol. **12:** 303–313.

41. JARVIKALLIO, A., I.T. HARVIMA & A. NAUKKARINEN. 2003. Mast cells, nerves and neuropeptides in atopic dermatitis and nummular eczema. Arch. Dermatol. Res. **295:** 2–7.
42. WIESNER-MENZEL, L., B. SCHULZ, F. VAKILZADEH, *et al.* 1981. Electron microscopical evidence for a direct contact between nerve fibers and mast cells. Acta Derm. Venereol. (Stockh) **61:** 465–469.
43. GOETZL, E.J., T. CHERNOV, F. RENOLD, *et al.* 1985. Neuropeptide regulation of the expression of immediate hypersensitivity. J. Immunol. **135:** 802s–805s.
44. FOREMAN, J.C. 1987. Neuropeptides and the pathogenesis of allergy. Allergy **42:** 1–11.
45. CHURCH, M.K., M.A. LOWMAN, P.H. REES, *et al.* 1989. Mast cells, neuropeptides and inflammation. Agents Actions **27:** 8–16.
46. GOETZL, E.J., P.P.J. CHENG, A. HASSNER, *et al.* 1990. Neuropeptides, mast cells and allergy: novel mechanisms and therapeutic possibilities. Clin. Exp. Allergy **20:** 3–7.
47. CARRAWAY, R., D.E. COCHRANE, J.B. LANSMAN, *et al.* 1982. Neurotensin stimulates exocytotic histamine secretion from rat mast cells and elevates plasma histamine levels. J. Physiol. **323:** 403–414.
48. WATT, F.M. 1991. Cell culture models of differentiation. FASEB J. **5:** 287–294.
49. FEWTRELL, C.M.S., J.C. FOREMAN, C.C. JORDAN, *et al.* 1982. The effects of substance P on histamine and 5-hydroxytryptamine release in the rat. J. Physiol. **330:** 393–411.
50. ODUM, L., L.J. PETERSEN, P.S. SKOV, *et al.* 1998. Pituitary adenylate cyclase activating polypeptide (PACAP) is localized in human dermal neurons and causes histamine release from skin mast cells. Inflamm. Res. **47:** 488–492.
51. TOYODA, M., T. MAKINO, M. KAGOURA, *et al.* 2000. Immunolocalization of substance P in human skin mast cells. Arch. Dermatol. Res. **292:** 418–421.
52. XIANG, Z. & G. NILSSON. 2000. IgE receptor-mediated release of nerve growth factor by mast cells. Clin. Exp. Allergy **30:** 1379–1386.
53. SLOMINSKI, A. & J. WORTSMAN. 2000. Neuroendocrinology of the skin. Endocr. Rev. **21:** 457–487.
54. SLOMINSKI, A., J. WORTSMAN, T. LUGER, *et al.* 2000. Corticotropin releasing hormone and proopiomelanocortin involvement in the cutaneous response to stress. Physiol. Rev. **80:** 979–1020.
55. SLOMINSKI, A., J. WORTSMAN, A. PISARCHIK, *et al.* 2001. Cutaneous expression of corticotropin-releasing hormone (CRH), urocortin, and CRH receptors. FASEB J. **15:** 1678–1693.
56. LYTINAS, M., D. KEMPURAJ, M. HUANG, *et al.* 2003. Acute stress results in skin corticotropin-releasing hormone secretion, mast cell activation and vascular permeability, an effect mimicked by intradermal corticotropin-releasing hormone and inhibited by histamine-1 receptor antagonists. Int. Arch. Allergy Immunol. **130:** 224–231.
57. DHABHAR, F. & B.S. MCEWEN. 1996. Stress-induced enhancement of antigenspecific cell-mediated immunity. J. Immunol. **156:** 2608–2615.
58. DHABHAR, F.S. & B.S. MCEWEN. 1999. Enhancing versus suppressive effects of stress hormones on skin immune function. Proc. Natl. Acad. Sci. USA **96:** 1059–1064.
59. KANEKO, K., S. KAWANA, K. ARAI, *et al.* 2003. Corticotropin-releasing factor receptor type 1 is involved in the stress-induced exacerbation of chronic contact dermatitis in rats. Exp. Dermatol. **12:** 47–52.

60. KIMATA, H. 2003. Enhancement of allergic skin wheal responses and *in vitro* allergen-specific IgE production by computer-induced stress in patients with atopic dermatitis. Brain Behav. Immun. **17:** 134–138.
61. KIMATA, H. 2003. Enhancement of allergic skin wheal responses in patients with atopic eczema/dermatitis syndrome by playing video games or by a frequently ringing mobile phone. Eur. J Clin. Invest **33:** 513–517.
62. CHOI, I.S., Y.I. KOH, S.W. CHUNG, *et al.* 2004. Increased releasability of skin mast cells after exercise in patients with exercise-induced asthma. J. Korean Med. Sci. **19:** 724–728.
63. THEOHARIDES, T.C., L.K. SINGH, W. BOUCHER, *et al.* 1998. Corticotropin-releasing hormone induces skin mast cell degranulation and increased vascular permeability, a possible explanation for its pro-inflammatory effects. Endocrinology **139:** 403–413.
64. SINGH, L.K., W. BOUCHER, X. PANG, *et al.* 1999. Potent mast cell degranulation and vascular permeability triggered by urocortin through activation of CRH receptors. J. Pharmacol. Exp. Ther. **288:** 1349–1356.
65. CLIFTON, V.L., R. CROMPTON, R. SMITH, *et al.* 2002. Microvascular effects of CRH in human skin vary in relation to gender. J. Clin. Endocrinol. Metab. **87:** 267–270.
66. KATSAROU-KATSARI, A., L.K. SINGH & T.C. THEOHARIDES. 2001. Alopecia areata and affected skin CRH receptor upregulation induced by acute emotional stress. Dermatology **203:** 157–161.
67. PAPADOPOULOU, N., D. KALOGEROMITROS, N.G. STAURIANEAS, *et al.* 2005. Corticotropin-releasing hormone receptor-1 and histidine decarboxylase expression in chronic urticaria. J. Invest. Dermatol. **125:** 952–955.
68. SINGH, L.K., X. PANG, N. ALEXACOS, *et al.* 1999. Acute immobilization stress triggers skin mast cell degranulation via corticotropin releasing hormone, neurotensin and substance P: a link to neurogenic skin disorders. Brain Behav. Immun. **13:** 225–239.
69. CARRAWAY, R.E., D.E. COCHRANE, W. BOUCHER, *et al.* 1989. Structures of histamine-releasing peptides formed by the action of acid proteases on mammalian albumin(s). J. Immunol. **143:** 1680–1684.
70. COCHRANE, D.E., R.E. CARRAWAY, R.S. FELDBERG, *et al.* 1993. Stimulated rat mast cells generate histamine-releasing peptide from albumin. Peptides **14:** 117–123.
71. SCHMIDLIN, F. & N.W. BUNNETT. 2001. Protease-activated receptors: how proteases signal to cells. Curr. Opin. Pharmacol. **1:** 575–582.
72. MOLINO, M., E.S. BARNATHAN, R. NUMEROF, *et al.* 1997. Interactions of mast cell tryptase with thrombin receptors and PAR-2. J. Biol. Chem. **272:** 4043–4049.
73. KATSAROU-KATSARI, A., A. FILIPPOU & T.C. THEOHARIDES. 1999. Effect of stress and other psychological factors on the pathophysiology and treatment of dermatoses. Int. J. Immunopathol. Pharmacol. **12:** 7–11.
74. GRAHAM, D.T. & S. WOLF. 1953. The relation of eczema to attitude and to vascular reactions of the human skin. J. Lab. Clin. Med. **42:** 238–254.
75. MURPHY, P.M. 2001. Chemokines and the molecular basis of cancer metastasis. N. Engl. J. Med. **345:** 833–835.
76. THEOHARIDES, T.C., C.P. SPANOS, X. PANG, *et al.* 1995. Stress-induced intracranial mast cell degranulation. A corticotropin releasing hormone-mediated effect. Endocrinology **136:** 5745–5750.

77. CAO, J., N. PAPADOPOULOU, D. KEMPURAJ, *et al*. 2005. Human mast cells express corticotropin-releasing hormone (CRH) receptors and CRH leads to selective secretion of vascular endothelial growth factor (VEGF). J. Immunol. **174:** 7665–7675.

78. POLLARD, H., S. BISCHOFF, C. LLORENS-CORTES, *et al*. 1976. Histidine decarboxylase and histamine in discrete nuclei of rat hypothalamus and the evidence for mast cells in the median eminence. Brain Res. **118:** 509–513.

79. PANULA, P., H.-Y.T. YANG & E. COSTA. 1984. Histamine-containing neurons in the rat hypothalamus. Proc. Natl. Acad. Sci. USA **81:** 2572–2576.

80. YAMATODANI, A., K. MAEYAMA, T. WATANABE, *et al*. 1982. Tissue distribution of histamine in a mutant mouse deficient in mast cells: clear evidence for the presence of non-mast cell histamine. Biochem. Pharmacol. **31:** 305–309.

81. BUGAJSKI, A.J., Z. CHLAP, A. GADEK-MICHALSKA, *et al*. 1995. Degranulation and decrease in histamine levels of thalamic mast cells coincides with corticosterone secretion induced by compound 48/80. Inflamm. Res. **44**(Supp.1): S50–S51.

82. GADEK-MICHALSKA, A., Z. CHLAP, M. TURON, *et al*. 1991. The intracerebroventricularly administered mast cells degranulator compound 48/80 increases the pituitary-adrenocortical activity in rats. Agents Actions **32:** 203–208.

83. MATSUMOTO, I., Y. INOUE, T. SHIMADA, *et al*. 2001. Brain mast cells act as an immune gate to the hypothalamic-pituitary-adrenal axis in dogs. J. Exp. Med. **194:** 71–78.

84. ROBERTS, F. & C.R. CALCUTT. 1983. Histamine and the hypothalamus. Neuroscience **9:** 721–739.

85. KJAER, A., P.J. LARSEN, U. KNIGGE, *et al*. 1998. Neuronal histamine and expression of corticotropin-releasing hormone, vasopressin and oxytocin in the hypothalamus: relative importance of H_1 and H_2 receptors. Eur. J. Endocrinol. **139:** 238–243.

86. KEMPURAJ, D., N.G. PAPADOPOULOU, M. LYTINAS, *et al*. 2004. Corticotropin-releasing hormone and its structurally related urocortin are synthesized and secreted by human mast cells. Endocrinology **145:** 43–480; Epub 2003 Oct. 23.

87. BETHIN, K.E., S.K. VOGT & L.J. MUGLIA. 2000. Interleukin-6 is an essential, corticotropin-releasing hormone-independent stimulator of the adrenal axis during immune system activation. Proc. Natl. Acad. Sci. USA **97:** 9317–9322.

88. BUSKE-KIRSCHBAUM, A. & D.H. HELLHAMMER. 2003. Endocrine and immune responses to stress in chronic inflammatory skin disorders. Ann. N. Y. Acad. Sci. **992:** 231–240.

89. PAUS, R., T.C. THEOHARIDES & P.C. ARCK. 2006. Neuroimmunoendocrine circuitry of the "brain-skin connection." Trends Immunol **27:** 32–39.

90. CRISP, A.J., C.M. CHAMPAN, S.E. KIRKHAM, *et al*. 1984. Articular mastocytosis in rheumatoid arthritis. Arthritis Rheum. **27:** 845–851.

91. KOLDEWIJN, E.L., O.R. HOMMES, W.A.J.G. LEMMENS, *et al*. 1995. Relationship between lower urinary tract abnormalities and disease-related parameters in multiple sclerosis. J. Urol. **154:** 169–173.

92. WOOLLEY, D.E. 1995. Mast cells in the rheumatoid lesion—ringleaders or innocent bystanders. Ann. Rheum. Dis. **54:** 533–534.

93. TETLOW, L.C. & D.E. WOOLLEY. 1995. Distribution, activation and tryptase/chymase phenotype of mast cells in the rheumatoid lesion. Ann. Rheum. Dis. **54:** 549–555.

94. DE PAULIS, A., A. CICCARELLI, I. MARINÒ, et al. 1997. Human synovial mast cells. II. Heterogeneity of the pharmacologic effects of antiinflammatory and immunosuppressive drugs. Arthritis Rheum. **40:** 469–478.
95. DE PAULIS, A., I. MARINO, A. CICCARELLI, et al. 1996. Human synovial mast cells. I. Utrastructural in situ and in vitro immunologic characterization. Arthritis Rheum. **39:** 1222–1233.
96. GOTIS-GRAHAM, I., M.D. SMITH, A. PARKER, et al. 1998. Synovial mast cell responses during clinical improvement in early rheumatoid arthritis. Ann. Rheum. Dis. **57:** 664–671.
97. CONTI, P., M. REALE, R.C. BARBACANE, et al. 2002. Differential production of RANTES and MCP-1 in synovial fluid from the inflamed human knee. Immunol. Lett. **80:** 105–111.
98. LEE, D.M., D.S. FRIEND, M.F. GURISH, et al. 2002. Mast cells: a cellular link between autoantibodies and inflammatory arthritis. Science **297:** 1689–1692.
99. MATTHEOS, S., S. CHRISTODOULOU, D. KEMPURAJ, et al. 2003. Mast cells and corticotropin-releasing hormone (CRH) are required for experimental inflammatory arthritis. FASEB J. **17:** C44.
100. WEBSTER, E.L., R.M. BARRIENTOS, C. CONTOREGGI, et al. 2002. Corticotropin releasing hormone (CRH) antagonist attenuates adjuvant induced arthritis: role of CRH in peripheral inflammation. J. Rheumatol. **29:** 1252–1261.
101. MCEVOY, A.N., B. BRESNIHAN, O. FITZGERALD, et al. 2001. Corticotropin-releasing hormone signaling in synovial tissue from patients with early inflammatory arthritis is mediated by the type 1a corticotropin-releasing hormone receptor. Arthritis Rheum. **44:** 1761–1767.
102. LOWRY, P.J., R.J. WOODS & S. BAIGENT. 1996. Corticotropin releasing factor and its binding protein. Pharmacol. Biochem. Behav. **54:** 305–308.
103. UZUKI, M., H. SASANO, Y. MURAMATSU, et al. 2001. Urocortin in the synovial tissue of patients with rheumatoid arthritis. Clin. Sci. **100:** 577–589.
104. KOHNO, M., Y. KAWAHITO, Y. TSUBOUCHI, et al. 2001. Urocortin expression in synovium of patients with rheumatoid arthritis and osteoarthritis: relation to inflammatory activity. J. Clin. Endocrinol. Metab. **86:** 4344–4352.
105. THOMASON, B.T., P.J. BRANTLEY, G.N. JONES, et al. 1992. The relation between stress and disease activity in rheumatoid arthritis. J. Behav. Med. **15:** 215–220.
106. HERRMANN, M., J. SCHOLMERICH & R.H. STRAUB. 2000. Stress and rheumatic diseases. Rheum. Dis. Clin. North Am. **26:** 737–763.
107. WEISS, S.T. 2001. Epidemiology and heterogeneity of asthma. Ann. Allergy Asthma Immunol. **87:** 5–8.
108. PAPIRIS, S., A. KOTANIDOU, K. MALAGARI, et al. 2002. Clinical review: severe asthma. Crit. Care **6:** 30–44.
109. LAUBE, B.L., B.A. CURBOW & R.W. COSTELLO. 2002. A pilot study examining the relationship between stress and serum cortisol concentrations in women with asthma. Respir. Med. **96:** 823–828.
110. SCHMALING, K.B., P.E. MCKNIGHT & N. AFARI. 2002. A prospective study of the relationship of mood and stress to pulmonary function among patients with asthma. J. Asthma **39:** 501–510.
111. KILPELAINEN, M., M. KOSKENVUO, H. HELENIUS, et al. 2002. Stressful life events promote the manifestation of asthma and atopic diseases. Clin. Exp. Allergy **32:** 256–263.
112. LAWRENCE, D.A. 2002. Psychologic stress and asthma: neuropeptide involvement. Environ. Health Perspect. **110:** A230–A231.

113. BIENENSTOCK, J. 2002. Stress and asthma: the plot thickens. Am. J. Respir. Crit. Care Med. **165:** 1034–1035.
114. JOACHIM, R.A., D. QUARCOO, P.C. ARCK, et al. 2003. Stress enhances airway reactivity and airway inflammation in an animal model of allergic bronchial asthma. Psychosom. Med. **65:** 811–815.
115. VON HERTZEN, L.C. 2002. Maternal stress and T-cell differentiation of the developing immune system: possible implications for the development of asthma and atopy. J. Allergy Clin. Immunol. **109:** 923–928.
116. DENDORFER, U., P. OETTGEN & T.A. LIBERMANN. 1994. Multiple regulatory elements in the interleukin-6 gene mediate induction by prostaglandins, cyclic AMP, and lipopolysaccharide. Mol. Cell Biol. **14:** 4443–4454.
117. LIU, L.Y., C.L. COE, C.A. SWENSON, et al. 2002. School examinations enhance airway inflammation to antigen challenge. Am. J. Respir. Crit. Care Med. **165:** 1062–1067.
118. GORDON, D.J. & B.M. RIFKIND. 1989. High-density lipoprotein—the clinical implications of recent studies. N. Engl. J. Med. **321:** 1311–1316.
119. CHEN, E., E.B. FISHER, L.B. BACHARIER, et al. 2003. Socioeconomic status, stress, and immune markers in adolescents with asthma. Psychosom. Med. **65:** 984–992.
120. WRIGHT, R.J., H. MITCHELL, C.M. VISNESS, et al. 2004. Community violence and asthma morbidity: the Inner-City Asthma Study. Am. J. Public Health **94:** 625–632.
121. FAGAN, J., S. GALEA, J. AHERN, et al. 2003. Relationship of self-reported asthma severity and urgent health care utilization to psychological sequelae of the September 11, 2001 terrorist attacks on the World Trade Center among New York City area residents. Psychosom. Med. **65:** 993–996.
122. CENTERS FOR DISEASE CONTROL AND PREVENTION (CDC). 2002. Self-reported increase in asthma severity after the September 11 attacks on the World Trade Center—Manhattan, New York, 2001 MMWR **51:** 781–784.
123. SMITH, A. & K. NICHOLSON. 2001. Psychosocial factors, respiratory viruses and exacerbation of asthma. Psychoneuroendocrinology **26:** 411–420.
124. HASLER, G., P.J. GERGEN, D.G. KLEINBAUM, et al. 2005. Asthma and panic in young adults: a 20-year prospective community study. Am. J. Respir. Crit. Care Med. **171:** 1224–1230.
125. WRIGHT, R.J., S. COHEN, V. CAREY, et al. 2002. Parental stress as a predictor of wheezing in infancy: a prospective birth-cohort study. Am. J. Respir. Crit. Care Med. **165:** 358–365.
126. KAPOOR, U., G. TAYAL, S.K. MITTAL, et al. 2003. Plasma cortisol levels in acute asthma. Indian J. Pediatr. **70:** 965–968.
127. BUSKE-KIRSCHBAUM, A., K. VON AUER, S. KRIEGER, et al. 2003. Blunted cortisol responses to psychosocial stress in asthmatic children: a general feature of atopic disease? Psychosom. Med. **65:** 806–810.
128. KIPS, J.C., G.P. ANDERSON, J.J. FREDBERG, et al. 2003. Murine models of asthma. Eur. Respir. J. **22:** 374–382.
129. LLOYD, C.M. & J.C. GUTIERREZ-RAMOS. 2004. Animal models to study chemokine receptor function: in vivo mouse models of allergic airway inflammation. Methods Mol. Biol. **239:** 199–210.
130. WILSON, J. 2000. The bronchial microcirculation in asthma. Clin. Exp. Allergy **30:** 51–53.

131. OLIVENSTEIN, R., T. DU, L.J. XU, *et al.* 1997. Microvascular leakage in the airway wall and lumen during allergen induced early and late responses in rats. Pulm. Pharmacol. Ther. **10:** 223–230.
132. VAN RENSEN, E.L., P.S. HIEMSTRA, K.F. RABE, *et al.* 2002. Assessment of microvascular leakage via sputum induction: the role of substance P and neurokinin A in patients with asthma. Am. J. Respir. Crit. Care Med. **165:** 1275–1279.
133. JOHNSON, J.R., R.E. WILEY, R. FATTOUH, *et al.* 2004. Continuous exposure to house dust mite elicits chronic airway inflammation and structural remodeling. Am. J. Respir. Crit. Care Med. **169:** 378–385.
134. NAURECKAS, E.T., I.M. NDUKWU, A.J. HALAYKO, *et al.* 1999. Bronchoalveolar lavage fluid from asthmatic subjects is mitogenic for human airway smooth muscle. Am. J. Respir. Crit. Care Med. **160:** 2062–2066.
135. SADAKANE, K., T. ICHINOSE, H. TAKANO, *et al.* 2002. Murine strain differences in airway inflammation induced by diesel exhaust particles and house dust mite allergen. Int. Arch. Allergy Immunol. **128:** 220–228.
136. FORSYTHE, P., C. EBELING, J.R. GORDON, *et al.* 2004. Opposing effects of short- and long-term stress on airway inflammation. Am. J. Respir. Crit. Care Med. **169:** 220–226.
137. CHO, S.H., A.J. ANDERSON & C.K. OH. 2002. Importance of mast cells in the pathophysiology of asthma. Clin. Rev. Allergy Immunol. **22:** 161–174.
138. BRADDING, P. 2003. The role of the mast cell in asthma: a reassessment. Curr. Opin. Allergy Clin. Immunol. **3:** 45–50.
139. BRIGHTLING, C.E., P. BRADDING, I.D. PAVORD, *et al.* 2003. New insights into the role of the mast cell in asthma. Clin. Exp. Allergy **33:** 550–556.
140. VARADARADJALOU, S., F. FEGER, N. THIEBLEMONT, *et al.* 2003. Toll-like receptor 2 (TLR2) and TLR4 differentially activate human mast cells. Eur. J. Immunol. **33:** 899–906.
141. MCCURDY, J.D., T.J. OLYNYCH, L.H. MAHER, *et al.* 2003. Cutting edge: distinct Toll-like receptor 2 activators selectively induce different classes of mediator production from human mast cells. J. Immunol. **170:** 1625–1629.
142. ROCK, F.L., G. HARDIMAN, J.C. TIMANS, *et al.* 1998. A family of human receptors structurally related to *Drosophila* Toll. Proc. Natl. Acad. Sci. USA **95:** 588–593.
143. AKIRA, S., K. TAKEDA & T. KAISHO. 2001. Toll-like receptors: critical proteins linking innate and acquired immunity. Nat. Immunol. **2:** 675–680.
144. ADEREM, A. & R.J. ULEVITCH. 2000. Toll-like receptors in the induction of the innate immune response. Nature **406:** 782–787.
145. HEINE, H. & E. LIEN. 2003. Toll-like receptors and their function in innate and adaptive immunity. Int. Arch. Allergy Immunol. **130:** 180–192.
146. CRISTOFARO, P. & S.M. OPAL. 2006. Role of toll-like receptors in infection and immunity: clinical implications. Drugs **66:** 15–29.
147. ANTHONY, M. & J.W. LANCE. 1971. Whole blood histamine and plasma serotonin in cluster headache. Proc. Aust. Assoc. Neurol. **8:** 43–46.
148. CAIRNS, J.A. & A.F. WALLS. 1996. Mast cell tryptase is a mitogen for epithelial cells. Stimulation of IL-8 production and intercellular adhesion molecule-1 expression. J. Immunol. **156:** 275–283.
149. MASUDA, A., Y. YOSHIKAI, K. AIBA, *et al.* 2002. Th2 cytokine production from mast cells is directly induced by lipopolysaccharide and distinctly regulated by c-Jun N-terminal kinase and p38 pathways. J. Immunol. **169:** 3801–3810.

150. SUPAJATURA, V., H. USHIO, A. NAKAO, *et al.* 2002. Differential responses of mast cell Toll-like receptors 2 and 4 in allergy and innate immunity. J. Clin. Invest. **109:** 1351–1359.
151. IKEDA, R.K., M. MILLER, J. NAYAR, *et al.* 2003. Accumulation of peribronchial mast cells in a mouse model of ovalbumin allergen induced chronic airway inflammation: modulation by immunostimulatory DNA sequences. J. Immunol. **171:** 4860–4867.
152. KULKA, M., L. ALEXOPOULOU, R.A. FLAVELL, *et al.* 2004. Activation of mast cells by double-stranded RNA: evidence for activation through Toll-like receptor 3. J. Allergy Clin. Immunol. **114:** 174–182.
153. O'SULLIVAN, S.M. 2005. Asthma death, CD8+ T cells, and viruses. Proc. Am. Thorac. Soc. **2:** 162–165.
154. DAKHAMA, A., Y.M. LEE & E.W. GELFAND. 2005. Virus-induced airway dysfunction: pathogenesis and biomechanisms. Pediatr. Infect. Dis. J. **24:** S159–S169, discussion.
155. VAN RIJT, L.S., C.H. VAN KESSEL, I. BOOGAARD, *et al.* 2005. Respiratory viral infections and asthma pathogenesis: a critical role for dendritic cells? J. Clin. Virol. **34:** 161–169.
156. SACKESEN, C., A. PINAR, B.E. SEKEREL, *et al.* 2005. Use of polymerase chain reaction for detection of adenovirus in children with or without wheezing Turk. J. Pediatr. **47:** 227–231.
157. PELAIA, G., A. VATRELLA, L. GALLELLI, *et al.* 2006. Respiratory infections and asthma. Respir. Med. **100:** 775–784.
158. MATSUSE, H., Y. KONDO, S. SAEKI, *et al.* 2005. Naturally occurring parainfluenza virus 3 infection in adults induces mild exacerbation of asthma associated with increased sputum concentrations of cysteinyl leukotrienes. Int. Arch. Allergy Immunol. **138:** 267–272.
159. WILLIAMS, J.V., J.E. CROWE JR., R. ENRIQUEZ, *et al.* 2005. Human metapneumovirus infection plays an etiologic role in acute asthma exacerbations requiring hospitalization in adults. J. Infect. Dis. **192:** 1149–1153.
160. LEMANSKE, R.F. JR., D.J. JACKSON, R.E. GANGNON, *et al.* 2005. Rhinovirus illnesses during infancy predict subsequent childhood wheezing J. Allergy Clin. Immunol. **116:** 571–577.
161. KRISTJANSSON, S., S.P. BJARNARSON, G. WENNERGREN, *et al.* 2005. Respiratory syncytial virus and other respiratory viruses during the first 3 months of life promote a local TH2-like response. J. Allergy Clin. Immunol. **116:** 805–811.
162. GUALANO, R.C., R. VLAHOS & G.P. ANDERSON. 2006. What is the contribution of respiratory viruses and lung proteases to airway remodelling in asthma and chronic obstructive pulmonary disease? Pulm. Pharmacol. Ther. **19:** 18–23.
163. EDWARDS, M.R., T. KEBADZE, M.W. JOHNSON, *et al.* 2006. New treatment regimes for virus-induced exacerbations of asthma. Pulm. Pharmacol. Ther. **19:** 320–334.
164. DEEDWANIA, P.C. 1995. Mental stress, pain perception and risk of silent ischemia. J. Am. Coll. Cardiol. **25:** 1504–1506.
165. FREEMAN, L.J., P.G.F. NIXON, P. SALLABANK, *et al.* 1987. Psychological stress and silent myocardial ischemia. Am. Heart J. **114:** 477–482.
166. DEANFIELD, J.E., M. SHEA, M. KENSETT, *et al.* 1984. Silent myocardial ischaemia due to mental stress. Lancet **2:** 1001–1005.

167. ROZANSKI, A., C.N. BAIREY, D.S. KRANTZ, et al. 1988. Mental stress and the induction of silent myocardial ischemia in patients with coronary artery disease. N. Engl. J. Med. **318:** 1005–1012.
168. PATELLA, V., G. DE CRESCENZO, A. CICCARELLI, et al. 1995. Human heart mast cells: a definitive case of mast cell heterogeneity. Int. Arch. Allergy Immunol. **106:** 386–393.
169. FORMAN, M.B., J.A. OATES, D. ROBERTSON, et al. 1985. Increased adventitial mast cells in a patient with coronary spasm. N. Engl. J. Med. **313:** 1138–1141.
170. KAARTINEN, M., A. PENTTILÄ & P.T. KOVANEN. 1994. Accumulation of activated mast cells in the shoulder region of human coronary atheroma, the predilection site of atheromatous rupture. Circulation **90:** 1669–1678.
171. CONSTANTINIDES, P. 1995. Infiltrates of activated mast cells at the site of coronary atheromatous erosion or rupture in myocardial infarction. Circulation **92:** 1083–1088.
172. LAINE, P., M. KAARTINEN, A. PENTTILÄ, et al. 1999. Association between myocardial infarction and the mast cells in the adventitia of the infarct-related coronary artery. Circulation **99:** 361–369.
173. JENNE, D.E. & J. TSCHOPP. 1991. Angiotensin II-forming heart chymase is a mast-cell-specific enzyme. Biochem. J. **276:** 567.
174. LEE, M., P.T. KOVANEN, G. TEDESCHI, et al. 2003. Apolipoprotein composition and particle size affect HDL degradation by chymase: effect on cellular cholesterol efflux. J. Lipid Res. **44:** 539–546.
175. LEE, M., L. CALABRESI, G. CHIESA, et al. 2002. Mast cell chymase degrades apoE and apoA-II in apoA-I-knockout mouse plasma and reduces its ability to promote cellular cholesterol efflux. Arterioscler. Thromb. Vasc. Biol. **22:** 1475–1481.
176. KOVANEN, P.T. 1996. Mast cells in human fatty streaks and atheromas: implications for intimal lipid accumulation Curr. Opin. Lipidol. **7:** 281–286.
177. LINDSTEDT, L., M. LEE, G.R. CASTRO, et al. 1996. Chymase in exocytosed rat mast cell granules effectively proteolyzes apolipoprotein AI-containing lipoproteins, so reducing the cholesterol efflux-inducing ability of serum and aortic intimal fluid. J. Clin. Invest. **97:** 2174–2182.
178. GRISTWOOD, R.W., J.C. LINCOLN, D.A. OWEN, et al. 1981. Histamine release from human right atrium. Br. J. Pharmacol. **74:** 7–9.
179. GENOVESE, A. & G. SPADARO. 1997. Highlights in cardiovascular effects of histamine and H1-receptor antagonists. Allergy **52:** 67–78.
180. CHRISTIAN, E.P., B.J. UNDEM & D. WEINREICH. 1989. Endogenous histamine excites neurones in the guinea pig superior cervical ganglion in vitro. J. Physiol. **409:** 297–312.
181. LAINE, P., A. NAUKKARINEN, L. HEIKKILA, et al. 2000. Adventitial mast cells connect with sensory nerve fibers in atherosclerotic coronary arteries. Circulation **101:** 1665–1669.
182. PANG, X., N. ALEXACOS, R. LETOURNEAU, et al. 1998. A neurotensin receptor antagonist inhibits acute immobilization stress-induced cardiac mast cell degranulation, a corticotropin-releasing hormone-dependent process. J. Pharm. Exp. Ther. **287:** 307–314.
183. HUANG, M., X. PANG, L. LETOURNEAU, et al. 2002. Acute stress induces cardiac mast cell activation and histamine release, effects that are increased in apolipoprotein E knockout mice. Cardiovasc. Res. **55:** 150–160.

184. HUANG, M., X. PANG, K. KARALIS, *et al*. 2003. Stress-induced interleukin-6 release in mice is mast cell-dependent and more pronounced in Apolipoprotein E knockout mice. Cardiovasc. Res. **59:** 241–249.
185. DELIARGYRIS, E.N., R.J. RAYMOND, T.C. THEOHARIDES, *et al*. 2000. Sites of interleukin-6 release in patients with acute coronary syndromes and in patients with congestive heart failure. Am. J. Cardiol. **86:** 913–918.
186. CLEJAN, S., S. JAPA, C. CLEMETSON, *et al*. 2002. Blood histamine is associated with coronary artery disease, cardiac events and severity of inflammation and atherosclerosis. J. Cell Mol. Med. **6:** 583–592.
187. SUZUKI, M., S. INABA, T. NAGAI, *et al*. 2003. Relation of C-reactive protein and interleukin-6 to culprit coronary artery plaque size in patients with acute myocardial infarction. Am. J. Cardiol. **91:** 331–333.
188. KOUNIS, N.G. & G.M. ZAVRAS. 1996. Allergic angina and allergic myocardial infarction. Circulation **94:** 1789.
189. KOUNIS, N.G., N.D. GRAPSAS & J.A. GOUDEVENOS. 1999. Unstable angina, allergic angina, and allergic myocardial infarction. Circulation **100:** e156.
190. THEOHARIDES, T.C., J.M. DONELAN, N. PAPADOPOULOU, *et al*. 2004. Mast cells as targets of corticotropin-releasing factor and related peptides. Trends Pharmacol. Sci. **25:** 563–568.
191. THEOHARIDES, T.C. 2003. Dietary supplements for arthritis and other inflammatory conditions: key role of mast cells and benefit of combining anti-inflammatory and proteoglycan products. Eur. J. Inflamm. **1:** 1–8.
192. THEOHARIDES, T.C., P. PATRA, W. BOUCHER, *et al*. 2000. Chondroitin sulfate inhibits connective tissue mast cells. Br. J. Pharmacol. **131:** 1039–1049.
193. MIDDLETON, E. JR., C. KANDASWAMI & T.C. THEOHARIDES. 2000. The effects of plant flavonoids on mammalian cells: implications for inflammation, heart disease and cancer. Pharmacol. Rev. **52:** 673–751.
194. HOGABOAM, C.M., A.D. BEFUS & J.L. WALLACE. 1993. Modulation of rat mast cell reactivity by IL-1 beta. Divergent effects on nitric oxide and platelet-activating factor release. J. Immunol. **151:** 3767–3774.
195. LEAL-BERUMEN, I., P. O'BYRNE, A. GUPTA, *et al*. 1995. Prostanoid enhancement of interleukin-6 production by rat peritoneal mast cells. J. Immunol. **154:** 4759–4767.
196. GUPTA, A.A., I. LEAL-BERUMEN, K. CROITORU, *et al*. 1996. Rat peritoneal mast cells produce IFN-γ following IL-12 treatment but not in response to IgE-mediated activation. J. Immunol. **157:** 2123–2128.
197. LIN, T.J., N. HIRJI, O. NOHARA, *et al*. 1998. Mast cells express novel CD8 molecules that selectively modulate mediator secretion. J. Immunol. **161:** 6265–6272.
198. GORDON, J.R., X. ZHANG, K. STEVENSON, *et al*. 2000. Thrombin induces IL-6 but not TNFα secretion by mouse mast cells: threshold-level thrombin receptor and very low level FceRI signaling synergistically enhance IL-6 secretion. Cell Immunol. **205:** 128–135.
199. LIN, T.J., T.B. ISSEKUTZ & J.S. MARSHALL. 2000. Human mast cells transmigrate through human umbilical vein endothelial monolayers and selectively produce IL-8 in response to stromal cell-derived factor-1 alpha. J. Immunol. **165:** 211–220.
200. KALESNIKOFF, J., M. HUBER, V. LAM, *et al*. 2001. Monomeric IgE stimulates signaling pathways in mast cells that lead to cytokine production and cell survival. Immunity 801–811.

201. COULOMBE, M., B. BATTISTINI, J. STANKOVA, *et al.* 2002. Endothelins regulate mediator production of rat tissue-cultured mucosal mast cells. Up-regulation of Th1 and inhibition of Th2 cytokines. J. Leukoc. Biol. **71:** 829–836.
202. MELLOR, E.A., K.F. AUSTEN & J.A. BOYCE. 2002. Cysteinyl leukotrienes and uridine diphosphate induce cytokine generation by human mast cells through an interleukin 4-regulated pathway that is inhibited by leukotriene receptor antagonists. J. Exp. Med. **195:** 583–592.
203. PAPADOPOULOU, N.G., L. OLESON, D. KEMPURAJ, *et al.* 2005. Regulation of corticotropin-releasing hormone receptor-2 expression in human cord blood-derived cultured mast cells. J. Mol. Endocrinol. **35:** R1–R8.
204. ZHU, F., K. GOMI & J.S. MARSHALL. 1998. Short-term and long-term cytokine release by mouse bone marrow mast cells and the differentiated KU-812 cell line are inhibited by brefeldin A. J. Immunol. **161:** 2541–2551.
205. LEAL-BERUMEN, I., D.P. SNIDER, C. BARAJAS-LOPEZ, *et al.* 1996. Cholera toxin increases IL-6 synthesis and decreases TNF-α production by rat peritoneal mast cells. J. Immunol. **156:** 316–321.
206. CALDERON, G.M., J. TORRES-LOPEZ, T.J. LIN, *et al.* 1998. Effects of toxin A from *Clostridium difficile* on mast cell activation and survival. Infect. Immun. **66:** 2755–2761.
207. GONZALEZ-ESPINOSA, C., S. ODOM, A. OLIVERA, *et al.* 2003. Preferential signaling and induction of allergy-promoting lymphokines upon weak stimulation of the high affinity IgE receptor on mast cells. J. Exp. Med. **197:** 1453–1465.

Immunomodulation

The Future Cure for Allergic Diseases

DAPHNE C. TSITOURA AND YANNIS TASSIOS

Department of Immunology, Foundation of Biomedical Research of the Academy of Athens, 115 27, Athens, Greece

ABSTRACT: Allergies are the result of aberrant immune reactivity against common innocuous environmental proteins (allergens). A pivotal component of allergic pathogenesis is the generation of allergen-specific Th cells with an effector phenotype. These Th cells activate a complex immune cascade that triggers the release of potent mediators and enhances the mobilization of several inflammatory cells types, which in turn elicit the acute allergic reactions and promote the development of chronic inflammation. The current therapies for allergic diseases focus primarily on pharmacological control of symptoms and suppression of inflammation. This approach is beneficial, but not curative, since the underlying immune pathology is not inhibited. In an attempt to develop more effective therapeutic strategies, the scientific interest has been directed toward methods down-modulating the immune mechanisms that initiate and maintain the allergic cascade. Today, the only widely used disease-modifying form of allergy treatment is the specific immunotherapy with allergen extracts. More recently the use of anti-IgE has been approved for patients with allergic asthma. Other immunomodulatory methods being currently explored are the administration of microbial adjuvants that inhibit Th2 reactivity and the design of molecules that interrupt the activity of key allergic cytokines, chemokines, or other Th2 effector mediators.

KEYWORDS: allergy; asthma; immunomodulation; T cells; IgE

Allergies affect approximately the 20% of the population in industrialized countries and cause a broad spectrum of problems ranging from mild inconvenience to severe respiratory distress and life-threatening anaphylactic shock. Over the past 40 years the prevalence and severity of allergic diseases has increased dramatically. For asthma in particular, the overall annual mortality and morbidity have almost doubled during the last decade. Today, despite the

Address for correspondence: Daphne Tsitoura, M.D., Ph.D., Department of Immunology, Foundation of Biomedical Research of the Academy of Athens, 4 Soranou tou Efesiou, 115 27 Athens, Greece. Voice: +210-6597335. Fax: +210-6597545

e-mail: daphne_tsitoura@dr.com

Ann. N.Y. Acad. Sci. 1088: 100–115 (2006). © 2006 New York Academy of Sciences.
doi: 10.1196/annals.1366.026

development of new "antiallergic" drugs, a permanent cure for most of the allergic diseases cannot be achieved. The problem with the current pharmacological regimes (antihistamines, antileukotrienes, and corticosteroids) is that they target primarily the control of symptoms and/or suppression of inflammation, without affecting significantly the allergic pathogenesis. Thus, these regimes cannot offer long-lasting effects and the patients' relief depends on the continuous use of medication. To overcome these shortcomings the academic and industrial research efforts have been directed toward the design of novel therapeutic approaches altering the dysregulated immune mechanisms that are responsible for the development of acute allergic reactions and chronic inflammation. To this end, the improvement of our knowledge of the pathophysiology of allergic diseases has provided a new arsenal of exciting opportunities for therapeutic intervention that promise to bring a permanent solution to the allergy problem.

ALLERGY, A DYSREGULATED IMMUNITY TO INNOCUOUS ENVIRONMENTAL PROTEINS

Allergic diseases arise as a result of aberrant immune responsiveness against innocuous environmental proteins (allergens) present in pollen, house dust, mites, fungal spores, animal danders, food, insect venom, etc. We are all exposed to allergens, but in healthy individuals the natural immune response to allergens is characterized by lack of effector reactivity and maintenance of a status of immune tolerance. In contrast, in allergic individuals the immune mechanisms that preserve the development of tolerance to allergens are disrupted and a window allowing the induction and perpetuation of active immune responses is generated. The pathologic immunity to allergens is orchestrated by the induction of allergen-specific CD4$^+$ T cells with an effector phenotype.[1–3] The presence of these cells is an essential requirement not only for allergen sensitization, but also for the full expression of the inflammatory characteristics of allergic diseases. Activated allergen-specific Th cells are present in high frequency in the peripheral blood of allergic patients. Moreover, there is severe infiltration of the organ targets, such as the nose, lungs, skin, and gut.[1,3] Depletion of T cells with a specific neutralizing Ab inhibits the development of disease in animal models of allergic sensitization.[4,5] Accordingly, asthma cannot be generated in RAG-deficient mice, whilst reconstitution of CD4$^+$ T cells restores the potential for induction of airway inflammation and airway hyperresponsiveness (AHR).[5,6] The allergen-specific CD4$^+$ T cells involved in the initiation of allergic reactivity have a distinctive cytokine profile (Th2 cells), characterized by the enhanced production of IL-4, IL-5, IL-9, and IL-13.[1,7] The presence of high levels of Th2 cytokines in the immune environment sets in motion a wide range of events that lead to the development and polarization of the features of allergic pathophysiology.[1,2,8] For example,

IL-4 and IL-13 drive the IgE isotype switching on B cells, IL-5 promotes the maturation and recruitment of eosinophils, and IL-9 triggers the activation of mast cell and basophils.[8,9] Moreover, some Th2 cytokines directly contribute to the generation of specific disease symptoms, such as the AHR and mucus hypersecretion in asthma.[3,10]

The differentiation of naïve Th cells toward the Th2 phenotype and the production of Th2 cytokines is regulated by a complex network of signaling molecules and transcription factors. Presence of bystander IL-4 in the local microenvironment is essential for the initiation of Th2 programming.[11] Triggering of the IL-4R stimulates the activation of several intracellular molecules that transduce the signal to the nucleus and promote the transcription of the Th2 cytokine genes.[11,12] Of these molecules, activation of STAT6 is of paramount importance for effective IL-4 signal transduction and Th2 differentiation.[12,13] Knockout of the *Stat6* gene leads to deficient Th2 cell development and failure to produce IL-4.[13] The key signaling event downstream of STAT6 activation is the upregulation of the two principal Th2 transcription factors: GATA-3 and c-maf.[13,14] During Th cell differentiation GATA-3 promotes selectively the acquisition of Th2 phenotype, not only by enhancing the Th2 cytokine gene transcription, but also by controlling the remodeling of chromatin structure and the opening of the IL-4 locus.[15] GATA-3 is suppressed during Th1 cell development.[15] On the contrary, overexpression of GATA-3 leads to increased Th2 cytokine synthesis.[15] In addition to GAT-3 and c-maf, members of the NF-AT family of transcription factors (NF-ATc and NF-ATp) are also involved in the molecular regulation of Th2 responses.[14]

The most catalytic immune event promoting the generation of allergic symptoms following the initial shift to Th2 responsiveness is the increased synthesis of allergen-specific IgE. The presence of high IgE levels is deterministic for the development of acute allergic reactions, but also contributes significantly to the development of chronic allergic inflammation.[16] In clinical practice allergic sensitization is defined by the presence of elevated serum levels of allergen-specific IgE antibodies. IgE sustains allergic reactivity primarily through its tendency to bind to high-affinity receptors (FcɛRI) on the surface of tissue mast cells and circulating basophils. Cross-linking of cell-bound IgE with the specific allergens causes degranulation of the cells and release of several proinflammatory mediators (e.g., histamine, leukotrienes, prostagladins, PAF) and cytokines that cause pathophysiological changes within minutes, such as smooth muscle contraction, mucus production, and vascular leakage, which are responsible for the acute allergic reactions.[16] In addition to the immediate symptoms, the release of allergic mediators triggers another more prolonged inflammatory process associated with the attraction of various immune cells at the sites of allergenic exposure, including Th2 lymphocytes, eosinophils, basophils, and monocytes.[16] The recruited cells secrete several inflammatory factors that exacerbate the symptoms of the early phase and injure the local tissues. Upon continuous exposure to allergens this immunopathologic process becomes resistant to resolution and leads to refractory inflammatory changes that can cause serious tissue damage and dysfunction of the organ-targets.

The role of allergens in driving and maintaining chronic allergic inflammation is well established. However, with age and recurrent challenge the inflammatory process in diseases such as asthma and atopic dermatitis may become IgE-independent and be perpetuated by a variety of other nonallergenic stimuli.[17] Infections play a particularly important role, since they not only transiently exacerbate the allergic symptoms, but they also shape the disease progression by enhancing the inflammation and aggravating the tissue damage.[17] Nonspecific irritants, intrinsic proteins cross-reacting with allergen-specific T cells, autocrine stimulation of inflammatory cells, and epithelial defects are also among the factors that appear to be implicated in the persistence of inflammation.[17,18] The complexity of the immune mechanisms involved in the chronic forms of allergic disorders is often reflected in the type of activated T cells accumulated in the inflamed tissues. Thus, in addition to Th2 cells, Th1 cells or Th cells secreting a mixture of Th1- and Th2-type cytokines (e.g., secretion of IL-5 and IFN-γ, with little IL-4) can be detected, while CD8$^+$ T cells can also be prominent.[18,19]

The recruitment of effector cells at the sites of allergen exposure is controlled by the chemokines and adhesion molecules expressed in the local immune environment. In susceptible individuals the early signals elicited after the allergen entry and stimulation of an immune response lead to rapid release of chemokines in the local tissues (namely eotaxin, RANTES, MCP-3, MCP-5 and MDC) that act as chemoattractants.[9,20] The secreted chemokines upregulate the expression of integrins in the blood vessels, which facilitates transmigration of leukocytes into the tissues.[21] Once in the tissues the leukocytes follow the chemokine gradient and move to the sites of immune reactivity.[21] Since each chemokine attracts only inflammatory cells that express the corresponding receptor, the chemokine profile induced in response to a particular immune stimulus dictates the type of inflammation that develops.[20,22] Recent data suggest that the expression of chemokines and chemokine receptors is under stringent developmental and organ-specific control.[23] In particular, it has been demonstrated that the various types of leukocytes differ in their capacity to express certain chemokine receptors and therefore to respond to local signals.[23] Th1 and Th2 cells express diverse sets of chemokine receptors and because of that they are differentially recruited to the sites of inflammation.[23,24] Thus, the secretion of CCL11, CCL22, and CCL17 in the allergen-inflamed tissues leads to preferential recruitment of the Th2 cells that selectively express the matching receptors CCR3, CCR4, and CCR8.[24] The importance of chemokines in the development of allergic inflammation is tremendous and this is highlighted by studies showing that experimental allergic diseases cannot be induced in animals with specific chemokine deficiencies.[9,22] Of all the known chemokine–chemokine receptor systems, the eotaxin system seems to play the most critical role in allergic inflammation.[25] Animals deficient in the

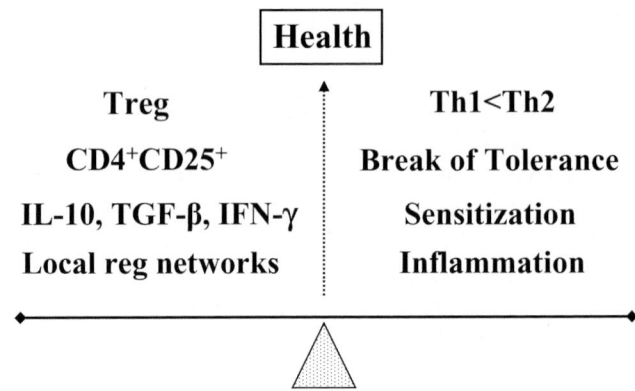

FIGURE 1. Tolerance to allergens. The natural immunity to allergens in characterized by the maintenance of a status of tolerance. Several mechanisms are involved, including T cell deletion, T cell anergy, Treg cell induction, and development of local regulatory networks. In allergic individuals the mechanisms preserving the immune tolerance to allergens are disrupted and effector Th2 reactivity leading to the development of disease is generated.

expression of eotaxin receptors (CCR3 and CCR2) have been found unable to develop lung and skin eosinophilia or disease features such as AHR in response to allergen challenge.[25]

In contrast to what happens in allergic individuals, in healthy subjects the maintenance of tolerance to allergens is the result of multiple systemic and local immune mechanisms that prevent or quickly eliminate the development of inappropriate reactivity (FIG. 1).[26,27] Studies in animals examining the natural immune responses to allergen exposure via the respiratory or gastrointestinal tract indicate that there is immediate activation of several mechanisms of immune tolerance including T cell deletion, T cell anergy, and T cell suppression.[28,29] The early activation of these mechanisms prevents the induction of allergen-specific T cell reactivity and protects from the development of allergic inflammation.[29,30] Exposure of healthy people to allergens is not associated with the rise of robust effector Th cell responses. Occasionally, few allergen-specific Th1 cells maybe detected in the peripheral blood of local tissues, but the dominant cell subset that is present consistently and expands after allergen challenge is the Treg cells.[26] The allergen-specific Treg cells are characterized by the production of high amounts of IL-10 and display strong immunosuppressive potential.[31] Data from experiments using Treg cells isolated from the peripheral blood of healthy individuals confirm that these cells suppress very effectively the proliferation and cytokine production of allergen-specific Th2 cells in an IL-10-dependent fashion.[31,32] Enhancement of the number and function of these cells has also been noticed in individuals who have overcome their allergies.[32] On the contrary, in atopic individuals only few allergen-specific Treg cells with reduced immunosuppressive capacity are present in the periphery.[32] It has been proposed that after exposure to allergens the ratio of allergen-specific effector Th2 cells and immunosuppressor Treg cells determines whether a healthy or allergic immune response will be generated. The naturally induced $CD4^+CD25^+$ Treg cells may also participate in the development of tolerance to allergens and protection from allergic diseases; however more investigations are needed to define their exact contribution.[32] Apart from the different types of peripheral T cells involved in tolerance induction, there are also indications that in the various organs additional local immunoregulatory mechanisms exist and provide an extra layer of protection against the development of aberrant immune reactivity. For example, it has been shown that the local epithelium, organ-specific cells, such as the alveolar macrophages in the lungs, and local immunosuppressive cytokines, such as TGF-β, favor the ablation of inflammatory responses and the maintenance of immune homeostasis.[33]

IMMUNOMODULATION: THE TARGET FOR EFFECTIVE THERAPEUTIC INTERVENTION

For the design of novel strategies for allergy prevention and therapy, several targets have emerged from the elucidation of the cellular and molecular mechanisms regulating the immunity to allergens. Theoretically, the ideal approach for a radical allergy therapy should include the eradication of reasons and mechanisms that sustain the development of effector reactivity to allergens and the redirection toward the induction of tolerogenic responses (FIG. 2). The

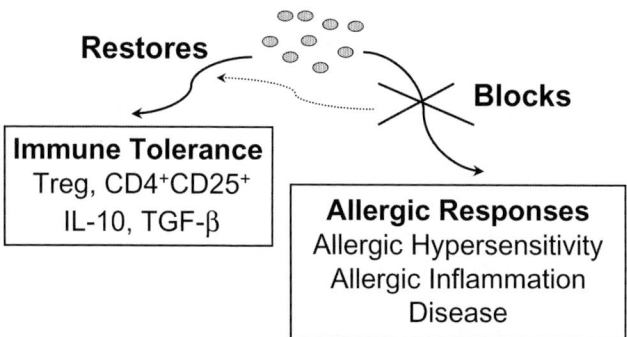

FIGURE 2. Ideal immunointervention. An ideal curative therapy for allergic diseases should include the suppression of the existing effector allergen-specific responses and the enhancement of mechanisms promoting the induction of tolerance to allergens.

TABLE 1. Immunomodulatory methods

Used in clincal practice	Under development
Allergen-specific immunotherapy	Th cell inhibition
Anti-IgE	Use of microbial adjuvants
	Inhibition of allergic cytokines
	Inhibition of allergic cell migration

break in immune tolerance to allergens is accompanied in most types of allergic diseases by generation of allergen-specific Th2 responses. Therefore, elimination of the existing pool of allergen-specific Th2 cells, deviation of the new responses away from the Th2 phenotype, and enhancement of the tolerance process are important goals for successful disease manipulation. Modulation of the phenotype of Th cell responses could be achieved with allergen-specific, as well as nonspecific methods. The various immunotherapy regimes using allergen extracts belong to the first category, while the methods aiming to alter the Th cell functions by blocking major molecules involved in Th cell differentiation (e.g., costimulatory molecules, cytokines, or transcription factors) represent examples of the second approach. An alternative strategy to suppress or reduce allergic reactivity is through inhibition of the key events of the allergic cascade. Blockade of IgE activity, inhibition of allergic second messengers, or suppression of the inflammatory cell migration are among the obvious targets. Downregulation of these immune events may not alter profoundly the nature of aberrant immune responsiveness to allergens, but it provides significant qualitative and quantitative restriction of allergic reactivity that prevents the full development and persistence of allergic features (TABLE 1).

IMMUNOMODULATORY THERAPIES USED IN CLINICAL PRACTICE

Allergen-Specific Immunotherapy

The goal of allergen immunotherapy is to eliminate allergic symptoms and achieve clinical desensitization through the exposure of patients to progressively increasing doses of extracts, made up of the allergens to which they are allergic. Subcutaneous allergen immunotherapy (SCIT) has been used in clinical practice for nearly 100 years and is the only widely used method of immunomodulatory treatment. It is highly effective in selected patients with IgE-mediated allergies and sensitivity to a limited number of allergens (e.g., patients with seasonal allergic rhinitis, asthma, or insect venom hypersensitivity). SCIT inhibits efficiently the early- and late-phase allergic responses and confers protection for several years after its discontinuation.[34] There is solid scientific evidence that SCIT exerts its therapeutic effects by altering the nature of immune responsiveness to allergens.[34,35] Successful SCIT induces an increase in the allergen-specific IgG (especially the IgG4 subtype), which results in diminished IgE-mediated immune activity.[36] This happens because the IgG antibodies compete with IgE for allergen binding to the surface of basophils and mast cells.[36] Furthermore, SCIT promotes the suppression of allergen-specific Th2 responses and enhances the generation of tolerant T cells.[35,37] In particular, it has been found that rapidly after the initiation of traditional, as well as rush protocols of SCIT there is significant rise of the IL-10-producing Treg cells in the peripheral blood and local tissues.[37] Some researchers believe that SCIT may also favor a shift of the allergen-induced Th cell responses toward the Th1 profile.[35]

Despite its efficacy SCIT has several drawbacks. The fact that it is allergen-specific restricts its use to patients with known and limited allergen-sensitivities. The compliance of the patients is also a common problem, since in order to achieve sustainable therapeutic results a long and expensive commitment is required (most SCIT protocols last for at least 3 years). More importantly, SCIT is not entirely free of side effects and there is the rare but existing risk of severe anaphylactic reaction, even when standardized extracts are used. To avoid these defects alternative forms of allergen-immunotherapy have been developed aiming to reproduce the immunomodulatory effects of SCIT, without bearing the potential risk of strong IgE-mediated reactions. Among them, sublingual and oral forms of allergen immunotherapy have been tested in clinical practice. Meta-analysis of the performed studies suggests that sublingual immunotherapy is probably safer than SCIT and equally effective for the treatment of allergic rhinitis and asthma.[38] However, much higher doses of sublingually administered allergens may be required to obtain beneficial results.[38] In an attempt to decrease the allergenicity (IgE reactivity) of allergen extracts and reduce the number of doses required to achieve clinical benefit (e.g., by prolonging the absorption), physical and chemical modification of the allergens have been employed. Thus, allergen absorption to alum hydroxide, calcium phosphate, tyrosine and liposomes, or chemical modification with polyethylenoglycol (PEG) or polymerization (allergoids) with formaldehyde, glutaraldehyde, or alginic salt have been tested with variable results.[34,39] An alternative option that has been recently discovered is the use of recombinant technology to produce large quantities of allergen derivatives genetically engineered to present reduced IgE binding capacity and therefore reduced allergenicity, but good ability to stimulate T cell responses.[40] An additional advantage of the recombinant allergens is that they are unable to generate new IgE antibodies, something that happens often when crude allergen extracts are used.[40] The efficacy of immunotherapy with recombinant allergens remains to be evaluated in the future. On the basis of the same rationale, immunotherapy using allergen-derived peptides that fail to bind to IgE, but are potent T cell stimulators has been proposed.[41] Preliminary trials assessing the subcutaneous administration of peptides derived from the cat allergen Feld 1 have shown modest reduction of the symptoms in cat-allergic patients.[41]

Anti-IgE

Since IgE is a key mediator of allergic pathogenesis, efforts to develop safe agents that block its activity have been going on for years. Recently a humanized recombinant monoclonal antibody (omalizumab) that is directed against IgE and inhibits its binding to FcεI receptor has reached the bedside.[42] Omalizumab cannot provoke undesirable IgE cross-linking because its design is such that it does not allow the interaction with IgE molecules already bound to the surface of mast cells or basophils.[42] Omalizumab was initially tested in patients with allergic asthma. The studies performed so far conclude that it is well-tolerated and effective in cases of both mild and severe allergic asthma.[42,43] In particular, they show that treatment with Omalizumab leads to diminished asthma symptoms and amelioration of lung function.[43] In parallel, Omalizumab reduces the frequency of asthma exacerbations and the need for rescue and other anti-inflammatory medication.[43] The improvement observed after therapy with Omalizumab seems to be associated with decline of the free IgE levels, downregulation of the FcεIR expression, and decrease of the early and late allergic reactivity following aeroallergen exposure.[44] Omalizumab has been recently launched in clinical practice; therefore further evaluations are required to exclude the potential development of long-term adverse effects, to better define the categories of patients that benefit most, and to evaluate the right use of anti-IgE in combination with other antiallergic therapies. Another question that remains to be answered is the cost-effectiveness of anti-IgE therapy compared to the current antiasthmatic drug regimes. Furthermore, the role of anti-IgE in the treatment of other allergic diseases, such as atopic eczema, allergic rhinitis, and food allergy needs to be investigated thoroughly.

IMMUNOMODULATORY METHODS UNDER EVALUATION

Inhibition of Th Cell Activation

The recognition of the central role of Th cells in allergic pathophysiology has propelled significant effort toward the development of anti-T cell therapeutic strategies. To this end a trial assessing the efficacy of a chimeric anti-CD4 monoclonal antibody to inhibit allergic Th cell responses and therefore to control the disease progress has been conducted in asthmatic patients.[3] Preliminary results suggest that a single intravenous administration of anti-CD4 leads to considerable decrease of $CD4^+$ T cell counts, alleviation of asthma symptoms, and increase in peak flow, but not in FEV1, measurements.[45] To avoid the side effects of generalized T cell suppression, other more elegant approaches targeting the qualitative restriction of Th2 responsiveness have been pursued. A lot of interest focused on the design of agents blocking the T cell costimulatory pathways that influence the acquisition of Th2 phenotype.[46] It has been proposed that selective interaction of CD28 with the CD86 molecule on the surface of antigen-presenting cells may preferentially promote Th2 cell differentiation.[47] Administration of antibodies blocking the binding of CD28 to CD80/CD86 in murine models of allergic airways disease has been shown to diminish the levels of Th2 cytokines, the degree of lung inflammation, and the development of AHR.[48] ICOS is another costimulatory molecule critically implicated in the regulation of Th2 responses to aeroallergens and thus an interesting candidate for therapeutic manipulation.[49] Some reports suggest that blocking the binding of ICOS to its ligand attenuates the development of experimental allergic diseases.[46,49] However, the issue remains controversial. The costimulatory activators OX40, CD30, or 4-1BB and the negative costimulator CTLA-4 are considered potential targets for allergy therapy.[46]

Immune Deviation Using Microbial Products

The observation that Th1 cells antagonize the proliferation and functions of Th2 cells led to the idea that preferential induction of Th1 immunity to allergens could have a protective effect in allergic patients. In this context, various experimental methods aiming to shift the immune responsiveness to allergens from a Th2- to a Th1-type have been examined. Exposure to microbes is the most efficient stimulus to activate Th1 immunity. For this purpose the use of attenuated microbes or other microbial components, alone or as adjuvants to allergen immunotherapy, has attracted considerable interest.[50] Experiments with heat-killed *Listeria* or attenuated mycobacterial strains (BCG vaccine or *Mycobacterium vaccae*) have demonstrated that these agents can protect against the development of allergic disease in mice, if used at the right time.[51–53] However, clinical studies have to be carried out to evaluate their real potential in allergy prevention and therapy. More data for the beneficial effect of microbial products have been accumulated from studies using the 3-deacylated monophosphoryl lipid A (MLP), an LPS-derived adjuvant that has been successfully used in viral vaccines.[50] Early trials with a combination of MLP with grass pollen allergen extracts have shown alleviation of allergic rhinitis symptoms and reduction of the need for supporting medication.[50] The Th2-modifying microbial adjuvants are potent promoters of Th1 responses through induction of IL-12 and IFN synthesis by antigen-presenting cells.[35,50] In parallel, they boost the activation of Treg cells secreting IL-10 and/or TGF-β.[35,50] An alternative approach to safely stimulate the generation of Th1/Treg cells is the use of DNA immunostimulatory sequences.[54] These sequences contain repeated dinucleotide cytosine-guanine (CpG) motifs and are highly preserved in microbial DNA, but are absent in mammals. The CpG motifs are universally recognized by the innate immune system of vertebrates through toll-like receptors and trigger the activation of protective immune responses.[54] Sole administration of synthetic oligodeoxynucleotides containing unmethylated CpG dinucleotides (ISS-ODN) have been found effective in preventing and reversing allergen-induced Th2 inflammation in murine models of asthma.[55,56] The protective effect of ISS-ODNs appears to be even higher when they are used directly conjugated to allergens.[55] An ISS-ODN-ragweed allergen (Amb1) conjugate has been proven to be a very effective suppressor of allergen-specific Th2 responses in mice as well as in humans.[56] Results from clinical trials in ragweed-sensitive adults have demonstrated that treatment with the ISS-ODN conjugate reduces the nasal eosinophilia and local expression of Th2-type cytokines.[57] Furthermore, there is significant lessening of rhinitis symptoms. The ISS-ODN conjugate appears to be 100-fold less allergenic than the conventional ragweed immunotherapy.[57] The successful results from the early phases of clinical trials have given rise to considerable enthusiasm about the development of DNA vaccines for allergy prevention, whereas an important caveat that remains to be delineated is the potential long-term stimulation of Th1 pathology that may lead eventually to severe deterioration of the inflammatory disease.

Inhibition of Allergy-Inducing Cytokine Networks

Cytokines play a deterministic role in the generation of allergic T and B cell responses, as well as in the maintenance of allergic inflammation. Therefore, it has been proposed that blocking key cytokines, such as IL-4, IL-13, and/or IL-5, may alter radically not only the phenotype of allergen-specific immune responses, but also the effector features of the disease. To examine this hypothesis several antiallergic cytokine agents have been developed, including humanized blocking antibodies against cytokines, antibodies against cytokine receptors, and soluble cytokine receptors.[11,58,59] Initial studies evaluating the effect of inhibiting the IL-4 activity with a humanized anti-IL-4 monoclonal antibody (pascolizumab) or a soluble recombinant IL-4 receptor had encouraging results. Administration of these agents in mice inhibited profoundly the development of allergen-mediated AHR and inflammation.[60] Unfortunately, the efficacy of the anti-IL-4 treatment has not been confirmed in large-scale clinical trials in patients with moderate to severe asthma.[60] Administration of anti-IL-4 in patients led to downregulation of several immune parameters, including IL-4 activity, Th2 cell activation, or IgE synthesis. However, these changes were not accompanied by a significant therapeutic benefit.[60] Mixed conclusions were also reached in the trials assessing the treatment of asthmatics with an anti-IL-5 monoclonal antibody (mepolizumab).[61] Thus, although reduction in the number of circulating eosinophils and prevention of their recruitment to the lungs were observed, marked improvement in lung function and airway reactivity was not achieved.[61] In contrast, therapy with anti-IL-5 had excellent results in other diseases primarily driven by eosinophils, such as the hypereosinophilic syndrome.[61] Agents blocking the pathways triggered by IL-13 are still under development (i.e., IL-13Ra2- IgGFc fusion protein) and their efficacy remains to be determined.[62] The failure to reach the therapeutic goals with the anti-IL-4 and anti-IL-5 agents has halted the initial optimism about the potential of anticytokine strategies. Nevertheless, this cannot preclude the possibility that the efforts to interrupt the cytokine pathways by using small molecules that block critical signal transduction events (e.g., suppressors of STAT6 or GATA3 activity) may not be more successful.[63] Another issue that needs to be examined is the use of multiple anticytokine agents in combination, as it is known that there is significant redundancy in the allergic cytokine network. Alternatively, the combination of anticytokine therapy with other disease-modifying approaches can also be evaluated.

Inhibition of Inflammatory Cell Transmigration

A new concept to treat allergic inflammation is by inhibiting the inappropriate recruitment of leukocytes at the sites of allergen exposure. This could be achieved by interfering selectively with the system of chemokines and adhesion molecules that regulate the trafficking of Th2 cells, eosinophils, basophils, and mast cells. For example, blocking the adhesion molecule LFA-1 or the binding to its ligand ICAM-1 has been shown effective in abrogating the early- and late-phase reactivity to allergens and the development of inflammation in animals.[64] Data from preliminary trials using an anti-LFA-1/CD11a monoclonal antibody (efalizumab) in allergic patients support this finding and show that following treatment the inflammatory infiltration at the sites of allergen challenge is attenuated.[64] Further studies are required to determine the therapeutic potential of this approach. Other suitable targets for suppressing the migration of allergic effector cells include the VLA-4, which serves as a receptor for VCAM-1, the eotaxin receptors, as well as several other chemokine–chemokine receptor interactions (e.g., CCL17/CCL22-CCR4, CCL1-CCR8, CXCL12-CXCR4) that appear to facilitate preferentially the development of Th2 inflammation.[20,25]

CONCLUSION

The immunomodulatory strategies provide a promising alternative for the treatment of allergic patients in the future. However, many questions remain to be answered before we have novel immunomodulatory tools in clinical practice. Apart from issues relevant to the efficacy, safety, and longevity of the novel forms of treatment, another point that needs to be clarified is the optimum timing for intervention in order to maximize the therapeutic benefit. It is probable that early intervention may be more successful in altering the disease pathogenesis and in preventing the progression beyond the stage of mild allergy. For this purpose, the development of prophylactic forms of immunotherapy targeting high-risk atopic children may have several merits. Further studies are also required to define the best therapeutic options for the treatment of the chronic forms of allergic inflammation where several allergen-independent mechanisms are involved (e.g., asthma, atopic dermatitis). In these cases, the design of comprehensive multilayer strategies targeting all the coexisting dysfunctional immune pathways may yield better results.

REFERENCES

1. ROMAGNANI, S. 2000. The role of lymphocytes in allergic disease. J. Allergy Clin. Immunol. **105:** 399–408.
2. KAY, A.B. 2001. Allergy and allergic diseases. First of two parts. N. Engl. J. Med. **344:** 30–37.
3. LARCHE, M., D.S. ROBINSON & A.B. KAY. 2003. The role of T lymphocytes in the pathogenesis of asthma. J. Allergy Clin. Immunol. **111:** 450–463.
4. LAMBERT, L.E., J.S. BERLING & E.M. KUDLACZ. 1996. Characterization of the antigen-presenting cell and T cell requirements for induction of pulmonary eosinophilia in a murine model of asthma. Clin. Immunol. Immunopathol. **81:** 307–311.
5. DE SANCTIS, G.T. *et al.* 1997. T-lymphocytes regulate genetically determined airway hyperresponsiveness in mice. Nat. Med. **3:** 460–462.
6. CORRY, D.B. *et al.* 1998. Requirements for allergen-induced airway hyperreactivity in T and B cell-deficient mice. Mol. Med. **4:** 344–355.
7. UMETSU, D.T. & R.H. DEKRUYFF. 1997. TH1 and TH2 CD4$^+$ cells in human allergic diseases. J. Allergy Clin. Immunol. **100:** 1–6.
8. BROIDE, D.H. 2001. Molecular and cellular mechanisms of allergic disease. J. Allergy Clin. Immunol. **108:** S65–S71.
9. ROMAGNANI, S. 2002. Cytokines and chemoattractants in allergic inflammation. Mol. Immunol. **38:** 881–885.
10. HERRICK, C.A. & K. BOTTOMLY. 2003. To respond or not to respond: T cells in allergic asthma. Nat. Rev. Immunol. **3:** 405–412.
11. LI-WEBER, M. & P.H. KRAMMER. 2003. Regulation of IL4 gene expression by T cells and therapeutic perspectives. Nat. Rev. Immunol. **3:** 534–543.
12. PERNIS, A.B. & P.B. ROTHMAN. 2002. JAK-STAT signaling in asthma. J. Clin. Invest. **109:** 1279–1283.
13. TAKEDA, K., T. KISHIMOTO & S. AKIRA. 1997. STAT6: its role in interleukin 4-mediated biological functions. J. Mol. Med. **75:** 317–326.
14. MOWEN, K.A. & L.H. GLIMCHER. 2004. Signaling pathways in Th2 development. Immunol Rev. **202:** 203–222.

15. ZHOU, M. & W. OUYANG. 2003. The function role of GATA-3 in Th1 and Th2 differentiation. Immunol Res. **28:** 25–37.
16. PLATTS-MILLS, T.A. 2001.The role of immunoglobulin E in allergy and asthma. Am. J. Respir. Crit. Care Med. **164:** S1–S5.
17. EL BIAZE, M. *et al.* 2003. T cell activation, from atopy to asthma: more a paradox than a paradigm. Allergy **58:** 844–853.
18. HOLGATE, S.T. 2002. Airway inflammation and remodeling in asthma: current concepts. Mol. Biotechnol. **22:** 179–189.
19. GIROLOMONI, G. *et al.* 2001. T-cell subpopulations in the development of atopic and contact allergy. Curr. Opin. Immunol. **13:** 733–737.
20. BISSET, L.R. & P. SCHMID-GRENDELMEIER. 2005. Chemokines and their receptors in the pathogenesis of allergic asthma: progress and perspective. Curr. Opin. Pulm. Med. **11:** 35–42.
21. ONO, S.J. *et al.* 2003. Chemokines: roles in leukocyte development, trafficking, and effector function. J. Allergy. Clin. Immunol. **111:** 1185–1199.
22. LUKACS, N.W. 2001. Role of chemokines in the pathogenesis of asthma. Nat. Rev. Immunol. **1:** 108–116.
23. SALLUSTO, F. & A. LANZAVECCHIA. 2000. Understanding dendritic cell and T-lymphocyte traffic through the analysis of chemokine receptor expression. Immunol. Rev. **177:** 134–140.
24. COSMI, L. *et al.* 2001. Chemoattractant receptors expressed on type 2 T cells and their role in disease. Int. Arch. Allergy Immunol. **125:** 273–279.
25. AMERIO, P. *et al.* 2003. Eotaxins and CCR3 receptor in inflammatory and allergic skin diseases: therapeutical implications. Curr. Drug Targets Inflamm. Allergy **2:** 81–94.
26. AKBARI, O. *et al.* 2003. Mucosal tolerance and immunity: regulating the development of allergic disease and asthma. Int. Arch. Allergy Immunol. **130:** 108–118.
27. KUIPERS, H. & B.N. LAMBRECHT. 2004. The interplay of dendritic cells, Th2 cells and regulatory T cells in asthma. Curr. Opin. Immunol. **16:** 702–708.
28. VAN PARIJS, L., V.L. PEREZ & A.K. ABBAS. 1998. Mechanisms of peripheral T cell tolerance. Novartis Found. Symp. **215:** 5–14.
29. TSITOURA, D.C. *et al.* 1999. Intranasal exposure to protein antigen induces immunological tolerance mediated by functionally disabled CD4$^+$ T cells. J. Immunol. **163:** 2592–2600.
30. TSITOURA, D.C. *et al.* 2000. Mechanisms preventing allergen-induced airways hyperreactivity: role of tolerance and immune deviation. J. Allergy Clin. Immunol. **106:** 239–246.
31. AKDIS, M., K. BLASER & C.A. AKDIS. 2005. T regulatory cells in allergy: novel concepts in the pathogenesis, prevention, and treatment of allergic diseases. J. Allergy Clin. Immunol. **116:** 961–968.
32. ROBINSON, D.S., M. LARCHE & S.R. DURHAM. 2004. Tregs and allergic disease. J. Clin. Invest. **114:** 1389–1397.
33. BLUMENTHAL, R.L. *et al.* 2001. Human alveolar macrophages induce functional inactivation in antigen-specific CD4 T cells. J Allergy Clin. Immunol. **107:** 258–264.
34. NELSON, H.S. 2004. Advances in upper airway diseases and allergen immunotherapy. J. Allergy Clin. Immunol. **113:** 635–642.
35. TILL, S.J. *et al.* 2004. Mechanisms of immunotherapy. J. Allergy Clin. Immunol. **113:** 1025–1034.

36. WACHHOLZ, P.A. & S.R. DURHAM. 2004. Mechanisms of immunotherapy: IgG revisited. Curr. Opin. Allergy Clin. Immunol. **4:** 313–318.
37. AKDIS, C.A., K. BLASER & M. AKDIS. 2006. Mechanisms of allergen-specific immunotherapy. Chem. Immunol Allergy. **91:** 195–203.
38. PASSALACQUA, G., C. LOMBARDI & G.W. CANONICA. 2004. Sublingual immunotherapy: an update. Curr. Opin. Allergy Clin. Immunol. **4:** 31–36.
39. WHEELER, A.W. & S.R. WORONIECKI. 2004. Allergy vaccines—new approaches to an old concept. Expert Opin. Biol. Ther. **4:** 1473–1481.
40. LINHART, B. & R. VALENTA. 2005. Molecular design of allergy vaccines. Curr. Opin. Immunol. **17:** 646–655.
41. LARCHE, M. & D.C. WRAITH. 2005. Peptide-based therapeutic vaccines for allergic and autoimmune diseases. Nat. Med. **11:** S69–S76.
42. BROWNELL, J. & T.B. CASALE. 2004. Anti-IgE therapy. Immunol. Allergy Clin. North Am. **24:** 551–568.
43. BUHL, R. 2005. Anti-IgE antibodies for the treatment of asthma. Curr. Opin. Pulm. Med. **11:** 27–34.
44. INFUHR, D. *et al.* 2005. Molecular and cellular targets of anti-IgE antibodies. Allergy. **60:** 977–985.
45. KON, O.M. *et al.* 2001. The effects of an anti-CD4 monoclonal antibody, keliximab, on peripheral blood CD4$^+$ T-cells in asthma. Eur. Respir J. **18:** 45–52.
46. KROCZEK, R. & E. HAMELMANN. 2005. T-cell costimulatory molecules: optimal targets for the treatment of allergic airway disease with monoclonal antibodies. J. Allergy Clin. Immunol. **116:** 906–909.
47. LARCHE, M. *et al.* 1998. Costimulation through CD86 is involved in airway antigen-presenting cell and T cell responses to allergen in atopic asthmatics. J. Immunol. **161:** 6375–6382.
48. CHEN, Y.Q. & H.Z. SHI. 2006. CD28/CTLA-4-CD80/CD86 and ICOS-B7RP-1 costimulatory pathway in bronchial asthma. Allergy. **61:** 15–26.
49. GONZALO, J.A. *et al.* 2001. ICOS is critical for T helper cell-mediated lung mucosal inflammatory responses. Nat. Immunol. **2:** 597–604.
50. FRANCIS, J.N. & S.R. DURHAM. 2004. Adjuvants for allergen immunotherapy: experimental results and clinical perspectives. Curr. Opin. Allergy Clin. Immunol. **4:** 543–548.
51. HANSEN, G. *et al.* 2000. Vaccination with heat-killed Listeria as adjuvant reverses established allergen-induced airway hyperreactivity and inflammation: role of CD8+ T cells and IL-18. J. Immunol. **164:** 223–230.
52. LI, X.M. *et al.* 2003. Engineered recombinant peanut protein and heat-killed *Listeria monocytogenes* coadministration protects against peanut-induced anaphylaxis in a murine model. J. Immunol. **170:** 3289–3295.
53. ZUANY-AMORIM, C. *et al.* 2002. Long-term protective and antigen-specific effect of heat-killed *Mycobacterium vaccae* in a murine model of allergic pulmonary inflammation. J. Immunol. **169:** 1492–1499.
54. CHU, R.S. *et al.* 1997. CpG oligodeoxynucleotides act as adjuvants that switch on T helper 1 (Th1) immunity. J. Exp. Med. **186:** 1623–1631.
55. HORNER, A.A. & E. RAZ. 2002. Immunostimulatory sequence oligodeoxynucleotide-based vaccination and immunomodulation: two unique but complementary strategies for the treatment of allergic diseases. J. Allergy Clin. Immunol. **110:** 706–712.
56. HUSSAIN, I. & J.N. KLINE. 2003. CpG oligodeoxynucleotides: a novel therapeutic approach for atopic disorders. Curr. Drug Targets Inflamm. Allergy. **2:** 199–205.

57. BROIDE, D.H. 2005. Immunostimulatory sequences of DNA and conjugates in the treatment of allergic rhinitis. Curr. Allergy Asthma Rep. **5:** 182–185.
58. FOSTER, P.S. *et al.* 2002. Interleukins-4, -5, and -13: emerging therapeutic targets in allergic disease. Pharmacol. Ther. **94:** 253–264.
59. CHUNG, K.F. 2003. Individual cytokines contributing to asthma pathophysiology: valid targets for asthma therapy? Curr. Opin. Investig. Drugs. **4:** 1320–1326.
60. STEINKE, J.W. 2004. Anti-interleukin-4 therapy. Immunol Allergy Clin. North Am. **24:** 599–614.
61. KAY, A.B. & A.D. KLION. 2004. Anti-interleukin-5 therapy for asthma and hypereosinophilic syndrome. Immunol. Allergy Clin. North Am. **24:** 645–666.
62. YANG, G. *et al.* 2004. Anti-IL-13 monoclonal antibody inhibits airway hyperresponsiveness, inflammation and airway remodeling. Cytokine **28:** 224–232.
63. NAKAMURA, Y. & M. HOSHINO. 2005. TH2 cytokines and associated transcription factors as therapeutic targets in asthma. Curr. Drug Targets Inflamm Allergy. **4:** 267–270.
64. GAUVREAU, G.M. *et al.* 2003. The effects of an anti-CD11a mAb, efalizumab, on allergen-induced airway responses and airway inflammation in subjects with atopic asthma. J. Allergy Clin. Immunol. **112:** 331–338.

Neural Correlates of IgE-Mediated Allergy

FREDERICO AZEVEDO COSTA-PINTO,[a]
ALEXANDRE SALGADO BASSO,[a] LUIZ CARLOS DE SÁ-ROCHA,[a]
LUIZ ROBERTO GIORGETTI BRITTO,[b] MOMTCHILO RUSSO,[c]
AND JOÃO PALERMO-NETO[a]

[a]Department of Pathology, School of Veterinary Medicine, University of São Paulo, São Paulo, Brazil

[b]Department of Physiology and Biophysics, Institute of Biomedical Sciences, University of São Paulo, São Paulo, Brazil

[c]Department of Immunology, Institute of Biomedical Sciences, University of São Paulo, São Paulo, Brazil

ABSTRACT: Although many authors have considered a direct interaction between allergic reactions and behavioral changes, supporting evidence has been elusive. In this series of studies we show that after oral or nasal ovalbumin (OVA) challenge, allergic mice present increased Fos expression in the paraventricular nucleus of the hypothalamus (PVN) and in the central nucleus of the amygdala (CeA). Mice with food allergy display higher levels of anxiety and increased serum corticosterone levels, and allergy-activated neurons express corticotropin-releasing factor (CRF) in the PVN and CeA. OVA-allergic mice develop aversion to an antigen-containing solution, and also avoid a dark compartment previously associated with nebulized OVA. Results on brain Fos expression and behavioral data seem compatible with adaptive responses. Removal of IgE by either antibody depletion or the development of oral tolerance precluded all responses analyzed here. C-sensitive fiber destruction by neonatal capsaicin inhibited the activation in the PVN, but not in the CeA, and decreased the magnitude of food aversion. Cromolyn, a mast cell stabilizer, completely blocked Fos expression in the PVN and CeA, and precluded the development of aversion to the dark compartment associated with nebulized OVA. Employing mice that do not develop an important inflammatory infiltrate following nasal OVA challenge, we found that inflammatory cells are not required at the site of challenge in order to trigger neural or behavioral correlates of murine experimental asthma. Altogether, we have built a solid foundation for understand-

Address for correspondence: Frederico Azevedo Costa-Pinto, Departamento de Patologia, Faculdade de Medicina Veterinária e Zootecnia, Universidade de São Paulo, Av. Dr. Orlando Marques de Paiva, 87, Cidade Universitária, São Paulo, SP, CEP 05508–000 Brazil,. Voice: 55-11-3091-1372; fax: 55-11-3091-7829.
e-mail: fpinto@usp.br

Ann. N.Y. Acad. Sci. 1088: 116–131 (2006). © 2006 New York Academy of Sciences.
doi: 10.1196/annals.1366.028

ing neuroimmune interactions during allergic responses that may contribute to the comprehension of psychological disorders associated with allergy.

KEYWORDS: neuroimmunomodulation; allergy; central nervous system; asthma; food; fos; mast cell; capsaicin; cromolyn; C-sensitive fiber; IgE; tolerance; ELISA, immunohistochemistry

INTRODUCTION

Allergic diseases have emerged as major public health problems on account of their dramatic increase over the past two to three decades.[1] The underlying mechanisms responsible for the development of allergies are complex and may vary according to individual, social, and geographical factors, but appear to be altogether mediated by an allergen-driven T-helper type 2 (Th2) response characterized by increased secretion of type 2 cytokines (mainly IL-4, IL-5, and IL-13) and participation of CD4+ T lymphocytes.[2]

Allergic reactions are responsible for a myriad of symptoms that involve the airways, the gastrointestinal (GI) tract, and the skin, among other organs.[3] Many of the early consequences of immediate allergic reactions are triggered by mast cell contents released following cross-linking of IgE antibodies bound to their high-affinity receptors (FcεRI) expressed in the membranes of these cells. The late phase of allergic reactions usually leads to an inflammatory milieu in which T lymphocytes, eosinophils, and cytokines play an important role.[4]

Although the pathophysiology of allergic reactions has been well characterized in humans and experimental models using rodents, little is known about its consequences on brain activity and behavior. Lack of supporting evidence for a direct effect of allergy on neural activity and behavior had always been the main argument against the acceptance of allergy-induced psychological symptoms.[5]

Over the history of medicine, several reports have suggested the presence of an association between allergic phenomena and emotional or behavioral changes. In a classical paper, Mackenzie described the "rose effect": asthmatic patients presenting bronchoconstriction when facing an artificial flower.[6] Changes in emotional status and increased levels of anxiety are commonly associated with asthma crises[7]; also, the distress caused by a recurrent, chronic disease might be responsible for generating pathological anxiety in patients suffering from long-term asthma.[8] Human patients admitted for food allergy present higher prevalence of trait anxiety or depression than healthy mates or unhealthy individuals with lactose intolerance.[9] Nonetheless, other investigators have failed to pinpoint this association, and have argued that it could be tracked to an artifact of referral bias.[10]

An experimental approach to understand the importance of the immune system on a highly conserved behavior, namely food ingestion, was provided by Denise Cara and colleagues, working in Nelson Vaz's laboratory, and published in 1994. The group developed a model of food selection based on a test thereafter referred to as the "two-bottle preference test," consisting of a choice between drinking from a bottle filled with tap water, or another containing a sweetened solution of egg white in water. When facing this choice, nonimmunized mice would prefer drinking the sweetened solution, while ovalbumin (OVA)-immunized animals would avoid the antigen-containing solution, drinking water instead.[11] It soon became clear that the immune system could drive a behavioral shift that lead to the avoidance of a potentially harmful molecule or context.

Several reports pointing to an interaction between immune responses and the activity of specific brain areas have piled up as a complex, sometimes controversial literature. Other studies have addressed the intimate relationship between mast cells and sensitive fibers,[12,13] in particular those of C-sensitive neurons, which probably constitute the shortest loop of cross-talk between the immune and the nervous systems, in action during an allergic response. In this regard, mast cell degranulation following peripheral nerve stimulation is a well-described phenomenon[14]; on the other hand, many studies report changes in the activity of particular afferents after IgE-mediated or independent mast cell degranulation.[15]

We compile here a series of studies on the neural and behavioral correlates of allergic reactions conducted in our laboratories, employing experimental models of food allergy and murine asthma. Our results present evidence of changes in the activity of specific brain nuclei in the hypothalamus and amygdala, along with behavioral changes associated with the exposure of allergic mice to the allergen.[16,17] Moreover, we focus on possible mechanisms underlying the responses described, including the importance of IgE and IgG1,[16–20] degranulation of mast cells,[20] signaling via capsaicin-sensitive C-fibers,[19,21] and the requirement of an inflammatory infiltrate.[20] We also provide evidence that neurons activated in the central nervous system (CNS) during an allergic reaction express the corticotropin-releasing factor (CRF) and lead to an increase in serum corticosterone.[18]

ANALYZING THE BEHAVIOR OF ALLERGIC MICE

Employing the two-bottle preference test used by Cara and colleagues,[11] we first aimed to confirm of their results with OVA-immunized mice. Nonimmunized mice choose a 20% egg white solution in water, artificially sweetened with 0.5% saccharin, when exposed to the two-bottle test[21,22]; OVA-immunized mice drink water instead, avoiding the supposedly preferable, allergen-containing solution (FIG. 1 A). No differences in total fluid intake were detected (FIG. 1 B).

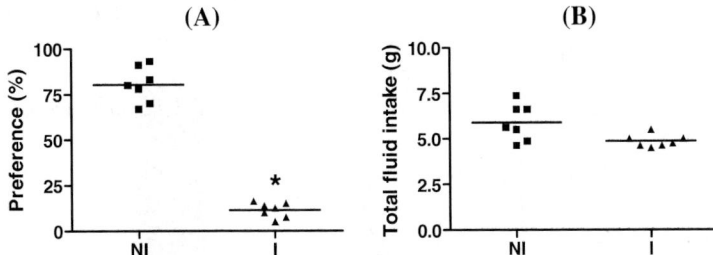

FIGURE 1. Feeding behavior of allergic mice. Animals immunized or not with OVA were submitted to the two-bottle preference test, choosing between tap water and a sweetened OVA-containing solution. (**A**) While nonimmunized mice (NI) show a clear preference for the sweetened solution, immunized animals (I) avoid drinking the OVA-containing solution, preferring water instead. (**B**) Total fluid intake is not altered by prior OVA immunization. Individual values are shown as solid *squares* or *triangles*, and *horizontal lines* represent the medians; $n = 7$ per group; *$P < 0.05$; Mann–Whitney test.

In order to compare the behavior of mice challenged by the oral route (food allergy) or through the airways (asthma), we adapted a passive avoidance test to analyze the behavior of immunized animals following exposure to airborne allergens. We built a transparent box consisting of two communicating compartments, one illuminated by a 60W bare bulb (making up one-third of its total length), and another painted black (the remaining two-thirds), referred to as a light–dark box (LDB). We then replaced the classic avoidance stimulus (electric shock) for nebulization with the allergen (OVA). Mice are placed on the training day in the lit side of the apparatus, and the delay for its first entry in the dark compartment is recorded (cutoff 5 min); the same animals are retested on the following day, without nebulization with OVA, and the delay for the first entry in the dark is recorded again (cutoff 1 min).[17]

Immunized animals that had gone into the dark compartment, and inhaled OVA on the training day, avoided this compartment on the following day (test session), 24 h later; nonimmunized mice continued to move quickly into that compartment on the following day (FIG. 2).[17,20]

Therefore, allergic mice display a shift in behavior capable of avoiding the source of the allergen that would trigger an immediate allergic reaction. We also found that, if forced to have contact with the allergen (e.g., by gavage), immunized mice display clear anxiety-related behaviors, such as decrease in time and number of entries in the plus-maze, an arena frequently employed for the assessment of anxiety in rodents (FIG. 3 A), without changes in motor activity in the open field (FIG. 3 B).[16,21,22]

At that point, we adopted the working hypothesis that allergy leads to the expression of emotionally related behaviors, such as anxiety and avoidance.

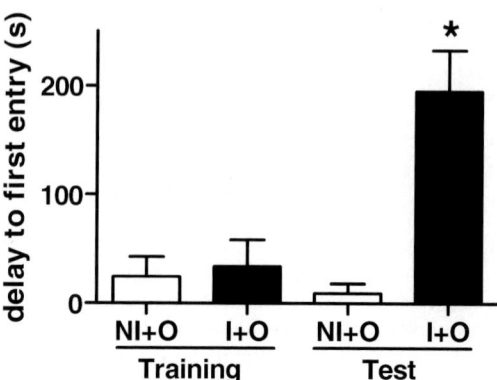

FIGURE 2. Avoidance behavior in the light–dark box. Animals immunized or not with OVA were submitted to a training session in the light–dark box (LDB) test, and nebulized with OVA upon moving into the dark compartment of the LDB; on the following day (test session) the delay for the first entry in the dark compartment was recorded. While immunized mice (I+O) behave like nonimmunized (NI+O) animals in the training session, they avoided the compartment previously associated with nebulized OVA on the test session. Results are mean $\pm$ SD; $*P < 0.01$ against NI+O on the test session, or I+O on the training session; $n = 5$–7 per group; ANOVA followed by Dunnet's *post hoc* test.

BRAIN ACTIVITY FOLLOWING CHALLENGE WITH THE ALLERGEN

We chose a relatively simple, albeit quite precise, method for assessing brain activity post mortem in rodents, the localization of Fos protein in neurons by

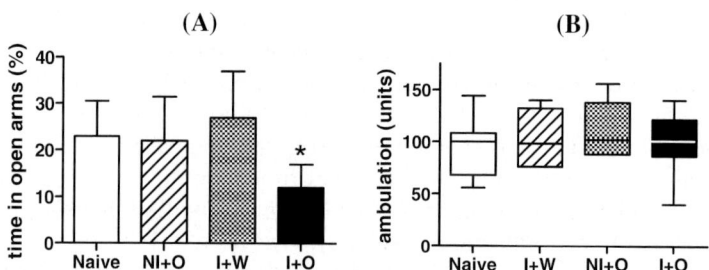

FIGURE 3. Behavioral changes in allergic mice. (**A**) Elevated plus-maze. One hour after OVA challenge, immunized mice (I+O) display increased levels of anxiety, expressed as a decrease in the time exploring the open arms of the apparatus, compared to naïve animals, nonimmunized animals challenged with OVA (NI+O), or immunized animals receiving water (I+W); results are mean $\pm$ SD; $*P < 0.05$ compared to all other groups; $n = 10$ per group; ANOVA followed by Student–Newman–Keuls *post hoc* test. (**B**) Ambulation in the open field. Number of entries in cells of the apparatus do not differ among groups, showing that motor activity is similar among animals; $n = 10$; *horizontal lines* represent medians.

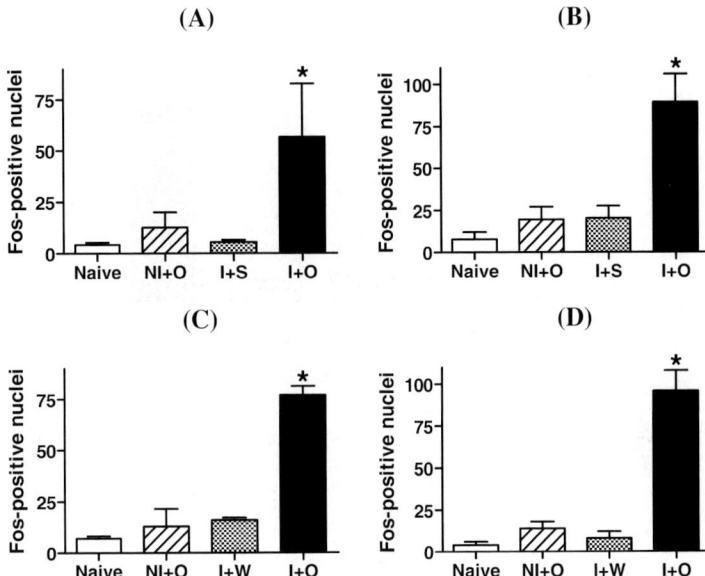

FIGURE 4. Fos staining in emotionality-related brain areas of allergic mice. Animals immunized and challenged with OVA (I+O) display an intense Fos staining in the paraventricular nucleus of the hypothalamus (PVN, *panels* **A** and **C**) and central nucleus of amygdala (CeA, *panels* **B** and **D**), 90 min after OVA challenge. (**A**) and (**B**) represent animals challenged by intranasal instillation of OVA; (**C**) and (**D**) express challenge with OVA by gavage; results are mean $\pm$ SD; *$P < 0.01$ compared to naïve animals, nonimmunized animals receiving OVA, or immunized mice receiving the vehicle (I+W, for water, or I+S, for saline); $n = 5$–7 per group; ANOVA followed by Tukey–Kramer *post hoc* test.

immunohistochemistry. Fos is the product of an immediate early gene (*fos*) that plays an important role as transcription factor in many cell types, including neurons. Nuclei that had been activated over the last hour prior to euthanasia will appear dark brown after staining, allowing for the quantification of Fos-positive nuclei, directly associated with the activity of that particular brain area.[23]

We reported an increase in the activity of the paraventricular nucleus of the hypothalamus (PVN) and central nucleus of the amygdala (CeA) triggered by OVA in allergic mice, by gavage (food allergy), or intranasal instillation (asthma) (FIG. 4).[16,17] These are important areas in the modulation of affective behaviors and participate in stress responses, including the activation of the hypothalamus-pituitary-adrenal (HPA) axis, containing the highest amounts of CRF in the CNS.

Through *in situ* hybridization double-labeling with Fos immunohistochemistry, we found that Fos-positive nuclei in the PVN and CeA also express transcripts for CRF,[18] and lead to a moderate, but significant increase in serum corticosterone (FIG. 5).[18]

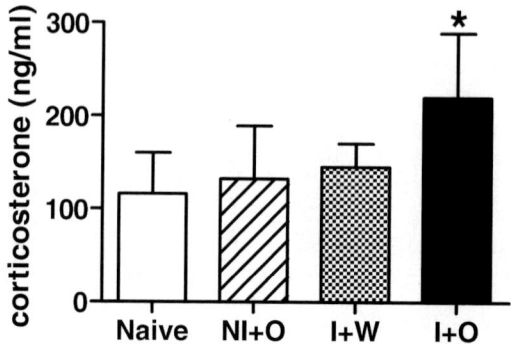

FIGURE 5. Secretion of corticosterone following OVA challenge in allergic mice. Animals previously immunized with OVA (I+O) present higher levels of serum corticosterone than naïve animals, nonimmunized mice receiving OVA by gavage (NI+O), or immunized animals given water (I+W); results are mean ± SD; *$P < 0.05$ for I+O compared to all other groups; $n = 7$–9 per group; ANOVA followed by Student–Newman–Keuls *post hoc* test.

Along with the results from behavioral tests, we believe, employing the models of experimental allergy used here, that allergic reactions evoke activation of specific brain areas compatible with the behavioral pattern displayed by allergic mice, including avoidance and anxiety.

ROLE OF ANTI-OVA ANTIBODIES

The role of anaphylactic antibodies (IgE and IgG1 in mice) was assessed by means of two different approaches. We used an anti-IgE antibody to completely deplete IgE in mice previously immunized, and we precluded its production using a protocol of immunological tolerance.

Immunological tolerance is accomplished by offering a solution of OVA in tap water prior to, or along with, the primary OVA immunization. The main difference between each protocol is that animals receiving oral OVA from days −7 to −2 (prior to OVA immunization) would not produce either class of antibody, while mice offered oral OVA from days 0 to +5 would generate anti-OVA IgG1, but not IgE.[20]

FIGURE 6 shows that removal of IgE, by anti-IgE or oral tolerance, was effective in preventing the development of food aversion (measured in the two-bottle preference test),[16] and avoidance of the dark compartment, previously associated with OVA nebulization (light–dark box),[17] respectively.

Activation of the PVN and CeA was also prevented by inhibiting anti-OVA IgE,[16] strongly suggesting that signaling these immune reactions to the brain uses an IgE-dependent mechanism (FIG. 7).

Since treatment with anti-IgE antibody, or the development of oral tolerance that only precludes IgE, totally prevented the increase in Fos staining following

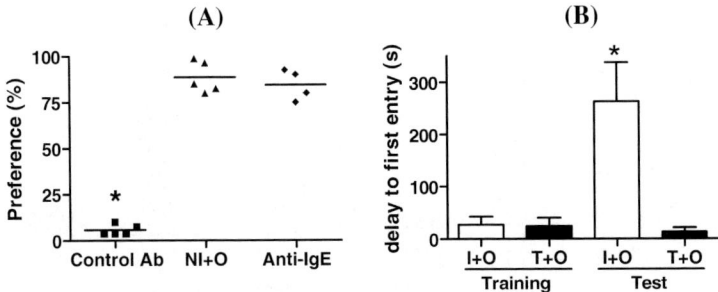

FIGURE 6. Role of IgE antibodies in allergy-induced behavioral changes. **(A)** Two-bottle preference test. Preference for the sweetened OVA-containing solution by individual mice shows that while nonimmunized mice (NI+O) receiving the antigen and immunized mice treated with an anti-IgE antibody (a-IgE) preferred the OVA-containing solution, immunized mice treated with the control antibody (C-Ab) developed food aversion, drinking water instead. $*P < 0.05$ for C-Ab compared to all others; $n = 4$–5 per group; Kruskall–Wallis followed by Kolgomorov–Smirnov two-sample test. **(B)** Avoidance behavior in the LDB test. During the training session, immune (I+O) or tolerant (T+O) mice behave in similar manner; nonetheless, on the test session, only animals immunized and challenged with OVA avoid the dark compartment associated with nebulized OVA; $*P < 0.05$ compared to T+O on the test session or to I+O on the training day; $n = 5$–7 per group; ANOVA followed by Tukey *post hoc* test.

allergic reactions, and the establishment of avoidance responses, we assumed that these phenomena are IgE-mediated, and IgG1-independent.

SIGNALING ALLERGY TO THE MOUSE BRAIN

Lessons from several groups working on neuroimmune interactions suggested to us that an important interface of these systems, namely the intimate contact between mast cells and peripheral nerves, should not be forgotten, since it is commonly described in many tissues; relevant to us were the reports on afferents responding to mast cell degranulation and signaling to relay stations in the brain (such as the vagus nerve–vagal complex in the brain stem) that ultimately reach the hypothalamus and extended limbic system, responsible for endocrine and behavioral changes.[24]

We employed neonatal destruction of capsaicin-sensitive fibers in order to analyze the role of these afferents in signaling an allergic reaction triggered in the GI tract by OVA in immunized animals. Capsaicin *per se* did not alter antibody production, or preference for the sweetened solution. Neonatal capsaicin selectively blocked activation of the PVN following OVA gavage in immunized animals, did not alter Fos staining in the CeA, and partially prevented activation of a putative relay station in the brain stem, the nucleus of the solitary tract (NTS) (FIG. 8) involved in conveying and integrating sensory information, particularly important in viscero–visceral reflexes.[25]

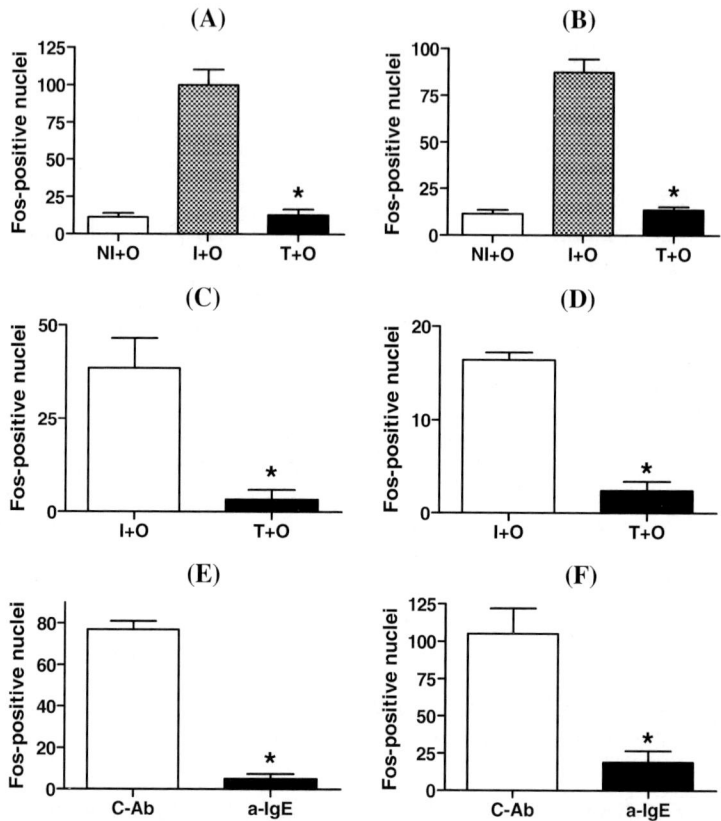

FIGURE 7. Role of IgE on the activity of the PVN and CeA following OVA challenge in immunized animals. While animals immunized and challenged intranasally with OVA (I+O) display a strong activity of the PVN (**A**) and CeA (**B**), tolerant mice (T+O) present a degree of Fos staining similar to that of nonimmunized mice (NI+O). Oral tolerance also prevents the increase in activity of the PVN (**C**) and CeA (**D**) in mice challenged with OVA by gavage, compared to group I+O. Depletion of IgE by the administration of an anti-IgE antibody (a-IgE) also precludes the increase in activity in the PVN (**E**) and CeA (**F**), when compared to the isotype control (C-Ab). *$P < 0.05$ compared to the immunized group (**A**–**D**) or the control antibody (**E**–**F**); $n = 5$–7 per group; ANOVA followed by Tukey–Kramer *post hoc* test.

Nonetheless, whereas capsaicin was unable to prevent the development of food aversion, there was a significant increase in the consumption of the sweetened OVA-containing solution by immunized mice, compared to those previously treated with the vehicle of capsaicin (FIG. 9).

Although we employed two different tests in order to evaluate the degree of C-sensitive fiber destruction by capsaicin (increase in skin vascular permeability by xylene, and number of abdominal contortions by i.p. injection of acetic

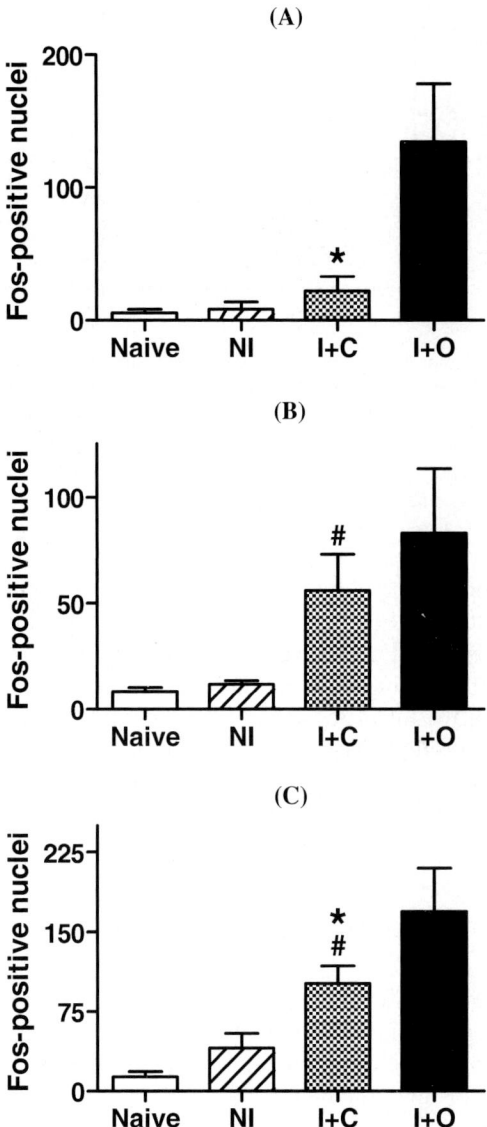

FIGURE 8. Effects of capsaicin on brain activation following OVA challenge in immunized animals. (**A**) Capsaicin completely abolished Fos staining in the PVN of animals immunized and challenged with OVA (I+C) compared to vehicle-treated mice; (**B**) Capsaicin did not significantly alter the patter of Fos staining in the CeA following OVA challenge in allergic mice compared to vehicle-treated animals; (**C**) Capsaicin diminished, but did not completely preclude the activation of the NTS: animals treated with capsaicin (I+C) show a moderate degree of activation (lesser than I+V), but still increased in comparison to nonimmunized or naïve mice. Results are mean ± SD; *$P < 0.05$ versus I+O, and #$P < 0.05$ versus NI+O; $n = 4$ per group; ANOVA followed by Tukey–Kramer *post hoc* test.

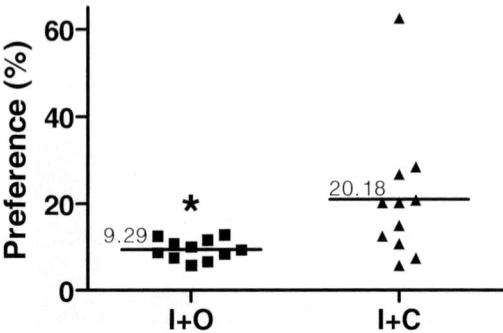

FIGURE 9. Effects of capsaicin on the preference for the sweetened OVA-containing solution. Individual values are shown as *squares* or *triangles*, and *horizontal lines* represent medians. Capsaicin caused a twofold increase in the consumption of the sweetened OVA-containing solution, compared to vehicle-treated mice. Note that aversion was not totally inhibited by capsaicin (compare to FIG.1A), but its magnitude was clearly attenuated, suggesting a partial role for C-sensitive fibers in this phenomenon. *$P < 0.05$ for I+O compared to I+C; $n = 11$ per group; Mann–Whitney test.

acid[18,22]), nonetheless, the loss of afferents that interfere with the outcome of the behavioral tests used here was not directly assessed in our condition.

Some authors reported that capsaicin destroys between 60 and 70% of C-sensitive fibers. This percentage can be even lower in the GI tract because of the existence of the intrinsic fibers of the enteric nervous system, particularly resistant to capsaicin. Therefore, the lack of, or decrease in, the magnitude of expected responses could be attributed, at least in part, to ineffective or incomplete depletion of C-sensitive fibers by our protocol of capsaicin treatment.

ROLE OF MAST CELLS

Regardless of the particular signaling pathways from a peripheral site presenting an ongoing allergic response to the brain, the first step in this process— triggering the early phase of an allergic reaction—is undoubtedly dependent on IgE-mediated (or IgG1-mediated) mast cell degranulation.[4]

Thus we subsequently aimed at the pharmacological inhibition of mast cell degranulation using dissodium cromoglycate (cromolyn), a mast cell membrane stabilizer commonly used in humans to prevent allergic reactions in the airways.

Mice in this model of experimental allergic asthma were treated with cromolyn prior to OVA challenge and used for the evaluation of PVN and CeA activity. Inhibition of mast cell degranulation by cromolyn totally precluded the increase in neuronal activity assessed in these two areas (FIG. 10). Moreover, immunized mice treated with cromolyn no longer developed the

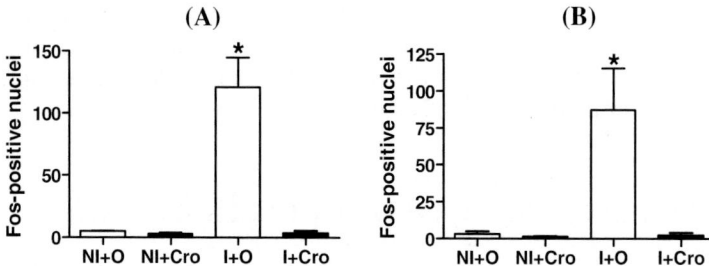

FIGURE 10. Role of mast cells on the activity of the PVN and CeA following OVA challenge in immunized mice. Prior treatment with the inhibitor of mast cell degranulation, cromolyn, precluded the increase in Fos staining in the PVN (**A**) and CeA (**B**) of mice immunized and challenged with OVA (I+O). While animals from group I+O displayed strong activity of these nuclei following OVA challenge, treatment with cromolyn (I+Cro) led to a pattern of Fos expression in the PVN and CeA similar to that found in nonimmunized mice (NI+O). Results are mean ± SD; *$P < 0.05$ for I+O compared to all other groups; $n = 5$ per group; ANOVA followed by Tukey *post hoc* test.

aversion to the dark compartment previously associated with OVA nebulization (FIG. 11).[20]

In order to test the efficacy of cromolyn in inhibition mast cell degranulation, we analyzed the increase in vascular permeability in the lungs of allergic mice following OVA challenge; animals pretreated with cromolyn had around 45% reduction in Evans blue dye extravasation to their lungs (data not shown), compatible to that described in literature.

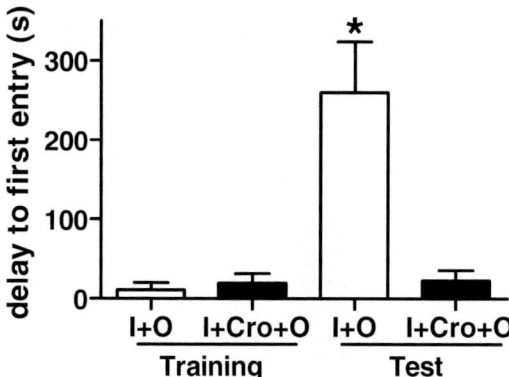

FIGURE 11. Avoidance behavior in the LDB test. During the training session, immunized animals treated (I+Cro+O) or not (I+O) with cromolyn, and challenged with OVA behaved in similar manner; nonetheless, on the test session, cromolyn-treated animals did not develop an aversion to the dark compartment, previously associated with nebulized OVA.*$P < 0.05$ for I+O compared to I+Cro+O on the test session, or to I+O on the training day; $n = 5$–7 per group; ANOVA followed by Tukey *post hoc* test.

Taking into account our previous results on behavior and brain activity, it is probable that we are dealing with IgE- and mast cell-dependent mechanisms, commonly associated with the early phase of the immediate allergic response characteristic of food allergy and asthma.

ROLE OF INFLAMMATORY CELL INFILTRATE

Since inflammation is commonly associated with CNS activation and behavioral changes in immune-driven phenomena of neuroimmunomodulation, we used C_3H/HeJ mice, known for being resistant to bacterial lipopolysaccharide (LPS) effects on cytokine production and behavioral changes due to a point mutation in the toll-like receptor 4 (TLR4) and downstream signaling. Relevant in our case is the fact that these animals, for some reason not particularly well understood, do not mount an important inflammatory response in the airways following OVA challenge in immunized animals. While immunized BALB/c mice accumulate an important inflammatory infiltrate composed mainly of mononuclear cells (specially CD4+ T lymphocytes) and eosinophils, C_3H/HeJ animals do not present cellular infiltration in the lungs even 48–72 h after OVA challenge.[20]

C_3H/HeJ mice had similar activation of the PVN and CeA following immunization and challenge with OVA (FIG. 12), suggesting that inflammatory cell infiltration in the lungs is not required for asthma signaling to the mouse brain in our conditions. Moreover, the avoidance assessed in the light–dark box test was displayed by C_3H/HeJ mice in a similar level of that observed in BALB/c animals (FIG. 13).[20]

It is noteworthy that C_3H/HeJ mice do mount an allergic response to OVA in terms of IgE production, and that the levels of this antibody reach similar titers as those found in BALB/c mice (data not shown).

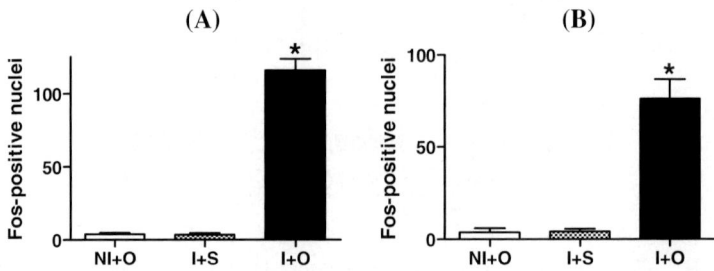

FIGURE 12. Allergy-induced activity in the PVN and CeA of C_3H/HeJ immunized mice. Immunization and challenge with OVA to C_3H/HeJ caused an increase in the activity of the PVN and CeA in a similar pattern to that found in BALB/c mice. Only immunized mice (I+O) present a strong Fos staining in the PVN (**A**) and CeA (**B**) following challenge with OVA. Results are mean $\pm$ SD; $^*P < 0.05$ for I+O compared to all other groups; $n = 5$ per group; ANOVA followed by Tukey *post hoc* test.

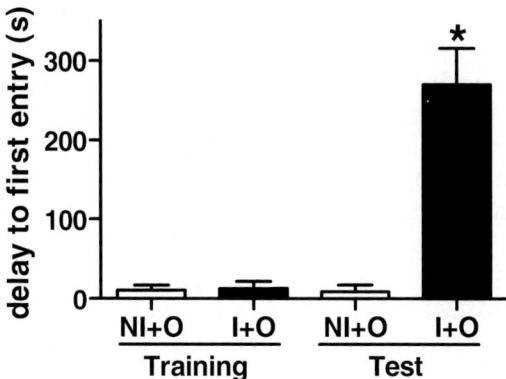

FIGURE 13. Avoidance behavior of C$_3$H/HeJ mice in the LDB test. Immunized mice (I+O) behaved like nonimmunized (NI+O) animals in the training session, but avoided the compartment previously associated with nebulized OVA on the test session. Results are mean ± SD; *$P < 0.05$ for I+O versus NI+O on the test session, or versus I+O on the test sessions; $n = 5$–7 per group; ANOVA followed by Dunnet's *post hoc* test.

CONCLUDING REMARKS

Considering our findings described here, the following facts guide our on-going research: Allergic reactions can, and will, lead to changes in neuronal activity, particularly in brain areas involved in processing emotionality and affective behaviors, and in the activation of the HPA axis and triggering of stress responses. These areas directly or indirectly participate in adaptive behavioral changes and control of endocrine pathways, such as secretion of glucocorticoids. These changes might be important in avoiding further contact with the allergen, and minimizing future allergic reactions.

Changes are very similar in food allergy and asthma, including behavior and brain activity, suggesting that these could share a conserved set of mechanisms with a common outcome. The CNS circuitry includes, at least, the hypothalamus and the amygdala. Hints on pathways and relay stations, such as the NTS for food allergy, need further elucidation for asthma in future studies.

Altogether, these responses depend on IgE and mast cells, partially involve C-sensitive fibers, and do not seem to require an important inflammatory infiltrate or the presence of IgG1 antibodies.

ACKNOWLEDGMENTS

We are in eternal debt to all people who indirectly contributed to the work described here. Technical assistance of Mr. Adilson Alves and Mrs. Eliane Gomes was greatly appreciated. We have enormous gratitude for Dr. Jackson Bittencourt and Dr. Carol Elias for their help with *in situ* procedures. We acknowledge the support from the Animal Facilities from the Department of Pathology–FMVZ–USP, providing the animals used throughout the Ph.D. work of F. A. Costa-Pinto and A. S. Basso. We are especially grateful to the Foundation for Supporting Science in the State of São Paulo (FAPESP) for several grants and scholarships (# 99/03778-3, 99/04228-7, 00/07126-0, 00/07127-6, 01/13510-0, 04/14128-0, 04/14297-2, 05/55966-0), without which these studies would certainly be impossible.

REFERENCES

1. UMETSU, D.T. *et al*. 2002. Asthma: an epidemic of dysregulated immunity. Nat. Immunol. **3:** 715–720.
2. DE SOUSA MUCIDA, D. *et al*. 2003. Unconventional strategies for the suppression of allergic asthma. Curr. Drug Targets Inflamm. Allergy **2:** 187–195.
3. CROWE, S.E. & M.H. PERDUE. 1992. Gastrointestinal food hypersensitivity: basic mechanisms of pathophysiology. Gastroenterology **103:** 1075–1095.
4. MADDOX, L. & D.A. SCHWARTZ. 2002. The pathophysiology of asthma. Annu. Rev. Med. **53:** 477–498.
5. PEARSON, D.J. 1988. Psychologic and somatic interrelationships in allergy and pseudoallergy. J. Allergy Clin. Immunol. **81:** 351–360.
6. MACKENZIE, J.N. 1886. The production of the so-called rose effect by means of an artificial rose, with remarks and historical notes. Am. J. Med. Sci. **91:** 45–57.
7. LEHRER, P.M., S. ISENBERG & S.M. HOCHRON. 1993. Asthma and emotion: a review. J. Asthma **30:** 5–21.
8. RIETVELD, S., W. EVERAERD & T.L. CREER. 2000. Stress-induced asthma: a review of research and potential mechanisms. Clin. Exp. Allergy **30:** 1058–1066.
9. ADDOLORATO, G. *et al*. 1998. Anxiety and depression: a common feature of health care seeking patients with irritable bowel syndrome and food allergy. Hepatogastroenterology **45:** 1559–1564.
10. PEVELER, R. *et al*. 1996. Psychiatric aspects of food-related physical symptoms: a community study. J. Psychosom. Res. **41:** 149–159.
11. CARA, D.C., A.A. CONDE & N.M. VAZ. 1994. Immunological induction of flavor aversion in mice. Braz. J. Med. Biol. Res. **27:** 1331–1341.
12. BIENENSTOCK, J. *et al*. 1988. Role of neuropeptides, nerves and mast cells in intestinal immunity and physiology. Monogr. Allergy **24:** 134–143.
13. BIENENSTOCK, J. *et al*. 1988. Inflammatory cells and the epithelium. Mast cell/nerve interactions in the lung in vitro and in vivo. Am. Rev. Respir. Dis. **138:** S31–S34.
14. KIERNAN, J.A. 1990. Degranulation of mast cells in the trachea and bronchi of the rat following stimulation of the vagus nerve. Int. Arch. Allergy Appl. Immunol. **91:** 398–402.
15. JOOS, G.F. 2003. Bronchial hyperresponsiveness: too complex to be useful? Curr. Opin. Pharmacol. **3:** 233–238.
16. BASSO, A.S. *et al*. 2003. Neural correlates of IgE-mediated food allergy. J. Neuroimmunol. **140:** 69–77.
17. COSTA-PINTO, F.A. *et al*. 2005. Avoidance behavior and neural correlates of allergen exposure in a murine model of asthma. Brain Behav. Immun. **19:** 52–60.
18. BASSO, A.S. 2004. Neural correlates of food allergy: role of IgE-mediated mechanisms and sensory C-fibers. Ph.D. thesis. University of São Paulo. São Paulo.

19. BASSO, A.S. *et al.* 2004. Neural pathways involved in food allergy signaling in the mouse brain: role of capsaicin-sensitive afferents. Brain Res. **1009:** 181–188.
20. COSTA-PINTO, F.A. 2004. Neural and behavioral correlates of experimental allergic asthma in mice. Ph.D. thesis. University of São Paulo. São Paulo.
21. BASSO, A.S., L.C. DE SA-ROCHA & J. PALERMO-NETO. 2001. Immune-induced flavor aversion in mice: modification by neonatal capsaicin treatment. Neuroimmunomodulation **9:** 88–94.
22. BASSO, A.S. 1999. Interactions between the nervous system and an immune-induced diet selection in mice. M.Sc. dissertation. University of São Paulo. São Paulo.
23. DRAGUNOW, M. & R. FAULL. 1989. The use of c-fos as a metabolic marker in neuronal pathway tracing. J. Neurosci. Methods **29:** 261–265.
24. MENZAGHI, F. *et al.* 1993. The role of limbic and hypothalamic corticotropin-releasing factor in behavioral responses to stress. Ann. N. Y. Acad. Sci. **697:** 142–154.
25. CASTEX, N. *et al.* 1995. c-fos expression in specific rat brain nuclei after intestinal anaphylaxis: involvement of 5-HT3 receptors and vagal afferent fibers. Brain Res. **688:** 149–160.

Dialogue between the Brain and the Immune System in Inflammatory Arthritis

DIMITRIOS VASSILOPOULOS AND DIMOSTHENIS MANTZOUKIS

Academic Department of Medicine, Athens University School of Medicine, Hippokration General Hospital, Athens, Greece

ABSTRACT: The crosstalk between the brain and the immune system in inflammatory arthritis is exerted mainly through the activation or downregulation of the hypothalamic-pituitary-adrenal (HPA), the hypothalamic-pituitary-gonadal (HPG), and the hypothalamic-autonomic nervous system (HANS) axes. In this review, we will present an overview of the most recent data regarding the regulation of these complex pathways of neuroendocrine response during the different phases of inflammatory arthritides such as rheumatoid arthritis (RA). Furthermore, the effect of the most recently available biologic therapies like anti-tumor necrosis factor (TNF-a) on the neuroendocrine function in patients with RA will be reviewed.

KEYWORDS: arthritis; hypothalamic-pituitary-adrenal; hypothalamic-pituitary-gonadal; hypothalamic-autonomic nervous system

INTRODUCTION

Inflammatory arthritides are common, affecting approximately 3% of the general population.[1] The majority of inflammatory arthritides run a chronic course with significant associated morbidity and mortality. The most common chronic form of inflammatory arthritis is rheumatoid arthritis (RA), which affects approximately 1% of the general population, without any significant geographic variation.[1] Other commonly encountered inflammatory arthritides include spondyloarthropathies (psoriatic arthritis, ankylosing spondylitis, arthritides associated with inflammatory bowel diseases, reactive arthritis, undifferentiated spondyloarthropathy), arthritides associated with various rheumatic disorders (such as systemic lupus erythematosus, Sjögren's syndrome, systemic sclerosis), and crystal-induced arthritides such as gout and pyrophosphate arthropathy.

Address for correspondence: Dimitrios Vassilopoulos, M.D., Academic Department of Medicine, Hippokration General Hospital, Athens University School of Medicine, 114 Vass. Sophias Ave., 115 27 Athens, Greece. Voice: +30-210-7774742; fax: +30-210-7481771.

e-mail: dvassilop@med.uoa.gr

Ann. N.Y. Acad. Sci. 1088: 132–138 (2006). © 2006 New York Academy of Sciences.
doi: 10.1196/annals.1366.031

The complex interactions between the neuroendocrine system and the localized and systemic inflammatory response that is characteristic of RA[2] will be the focus of this review, since RA represents the most common and best-studied form of inflammatory arthritis. Furthermore, the latest data regarding the effect of biologic therapies that target specific pro-inflammatory cytokines, such as tumor necrosis factor (TNF-α), on the neuroendocrine response will be discussed.

RA PATHOGENESIS—POTENTIAL ROLE OF THE NEUROENDOCRINE SYSTEM

RA is chronic destructive inflammatory arthritis of unknown etiology that affects mainly middle-aged women and men.[1,2] Recent epidemiological data have shown that this chronic disease is associated with increased cardiovascular morbidity and mortality, indicating the systemic nature of the inflammatory process.

The neuroendocrine system could affect different stages of RA including the preclinical or asymptomatic phase, the transition of early acute inflammatory arthritis to chronicity, and the chronic arthritis phase (FIG. 1).

PRECLINICAL PHASE—ANIMAL MODELS

It is evident from recent data that a long asymptomatic phase precedes the onset of RA.[3] During this phase, which may last up to 15 years, antibodies against cyclic citrullinated peptides (anti-CCP) and rheumatoid factor (RF) are detected in approximately half of the patients. Signals delivered by the

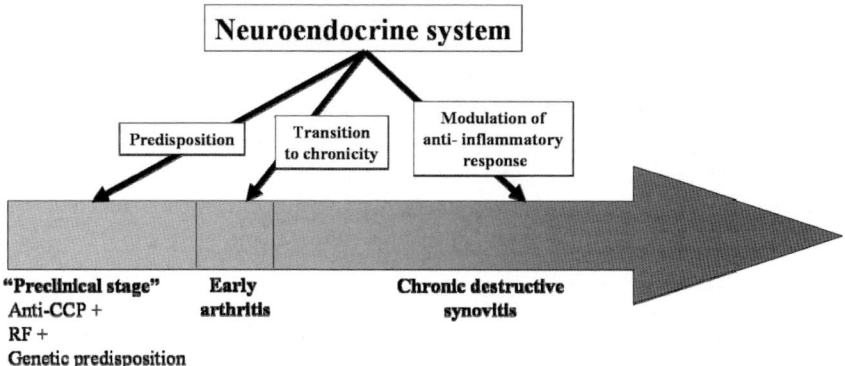

FIGURE 1. The potential effects of the neuroendocrine system response during the different phases (preclinical and clinical) of rheumatoid arthritis is depicted. Anti-CCP = antibodies against cyclic citrullinated peptides; RF = rheumatoid factor.

neuroendocrine system could potentially increase the risk of such predisposed individuals to RA development. Data suggesting such interaction are derived from animal models of inflammatory arthritis, epidemiological studies suggesting a role of hormonal factors in the development of human RA, as well as by large genomic analyses of genes related to the neuroendocrine axis that could predispose to RA.

Animal models that indicate an interaction between the neuroendocrine system and inflammatory arthritis are mainly based on animals with an altered hypothalamic-pituitary-adrenal (HPA) axis.[4] The best studied model is that of arthritis developing in certain strains of Lewis (LEW/N) and Fischer (F344/N) rats. LEW/N rats that display a blunted HPA response to a number of stimuli develop chronic arthritis after exposure to streptococcal cell wall (SCW) antigen. On the contrary, F344/N rats exhibiting a strong hypothalamic corticotrophin-releasing hormone (CRH) response are resistant to SCW-induced arthritis. Treatment of arthritis-resistant F344/N rats with a glucocorticoid antagonist (RU 486) increases their susceptibility to arthritis development, while treatment of arthritis-susceptible LEW/N rats with glucocorticoids ameliorates the inflammatory response.[4] These findings signify the importance of an intact versus a defective HPA axis in experimental arthritis susceptibility. However, it should be noted that inflammatory arthritis in these animal models is a polygenic disease in which genetic variability accounts for only one third of the phenotypic disease expression.[4] Candidate genes have been mapped on rat chromosome 10, where a number of genes closely linked to the HPA axis and immune response have been identified. These include the CRH receptor type 1, the angiotensin-converting enzyme (ACE), and transcription factors (STATs).

In human RA, large-scale genome-wide linkage analyses looking for disease susceptibility genes have been performed in different parts of the world.[5] Disease predisposition has been shown to be attributed to HLA-related genes (located in chromosome 6) in about one third of the cases whereas the other two thirds involve non-HLA regions. Approximately 16 candidate non-HLA regions have been identified, including the PAD-14 (chromosome 1), TNF receptor II (chromosome 1), SLC22A4 (chromosome 5), and RANK (chromosome 18) encoding genes.[5] None of these regions identified so far is closely related to the HPA axis. Ongoing studies using newer gene identification techniques are expected to clarify whether genes involved in neuroendocrine axis regulation are playing a role in RA predisposition.

CLINICAL PHASE (EARLY AND CHRONIC PHASE)

RA is predominantly an inflammatory disease affecting the synovial membrane of multiple joints in a symmetrical fashion.[1,2] Histological analysis of involved joints reveals an infiltration of the synovium by T and B cells as well as macrophages.[2] Activation of these cells is followed by activation of chondrocytes, fibroblasts, and osteoclasts leading to pannus formation and bone and cartilage destruction. Exciting experimental and human data over the last 15 years have pointed to the significant role of cytokines such as TNF-α and IL-1 in joint inflammation and bone destruction.[6] Although the immune response appears to be localized predominantly in the synovial microenviroment, a systemic inflammatory response is also evident.

The "physiologic" neuroendocrine response to the pro-inflammatory signals delivered by the inflamed joints has been investigated in a number of animal and human studies over the last decades.[7,8] The mediators of such pro-inflammatory signals include substance P released by sensory fibers in the inflamed synovium, cytokines such as TNF-α, IL-2, IL-6, IL-8, and IL-12 produced by different cells in inflamed joints that are released either locally or systemically, and finally circulating activated immune cells like lymphocytes and monocytes.[8] These signals collectively lead to the activation of the HPA and the hypothalamic-autonomic nervous system (HANS) axis, while at the same time the response of the hypothalamic-pituitary-gonadal (HPG) axis is downregulated. The activated HPA axis, through the action of cortisol and androgens released by the adrenals, has a direct anti-inflammatory effect in arthritic joints. Similarly, activated sympathetic fibers in the synovium release high levels of anti-inflammatory mediators such as epinephrine, norepinephrine, and adenosine.[8]

Extensive studies have examined the magnitude and the specificity of this "physiologic" response in RA patients during the early or chronic disease phase. The overall prevailing theory is that the response of these homeostatic mechanisms is inappropriately inadequate for the degree of the localized and systemic inflammation characterizing RA.[8] An inadequate neuroendocrine response could contribute to the transition of the early inflammatory arthritis to a chronic one or to the persistence of a chronic inflammatory process (see Fig. 1).

In regards to the HPA axis, a number of studies have shown a relatively normal ACTH and cortisol response,[9] although these levels are inappropriately low for the degree of inflammation seen in inflammatory arthritides.[10] In a recent study, Straub et al. showed that untreated RA patients with early arthritis had higher cortisol and similar ACTH levels compared to healthy controls.[11] However, when these levels were corrected for the levels of TNF-α and IL-1 in the serum, they were significantly lower than those of healthy individuals. Similar results were obtained in patients with other forms of inflammatory arthritis such as reactive arthritis.[11] Adrenal androgens such as dehydroepiandrosterone (DHEA), DHEA sulfate (DHEAS), and androstenedione (ASD) possess significant anti-inflammatory properties.[8] Their levels in RA patients are relatively low, which could also be a contributing factor leading to an inadequate host anti-inflammatory response. It is though unclear whether this is a disease-specific event, since similarly low adrenal androgen levels have been observed in other chronic inflammatory diseases such as systemic lupus erythematosus (SLE), Crohn's disease, and psoriasis.

The stimulation of sensory fibers in the synovial tissue leads to an increased sympathetic system response in RA patients.[8] Despite this increased central response, a study by Miller *et al.* has shown that the number of sympathetic fibers in the inflamed RA joints are decreased, whereas the number of sensory fibers are increased compared to non-inflammatory joints from patients with osteoarthritis.[12] This secondary localized loss of sympathetic fibers could prevent the host from conveying its anti-inflammatory actions through the sympathetic system.

The alterations of the HPG axis observed during the course of RA is far more complicated.[8] Overall, it appears that estrogen levels remain normal in RA patients, while at the same time the levels of gonadal androgens such as testosterone are significantly lower in these patients.[8] Testosterone has been shown to exert a direct anti-inflammatory effect, mainly by inhibiting IL-1 production from immune cells such as peripheral blood mononuclear cells and synovial macrophages. Although the exact mechanisms that lead to decreased gonadal androgen levels in RA have not been delineated, their role in disease progression could be significant.

BIOLOGIC THERAPIES AND NEUROENDOCRINE FUNCTION

Over the last decade, there has been an explosion in the number of available biologic agents for the treatment of various autoimmune diseases.[13] These agents specifically target either pro-inflammatory mediators such as TNF-α, IL-1, IL-6, or IL-15 or cells of the immune system and their interactions (e.g., anti-B cell agents, agents targeting T–B cell interaction or costimulatory molecules such as LFA-1 or LFA-3).[13] These agents have been proved extremely useful in the treatment of patients with RA, psoriasis, proriatic arthritis, ankylosing spondylitis, autoimmune cytopenias, and Crohn's disease.[13] Aside from their obvious therapeutic effect, these agents could prove to be valuable tools in the study of neuroendocrine–joint interaction in complex inflammatory diseases such as RA.

Preliminary data about the effects of these agents on synovial inflammation and neuroendocrine response are starting to emerge.[14–16] Straub *et al.* studied the role of anti-TNF-α administration on HPA axis in RA patients with or without the concomitant use of corticosteroids.[16] In this study infliximab, a chimeric monoclonal antibody targeting soluble and membrane-bound TNF-α, was used. The authors found that infliximab administration was associated with increased absolute ACTH levels in corticosteroid-naïve patients, while at the same time ACTH and cortisol levels relative to serum TNF-α levels increased gradually during the three-month treatment period.[16] Furthermore, they observed that the serum cortisol to ACTH ratio decreased, indicative of a sensitization of the hypothalamic-pituitary gland during treatment.

The effects of anti-TNFα agents on androgen production appear more complicated. Short-term administration of two different anti-TNF-α agents, infliximab and adalimumab, in corticosteroid-naïve RA patient, did not lead to significant changes in serum adrenal (DHEA, DHEAS, ASD) and gonadal (testosterone) androgen levels.[14–16] Nevertheless, it was found that the ratio of serum ASD to serum cortisol increased during treatment with both agents.[14,16] These findings could suggest that there is a trend towards normalization of adrenal androgen production during effective RA treatment. Obviously, further long-term studies are needed in order to fully explore these potential effects of anti-TNF-α treatment.

CONCLUSIONS

This is an exciting era for the study of the complex interactions between the neuroendocrine axis and the aberrant immune response characterizing inflammatory arthritides like RA. Building on the data available from experimental, animal, and human studies in the past, one could expect that the careful study of patients undergoing treatment with the newly available biologic agents would provide valuable additional information for this complex homeostatic mechanisms. Better knowledge of these mechanisms could prove to be useful in the design of more appropriate and specific therapeutic interventions aiming at the restoration of these imbalances.

REFERENCES

1. LEE, D.M. & M.E. WEINBLATT. 2001. Rheumatoid arthritis. Lancet **358:** 903–911.
2. GORONZY, J.J. & C.M. WEYAND. 2005. Rheumatoid arthritis. Immunol. Rev. **204:** 55–73.
3. NIELEN, M.M., D. VAN SCHAARDENBURG, H.W. REESINK, *et al.* 2004. Specific autoantibodies precede the symptoms of rheumatoid arthritis: a study of serial measurements in blood donors. Arthritis Rheum. **50:** 380–386.
4. JAFARIAN-TEHRANI, M. & E.M. STERNBERG. 2000. Neuroendocrine and other factors in the regulation of inflammation. Animal models. Ann. N.Y. Acad. Sci. **917:** 819–824.
5. STEINSSON, K. & M.E. ALARCON-RIQUELME. 2005. Genetic aspects of rheumatic diseases. Scand. J. Rheumatol. **34:** 167–177.
6. FELDMANN, M. & R.N. MAINI. 2003. Lasker Clinical Medical Research Award: TNF defined as a therapeutic target for rheumatoid arthritis and other autoimmune diseases. Nat. Med. **9:** 1245–1250.
7. HARLE, P., T. BONGARTZ, J. SCHOLMERICH, *et al.* 2005. Predictive and potentially predictive factors in early arthritis: a multidisciplinary approach. Rheumatology (Oxford). **44:** 426–433.

8. STRAUB, R.H. & M. CUTOLO. 2001. Involvement of the hypothalamic–pituitary–adrenal/gonadal axis and the peripheral nervous system in rheumatoid arthritis: viewpoint based on a systemic pathogenetic role. Arthritis Rheum. **44:** 493–507.
9. HARBUZ, M.S. & D.S. JESSOP. 1999. Is there a defect in cortisol production in rheumatoid arthritis? Rheumatology (Oxford) **38:** 298–302.
10. CROFFORD, L.J., K.T. KALOGERAS, G. MASTORAKOS, *et al.* 1997. Circadian relationships between interleukin (IL)-6 and hypothalamic-pituitary-adrenal axis hormones: failure of IL-6 to cause sustained hypercortisolism in patients with early untreated rheumatoid arthritis. J. Clin. Endocrinol. Metab. **82:** 1279–1283.
11. STRAUB, R.H., L. PAIMELA, R. PELTOMAA, *et al.* 2002. Inadequately low serum levels of steroid hormones in relation to interleukin-6 and tumor necrosis factor in untreated patients with early rheumatoid arthritis and reactive arthritis. Arthritis Rheum. **46:** 654–662.
12. MILLER, L.E., H.P. JUSTEN, J. SCHOLMERICH & R.H. STRAUB. 2000. The loss of sympathetic nerve fibers in the synovial tissue of patients with rheumatoid arthritis is accompanied by increased norepinephrine release from synovial macrophages. FASEB J. **14:** 2097–2107.
13. FELDMANN, M. & L. STEINMAN. 2005. Design of effective immunotherapy for human autoimmunity. Nature **435:** 612–619.
14. STRAUB, R.H., P. SARZI-PUTTINI, F. ATZENI, *et al.* 2005. Anti-tumour necrosis factor antibody treatment does not change serum levels of cortisol binding globulin in patients with rheumatoid arthritis but it increases androstenedione relative to cortisol. Ann. Rheum. Dis. **64:** 1353–1356.
15. STRAUB, R.H., P. HARLE, F. ATZENI, *et al.* 2005. Sex hormone concentrations in patients with rheumatoid arthritis are not normalized during 12 weeks of anti-tumor necrosis factor therapy. J. Rheumatol. **32:** 1253–1258.
16. STRAUB, R.H., G. PONGRATZ, J. SCHOLMERICH, *et al.* 2003. Long-term anti-tumor necrosis factor antibody therapy in rheumatoid arthritis patients sensitizes the pituitary gland and favors adrenal androgen secretion. Arthritis Rheum. **48:** 1504–1512.

Neurosteroids as Endogenous Inhibitors of Neuronal Cell Apoptosis in Aging

IOANNIS CHARALAMPOPOULOS,[a] VASSILIKI-ISMINI ALEXAKI,[b]
CHRISTOS TSATSANIS,[c] VASSILIS MINAS,[a] ERENE DERMITZAKI,[c]
IAKOVOS LASARIDIS,[a] LINA VARDOULI,[d] CHRISTOS STOURNARAS,[d]
ANDREW N. MARGIORIS,[c] ELIAS CASTANAS,[b]
AND ACHILLE GRAVANIS[a]

[a]Department of Pharmacology, School of Medicine, University of Crete, Heraklion 71110, Greece

[b]Department of Experimental Endocrinology, School of Medicine, University of Crete, Heraklion 71110, Greece

[c]Department of Clinical Chemistry, School of Medicine, University of Crete, Heraklion 71110, Greece

[d]Department of Biochemistry, School of Medicine, University of Crete, Heraklion 71110, Greece

ABSTRACT: The neuroactive steroids dehydroepiandrosterone (DHEA), its sulfate ester DHEAS, and allopregnanolone (Allo) are produced in the adrenals and the brain. Their production rate and levels in serum, brain, and adrenals decrease gradually with advancing age. The decline of their levels was associated with age-related neuronal dysfunction and degeneration, most probably because these steroids protect central nervous system (CNS) neurons against noxious agents. Indeed, DHEA(S) protects rat hippocampal neurons against NMDA-induced excitotoxicity, whereas Allo ameliorates NMDA-induced excitotoxicity in human neurons. These steroids exert also a protective role on the sympathetic nervous system. Indeed, DHEA, DHEAS, and Allo protect chromaffin cells and the sympathoadrenal PC12 cells (an established model for the study of neuronal cell apoptosis and survival) against serum deprivation–induced apoptosis. Their effects are time- and dose-dependent with EC_{50} 1.8, 1.1, and 1.5 nM, respectively. The prosurvival effect of DHEA(S) appears to be NMDA-, $GABA_A$- sigma1-, or estrogen receptor-independent, and is mediated by G-protein-coupled-specific membrane binding sites. It involves the antiapoptotic Bcl-2 proteins, and the activation of prosurvival transcription factors CREB and NF-κB, upstream effectors of the antiapoptotic Bcl-2 protein expression, as well as prosurvival kinase PKCα/β, a posttranslational activator of Bcl-2. Furthermore, they directly stimulate biosynthesis and release of neuroprotective catecholamines, exerting a

Address for correspondence: Achille Gravanis, Department of Pharmacology, School of Medicine, University of Crete, Heraklion 71110, Greece. Voice: +30-2810-394521; fax: +30-2810-394530.
e-mail: gravanis@med.uoc.gr

Ann. N.Y. Acad. Sci. 1088: 139–152 (2006). © 2006 New York Academy of Sciences.
doi: 10.1196/annals.1366.003

139

direct transcriptional effect on tyrosine hydroxylase, and regulating actin depolymerization and submembrane actin filament disassembly, a fast-response cellular system regulating trafficking of catecholamine vesicles. These findings suggest that neurosteroids may act as endogenous neuro-protective factors. The decline of neurosteroid levels during aging may leave the brain unprotected against neurotoxic challenges.

KEYWORDS: neurosteroids; apoptosis; neurons; catecholamines; neuro-protection

INTRODUCTION

Dehydroepiandrosterone (DHEA) and its sulfate ester DHEAS are the most abundant steroids in humans. They are mainly produced in zona reticularis of the human adrenal cortex. Adrenal secretion of DHEA(S) increases during adrenarche. Maximal values of circulating DHEA(S) are reached between the ages of 20 and 30 years; thereafter, their levels decrease markedly[1–4] and in persons 70 years of age, they are at approximately 20% of their peak values. Furthermore, stressful conditions, such as major depression, chronic psychological stress, or chronic inflammatory diseases result in decreased levels of adrenal DHEA(S).[5,6]

These steroids are also synthesized *de novo* in various regions of the central and peripheral nervous system (CNS and PNS), respectively of humans and other species.[7–9] Indeed, recent experimental and clinical evidence supports the hypothesis that the brain is a steroidogenic organ. Neurosteroids are still found in the brain after steroidogenic glands are removed, indicating that they are synthesized either *de novo* or from endogenous precursors by enzymes present in the CNS. In fact, steroidogenic acute regulatory protein and the most important steroidogenic enzymes are expressed in the brain. These enzymes are expressed in both neurons and glia, suggesting that these two cell types must work in concert to produce the appropriate active neurosteroid. Neurosteroids are synthesized either from CNS cholesterol or from peripheral steroid precursors and exhibit a wide variety of diverse functions. The functions attributed to specific neurosteroids include modulation of $GABA_A$, NMDA, and sigma receptor function, regulation of myelinization, neuroprotection, and growth of axons and dendrites.[9] Additionally, neurosteroids have also been shown to modulate the expression of particular subunits of $GABA_A$ and NMDA receptors, providing additional sites at which these compounds can regulate neural function.

The decline of neurosteroid levels during aging was associated with neuronal dysfunction and degeneration,[10–12] most probably because these steroids protect CNS neurons against noxious agents.[13–15] Indeed, DHEA protects rat hippocampal neurons against NMDA-induced excitotoxicity,[16] whereas al-lopregnanolone (Allo) ameliorates NMDA-induced excitotoxicity in human neurons.[17] The decline of brain concentrations of neurosteroids was also associated with age-related neurodegenerative conditions. Indeed, recent studies investigating the physiopathological significance of neurosteroids in Alzheimer's disease (AD) have shown a significant decline of neurosteroid concentrations in individual brain regions of AD patients compared to aged nondemented controls.[18,19] Pregnenolone sulfate (PREGS) and DHEAS were significantly lower in the striatum and cerebellum, and DHEAS was also significantly reduced in the hypothalamus in these patients. Additionally, a significant negative correlation was found between the levels of cortical β-amyloid peptides and those of PREGS in the striatum and cerebellum and between the levels of phosphorylated tau proteins and DHEAS in the hypothalamus.[18] These studies suggest a possible endogenous neuroprotective role of these neurosteroids in AD. It is also of interest that DHEA is able to potentiate locomotor activity of hemiparkinsonian monkeys, improving symptomatic treatment of the moderately and severely impaired MPTP animals.[20,21]

DHEA AND ALLO PREVENT APOPTOSIS OF SYMPATHOADRENAL CELLS VIA INDUCTION OF ANTIAPOPTOTIC BCL-2 PROTEINS

Recent experimental evidence indicates that neurosteroids, such as DHEA, DHEAS, and Allo, may protect against apoptosis of the neural crest–derived sympathoadrenal medulla cells, adjacent to their primary site of production in adrenals. Adrenomedullary cells are ganglion-like cells, share a common precursor with sympathetic neurons, possessing a mixed neuronal–epithelial phenotype, and play a crucial role in the physiology of the peripheral sympathetic nervous system. All three steroids protect, in a time- and dose-dependent fashion, PC12 sympathoadrenal cells from serum deprivation–induced apoptosis, with EC_{50} at 1.8, 1.1, and 1.5 nM for DHEA, DHEAS, and Allo, respectively.[22]

Structure–activity relation (SAR) analysis of the antiapoptotic effects of neurosteroids revealed the following: (*a*) *Androstenes*: (i) Conformations 3α-OH, 3-keto, Δ^4 (double bond at C4–C5) are inactive. Thus, the Δ^4-3-keto steroids including testosterone, progesterone, corticosterone, and 4-androsten-3β-ol-17-one, 5-androsten-3α-ol-17-one, and 5-androsten-3,17-dione do not have any antiapoptotic activity in serum-starved cells. (ii) Hydroxylation at C7 (7α-hydroxy-DHEA, 7β-hydroxy-DHEA) or at C17 (hermaphrodiol) resulted in a loss of antiapoptotic activity. (*b*) *Pregnanes:* Conformation 3α-OH is crucial since the 3β-OH analogue of Allo, epiallopregnanolone had no effect. On the other hand, the α or β conformation of C5 is not critical for antiapoptotic activity since pregnanolone and its sulfate ester are effective.

The prosurvival effect of DHEA(S) and Allo use the major prosurvival pathway in sympathoadrenal cells, the antiapoptotic Bcl-2 proteins. Indeed, DHEA(S) and Allo induce the expression of the antiapoptotic Bcl-2 and Bcl-xL proteins.[22] The role of these proteins appears to be crucial since inhibition of their production by antisense oligonucleotides (directed toward the translation initiation site of the Bcl-2 transcript) resulted in an almost complete abolition of the protective effect of neuroactive steroids. The promoter regions of antiapoptotic Bcl-2 and Bcl-xL genes contain the cAMP-response element (CRE) and the NF-κB sensitive motif, and transcription factors CREB and NF-κB[23,24] have been identified as positive regulators of Bcl-2 and Bcl-xL gene expression, and have been involved in neuroprotective and survival mechanisms of central and peripheral neurons. Confocal laser scanning microscopy localization of p65 NF-κB shows that in PC12 cells cultured in serum-supplemented media NF-κB is almost exclusively localized within the nucleus, while in cells maintained in serum-free media NF-κB is found in the cytoplasm. In serum-deprived cells exposed to DHEA or Allo, NF-κB staining is mainly seen within the nucleus, as in the case of serum-supplemented cells. These neurosteroids affect also the phosphorylation/activation of CREB protein. Indeed, Western blot analysis, using cell extracts from serum-deprived PC12 cells, treated for 1 h with DHEA, DHEAS, and Allo, and antibodies specific for the phosphorylated and total forms of CREB, shows that serum deprivation results in a sharp, within 1 h, decrease of phosphorylated CREB, compared to serum-supplemented cells. However, in serum-deprived cells exposed to neuroactive steroids, levels of phosphorylated CREB are almost completely restored to those seen with serum supplementation. Phosphorylation of Bcl-2 at serine 70 is required for its antiapoptotic function.[25] It is now well documented in various biological systems that phosphorylation of Bcl-2 is afforded by αβ forms of PKC. Western blot analysis, performed on cell extracts from serum-deprived PC12 cells, treated for various time periods with DHEA, DHEAS, and Allo, using antibodies specific for the phosphorylated and total forms of PKCαβ, shows that in serum-deprived cells exposed to steroids for 10 and 20 min, levels of phosphorylated PKCαβ are highly induced, compared to those seen in serum-deprived cells cultured in the absence of adrenal steroids.[22]

These data suggest that DHEA and Allo may protect neural crest–derived cells against apoptosis, by tightly controlling the expression of antiapoptotic Bcl-2 proteins, both at transcriptional and posttranslational levels, activating the prosurvival transcription factors CREB and NF-κB, as well as the PKCαβ kinase (FIG. 1).

DHEAS AND ALLO DIRECTLY STIMULKATE THE BIOSYNTHESIS AND SECRETION OF NEUROPROTECTIVE CATECHOLAMINES

A deficiency in the noradrenergic system of the brain, originating largely from cells in the locus coeruleus (LC), is theorized to play a critical role in the

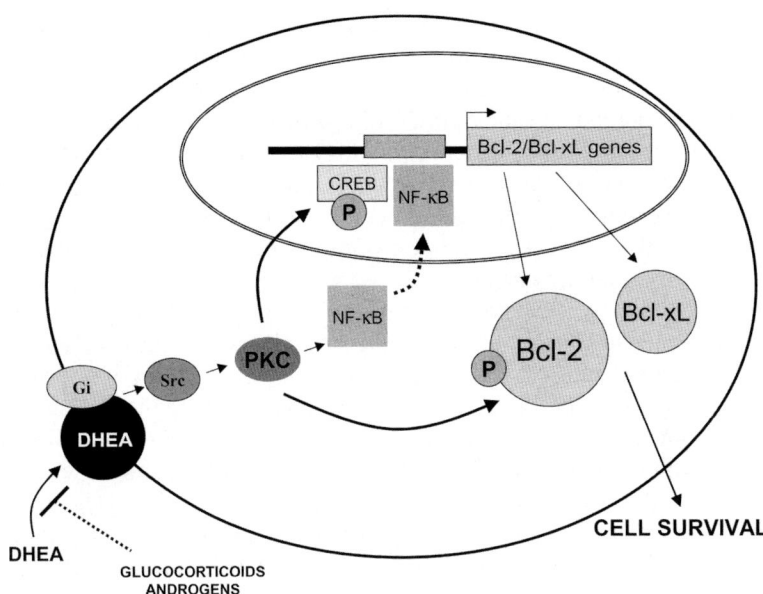

FIGURE 1. Hypothetical mechanism of the neuroprotective actions of neurosteroids. DHEA protects neural crest–derived cells against apoptosis by tightly controlling the expression of antiapoptotic Bcl-2 proteins, both at transcriptional and posttranslational levels. They bind on G-protein-associated binding sites, downstream activating the prosurvival Src-PKC kinases, which then activate the prosurvival transcription factors CREB and NF-κB, and stimulate the expression of antiapoptotic Bcl-2 proteins. Glucocorticoids and androgens act as endogenous antagonists of the DHEA actions, via competition on the G-protein membrane binding sites.

progression of a family of neurodegenerative disorders that includes Parkinson's disease (PD) and AD. Findings in animal models of PD indicate that the modification of LC-noradrenergic activity alters electrophysiological, neurochemical, and behavioral indices of neurotransmission in the nigrostriatal dopaminergic system, and influences the response of this system to experimental lesions. In models related to AD, noradrenergic mechanisms appear to play important roles in modulating the activity of the basalocortical cholinergic system and its response to injury, and to modify cognitive functions including memory and attention. Catecholamines promote recovery from neural damage by affecting neuroplasticity, neurotrophic factors (BDNF), neurogenesis, inflammation, cellular energy metabolism, excitotoxicity, and oxidative stress.

Recent experimental evidence suggests that neuroactive steroids, such as DHEA, DHEAS, and Allo, have indirect modulatory effects on brain catecholamine turnover. Indeed, DHEAS has been shown to potentiate NMDA-evoked norepinephrine secretion in rat hippocampal cells,[27] while in the mouse, DHEA prevents MPTP-induced dopamine depletion in striatal neurons.[28]

It now appears that neurosteroids may exert part of their neuroprotective effects by directly regulating neuroprotective catecholamines. Indeed, DHEA, DHEAS, and Allo may increase rapidly (within 10 min) the secretion of dopamine and norepinephrine from PC12 sympathoadrenal cells.[29] The effect of all three steroids is dose-dependent, with EC_{50} at the nM level. It appears that the acute effect of these steroids involves actin filament disassembly, a fast-response cellular system regulating trafficking of catecholamine vesicles. Specifically, 10^{-6} M of phallacidin, an actin filament stabilizer, completely prevents steroid-induced catecholamine secretion.[29]

In addition to their effect on catecholamine secretion, neurosteroids also directly affect catecholamine synthesis. Indeed, DHEAS and Allo exert a chronic effect on catecholamines *in vitro*, by stimulating the expression of tyrosine hydroxylase (TH), the rate-limiting enzyme of catecholamine biosynthesis. RT-PCR, real-time PCR, and Western blot experiments have shown that DHEAS and Allo result in a strong fourfold induction of both mRNA and protein levels of tyrosine hydroxylase (TH), within 6 h and 8 h, respectively, suggesting a direct transcriptional effect on TH expression.[29] The effects of DHEAS and Allo are completely blocked by AMPT and NSD-1015, inhibitors of TH and L-aromatic amino acid decarboxylase, respectively, further supporting the hypothesis that their effect involves catecholamine synthesis. It is thus possible that DHEAS and Allo exert multiple effects on catecholamines, closely monitoring their *de novo* synthesis and secretion (FIG. 2).

The possible physiological significance of these findings can be based on several published reports showing that with advancing age, the intra-adrenal and circulating levels of DHEAS decline in humans.[1–4] Indeed, it has been calculated that by the age of 70 years the circulating levels of DHEAS decrease by about 20% compared to young adults. It is of note that the release of epinephrine from the human adrenal medulla at rest was found to be lower in older men, 112 ng/mL compared to 248 ng/mL in younger men.[12,30] Furthermore, in younger men, the secretion of epinephrine doubles or even triples with mental stress, with isometric or dynamic exercise, compared to older men, who can master only 33% of the corresponding responses of younger men.[30] Thus, the decline of DHEAS and Allo production from zona reticularis of the adrenal cortex may affect catecholamine levels and the effectiveness of adrenal medulla to respond to sympathetic stimuli, particularly with advancing age. These findings suggest that an intra-adrenal paracrine regulatory loop is in action between adrenal neuroactive steroids and catecholamines, which may be deregulated with advancing age. This hypothesis is supported by recent experimental findings in H295R human adrenocortical cells showing that the synthetic catecholamine isoproterenol increases dose-dependently the secretion of DHEA.[31] Similarly, isoproterenol stimulates DHEAS production from human fetal adrenocortical cells in culture.[32] As mentioned before, DHEA affects brain catecholamines, potentiating NMDA-evoked norepinephrine secretion in rat hippocampal cells,[27] while in the mouse DHEA prevents MPTP-induced

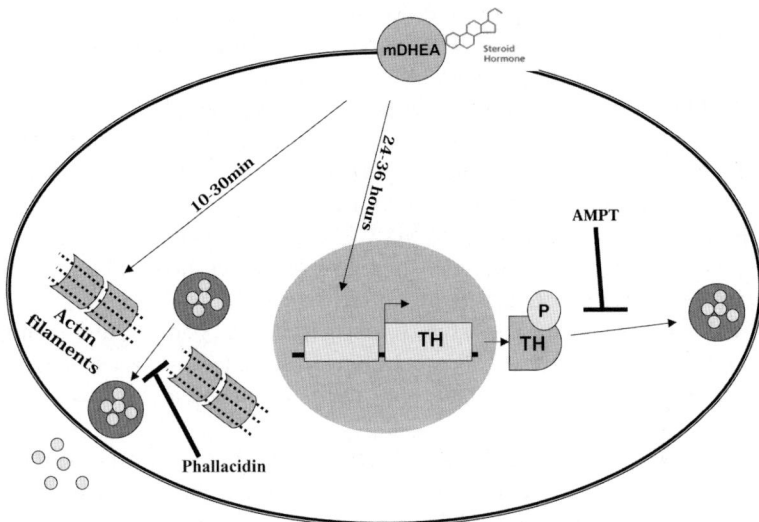

FIGURE 2. Hypothetical model of the stimulatory effects of neurosteroids on synthesis and secretion of neuroprotective catecholamines. DHEA sulfate and allopregnanolone directly stimulate biosynthesis and release of neuroprotective catecholamines, exerting a direct transcriptional effect on tyrosine hydroxylase, and regulating actin depolymerization and submembrane actin filament disassembly, a fast-response cellular system regulating trafficking of catecholamine vesicles. Phallacidin, a stabilizer of the submembrane actin cytoskeleton, inhibits the effects of DHEAS and Allo on catecholamine secretion. AMPT, a tyrosine hydroxylase inhibitor, blocks the effect of neurosteroids on catecholamine biosynthesis.

dopamine depletion in striatal neurons.[28] These findings suggest that DHEAS and Allo may directly augment dopamine and norepinephrine levels in the brain too. Induction of dopamine or norepinephrine secretion and production by DHEAS and Allo might contribute to the neuroprotective effects of these neurosteroids, further suggesting their involvement in the pathophysiology of aging-related neurodegenative processes, such as PD and AD.[20,21,33]

DHEA EXERTS ITS NEUROPROTECTIVE EFFECTS BY BINDING ON G-PROTEIN-COUPLED MEMBRANE BINDING SITES

The antiapoptotic effect of DHEA(S) in sympathoadrenal cells appears to be independent of most known receptors, associated with neurodegenerative/neuroprotective processes. It is known that part of the effects of DHEA depends on the conversion to estrogens and androgens and on the recruitment of the respective intracellular receptors. It is of note that PC12 cells do not express functional NMDA and GABA$_A$ receptors, while estrogen receptor (ER) and sigma1 (σ1)-receptor antagonists failed to reverse the antiapoptotic actions of DHEA(S).[22] The possibility of DHEA and estradiol acting through the same membrane binding is weak, since DHEA(S) failed to displace tritiated estradiol from its binding on PC12 cell membranes.[22] DHEA and DHEAS were shown to exert most of their actions on neural cells at micromolar concentrations, modulating NMDA, GABA$_A$, and sigma1 receptors.[5–7] However, DHEA and DHEAS, at low concentrations (1 nM), may protect NMDA- and GABA$_A$-receptor negative neural crest–derived PC12 rat sympathoadrenal cells against apoptosis, activating within minutes the prosurvival factors NF-κB and CREB, two upstream effectors of antiapoptotic Bcl-2 proteins.[22] Furthermore, in the same cell system, these neurosteroids, at nanomolar concentrations stimulate acutely (within 10 min) the secretion of catecholamines via induction of the depolymerization and disassembly of the submembrane actin cytoskeleton.[29]

The rapid onset of these actions supports the hypothesis that DHEA may use a membrane receptor system, although an intracellular receptor cannot be excluded. Membrane-impermeable DHEA conjugated to bovine serum albumin (BSA), a molecule with no intracellular penetrance abilities, can protect PC12 cells against serum deprivation-induced apoptosis with an apparent IC$_{50}$ of 1.5 nM, in a manner similar to that of unconjugated DHEA/DHEAS (1.8 nM), strongly suggesting the involvement of specific membrane binding sites.[34] Furthermore, DHEA-BSA effectively mimicked DHEA/DHEAS actions on antiapoptotic Bcl-2 proteins, by preventing their downregulation by serum deprivation. Saturation binding assays of [^{3}H]-DHEA on isolated PC12 cell membranes revealed a rapidly saturable (30 min) binding of DHEA, with an apparent K$_D$ of 0.9 nM. Similar binding assays indicate DHEA binding at high affinity on membranes isolated from rat hippocampal cells (K$_D$: 61.9 nM) and from human normal adrenal chromaffin cells (K$_D$: 0.1 nM). DHEA-specific membrane binding to PC12 plasma membranes was also confirmed with the DHEA-BSA-FITC conjugate using flow cytometry and confocal laser microscopy. Thus, our findings suggest the presence on neural crest–derived cells of DHEA-specific high-affinity membrane binding sites that mediate the neuroprotective effect of DHEA.

Experimental evidence suggests the involvement of Gi protein in the DHEA- and DHEA-BSA-induced protection of PC12 cells against serum deprivation-induced apoptosis, since their beneficial effect was abolished in the presence of 10^{-6}M pertussis toxin (PTX).[34] The ability of DHEA and DHEA-BSA to protect against serum deprivation-induced suppression of the antiapoptotic and prosurvival Bcl-2/Bcl-xL proteins was also completely abolished in the presence of PTX. Furthermore, DHEA increased the specific binding of [^{35}S]-GTPγS on PC12 cell membrane preparations in a dose-dependent manner. Taken together, these findings provide further support for previous observations that link membrane DHEA binding to Gi proteins. Indeed, recent experimental findings suggest that the DHEA binding on plasma membranes of bovine aortic endothelial cells may be functionally coupled to Gi proteins.[35] Furthermore, on the basis of recent findings showing phosphorylation activation of Src tyrosine kinase by direct interaction with $G\alpha i$,[36] it was hypothesized that DHEA activates Src kinase by a Gi-dependent pathway.[35] Interestingly, both DHEA and DHEA-BSA rapidly increased the phosphorylation of Src (within 5 min of exposure), an effect that was completely reversed by the Gi inhibitor PTX.[35] It should be noted here that activation of the Src-PKC pathway induces NF-κB activity and PC12 cell survival.[37] These observations considered together suggest that DHEA may exert its protective effects, activating G-protein-associated membrane binding sites, and the subsequent activation of prosurvival Src-PKC kinases, leading finally to mobilization of transcription factor NF-κB and the production of antiapoptotic Bcl-2 proteins (FIG. 1).

Several structurally related steroids, including the synthetic estrogen diethylstilbestrol, progestin ORG2058, and the pregnane Allo, are unable to compete with [³H]-DHEA for binding at concentrations ranging from 1 pM to 1 μM. On the other hand, the DHEA sulfate ester (DHEAS) is an efficient competitor with an IC_{50} of 1.3 nM, that is, similar to that of DHEA (1.5 nM) and to the K_D of DHEA binding (0.9 nM). Interestingly, glucocorticoids and androgens showed a 10–15-fold lower affinity for the DHEA membrane binding sites, displacing 70% and 60% of [³H]-DHEA binding at a concentration of 1 μM. However, these steroids completely lacked protective antiapoptotic effects on PC12 cells.[22] These observations support the hypothesis that androgens and glucocorticoids may act as endogenous antagonists of DHEA. Indeed, priming of PC12 cells for 30 min with DEX or DHT followed by exposure to DHEA with a molar excess of DEX or DHT completely reverses the protective effects of DHEA, as well as its stimulatory effect on the antiapoptotic Bcl-2 proteins and prosurvival Src activation.[34] It is thus logical to assume that glucocorticoids and androgens act as antagonists of DHEA by binding to common membrane binding sites.

Glucocorticoids and testosterone can exert neurotoxic effects on a range of tissues.[38–40] Indeed, chronic exposure to glucocorticoids has been associated with decreased cognitive performance, attenuation of synaptic efficacy, and neuronal atrophy. Elevation of glucocorticoids during aging is also associated with cognitive impairment and hippocampal atrophy. Furthermore, earlier animal experiments have shown that overexposure to glucocorticoids during prolonged periods of stress is detrimental to CNS neurons, especially in aged animals, affecting mainly the hippocampus. Cumulative exposure to corticosteroids or to chronic stress, with its ensuing increase in corticosteroid levels, caused degenerative loss of pyramidal neurons in the hippocampus, and reduced cell numbers in CA1 and CA3 and subsequent deficits in memory function and cognition in rats. Meanwhile, the greater tendency to nigrostriatal dopaminergic neurotoxicity and neurodegeneration in PD observed in males[41]

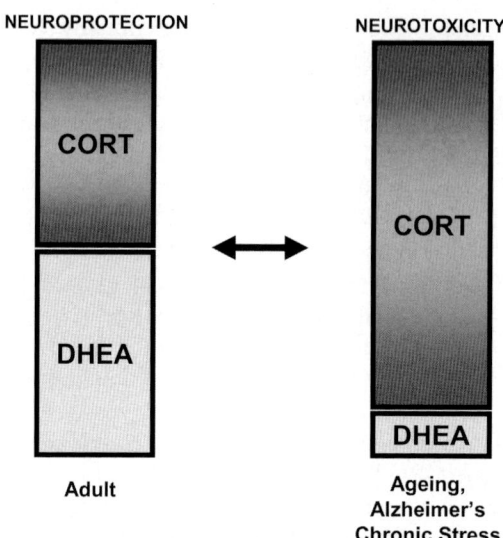

FIGURE 3. Glucocorticoids exert neurotoxic effects. Chronic exposure to glucocorticoids is associated with decreased cognitive performance, attenuation of synaptic efficacy, and neuronal atrophy. Elevation of glucocorticoids during aging is also associated with cognitive impairment and hippocampal atrophy. It is possible that part of neurotoxic effects of glucocorticoids could be attributed to their antagonistic effect on the neuroprotective effect of endogenous DHEA. The decline of brain DHEA levels during aging and in AD might exacerbate this phenomenon, rendering neurons more vulnerable to glucocorticoid toxicity.

may be partially attributed to the neurotoxic effect of testosterone. In recent studies, testosterone has been shown to possess a deleterious effect on ischemic stroke in a focal ischemia model, whereas acute testosterone depletion exerts a neuroprotective effect, suggesting that testosterone could also contribute to gender differences in the outcome of stroke.[42] These findings considered together suggest that part of neurotoxic effects of glucocorticoids (FIG. 3) and testosterone (FIG. 4) could be attributed to their antagonistic effect on the neuroprotective effect of endogenous DHEA. Indeed, it was recently shown that corticosterone and testosterone displace [^{3}H]-DHEA binding on isolated PC12 plasma membranes and at the same time prevent DHEA and DHEA-BSA, protecting against serum deprivation-induced apoptosis.[34] Effects on the antiapoptotic Bcl-2 proteins and the prosurvival Src support further this hypothesis. The decline of brain DHEA levels during aging and in AD[1–4] might exacerbate this phenomenon, rendering neurons more vulnerable to glucocorticoid and androgen toxicity. Furthermore, glucocorticoid neurotoxicity becomes more pronounced in aged subjects since cortisol levels in the CSF increase in the course of normal aging, as well as in relatively early stages of AD.[43,44]

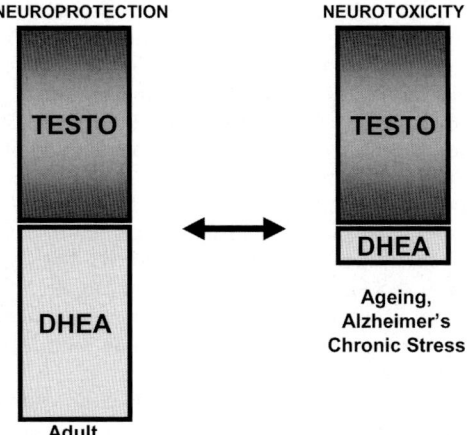

FIGURE 4. Testosterone exerts neurotoxic effects. Greater tendency to nigrostriatal dopaminergic neurotoxicity and neurodegeneration in PD is observed in males. Testosterone has deleterious effects on ischemic stroke, whereas acute testosterone depletion exerts a neuroprotective effect. We hypothesize that part of the neurotoxic effects of testosterone could be attributed to their antagonistic effect on the neuroprotective effect of endogenous DHEA. The decline of brain DHEA levels during aging and in AD might exacerbate this phenomenon, rendering neurons more vulnerable to testosterone toxicity.

ACKNOWLEDGMENTS

This work is supported by a grant from GGET (General Secretariat of Research and Technology) (PENED2001- ED258).

REFERENCES

1. ORENTREICH, N., J.L. BRIND, R.L. RIZER & J.H. VOGELMAN. 1984. Age changes and sex differences in serum dehydroepiandrosterone sulfate concentrations throughout adulthood. J. Clin. Endocrinol. Metab. **59:** 551–555.
2. BE'LANGER, A., B. CANDAS, A. DUPONT, *et al.* 1994. Changes in serum concentrations of conjugated and unconjugated steroids in 40- to 80-year old men. J. Clin. Endocrinol. Metab. **79:** 1086–1090.
3. GENAZZANI, A.R., F. PETRAGLIA, F. BERNARDI, *et al.* 1998. Circulating levels of allopregnanolone in humans: gender, age, and endocrine influences. J. Clin. Endocrinol. Metab. **83:** 2099–2103.
4. BERNARDI, F., C. SALVESTRONI, E. CASAROSA, *et al.* 1998. Aging is associated with changes in allopregnanolone concentrations in brain, endocrine glands and serum in male rats. Eur. J. Endocrinol. **138:** 316–321.
5. WOLKOWITZ, O.M., E.S. EPEL & V.I. REUS. 2001. Stress hormone-related psychopathology: pathophysiological and treatment implications. World J. Biol. Psychiatry **2:** 115–143.

6. STRAUB, R.H., K. LEHLE, H. HERFARTH, *et al.* 2002. Dehydroepiandrosterone in relation to other adrenal hormones during an acute inflammatory stressful disease state compared with chronic inflammatory disease: role of interleukin-6 and tumour necrosis factor. Eur. J. Endocrinol. **146:** 365–374.

7. BAULIEU, E.E. & P. ROBEL. 1998. Dehydroepiandrosterone (DHEA) and dehydroepiandrosterone sulfate (DHEAS) as neuroactive neurosteroids. Proc. Natl. Acad. Sci. USA **95:** 4089–4091.

8. MENSAH-NYAGAN, A.G., J.L. DO-REGO, D. BEAUJEAN, *et al.* 1999. Neurosteroids: expression of steroidogenic enzymes and regulation of steroid biosynthesis in the central nervous system. Pharmacol. Rev. **51:** 63–81.

9. COMPAGNONE, N.A. & S.H. MELLON. 2000. Neurosteroids: biosynthesis and function of these novel neuromodulators. Front. Neuroendocrinol. **21:** 1–56.

10. SAPOLSKY, R.M. 1992. Stress, the Aging Brain and the Mechanism of Neuron Death. MIT Press, Cambridge, MA.

11. SEALS, D.R. & M. ESLER. 2000. Human ageing and the sympathoadrenal system. J. Physiol. **528:** 407–417.

12. ESLER, M., G. LAMBERT, D. KAYE, *et al.* 2002. Influence of ageing on the sympathetic nervous system and adrenal medulla at rest and during stress. Biogerontology **3:** 45–49.

13. BASTIANETTO, S., C. RAMASSAMY, J. POIRIER & R. QUIRION. 1999. Dehydroepiandrosterone (DHEA) protects hippocampal cells from oxidative stress-induced damage. Brain Res. Mol. Brain Res. **66:** 35–41.

14. CARDOUNEL, A., W. REGELSON & M. KALIMI. 1999. Dehydroepiandrosterone protects hippocampal neurons against neurotoxin-induced cell death: mechanism of action. Proc. Soc. Exp. Biol. Med. **22:** 145–149.

15. LAPCHAK, P.A., D.F. CHAPMAN, S.Y. NUNEZ & J.A. ZIVIN. 2000. Dehydroepiandrosterone sulfate is neuroprotective in a reversible spinal cord ischemia model: possible involvement of GABA(A) receptors. Stroke **31:** 1953–1956.

16. KIMONIDES, V.G., N.H. KHATIBI, C.N. SVENDSEN, *et al.* 1998. Dehydroepiandrosterone (DHEA) and DHEA-sulfate (DHEAS) protect hippocampal neurons against excitatory amino acid-induced neurotoxicity. Proc. Natl. Acad. Sci. USA **95:** 1852–1857.

17. LOCKHART, E., D. WARNER, R. PEARLSTEIN, *et al.* 2002. Allopregnanolone attenuates N-methyl-D-aspartate-induced excitotoxicity and apoptosis in the human NT2 cell line in culture. Neurosci. Lett. **238:** 33–36.

18. WEILL-ENGERER, S., J.P. DAVID, V. SAZDOVITCH, *et al.* 2002. Neurosteroid quantification in human brain regions: comparison between Alzheimer's and nondemented patients. J. Clin. Endocrinol. Metab. **87:** 5138–5143.

19. SCHUMACHER, M., S. WEILL-ENGERER, P. LIERE, *et al.* 2003. Steroid hormones and neurosteroids in normal and pathological aging of the nervous system. Prog. Neurobiol. **71:** 3–29.

20. BELANGER, N., L. GREGOIRE, P. BEDARD & T. DI PAOLO. 2003. Estradiol and dehydroepiandrosterone potentiate levodopa-induced locomotor activity in 1-methyl-4-phenyl-1,2,3,6-tetrahydropyridine monkeys. Endocrine **1:** 97–101.

21. BELANGER, N., L. GREGOIRE, P.J. BEDARD & T. DI PAOLO. 2005. DHEA improves symptomatic treatment of moderately and severely impaired MPTP monkeys. Neurobiol Aging. 2005 Oct 24; e-pub ahead of print.

22. CHARALAMPOPOULOS, I., C. TSATSANIS, E. DERMITZAKI, *et al.* 2004. Dehydroepiandrosterone and allopregnanolone protect sympathoadrenal cells against

apoptosis, via Bcl-2 antiapoptotic proteins. Proc. Natl. Acad. Sci. USA **101:** 8209–8214.

23. RICCIO, A., S. AHN, C.M. DAVENPORT, *et al.* 1999. Mediation by a CREB family transcription factor of NGF-dependent survival of sympathetic neurons. Science **286:** 2358–2361.

24. TAMATANI, M., Y.H. CHE, H. MATSUZAKI, *et al.* 1999. Tumor necrosis factor induces Bcl-2 and Bcl-x expression through NFkappaB activation in primary hippocampal neurons. J. Biol. Chem. **274:** 8531–8538.

25. RUVOLO, P., X. DENG, B. CARR & W.S. MAY. 1998. A functional role for mitochondrial protein kinase C alpha in Bcl2 phosphorylation and suppression of apoptosis. J. Biol. Chem. **273:** 25436–25442.

26. MARIEN, M., F.C. COLPAERT & A. ROSENQUIST. 2004. Noradrenergic mechanisms in neurodegenerative diseases: a theory. Brain Res. Rev. **45:** 38–78.

27. MONNET, F., V. MAHE, P. ROBEL & E.E. BAULIEU. 1995. Neurosteroids via σ receptors modulate the [3H]norepinephrine release evoked by NMDA in the rat hippocampus. Proc. Natl. Acad. Sci. USA **92:** 3774–3778.

28. D'ASTOUS, M., M. MORISSETTE, B. TANGUAY, *et al.* 2003. Dehydroepiandrosterone (DHEA) such as 17beta estradiol prevents MPTP-induced dopamine depletion in mice. Synapse **47:** 10–14.

29. CHARALAMPOPOULOS, I., E. DERMITZAKI, L. VARDOULI, *et al.* 2005. Dehydroepiandrosterone and allopregnanolone directly stimulate catecholamine production via induction of tyrosine hydroxylase and secretion by affecting actin polymerization. Endocrinology **146:** 3309–3318.

30. ESLER, M., D. KAYE, J. THOMPSON, *et al.* 1995. Effects of ageing on epinephrine secretion and regional release of epinephrine from the human heart. J. Clin. Endocrinol. Metab. **80:** 435–442.

31. KOSTI, O., P.J. KING & J.P. HINSON. 2002. Tumor-derived human adrenocortical cells express beta adrenergic receptors: steroidogenic effects of beta-adrenergic input. Endocr. Res. **28:** 363–367.

32. BREAULT, L., L. YON, M. MONTERO, *et al.* 2000. Occurrence and effect of PACAP in the human fetal adrenal gland. Ann. N.Y. Acad. Sci. **921:** 429–433.

33. TOMAS-CAMARDIEL, M., M.C. SANCHEZ-HIDALGO, M.J. SANCHEZ DEL PINO, *et al.* 2002. Comparative study of the neuroprotective effect of dehydroepiandrosterone and 17beta-estradiol against 1-methyl-4-phenylpyridium toxicity on rat striatum. Neuroscience **109:** 569–584.

34. CHARALAMPOPOULOS, I., V.I. ALEXAKI, I. LAZARIDIS, *et al.* 2006. G protein-associated, specific membrane binding sites mediate the neuroprotective effect of dehydroepiandrosterone. FASEB J. **20:** 577–579.

35. LIU, D. & J.S. DILLON. 2002. Dehydroepiandrosterone activates endothelial cell nitric-oxide synthase by a specific plasma membrane receptor coupled to G alpha(i2,3). J. Biol. Chem. **277:** 21379–21388.

36. MA, Y.C., J. HUANG, S. ALI, *et al.* 2000. Src tyrosine kinase is a novel direct effector of G proteins. Cell **102:** 636–646.

37. WOOTEN, M., M.L. SEIBENHENER, K. NEIDICH & M. VANDENPLAS. 2000. Mapping of atypical protein kinase C within the nerve growth factor signaling cascade: relationship to differentiation and survival of PC12 cells. Mol. Cell. Biol. **20:** 4494–4504.

38. SWAAB, D.F., A.M. BAO & P.J. LUCASSEN. 2005. The stress system in the human brain in depression and neurodegeneration. Ageing Res. Rev. **2:** 141–194.

39. SAPOLSKY, R.M. 1986. Glucocorticoid toxicity in the hippocampus: reversal by supplementation with brain fuels. J. Neurosci. **6:** 2240–2244.
40. SAPOLSKY, R.M., L.C. KREY & B.S. MCEWEN. 1986. The neuroendocrinology of stress and aging: the glucocorticoid cascade hypothesis. Endocrine Revs **7:** 284–301.
41. MARDER, K., M.X. TANG, H. MEJIA, et al. 1996. Risk of Parkinson's disease among first-degree relatives: a community-based study. Neurology **47:** 155–160.
42. YANG, S.H., E. PEREZ, J. CUTRIGHT, et al. 2002. Testosterone increases neurotoxicity of glutamate in vitro and ischemia-reperfusion injury in an animal model. J. Appl. Physiol. **1:** 195–201.
43. SWAAB, D.F., F.C. RAADSHEER, E. ENDERT, et al. 1994. Increased cortisol levels in aging and Alzheimer's disease in postmortem cerebrospinal fluid. J. Neuroendocrinol. **6:** 681–687.
44. UMEGAKI, H., H. IKARI, H. NAKAHATA, et al. 2000. Plasma cortisol levels in elderly female subjects with Alzheimer's disease: a cross-sectional and longitudinal study. Brain Res. **881:** 241–243.

Role of Thymulin or Its Analogue as a New Analgesic Molecule

MIREILLE DARDENNE,[a] NAYEF SAADE,[b] AND BARED SAFIEH-GARABEDIAN[c]

[a]CNRS UMR 8147, Hôpital Necker, University Paris V, Paris, France

[b]Department of Human Morphology, American University of Beirut, Beirut, Lebanon

[c]Department of Biology, American University of Beirut, Beirut, Lebanon

ABSTRACT: The thymic peptide thymulin is known for its immunomodulatory role. However, several recent reports have indicated that thymulin is capable of interacting directly and/or indirectly with the nervous system. One of the first lines of evidence of this interaction was obtained in a series of experiments showing the hyperalgesic actions of this peptide. We demonstrated that, at low doses (ng), local (intraplantar) or systemic (intraperitoneal) injections of thymulin resulted in hyperalgesia with an increase in proinflammatory mediators, and that this peptide could act directly on the afferent nerve terminals through prostaglandin-E2 (PGE2)-dependent mechanisms, thus forming a neuroimmune loop involving capsaicin-sensitive primary afferent fibers. In further experiments, systemic injections of relatively high doses (1–25 μg) of thymulin or of an analogue peptide (PAT) deprived of hyperalgesic effect, have been shown to reduce the inflammatory pain and the upregulated levels of cytokines induced by endotoxin (ET) injection. In addition, PAT treatment appeared to alleviate the sickness behavior (motor behavior and fever) induced by systemic inflammation. These effects could be attributed, at least partly, to the downregulation of proinflammatory mediators. Furthermore, when compared with the effects of other anti-inflammatory drugs, PAT exerted equal or even stronger analgesic effects, and at much lower concentrations. Subsequent experiments were designed to examine the effects of intracerebroventricular (i.c.v.) injections of thymulin on cerebral inflammation induced by i.c.v. injection of ET. Pretreatment with thymulin reduced, in a dose-dependant manner, the ET-induced hyperalgesia, and exerted differential effects on the upregulated levels of cytokines in different areas of the brain, suggesting a neuroprotective role for thymulin in the central nervous system (CNS). Preliminary results demonstrate that thymulin inhibits in the hippocampus the ET-induced nuclear activation of NF-κB, the transcription factor required for the expression of proinflammatory cytokines genes. Although the

Address for correspondence: Mireille Dardenne, CNRS UMR 8147–Université Paris V, Hôpital Necker, 161 rue de Sèvres, 75015 Paris, France. Voice: 33-1-44-49-53-91; fax: 33-1-44-49-06-76.
e-mail: dardenne@necker.fr

Ann. N.Y. Acad. Sci. 1088: 153–163 (2006). © 2006 New York Academy of Sciences.
doi: 10.1196/annals.1366.006

mechanism of action of these molecules is not totally elucidated, our results indicate a possible therapeutic use of thymulin or PAT as analgesic
and anti-inflammatory drugs.

KEYWORDS: thymulin; PAT (peptide analogue of thymulin); hyperalgesia; analgesics; inflammation; cytokines; thymus

INTRODUCTION

Thymulin, a highly conserved nonapeptide synthesized by two discrete populations of thymic epithelial cells, has been characterized mainly for its role in
the immune system.[1] It has been shown to have two major actions on T cells
and their immature precursors; first, induction of differentiation markers and
second, enhancement of various T and NK cell activities.[2] Thymulin requires
the presence of zinc to express its biological activity.[3]

More recent evidence points to an important role for thymulin as a signaling molecule for interaction between the immune, endocrine, and the nervous
system.[4] Immunohistochemical techniques have shown the presence of this
peptide in astrocytic glial cells in the brain and skin basal keratinocytes.[5] Several studies have described a bidirectional communication between the thymic
epithelium and the hypothalamus-pituitary axis.[6] For example, thymulin has
been shown to be released into the blood with a circadian rhythm coinciding
with the activity of the hypothalamus-pituitary axis.[7] Moreover, adrenocorticotrophic hormone (ACTH), at physiological levels, injected into rats elevates
plasma thymulin, whereas ACTH, administered *in vitro*, stimulates thymulin
release from cultured thymic fragments.[8] Other hormones, including prolactin,
growth, and thyroid hormones, also exert regulatory effects on thymulin release.[6] All these observations support the existence of a bidirectional communication between the immune and the nervous system, which is believed
to represent an important homeostatic mechanism. Cytokines and other products of immunocompetent cells are known to play a crucial role as signaling
molecules in these interactions.[9] During inflammation, interactions between
the immune and the nervous system become more apparent. In this review, we
provide further evidence that strongly supports the hypothesis that thymulin
can interact with the nervous system either directly or indirectly, thus forming
an afferent component in a neuroendocrine immune loop.

HYPERALGESIC ACTIONS OF THYMULIN

One of the first lines of evidence indicating that thymulin interacts with the
nervous system was obtained in a series of experiments showing the hyperalgesic actions of this peptide. Various doses of thymulin were administered
either via intraperitoneal (i.p.) or intraplantar (i.pl.) injections, and their effects

on pain-related behavior and cytokine levels were assessed. Intraperitoneal injection of low doses of thymulin resulted in both mechanical hyperalgesia, as assessed by the paw pressure (PP) test, and thermal hyperalgesia, as assessed by the hot plate (HP) and tail-flick (TF) tests. The effect was apparent at doses ranging between 20–150 ng.[10] Similar observations were obtained with i.pl. injections of thymulin (0.5 ng, 1 ng, 5 ng, and 10 ng), which resulted in a significant reduction in nociceptive thresholds, localized to the injected hind paw of the rats, as assessed by the different pain tests.[11]

Thymulin-induced hyperalgesia, of either somatic or visceral origin, was not accompanied by any signs of inflammation (redness, swelling, edema). It is interesting to note here that thymulin-induced hyperalgesia was significantly reduced by pretreatment with the tripeptide Lys-D-pro-val,[10] known to antagonize interleukin-1β (IL-1β) and prostaglandin-E2 (PGE2)–induced hyperalgesia.[12] On the other hand, lys-D-pro-thr, known to antagonize IL-1β-induced hyperalgesia,[13] was significantly less effective.[10]

Furthermore, thymulin-induced hyperalgesia was prevented by pretreatment with dexamethasone and indomethacin.[11] Subsequent evidence indicating an important role for PGE2 was obtained with experiments using the cyclooxygenase (COX) inhibitor meloxicam, with a preferential effect on COX-2.[14] Pretreatment with meloxicam produced a complete reversal of both mechanical and thermal hyperalgesia as assessed by the different pain tests. These results suggest that thymulin may be acting directly or indirectly on nerve terminals of the CNS. The results also indicate that PGE2 might be a key mediator in these actions.

Role of Proinflammatory Cytokines

We investigated the role of cytokines in thymulin-induced hyperalgesia. The effect of antitumor necrosis factor α (TNF-α), interleukin-1 receptor antagonist (IL-1ra), and antinerve growth factor (NGF) antiserum on thymulin-induced hyperalgesia was studied either with pretreatment with each of these reagents, 30 min before thymulin injection, or with a mixture of all three (the cocktail). Our results indicated that a mild reduction in thymulin-induced hyperalgesia was obtained by IL-ra, even when used at relatively high doses. On the other hand, anti-NGF antiserum, used at concentrations shown to be effective in reducing inflammatory hyperalgesia induced by complete Freund's adjuvant,[15] was only effective in reducing mechanical hyperalgesia as assessed by the PP test. A more effective reduction in thymulin-induced mechanical and thermal hyperalgesia was obtained by the anti-TNF-α antiserum, at doses used previously to neutralize endogenous TNF-α and resulting in the reduction of carrageenan-induced hyperalgesia.[16] These results demonstrate that each of these cytokines contribute, to some extent, to the thymulin-induced hyperalgesia. This assumption receives further support from the fact that pretreatment with a "cocktail" of the antisera and antagonists resulted in an almost complete

reversal of the thymulin-induced hyperalgesia. Further proof for the involvement of proinflammatory cytokines and other mediators was obtained with
experiments in which thymulin injection both i.p. and i.pl. resulted in a significant elevation in the level of proinflammatory mediators NGF and PGE2
as measured by specific ELISA.[17] For the experiments in which thymulin was
injected i.p. into a group of rats, the level of IL-1β, IL-6, TNF-α, NGF, and
PGE2 was determined in the liver of these animals and was found to be significantly elevated as compared to saline-treated controls.[10] Similarly, in rats
treated with thymulin (5 ng , i.pl.), there was a significant elevation in the level
of IL-1β and NGF in the injected paw as compared to the noninjected paw.[11]
When the effect of pretreatment with meloxicam was investigated, our results
showed that the increased levels of IL-1β, TNF-α, and NGF, due to thymulin
injection, recovered their control levels.

We can conclude, therefore, that the proinflammatory mediators play an important role in thymulin-induced hyperalgesia with PGE2 having a prominent
role.

Potential Action of Thymulin on the Nervous System

Previous results provide evidence for a possible direct and dual action of
thymulin on the peripheral (PNS) and central nervous systems (CNS).

On the one hand, it has been shown that the hyperalgesic effects of either i.p.
or i.pl. injections of thymulin are almost abolished in rats neonatally treated
with capsaicin.[18] Similar attenuation of thymulin-induced hyperalgesia (i.p.)
was observed in rats subjected to either subdiaphragmatic vagotomy or to ablation of the vagal capsaicin-sensitive fibers (CSPA). The residual hyperalgesic
effects of thymulin were attributed to either the mediation of thymulin effect
by non-CSPA fibers or to a possible humoral action of thymulin on the CNS.
On the other hand, more recently, the induction of fos-like immunoreactivity
(FLI) in the dorsal horn of the lumbosacral spinal cord of rats subjected to
i.pl. injections of thymulin has been reported.[19] Several lines of evidence are
in favor of the hypothesis that the FLI induced by thymulin may involve other
mechanisms than nociceptive processing[19]: (*a*) fos-labeled neurons showed
a temporal and spatial distribution different from those observed following
injection of endotoxin (ET) or other irritants; (*b*) morphine pretreatment reduced FLI induced by i.pl. injection of thymulin at a concentration of 4 mg/kg,
twice the amount needed to abolish FLI and hyperalgesia induced by i.pl. ET
injections[18,20]; (*c*) pretreatment with meloxicam, a cyclooxygenase inhibitor,
reduced thymulin-induced FLI at concentration of 2 mg/kg, while a dose of
0.4 mg/kg was sufficient to produce a significant reduction of the hyperalgesia
induced by similar injections of thymulin.[19]

All these data are in favor of the hypothesis of a possible action of thymulin on the PNS and the CNS, either directly or through PGE2-dependent
mechanisms.

TABLE 1. Effect of PAT on cytokine upregulation by i.pl. injection of ET (1.25 μg)

Treatment	IL-1 (pg/hind paw)	IL-6 (pg/hind paw)	NGF (ng/hind paw)	TNFα (pg/hind paw)
ET (1.25 μg) i. pl.	$2,850 \pm 255$	$2,831 \pm 285$	23 ± 1.73	350 ± 50
PAT (25 μg) + ET (1.25 μg)	$1,686 \pm 266$	$1,158 \pm 197$	16.73 ± 2.70	104 ± 12
P-value	< 0.05	< 0.01	< 0.01	< 0.001

Levels of each cytokine and NGF in the skin tissues of the hind paws are shown of a separate group of five rats for the indicated treatment. The levels of mediators were measured at the time peak of the upregulation by ET, which corresponds to 1 h for TNF and 3 h for the other mediators.

ANALGESIC AND ANTI-INFLAMMATORY EFFECTS OF THYMULIN AND ITS ANALOGUE, PAT

Two models of ET-induced inflammatory hyperalgesia have been characterized during the last decade. The first was based on systemic inflammation induced by i.p. injection of high doses of ET,[21] and the observed hyperalgesia, fever, and illness were attributed to the upregulation of cytokine levels, especially IL-1β and PGE2.[22] The second described inflammatory hyperalgesia that was induced by local (i.pl.) injection of a small dose of ET in rats and mice.[23] Further investigations showed that this localized inflammatory hyperalgesia was preceded by significant upregulation of proinflammatory cytokines and NGF[24,25] and that pretreatment with either anti-inflammatorey drugs or anti-inflammatory cytokines (IL-10) prevented the ET-induced hyperalgesia.[24,25] The present study was based on the use of both models, and showed significant inhibitory effects exerted by thymulin and PAT on the ET-induced hyperalgesia and upregulation of cytokine levels (TABLE 1).

Effects of High Doses of Thymulin on Inflammatory Hyperalgesia

In a first series of experiments, the possible effects of thymulin on pain behavior in normal animals and in animals with localized inflammation were investigated. The classical tests for mechanical (PP test) and thermal (HP, and TF tests) hyperalgesia were used. Different groups of rats and mice were subjected to pain tests for three consecutive days before and 1 day after intraperitoneal (i.p.) thymulin injections (0.5, 1, and 2 μg in 100 μL saline). Baseline values of the various pain tests in thymulin-injected animals were comparable to those of saline-injected rats. In a second group of experiments, the animals also received i.p. injections of thymulin (0.5, 1, and 2 μg in 100 μL saline) prior to intraplantar (i.pl.) ET injections (1.25 μg). At this dose level, ET has been shown to induce local inflammation and hyperalgesia, which peaks at 9 h in rats and 24 h in mice and subsequently recovers by 24 and 48 h, respectively.[23]

Thymulin injections reduced, in a dose-dependent manner, the ET-induced mechanical and thermal hyperalgesia. It was thus concluded that thymulin in supraphysiological doses can reverse inflammatory hyperalgesia without altering pain thresholds in intact animals. Further experiments were carried out to investigate whether this analgesic effect of thymulin correlates with changes in the levels of the proinflammatory cytokines IL-1β and nerve growth factor (NGF), specially in view of the recent demonstrations of a major role for the neurotrophin NGF in mediating inflammatory hyperalgesia.[26,27] During ET-induced hyperalgesia there was a significant increase in the levels of IL-1β and NGF, and pretreatment with steroidal and nonsteroidal anti-inflammatory drugs reversed the ET-induced hyperalgesia and downregulated the levels of IL-1β and NGF.[25] Pretreatment of rats with thymulin (1 μg in 100 μg saline, i.p.) prior to ET injection, downregulated IL-1β and NGF levels in a manner comparable to that observed with the anti-inflammatory drugs.[28] These findings strongly suggest that the attenuation of hyperalgesia by high doses of thymulin involve the downregulation of the proinflammatory cytokines.

Effect of PAT on Inflammatory Hyperalgesia

In a further study, we analyzed the analgesic and anti-inflammatory actions of a synthetic peptide analogue of thymulin (PAT), which was initially synthesized with the potential for clinical applications as an immunomodulating agent.[29] To characterize the analgesic and anti-inflammatory actions of PAT, we used the two animal models of inflammation and hyperalgesia already described using i.pl. and i.p. ET injections, the aim of this study being to investigate whether PAT could affect the inflammatory hyperalgesia and to compare the efficacy of this molecule to that of steroids, NSAIDs, and peptides with known anti-inflammatory and antihyperalgesic actions.

PAT in a single dose, was effective in decreasing the level of several inflammatory mediators, which may prove to be an important effect not shown by other anti-inflammatory molecules. As an illustration, PAT exerted stronger inhibition of ET-induced hyperalgesia than K (D)PV or K (D)PT and at a dosage at least 10 times lower than that used for both peptides.

Another interesting aspect in the effects of PAT treatment was the amelioration of the symptoms of illness behavior induced by systemic injection of ET. This amelioration took the form of reversal of the hyperalgesia, improvement of the motor behavior, and prevention of febrile reactions to ET. Cumulative evidence has shown that ET does not cross the blood–brain barrier[30] and can induce the illness behavior and fever through PGE2-dependent mechanisms.[22] Therefore, the antifebrile effect of PAT can be attributed to the inhibition of COX-2 mechanisms leading to PGE2 formation. This assumption can be correlated with the observed downregulation of the levels of cytokine and PGE2, which were shown to be upregulated in the liver following systemic injection of ET. However, we cannot exclude possible action of PAT, like thymulin, on the afferent nerve fibers involved in nociception and neuroimmune regulations.[18] Recent evidence demonstrates that PAT exerts strong inhibition of neuropathic manifestations, which are not necessarily the end product of inflammatory mechanisms.[31]

The observed antihyperalgesic action of PAT can be ascribed to its inhibitory effects on the inflammatory cascade through the downregulation of the levels of proinflammatory cytokines and NGF. This inhibition may be attributed, at least in part, to the inhibition of COX-2 mechanisms targeted by the NSAIDs. Thus, PAT may exert its antihyperalgesic effects, at least partially, as do NSAIDs, by reducing the inflammatory reactions.

ANTI-INFLAMMATORY EFFECTS OF THYMULIN-INJECTED INTRACEREBROVENTRICULARLY

Ample evidence implicates inflammatory processes in the development of a number of neurodegenerative diseases and demonstrates that neurons and microglia can serve as targets and/or sources for various cytokines, which are believed to be involved in the neuropathology.[32,33] An important aspect of brain injury is its association with increased production of cytokines.[34] Moreover, it is now established that many of these inflammatory molecules, commonly associated with the peripheral immune system, are also produced within the CNS.[35] The proinflammatory cytokines, including IL-1β, TNF-α, and IL-6, have been shown to play important roles in the development of sickness behavior and to the ensuing hyperalgesia.[36]

Considerable research is currently directed at targeting proinflammatory mediators like cytokines and the transcription factors responsible for their expression as a possible novel therapeutic approach for inflammation-associated neurodegeneration.[38]

The following experiments were designed, first, to characterize the effect of i.c.v. injection of ET in awake rats by assessing its nocipeptide effect using the paw withdrawal (PW) and the HP tests and to determine the effects of pretreatment with thymulin on the observed hyperalgesia; second, to determine the changes in the concentrations of proinflammatory cytokines in different areas of the brain following i.c.v. injections of either thymulin alone, ET alone, or ET preceded by thymulin. Knowledge gained by this investigation could allow the use of the rat model in question to study neuroimmune interactions and to investigate the effect of substances that modulate factors contributing to neurodegeneration.

Injection of relatively small doses of ET (1 μg) was sufficient to produce early and significant reduction in the latencies of the nociceptive (PW and HP) tests, which recovered within 24 h. This effect was more pronounced on the HP than on the PW test, which suggests a centrally triggered hyperalgesia affecting more selectively the supraspinally coordinated behavior (i.e., HP test).

Furthermore, the observed hyperalgesia was not accompanied by other evident signs of sickness behavior including motor disturbances, fever, or diarrhea observed with the higher doses of ET or other proinflammatory agents injected either via the i.p. or i.c.v. routes.[35]

Significant increases in the concentrations of IL-1β, IL-6, and TNF-α in the brain were observed following i.c.v. injection of a relatively small dose of ET. Similar results have been reported following the injection of ET or other inflammatory agents either in the CNS or peripherally.[39,40] The presence of proinflammatory cytokines at increased concentrations has been considered as responsible for the observed illness-induced behavior in general[35,41] and for the increased nociceptive reactivity or hyperalgesia.[37]

Effect of Intracerebroventricular Injections of Thymulin on ET-Induced Hyperalgesia and Upregulation of Cytokine Levels

Intracerebroventricular administration of different doses of thymulin did not result in significant changes in pain-related behavior in rats or in the levels of IL-1β, IL-6, and TNF-α in different brain areas, with the exception of mild alterations of TNF-α level in the diencephalon.

However, pretreatment (i.c.v.) with different doses of thymulin (0.1, 0.5, and 1 μg) 20 min before the ET (1 μg) injection (i.c.v.) reduced, the ET- induced hyperalgesia in a dose-dependent manner. In addition, this pretreatment exerted differential effects on the upregulated levels of cytokines in the brain. Measured 3–4 h after ET injection, the levels of IL-1 were reduced in the cerebellum and hippocampus, but not in the diencephalon. IL-6 levels recovered their normal values in all the examined brain areas following thymulin pretreatment.

Thus, thymulin appears to play a protective role against inflammation in the CNS similar to the action previously described against the inflammatory effects of i.p. injection of ET.[42] This protective effect appears to be exerted directly at the level of the CNS since i.p. administration of equivalent or greater (1–5 μg) doses of thymulin failed to reverse the effects of i.c.v. injection of ET.

These results provide behavioral and immunochemical characterization of a rat model for intracerebral inflammation. Also, it demonstrates the neuroprotective role of thymulin in the CNS, which becomes evident during inflammatory states. Although the mode of action of this molecule in the brain is not totally elucidated, these results indicate a potential therapeutic use of thymulin as an analgesic and anti-inflammatory drug.

REFERENCES

1. BACH, J.F., M. DARDENNE, J.M. PLEAU & J. ROSA. 1977. Biochemical characterization of a serum thymic hormone. Nature **266**: 55–56.

2. BACH, J.F. 1983. Thymulin (FTS-Zn). Clin. Immunol. Allergy **3**: 133–156.
3. DARDENNE, M., J.M. PLEAU, B. NABARRA, *et al.* 1982. Contribution of zinc and other metals to the biological activity of the serum thymic factor (FTS). Proc. Natl. Acad. Sci. USA **79**: 5370–5375.
4. DARDENNE, M., B. SAFIEH-GARABEDIAN & J.M. PLEAU. 2000. Thymic peptides: transmitters between the neuroendocrine and immune system. *In* Pain and Neuroimmune Interactions. N.E. Saade, A.V. Apkarian & S.J. Jabbur, Eds.: 127–137. Kluwer Academic/Plenum. New York.
5. VON GAUDECKER, B., M.D. KENDALL & M.A. RITTER. 1997. Immuno-electron microscopy of the thymic microenvironment. Micros. Res. Tech. **38**: 237–249.
6. SAVINO, W. & M. DARDENNE. 2000. Neuroendocrine control of thymus physiology. Endocrine Rev. **21**: 412–443.
7. SAFIEH, B., G.E. VENN, M. RITTER, *et al.* 1991. Plasma thymulin concentrations in cardiac patients: involvement with the hypothalamo-pituitary-adrenal axis. J. Physiol. (Paris) **438**: 50.
8. BUCKINGHAM, J.C., B. SAFIEH-GARABEDIAN, S. SINGH, *et al.* 1992. Interactions between the hypothalamus-pituitary adrenal axis and the thymus in the rat: a role for corticotrophin in the control of thymulin release. J. Neuroendocrinol. **4**: 295–301.
9. BLALOCK, J.E. 1994. The syntax of immune-neuroendocrine communication. Immunol. Today **15**: 504–511.
10. SAFIEH-GARABEDIAN, B., S.A. KANAAN, R.H. JALAKHIAN, *et al.* 1997. Hyperalgesia induced by low doses of thymulin injections: possible involvement of prostaglandin E2. J. Neuroimmunol. **73**: 162–168.
11. POOLE, S., A.F. BRISTOW, B.B. LORENZETTI, *et al.* 1992. Peripheral analgesic activities of peptides related to alpha-melanocyte stimulating hormone and interleukin-1β193-195. Br. J. Pharmacol. **106**: 489–492.
12. SAFIEH-GARABEDIAN, B., S.A. KANAAN, J.J. HADDAD, *et al.* 1997. Involvement of interleukin 1β, nerve growth factor and prostaglandin-E2 in endotoxin induced localized inflammatory hyperalgesia. Br. J. Pharmacol. **121**: 1619–1626.
13. FERREIRA, S.H., B.B. LORENZETTI, A.F. BRISTOW & S. POOLE. 1988. Interleukin-1 as a potent hyperalgesic agent antagonized by a tripeptide analogue. Nature **334**: 698–700.
14. VANE, J.R., J.A. MITCHELL, I. APPLETON, *et al.* 1994. Inducible isoforms of cyclooxygenase and nitric-oxide synthase in inflammation. Proc. Natl. Acad. Sci. USA **91**: 2046–2050.
15. WOOLF, C.J., B. SAFIEH-GARABEDIAN, Q.P. MA, *et al.* 1994. Nerve growth factor contributes to the generation of inflammatory sensory hypersensitivity. Neuroscience **62**: 327–331.
16. CUNHA, F.Q., S. POOE, B.B. LORENZETTI & S.H. FERREIRA. 1992. The pivotal role of tumour necrosis factor alpha in the development of inflammatory hyperalgesia. Br. J. Pharmacol. **107**: 660–664.
17. SAFIEH-GARABEDIAN, B., M. DARDENNE, S.A. KANAAN, *et al.* 2000. The role of cytokines and prostaglandin-E2 in thymulin induced hyperalgesia. Neuropharmacology **39**: 1653–1661.
18. SAADE, N.E., S.C. MAJOR, S.J. JABBUR, *et al.*, 1998. Involvement of capsaicin sensitive primary afferents in thymulin-induced hyperalgesia. J. Neuroimmunol. **91**: 171–179.

19. SAADE, N.E., H.F. LAWAND, B. SAFIEH-GARABEDIAN, *et al*. 1999. Thymulin induces c-Fos expression in the spinal cord of rats, which is reversed by meloxicam and morphine. J. Neuroimmunol. **97:** 16–24.

20. SAADE, N.E., P.G. ABOU JAOUDE, F.A. SAADEH, *et al*. 1997. Fos-like immunoreactivity induced by intraplantar injection of endotoxin and its reduction by morphine. Brain Res. **769:** 57–65.

21. MAIER, S.F., E.P. WIERTELAK, L. GOEHLER, *et al.*, 1993. Interleukin-1 mediates the behavioral hyperalgesia produced by lithium chloride and endotoxin. Brain Res. **623:** 321–325.

22. KONSMAN, J.P., P. PARNET & P. DANTZER. 2002. Cytokine-induced sickness behaviour: mechanisms and implications. Trends Neurosci. **25:** 154–159.

23. KANAAN, S.A., N.E. SAADE, J.J. HADDAD, *et al.*, 1996. Endotoxin-induced local inflammation and hyperalgesia in rats and mice: a new model of inflammatory pain. Pain **66:** 373–379.

24. KANAAN, S.A., S. POOLE, N.E. SAADE, *et al.*, 1998. Interleukin-10 reduces the endotoxin induced hyperalgesia in mice. J. Neuroimmunol. **86:** 142–150.

25. SAFIEH-GARABEDIAN, B., S.A. KANAAN, R.H. JALAKHIAN, *et al.*, 1997. Involvement of interleukin-1ß, nerve growth factor, and prostaglandin-E2 in the hyperalgesia induced by intraplantar injections of low doses of thymulin. Brain Behav. Immun. **11:** 185–200.

26. LEWIN, G.R., A.M. RITTER & L.M. MENDELL. 1993. Nerve growth factor-induced hyperalgesia in the neonatal and adult rat. J. Neurosci. **13:** 2136–2148.

27. WOOLF, C.J., B. SAFIEH-GARABEDIAN, Q.A. MA, *et al.*, 1994. Nerve growth factor contributes to the generation of inflammatory sensory hypersensitivity. Neurosci. **62:** 327–331.

28. SAFIEH-GARABEDIAN, B., R.H. JALAKHIAN, S.J. JABBUR, *et al.*, 1998. Thymulin at high doses reduces endotoxin-induced hyperalgesia by reducing interleukin-1β and nerve growth factor levels in the hind paw of rats. *In* Pain Mechanisms and Management. A.V. Apkarian & S. Ayrapetian, Eds.: 131–138. Kluwer Academic/Plenum. New York.

29. PLEAU, J.M., M. DARDENNE, D. BLANOT, *et al.*, 1979. Antagonistic analogue of serum thymic factor (FTS) interacting with FTS cellular receptor. Immunol. Lett. **1:** 179–182.

30. DASCOMBE, M.J. & A.S. MILTON. 1979. Study on the possible entry of bacterial endotoxin and prostaglandin E2 into the central nervous system from the blood. Br. J. Pharmacol. **66:** 565–572.

31. SAADE, N.E., S.F. ATWEH, S.J. JABBUR, *et al.* 2003. A thymulin analogue peptide with powerful inhibitory effects on pain of neurogenic origin. Neuroscience **119:** 155–165.

32. SPRANGER, M. & A. FONTANA. 1996. Activation of microglia: a dangerous interlude in immune function in the brain. Neuroscientist **2:** 293–299.

33. LEMKE, R., M. HARTLAGE-RUBSAMER & R. SCHLEIBS. 1999. Differential injury-dependent glial expression of interleukin-1 alpha, beta, and interleukin-6 in rat brain. Glia **27:** 75–87.

34. BALASINGAM, V., T. TEJADA-BERGES, E. WRIGHT, *et al.* 1994. Reactive astrogliosis in the neonatal mouse brain and its modulation by cytokines. J. Neurosci. **14:** 846–856.

35. KONSMAN, J.P., P. PARNET & R. DANTZER. 2002. Cytokine-induced sickness behavior: mechanisms and implications. Trends Neurosci. **25:** 154–159.

36. POOLE, S., F.Q. CUNHA & S.H. FERREIRA. 2000. Bradykinin, cytokines and inflammatory hyperalgesia. *In* Pain and Neuroimmune Interactions. N.E. Saade, A.V. Apkarian, S.J. Jabbur, Eds.: 31–45. Kluwer Academic/Plenum Pub. New York.
37. HORI, T., T. OKA, M. HOSOI, *et al.*, 2000. Biphasic modulation of pain by hypothalamic cytokines. *In* Pain and Neuroscience Interactions. N.E. Saade *et al.*, Eds.: 171–189. Kluwer Academic/Plenum Pub. New York.
38. DINARELLO, C.A., J.A. GELFAND & S.M. WOLFF. 1993. Anticytokine strategies in the treatment of the systemic inflammatory response syndrome. JAMA **269:** 1829–1835.
39. DE SIMONI, M.G., R. DEL BO, A. DE LUIGI, *et al.*, 1995. Central endotoxin induces different patterns of interleukin (IL)-1ß and IL-6 messenger ribonucleic acid expression and IL-6 secretion in the brain and periphery. Endocrinology **136:** 897–902.
40. TURRIN, N.P., D.A. GAYLE, S.E. ILYIN, *et al.*, 2001. Pro-inflammatory and antiinflammatory cytokine mRNA induction in the periphery and brain following intra-peritoneal administration of bacterial lipopolysaccharide. Brain Res. Bull. **54:** 443–453.
41. DANTZER, R.R., M. BLUTHE, J.L. SLAYE, *et al.*, 1998. Cytokines and sickness behavior. Ann. N.Y. Acad. Sci. **840:** 586–590.
42. SAFIEH-GARABEDIAN, B., S.A. KANAAN, S.J. JABBUR & N.E. SAADE. 1999. Cytokine mediated or direct effects of thymulin on the nervous system. Neuroimmunomodulation **6:** 39–44.

Therapeutic Management of Chronic Neuropathic Pain

An Examination of Pharmacologic Treatment

ATHINA VADALOUCA,[a] IOANNA SIAFAKA,[a] ERIPHYLLI ARGYRA,[a] EVI VRACHNOU,[b] AND ELENI MOKA[c]

[a] 1st Anaesthesiology Clinic, Pain Relief and Palliative Care Unit, Aretaieion University Hospital, University of Athens, Athens, Greece

[b] Anaesthesiology Department and Pain Relief and Palliative Care Unit, 7th IKA Hospital, Athens, Greece

[c] Anaesthesiology Department, Creta Interclinic Hospital, Heraklion, Crete, Greece

ABSTRACT: Neuropathic pain is defined as pain caused by a lesion in the nervous system and is common in clinical practice. Diagnosis can be difficult. Recommendations for first-line pharmacologic treatments are based on positive results from multiple, randomized, controlled trials, and recommendations for second-line pharmacologic treatments are based on the positive result of a single, randomized, controlled trial or inconsistent results of multiple, randomized, controlled trials. The results of published trials and clinical experience provide the foundation for specific recommendations for first-line treatments, which include gabapentin, 5% lidocaine patch, opioid analgesics, tramadol hydrochloride, and tricyclic antidepressants (TCAs). Gabapentin (up to 3,600 mg/day) significantly reduced pain compared with placebo; improvements in sleep, mood, and quality of life were also demonstrated. Adverse effects of gababentin include somnolence and dizziness, and, less commonly, gastrointestinal symptoms and mild peripheral edema. Thus, monitoring and dosage adjustment are required, without discontinuation of the drug. Gabapentin combined with morphine achieved better analgesia at lower doses of each drug than each drug alone, with only mild adverse effects. The first medication that proved effective for neuropathic pain in placebo-controlled trials was TCAs. Treatment decisions for patients with neuropathic pain can be difficult. Interest in the mechanisms and treatment of chronic neuropathic pain has increased during the past years, resulting in significant treatment advances in the future. In this article all recent knowledge on therapeutic management of chronic neuropathic pain is presented.

Address for correspondence: Athina Vadalouca, Department of Anaesthesiology, Pain Relief and Palliative Care, Aretaieion University Hospital, Lefkon Oreon Street, Gerakas, Athens, Greece. Voice: +306936718181; fax: +302107286168.

e-mail: athinajv@ath.forthnet.gr

Ann. N.Y. Acad. Sci. 1088: 164–186 (2006). © 2006 New York Academy of Sciences.

doi: 10.1196/annals.1366.016

KEYWORDS: neuropathic pain; mechanisms; diagnosis; therapy; guidelines treatment algorithms; randomized controlled trials; meta-analysis; antiepileptic drugs; antidepressive drugs; topical antineuralgics; opioids; tramadol

In this world nothing can be said to be certain,
except death and taxes.

—BENJAMIN FRANKLIN, *1706–1790*

Today, in 2006, more than two centuries after what Benjamin Franklin had so simply expressed, one could agree that death and taxes still remain two certainties of life, but, with the definite addition of a third one: suffering. Even if suffering is a sad, yet acceptable reality, according to EFIC's (European Federation of IASP Chapters) declaration in 2001, pain, indeed, is not a symptom but a disease in its own right, which undoubtedly will always need appropriate treatment. Pain is a diverse set of complex perpetual events that are characterized by their unpleasant or distressing nature. Its introduction encompasses multiple different neurobiologic components, originating in a complex fashion from mechanisms that may manifest and interact at many different levels of the neuraxis and that are inherently dynamic or changeable.[1]

Enormous progress is currently being made by the exploitation of modern neurobiological techniques in the elucidation of mechanisms that may contribute to the pathogenesis of pain.[2–4] This indicates that pain can be generated in multiple ways at a number of different sites that may coexist between and across diverse disease states.[5,6] Molecular biologic techniques are contributing to the analysis of pain mechanisms and are leading to the discovery of new targets, specific to particular pain mechanisms.[1]

Neuropathic pain has dated back for centuries, but it was not until the International Association for the Study of Pain (IASP) was founded in 1973 that attention was focused on the causes and treatment of neuropathic pain.[7] IASP published its first list of pain terms in 1979 [8,9] however, neuropathic pain was not included in the list until 1994. According to the definition of IASP, the term *neuropathic pain* refers to all pain initiated or caused by a primary lesion or dysfunction or transitory perturbation in the peripheral or central nervous system (CNS).[8,9] It is a subentity where transitory perturbation is omitted, and hence it refers to irreversible, long-term conditions. This very broad definition encapsulates the concept that, when a nerve becomes damaged, changes within the neural pathways can result in chronic pain even in the absence of continuing stimulus. Although this theory has now gained general acceptance, it was initially a revolutionary idea that repudiated the Cartesian model of nociception and pain.[7]

Nevertheless, this definition has long been a subject of discussion and still remains a matter of controversy, mostly due to the term "dysfunction," by not clarifying the nature of the lesion. However, it is generally understood that the lesion must involve the somatosensory pathways with damage to small fibers in peripheral nerves or to the spino-thalamo-cortical system in the CNS.[10] If the IASP definition is strictly applied, the clinician needs only to demonstrate nerve damage or dysfunction in a patient experiencing pain to make the diagnosis of neuropathic pain. However, nerve damage and/or dysfunction may manifest itself as negative symptoms (e.g., sensory, loss), as well as positive symptoms (e.g., hyperalgesia). Although the sensitivity of the IASP definition is potentially high, the specificity is low, since not all patients with nerve damage experience neuropathic pain. This may lead to a situation in which a patient with nerve damage and coincidental pain from another source could be misdiagnosed with neuropathic pain and subsequently mistreated. Conversely, neuropathic pain may be underdiagnosed when the signs and symptoms of neuronal dysfunction are not recognized.[7] The issue of definition became even more demanding following the suggestion of a mechanism-based classification.[1]

In 2002 and 2004 a new definition for neuropathic pain was developed and became established. Gruccu *et al.* and Hansson *et al.* defined neuropathic pain as a form of pain caused by a lesion in the peripheral or CNS.[10,11] Although this narrow definition is easier to understand as it refers to the site of the lesion, complying with current disease-based treatment indications, the broad definition of the IASP may be rewarding for some reason.[10] By focusing on the mechanism, it is clear that hyperexcitability and plasticity of the nervous system are key phenomena in chronic pain, and that treatment efficacy depends more on the underlying mechanism than etiology.[1,3,6,10] Testing the validity of a narrow versus broad definition of neuropathic pain may prove to be a major goal in future studies. In the meanwhile, nevertheless, according to the guidelines of the EFNS (European Federation of Neurological Societies) the use of a narrower definition of Gruccu *et.al.* has also been adopted from the EFNS as it is more easily understood and does not overestimate neuropathic pain.[10]

Chronic neuropathic pain is common in clinical practice, causing considerable suffering and substantial reduction in the patients' health-related quality of life.[12,13] Neuropathic pain, as part of the neurological disease spectrum, is a common disability and may be an expression of severe medical pathology. Apart from traumatic nerve damage, a number of diseases may be accompanied by neuropathic pain. For example, patients with conditions as diverse as diabetic polyneuropathy, human immunodeficiency virus (HIV), sensory neuropathy, poststroke syndromes, herpes zoster, myelopathy, and multiple sclerosis frequently experience daily pain that greatly impairs their quality of life. Neuropathic pain may also be cancer related, as it may result from tumor invasion of nervous tissue, surgical nerve damage during tumor removal, radiation-induced nerve damage, or chemotherapy-related neuropathy. Neuropathic pain has multiple disguises and may also be mimicked by non-neurological pain conditions.[10,11]

The true prevalence of neuropathic pain is largely unknown, as comprehensive epidemiological studies have not been performed. It has already been suggested that 1–1.5% of the general population is affected, but even this might be an underestimate. In the United States, 1 and 3 million people suffer from postherpetic neuralgia and diabetic peripheral neuropathy, respectively, whereas in Europe 6–7.7% of the population experiences chronic neuropathic pain at some point.[14,15] Approximately 5% of patients with traumatic nerve injury suffer from neuropathic pain,[16] whereas this specific type of central pain has been reported with multiple sclerosis, syringomyelia, spinal cord injury, and stroke in 28%, 75%, 60–70%, and 8% patients, respectively.[17–19]

These figures are probably an underestimate,[20] as the pain experienced by patients with cancer, degenerative diseases, or neurological conditions (such as Parkinson's disease) could have a neurologic components, which has so far gone unnoticed. These conditions are most prevalent in the aging population; since the size of this population is increasing worldwide, it is inevitable that neuropathic pain will place a progressively demanding burden on health care resources.[7]

What makes seemingly similar nerve injuries painful or painless is still unknown, and there are no systematic studies on the correlation between the intensity of the symptoms and the nature and severity of the nerve injury in patients with neuropathic pain. In highly specialized units for neuropathic pain, patients with partial nerve injury and pain far outnumber patients with complete deafferentation and pain. Whether this indicates a lower incidence of painful sequelae in total deafferentation or reflects the lower frequency of total deafferentation in the population is also unknown.[11]

The diagnosis of neuropathic pain is based on a detailed medical history, analytical systems' review, meticulous physical and neurological examination, appropriate laboratory studies, including blood and serological tests, magnetic resonance imaging, and electrophysiological studies. In some instances, nerve or skin biopsy is necessary to directly visualize the nerve fibers.[11,21] The diagnosis of peripheral or central neuropathic pain should be made only when the history and signs are indicative of neuropathy, in conjunction with neuroanatomically correlated pain distribution and sensory abnormalities within the area of pain. Cornerstones of the diagnostic workup in neuropathic pain, which also aim at disclosing the etiology of the pain, are listed in TABLE 1.[10,11,22] Proper diagnosis is the cornerstone of effective treatment, and complex patterns of signs and symptoms may demand the involvement of multiple medical specialties.[7,10,11,22]

Historically, the earliest treatment strategies for neuropathic pain were invasive in nature. By applying the Cartesian model for pain, it was hoped that blocking neural transmission, either temporarily by using local anaesthetics, or permanently by surgical nerve ablation and periarterial sympathectomy, would alleviate pain. However, none of these therapies was found to be consistently successful.[7]

Unfortunately, neuropathic pain poorly responds to conventional analgesics but is, nevertheless, a challenging condition to treat, in part because of the

TABLE 1. Cornerstones of the neuropathic pain diagnostic workup

Basic components of diagnostic workup	Detailed workup— Neurophysiological testing
Careful medical history	Electroneurography
Patients' coping skills	Electromyography
Specific characteristics of pain	Microneurography
Patients' functional condition–status	Somatosensory evoked potentials
Previous therapy	Quantitative sensory testing
Detailed clinical examination	Quantitative sudomat axon reflex test
Motor, sensory, autonomic system	Magnetic resonance imaging (MRI)
Pain drawing	Positron emission tomography (PET)
Comprehensive neurologic examination	Functional MRI (fMRI)
Survey of somatosensory functions	Pharmacological fMRI
	Laser-evoked potentials (LEP)

heterogeneity of etiologies, symptoms, and underlying mechanisms. Awareness among clinicians of evidence-based therapeutic options is less than optimum, probably because the complexity of the phenomenon makes the available data difficult to interpret.[23]

Another important reason for the difficulty confronted might be the fact that the drugs used to treat neuropathic pain are commonly classified according to their original therapeutic category (antidepressants, anticonvulsants, etc.), a mistake frequently made by clinicians who are not familiar with neuropathic pain treatment. Unfortunately, this may be misleading, since it might suggest that the use of other drugs belonging to the same category (antidepressants, anticonvulsants), as those with proven efficacy, are also equally effective.[23]

Recent studies have shown that most of the patients treated for neuropathic pain were receiving medication of unproven efficacy or suboptimum doses of the appropriate medication.[24,25] Nonetheless, it is true that with appropriate therapy of neuropathic pain a significant proportion of patients experiences substantial pain reduction.[23]

Another reason why the neuropathic pain treatment often fails is that it tends to be used in a uniform fashion across the patient population. In other words, a drug shown to be useful in one group of patients is actually used to treat patients whose neuropathic pain is caused by a completely different pathology. The current data indicate that from a therapeutic point of view, at least four distinct etiologic groups should be considered when a treatment decision is made: peripheral neuropathic pain (PNP), complex regional pain syndrome (CRPS), trigeminal neuralgia (TN), and central neuropathic pain (CNP).[23]

Most authors agree that a major breakthrough in the pharmacological treatment of neuropathic pain can be achieved only with therapy tailored to the individual patient on the basis of the mechanisms underlying the pain of that particular patient.[6] The ideal for pain management is to treat the mechanisms (apart from disease-modifying therapy). However, at present, this is not achievable since the underlying mechanisms have not been identified as yet. At present, our only indication is the symptoms generated by the mechanisms, which, however, are not equivalent to the mechanisms. Specific and sensitive diagnostic tools providing clear-cut evidence of the nature of the particular pathophysiological process involved are lacking.[1,23]

Up to 2000, no official consensus on the optimal therapeutic management of neuropathic pain existed and practices varied greatly worldwide. Possible explanations for this included difficulties in developing agreed-upon diagnostic protocols and the coexistence of neuropathic, nociceptive, and, occasionally, idiopathic pain in the same patient. Also, up to that period of time, neuropathic pain had historically been classified according to its etiology without regard for the presumed mechanism(s) underlying the specific symptoms. Treatment was largely empirical, with several treatment strategies for managing neuropathic pain, including both invasive and noninvasive therapies.[7]

In 2000 and early in 2003, as is demonstrated in TABLE 2, treatment strategies and algorithms were published.[7,26] Currently, published guidelines exist for the treatment of neuropathic pain in general, as well as for the management of neuropathic pain associated with specific syndromes, such as painful diabetic neuropathy[27,28] and trigeminal neuralgia.[29] However, these recommendations were usually based on anecdotal evidence or clinical trials showing efficacy of a therapy in some patients with a particular causative condition for their neuropathic pain. Additionally, many of these early trials randomized small numbers of patients and were often poorly designed.[7]

It is generally accepted that pharmacotherapy remains the mainstay of neuropathic pain management. Since neuropathic pain may be partially or completely

TABLE 2. Suggested treatment strategies for neuropathic pain management

A. Medical management		B. Surgical management
I. Membrane stabilizing agents		Decompression
Antiepileptic Drugs(AEDs)		Neuroaugmentation
Oxcarbazepine		
Carbamazepine		
Phenytoin		
Valproate		
Antiarrythmics		
Lidocaine		
Mexiletine		
Corticosteroids		
II. Drugs that enhance dorsal horn inhibition		**C. Nerve blocks**
Antidepressants	*Antiepileptic drugs*	Local anesthetics
Amitryptiline	Oxcarbazepine	Corticosteroids
Desipramine	Clonazepam	
Fluoxetine	Gabapentin	
Imipramine	GABA–B agonists	
Nortryptiline	Baclofen	
Paroxetine		

unresponsive to primary analgesic treatments, medical therapies for neuropathic pain tend to involve adjuvant analgesics (i.e., drugs whose primary indication is not analgesia), such as antiepileptic drugs (AEDs), antiarrythmics, and antidepressants.[7]

On the basis of the assumption referred to above, later on in 2003, members of the faculty of the Fourth International Conference of the Mechanisms and Treatment of Neuropathic Pain participated in a meeting where a number of specialties were included. MEDLINE searches, examination of reference lists of published articles and book chapters, and personal knowledge of the literature were used to identify material relevant to developing treatment recommendations for patients with neuropathic pain. This material included systematic literature reviews, reports of randomized controlled trials, and publications discussing the development and evaluation of clinical guidelines. The faculty members finally concluded on first-line and second-line pharmacological treatment guidelines, as well as beyond second-line recommended medication, which are all summarized and presented in TABLE 3.[22]

Recommendations for first-line pharmacological treatments were based on positive results from multiple randomized controlled trials, and recommendations for second-line pharmacological treatments were based on the positive results of a single randomized controlled trial or inconsistent results of multiple randomized controlled trials. The results of published trials and clinical experience provided the foundation for specific recommendations for first-line treatments, thus leading to the inclusion of gabapentin, 5% lidocaine patch, opioids, tramadol, and trycyclic antidepressants (TCAs).[22] It should be noted, though, that these recommendations were made before the Food and Drugs Administration's (FDA) approval of duloxetine and pregabalin.[21]

TABLE 3. First-line, second-line, and beyond second-line treatment recommendations for neuropathic pain

First-line	Second-line	Beyond second-line
Gabapentin	*Other antiepileptics (AED)*	Capsaicin
	Lamotrigine	Clonidine
	Carbamazepine	Dextromethorphan
	Levetiracetam	Mexiletine
	Oxcarbazepine	
	Tiagabine	
	Topiramate	
	Zonisamide	
5% Lidocaine patch	*Other antidepressants*	
Opioid analgesics	Paroxetine	
Tramadol hydrochloride	Citalopram	
Tricyclic antidepressants (TCAs)	Bupropion hydrochloride	
Nortryptiline hydrochloride	Venlafaxine hydrochloride	
Desipramine hydrochloride		

The efficacy of gabapentin, 5% lidocaine patch, tramadol, opioids, and TCAs has been consistently demonstrated in multiple randomized controlled trials. Each one can be used as an initial treatment for neuropathic pain in certain clinical circumstances. Opioids and TCAs generally require greater caution than other options.[22] For each of these five medications brief reviews follow.

FIRST-LINE TREATMENT MEDICATIONS

Gabapentin

As with epilepsy, the hallmark characteristic of neuropathic pain is neuronal excitability. As a result, many AEDs have been effectively used in the management of neuropathic pain because of their inherent ability to suppress neuronal hyperexcitability through one or more mechanisms, which ultimately results in pain alleviation.[30] AEDs, as an important treatment option for neuropathic pain management, were used for the treatment of trigeminal neuralgia before the 1960s. The first published trial of an AED for neuropathic pain therapy was in 1942, when Bergouignan used phenytoin to treat patients with trigeminal neuralgia, based on the condition's resembling the neuronal hyperexcitability seen in some epilepsy models.[31,32] Later on, in 1962, carbamazepine was used by Blom for trigeminal neuralgia alleviation and in 1968 Ellenberg published his experience with using phenytoin in diabetic neuropathy.[32]

Gabapentin is an AED that acts on neuropathic pain, probably by reducing central sensitization. There are eight published double-blind, placebo-controlled, randomized clinical trials of gabapentin for chronic neuropathic pain. These studies examined patients with PHN, PDN, mixed neuropathic pain syndromes, phantom limb pain, Guillan–Barré syndrome, and acute and chronic pain from spinal cord injury.[33–40] Gabapentin at dosages up to 3,600 mg/day significantly reduced pain compared with placebo; improvements in sleep, mood, and quality of life were also demonstrated in some trials.[22] Gabapentin has the broadest evidence for efficacy against neuropathic pain. It has an FDA-approved indication for PHN in the United States and is licensed for the treatment of neuropathic pain in the UK.[21] This agent yielded positive results not only in PHN and PDN, as has already been mentioned,[41,42] but also in a wide range of neuropathic pain syndromes, such as CRPS, radiculitis, post-stroke pain, postoperative pain, and postthoracotomy pain,[43] as well as cancer-related and multiple sclerosis–related neuropathic pain (up to 3,600 mg/day).[44,45]

For neuropathic pain, dosing up to 600 mg three times a day is suggested. If this dosage provides partial benefit, it can be further increased to 3,600 mg/day in divided doses. Attempted suicide with overdose amounts in excess of 40 g have not resulted in cardiac, respiratory, or long-term sequelae, nor have there been any fatalities.[21] The adverse effects of gabapentin include somnolence, dizziness, and less commonly gastrointestinal symptoms, and mild peripheral edema. All these effects require close monitoring and dosage adjustment but usually not discontinuation of the drug. To decrease adverse effects and increase patient adherence to treatment, gabapentin should be initiated at low dosages—100 to 300 mg in a single dose at bedtime or 100 to 300 mg three times daily—and then titrated every 1 to 7 days by 100 to 300 mg as tolerated. Although three times daily is the target dosage, more rapid titration may be accomplished if most of the daily dose is initially given at bedtime to limit daytime sedation. The final dosage should be determined either by achieving complete pain relief or by the development of unacceptable adverse effects that do not resolve promptly. Dworkin *et al.* suggest that gabapentin should be used as a first-line medication for neuropathic pain with a 3- to 8-week titration period to allow the development of tolerance to adverse effects, plus 1 to 2 weeks at the maximal tolerated dosage.[22]

Topical Antineuralgics—5% Lidocaine Patch

Three published studies of the 5% lidocaine patch for neuropathic pain have yielded positive results, two in PHN,[46,47] for which the patch is FDA-approved, and one in focal neuropathic pain syndromes.[48] In these studies patients obtained statistically significantly greater pain relief with a lidocaine patch compared with vehicle-controlled patches containing no lidocaine.

Notably, the efficacy of this treatment has been demonstrated only in patients with PHN and focal neuropathic pain syndromes, expressed with allodynia, and no controlled studies have been conducted for other pain conditions. Anecdotal evidence of a beneficial effect in patients who have other types of neuropathic pain with allodynia has been published lately.[49] In addition, in our department, we have used the 5% lidocaine patch in 36 patients (17 PHN, 6 postthoracotomy syndrome, 4 postmastectomy pain, 2 PDN, 5 CRPS, 2 peripheral ischemia) in an open, observational study for the treatment of neuropathic pain of diverse origin. The therapy had a duration of 2 months to 4 years with good and/or very good analgesia in 50% of patients.[50]

Although systemic absorption from the patch is minimal, local skin absorption is believed to modulate sodium channels, by blocking them at the periphery. Blood levels of the drug are minimal and accumulation does not occur, even with the application of three patches for 12 h daily (12 h on and 12 h off). The only adverse effects appear to be mild skin reactions (such as erythema and rash) in some patients. Systemic absorption from the patch must be considered in patients receiving oral class I antiarrythmic drugs (e.g., mexiletine). Titration of the patch is not necessary, and an adequate trial should last 2 weeks.[21–23]

Opioid Analgesics

Opioids act through the descending inhibitory pathways modulating nociceptive impulses in the dorsal horn. There is increasing evidence of the efficacy of oral opioids in the treatment of chronic neuropathic pain.[22,23] Several trials of oral opioids for neuropathic pain have been published since 1998, presenting positive results.[51–57] If an adequate dose is used, at least a partial result may be observed.[51,53,55]

In patients with PHN, controlled-release oxycodone hydrochloride titrated to a maximum dosage of 60 mg/day significantly relieved pain, disability, and allodynia compared to placebo.[53] In patients with PDN, controlled-release oxycodone titrated to a maximum dosage of 120 mg/day significantly improved pain, performance of daily activities, and sleep compared to placebo, with an average dose of 37 mg/day,[51] whereas a maximum dose of 40 mg/day in PDN proved to be effective by improving pain and quality of life.[52] Controlled-release morphine titrated to a maximum dose of 300 mg/day was superior to placebo in patients with phantom limb pain.[54] The efficacy of methadone and levorphanol in the treatment of neuropathic pain was demonstrated in trials on patients with mixed peripheral and central etiologies.[56,57] Gabapentin combined with morphine achieved better analgesia at lower doses of each drug than either as a single agent, with constipation, sedation, and dry mouth as the most frequent adverse effects.[58] According to Dworkin *et al.*, all the results mentioned above provide a reliable base of evidence for considering opioids to be a first treatment for neuropathic pain.[22]

The most common adverse effects of opioids are constipation, sedation, and nausea. These effects most likely contributed to the relatively high withdrawal rates found in the placebo-controlled trials. In elderly patients cognitive impairment and problems with mobility can occur. Most patients become tolerant to the adverse effects, although constipation often persists. Opioids must be cautiously used in patients with a history of substance abuse or attempted suicide, whereas accidental death or suicide can occur with overdose. Opioid abuse must be distinguished from the appropriate desire to continue taking medication that effectively relieves pain and from apprehension about not having adequate access to medications that are often difficult to obtain. Concerns about causing a substance abuse disorder when there is no history of one do not justify refraining from using opioid analgesics in patients with chronic neuropathic pain. Although patients treated with opioid analgesics may develop analgesic tolerance, in responsive patients a stable dosage can usually be achieved. All patients receiving opioids develop physical dependence and must be advised not to abruptly discontinue their medication.[21,22,30]

Numerous short- and long-acting opioid analgesics are available besides diverse opinions regarding the algorithm for its administration. One approach recommends beginning with a short-acting opioid (oxycodone, hydrocodone) at dosages equianalgesic to the oral administration of morphine at 5–15 mg every 4 h as needed, in combination with acetaminophen, aspirin, or ibuprofen. After 1–2 weeks of therapy, the patient's total dosage of the short-acting opioid can be converted to an equianalgesic daily dosage of the long-acting one (CR-morphine, CR-oxycodone, TTS fentanyl, levorphanol, methadone).

Limited access to short-acting medication for breakthrough pain may be appropriate. Once the patient is receiving a stable dosage of a long-acting opioid, an adequate trial requires 4 to 6 weeks to access both pain and function. After careful titration and monitoring, it is clear that there is no clear maximum dosage of opioids. However, evaluation by a pain specialist may be considered when morphine equianalgesic dosages exceeding 120–180 mg/day are contemplated. The benefits of doses higher than 180 mg/day in patients with neuropathic pain have not been established in double-blind trials.[21,22,30]

Nonetheless, and despite all the already mentioned positive results, the use of opioids for neuropathic pain remains controversial, partly because studies have been small, have yielded equivocal results, and have not established the risk–benefit ratio of this treatment. Large variability in trial design in terms of the type of neuropathic pain treated, the type of opioid administered, and the duration of treatment has yielded contradictory results. Concerns about adverse effects and potential for abuse, addiction, hormonal abnormalities, dysfunction of the immune system, and sometimes paradoxical hyperalgesia often discourage use of opioids in the treatment of neuropathic pain.[59,60] Short-term studies provide only equivocal evidence regarding the efficacy of opioids in reducing the intensity of neuropathic pain. Intermediate-term studies demonstrate significant efficacy of opioids over placebo, which is likely to be clinically important. Reported adverse effects are common but not life-threatening. It is suggested that the practitioner who prescribes opioids obtain a signed opioid agreement and uses random urine screening to check for compliance. Follow-up discussions on side effects and functional improvement with the use of the opioid should be documented. Further randomized controlled trials are needed to establish their long-term efficacy, safety (including addiction potential), and effects on the quality of life.[21,59]

Tramadol Hydrochloride

Tramadol is a norepinephrine and serotonin reuptake inhibitor (SNRI), centrally acting analgesic, which has both direct opioid action (has a metabolite with major μ-opioid agonist effect) and indirect monoaminergic action (like TCAs). Randomized controlled trials have yielded positive results in painful diabetic neuropathy,[61] different neuropathic pain states,[62] and PHN.[63] In all trials, tramadol titrated to a maximum dosage of 400 mg/day significantly relieved pain compared to placebo, whereas beneficial effects of tramadol treatment on allodynia and quality of life were also reported.

Tramadol is usually started at 100 mg/day and titrated up to 200–400 mg/day (in divided doses, four times daily). Efficacy in neuropathic pain treatment is usually evident at 250 mg/day in divided doses. It has a low abuse liability, and the development of tolerance and dependence during long-term treatment is usually uncommon. The most frequent side effects of tramadol include dizziness, nausea, constipation, somnolence, and orthostatic hypotension. These occur more frequently when the dosage is escalated rapidly and with concurrent administration of other drugs that have similar side effects. Seizures can also occur, whereas serotonin syndrome can occur with simultaneous prescription of selective serotonin reuptake inhibitors (SSRIs such as fluoxetine or centraline) or MAOIs (monoamine oxidase inhibitors). Tramadol may also cause or exacerbate cognitive dysfunction in the elderly.[21–23] According to Dworkin *et al.*, to decrease the likelihood of adverse effects and increase patients' adherence to treatment, tramadol should be initiated at low dosages (50 mg once or twice daily) and then titrated every 3–7 days by 50–100 mg/day in divided doses as tolerated. The maximum dosage of tramadol is 100 mg four times/day (in patients over the age of 75 years, 300 mg/day) and an adequate trial requires 4 weeks.[22]

Tricyclic Antidepressants

TCAs increase the activity of biogenic amines (norepinephrine and serotonin) by inhibiting their reuptake. They also modulate sodium channels peripherally and act as NMDA antagonists. Thus TCAs may act both by enhancing dorsal horn inhibition and by diminishing peripheral sensitization.[64,65]

The first medication category that proved to be effective for neuropathic pain in various trials for over 30 years was TCAs. Paoli *et al.* were the first who used antidepressants for chronic pain relief in 1960. All those trials suggested that TCAs might have direct analgesic action; however, many of these trials were uncontrolled or complicated by the presence of an adjuvant pain-relieving drug.[7] Nevertheless, the evidence for the efficiency for TCAs in treating neuropathic pain of peripheral origin comes from a meta-analysis of many old and relatively small-scale trials, which demonstrated that approximately 30% of patients responded (>50% relief), 30% exhibited minor side effects, and 4% suffered from major side effects that led to discontinuation of therapy.[66–68] Clinical trials of patients with HIV sensory neuropathy, pain from spinal cord injury, and cisplatin-induced neuropathy found little benefit using amitryptiline when compared with placebo. A summary of the overall efficacy of TCAs in neuropathic pain is provided by the title of a review by Max *et al.* in 1995.[22,66]

TCAs are initiated in a low bedtime dose (10–25 mg) that is gradually increased on a weekly basis (by 10–25 mg/day), usually up to 150 mg or until the side effects interfere with a further increase of the dose.[23] Although the analgesic effect of TCAs has been thought to occur at lower dosages than those for the antidepressant effect, there is no systematic evidence of this. However, some data are consistent with a dose–response relationship. An adequate trial of a TCA would last 6 to 8 weeks with at least 1 to 2 weeks at the maximum tolerated dosage. For neuropathic pain dosing up to antidepressant blood levels is suggested for 4–6 weeks.[21,22]

The most frequent side effects of TCAs are sedation, anticholinergic effects like dry mouth, constipation and postural hypotension, and weight gain.[23] In one large-scale study, the long-term use of TCAs was found to be associated with a 2.2-fold greater relative risk of myocardial infarction and a 1.7-fold increase in overall mortality, as compared with placebo.[69] Thus, caution is demanded when TCAs are prescribed for older patients, especially those with cardiovascular risk factors, and a screening electrocardiogram is recommended before therapy is started. The secondary amines, nortryptiline and desipramine, are safer than the parent drugs, amitryptiline and imipramine, respectively. TCAs are contraindicated in patients with a history of glaucoma, urinary retention, or autonomic neuropathy.[7,21-23]

The percentage of patients with neuropathic pain who do not respond to one of the five first-line medications, but who then experience satisfactory pain relief from a different medication is not known. Even within a class of drugs, patients fail to respond to one medication but then respond to another. The selection of a particular drug may depend on the experiences of the clinician and the patient, as well as the expected side effects. The current understanding of neuropathic pain mechanisms is consistent with the existence of multiple mechanisms, each of which may respond differently to medications with different ways of action. Therefore, there is both an empiric and a theoretical basis for recommending that patients who do not respond to one of these five first-line medications be treated with another one.[22,30]

When partial response to a single drug occurs, then their combination should be considered, in order to optimize pain control. Unfortunately, existing data on combination drug therapy for neuropathic pain are scanty and inadequate; pain management by combining drugs is entirely empirical and the guiding principle is to choose drugs according to their additional therapeutic effects rather than their adverse effects. Combination therapy could also be applied at the beginning of the treatment, in order to increase the likelihood of a beneficial response or to reach an effective dosage of the drugs used. Disadvantages of combination therapy include an increased risk of adverse effects, as the number of medications is increased, and difficulty in identifying which of several drugs is responsible for the side effects.[7,22]

SECOND-LINE TREATMENT MEDICATIONS

When patients do not have a satisfactory response to treatment with the five first-line medications, alone or in combination, several drugs can be considered second line. Unfortunately, since they are not used so often by physicians, fewer trials have examined their efficacy and their use is not described or presented in detail in the international literature.[22] All second-line medications, according to Dworkin et al., are presented in TABLE 3.

Other Anticonvulsants

Lamotrigine is the first second-line pharmacologic treatment for which there is evidence of efficacy for HIV sensory neuropathy, PDN, central poststroke pain, as well as in a subgroup of patients with incomplete spinal cord lesions, with pain from spinal cord injury, when gabapentin is ineffective.[70–74] Lamotrigine is not considered a first-line treatment for neuropathic pain because of the slow and careful titration required and the risk of both severe rash and Stevens–Johnson syndrome associated with its use (occurring in up to 10% of patients). Dosage of lamotrigine for neuropathic pain is less than 200 mg twice a day.[21,22]

Carbamazepine has a well-established beneficial effect for trigeminal neuralgia and is approved by the FDA for the treatment of this neuropathic pain syndrome. However, this drug has a number of drawbacks. It produces a toxic epoxide metabolite and regular blood tests are therefore recommended. It is associated with 10% incidence of rashes and has a negative effect on bone density, as well as significant drug interactions. It is suggested as a second-line anticonvulsant for neuropathic pain when there is no response to gabapentin. It is used in a dosage of less than 400 mg twice a day.[21–23,75]

Pregabalin has been FDA-approved for PHN and painful diabetic polyneuropathy, but has only recently been marketed. The action of pregabalin is similar to that of gabapentin (alpha 2-delta ligand), although it has linear absorption kinetics from the small bowel through a passive absorption mechanism and has a significantly greater affinity for the $\alpha2\delta$ subunit of voltage-gated calcium channels than does gabapentin. Pain alleviation is noted by the second day at full dosage. As it is not metabolized, so drug–drug interactions occur, but the dosage must be adjusted for patients with renal dysfunction. Its side effects are mild to moderate (dizziness, somnolence, headache, dry mouth, and peripheral edema). During the first 3 days 150 mg/day is administered (50 mg three times daily), followed by 300 mg/day for the next 4 days. From the beginning of the second week 600 mg/day is administered to those patients whose creatinine clearance is more than 60 mL/min (maximal dose 300 mg twice a day).[21,23,76,77]

Evaluation of the role of other second-generation anticonvulsants (levetiracetam, oxcarbazepine, tiagabine, topiramate, zonisamide) for the treatment of neuropathic pain must await publication of the results of randomized placebo-controlled trials. Although several anticonvulsant medications block sodium channels, available anticonvulsants have different and often multiple mechanisms of action. Therefore, lack of response to a single anticonvulsant does not necessarily predict lack of response to the category as a whole.[22]

Other Antidepressant Medications

SSRIs have fewer adverse effects and are generally better tolerated than TCAs. In studies of patients with PDN paroxetin and citalopram were associated with statistically significantly greater pain relief than placebo, whereas fluoxetine was found to be no more effective than placebo. SSRIs are probably less effective against neuropathic pain than antidepressants that increase the activity of both norepinephrine and serotonin.[21–23,78]

Sustained release bupropion, a norepinephrine and dopamine inhibitor (NDRI), was more effective than placebo in patients with different peripheral and central neuropathic pain states. It has a low incidence of sexual dysfunction and is associated with weight loss. Side effects include agitation and insomnia. For neuropathic pain it is given at a dosage of 150–300 mg daily.[21,22,79]

Venlafaxine, which has a chemical structure different from that of TCAs and SSRIs, inhibits norepinephrine and serotonin reuptake (SNRI) at a dose greater than 150 mg daily.[21] In a randomized, three-period crossover trial of venlafaxine and imipramine in patients with painful polyneuropathy, both antidepressants demonstrated superior pain relief compared to placebo but did not differ from each other.[80] In another study at doses greater than 150 mg daily venlafaxine essened pain associated with diabetic neuropathy, although a lower dose of 75 mg daily was ineffective.[81] Additionally, in a placebo-controlled, crossover trial of 13 patients with chronic neuropathic pain following breast cancer therapy (including surgery, chemotherapy, radiotherapy), the investigators failed to find a significant benefit of venlafaxine (18.75–187.5 mg/10/ weeks) versus placebo for the primary end point (daily pain diary ratings). However, a greater relief associated with venlafaxine treatment for two secondary pain end points (maximum intensity of everyday pain at rest and in movement) was found. No differences were found in adverse effects versus placebo.[82] Side effects of venlafaxine mostly include hypertension, which may be a concern if a patient is already hypertensive. More research is needed to find how titration of venlafaxine could succeed and if a combination of an antiepileptic with such an antidepressant has better results than each drug alone.[21]

Duloxetin is FDA-approved for the treatment of diabetic peripheral neuropathy. It has minimal or no effect on blood pressure and body weight and few sexual adverse effects in the studies have been reported so far. Dosing of duloxetin for such conditions is 60 mg or 120 mg daily, without any significant differences between the two doses, although with superior results versus placebo. Improvement should be noted in 1 to 2 weeks at 60 mg before increasing the dose further is considered.[21,83]

Results of all the above trials indicate that citalopram, paroxetine, bupropion, venlafaxine, and duloxetin can be recommended for patients who have not responded to an adequate trial of nortryptiline or another TCA, when additional treatment with an antidepressant is being considered. Any physician who prescribes an antidepressant should be aware that a recent "black box" warning, as well as other new labeling, has been issued by the FDA for all antidepressants regarding the increased risk for suicidality in some depressed patients, particularly children and adolescents, after the initiation of antidepressant drug therapy. Physicians who prescribe these medications for pain should also be aware of the possibility of comorbid pain and depression. A careful history, including that of suicidal ideation, should be taken. Signs of agitation or increased depression after the start of treatment with an antidepressant may warrant the involvement of a mental health care practitioner.[21]

BEYOND SECOND-LINE MEDICATIONS

Other medications sometimes used for the treatment of patients with neuropathic pain include capsaicin, clonidine, dextromethorphan, and mexiletine. According to the clinical experience that exists and the inconsistent results of clinical trials, these medications may occasionally be effective in individual circumstances.[21–23]

The interest in pharmacologic treatment of neuropathic pain is shown by the increase of the number of neuropathic pain medication patents filed. Before 2000 there were fewer than 27, in 2002 there were 54, in 2003 there were 104; and in 2004 about 100 applications were filed. These medications include cannabinoid receptor antagonists, $\alpha 2$-adrenergic agonist (clonidine, dexmetomidine, tizanidine), NMDA receptor antagonists (ketamine), lysine B antagonists, NR2B-selective agents, glycine antagonists, nicotinic receptor agonists, NK1 receptor antagonists, bradykinin B1 receptor antagonists, vanilloid VR1 receptor antagonists, cholecystokinin antagonists, oral TNF (tumor necrosis factor) antagonists, interleukin antagonists, neuroimmunomodulators, and others.[21,84,85] Completely new drug classes derived from exotic animal sources like conotoxins from a marine snail family and epitadine from a species of frog seem to modulate neuronal transmission in pain pathways.[86] New ways of approaching therapy include the development of GABA and serotonin-secreting neuron grafts for spinal cord injury pain and the use of herpes simplex or HIV-like viruses as drug or gene vectors to transport therapeutic agents into the dorsal root ganglion or dorsal horn. Although efficacy, side effects, and cost will be important, it will be fascinating to see whether we can achieve better pain relief in comparison to the present generation of medications.[21]

But even with all these analgesic modalities clinicians have in their armamentarium, what really happens if chronic neuropathic pain persists? Approximately 10% to 15% of all neuropathic pain patients are truly refractory to pharmacotherapy. After exhausting all available monotherapy options for refractory neuropathic pain, combination therapy from within and/or between drug classes may be tried with caution. Judicious monitoring of patients in whom combination therapy is initiated is strongly recommended to prevent the occurrence of serious adverse effects and drug interactions. Such patients should be referred to a pain clinic, where more invasive pain management interventions, such as intrathecal drug delivery, may be used.[30] Other specialized procedures, such as transelectrical nerve stimulation, have also been used to relieve pain by desensitizing sensory afferents through mechanisms similar to those of topical antineuralgics.[87] The administration of epidurals as well as dorsal root rhizotomy is also thought to be beneficial for severe refractory pain associated with chronic syndromes, such as CRPS. Despite their potential benefit, these procedures are often invasive and associated with their own inherent risks. However, the use of spinal cord stimulation has demonstrated some promise for patients with a variety of chronic neuropathic conditions, including CRPS, chronic low back pain, and severe ischemic limb pain, with a pain intensity reduction greater than 50% in more than 60% of such patients.[88] These highly specialized treatment strategies will no doubt entail longer waiting list times.[30]

Having all the above information in mind and taking into account the potential for variability in efficacy of the various therapeutic modalities (pharmacological and/or invasive), a succinct, logical treatment algorithm is required to successfully manage the symptoms of chronic neuropathic pain. In 2004, Namaka et al. published such an algorithm.[30] This algorithm was developed to provide a sequential guide to therapeutic planning strategies, bearing in mind that the multifaceted nature of neuropathic pain, together with dynamic needs of the patient, may alter the available therapeutic options (FIG. 1).

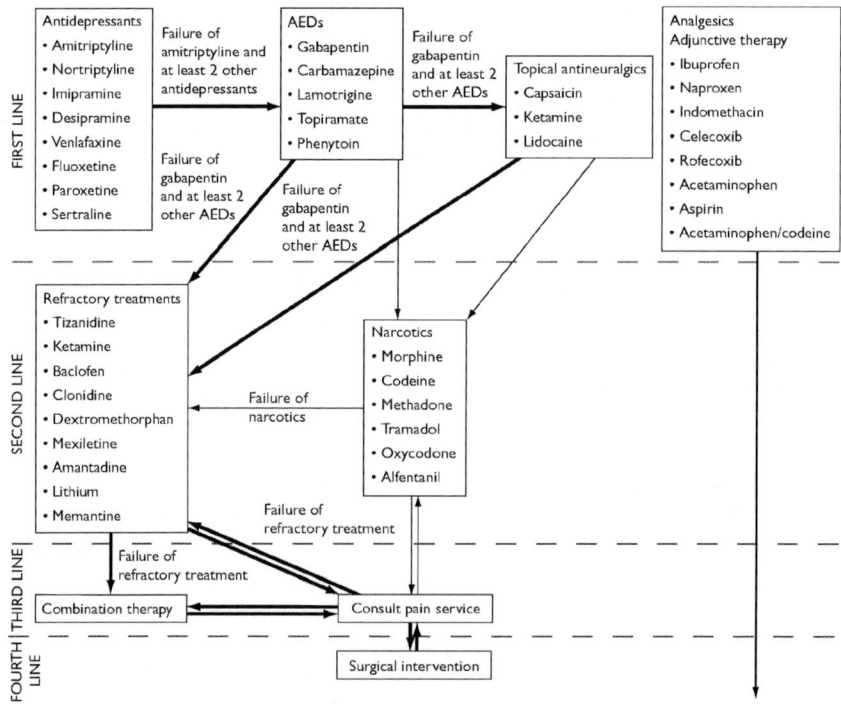

FIGURE 1. Treatment algorithm for neuropathic pain. (From Namaka et al.[30])

As a result the treatment algorithm was designed to be used not only with flexibility but also with universal application. Thus it might serve as a template from which clinicians can logically justify and track current and future treatment selections. It also serves as a means for clinicians to determine when the appropriate stage in treatment has been reached to make a referral to a pain clinic. Simply stated, this algorithm provides the clinician with the knowledge to ensure that all feasible pharmacological methods have been exhausted before resorting to such a referral. This idea would ensure that only patients with truly refractory chronic neuropathic pain are referred to a pain clinic, thus allowing better use of health care resources and more expedient care for individuals who may benefit from this specialized service.[30]

This year Finnerub *et al.* basing their work on the available randomized clinical trials, published a new, evidence-based treatment algorithm for peripheral neuropathic pain, which deals only with pharmacological considerations.[89] Approximately 105 studies were included in this algorithm and the numbers needed to treat (NNT) as well as numbers needed to harm (NNH) were used to compare efficacy and safety of the various treatments in different neuropathic pain syndromes. The quality of the trials used was assessed and a set of criteria was established before choice of treatment. Under these circumstances,

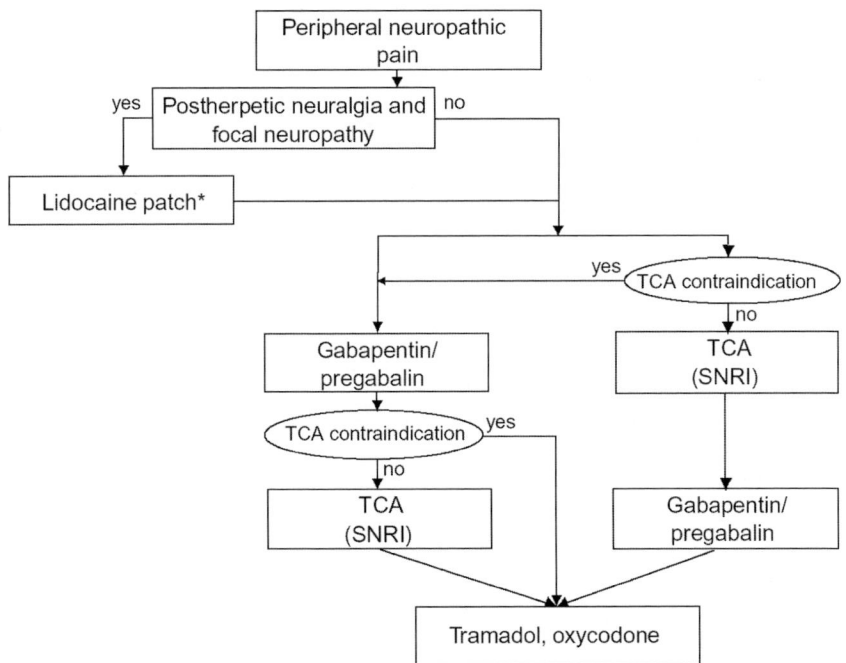

FIGURE 2. Suggested algorithm for the treatment of peripheral neuropathic pain. (From Finnerup *et al.*[89])

the algorithm for peripheral neuropathic pain treatment was constructed (FIG. 2). Since for central neuropathic pain few studies exist, a treatment algorithm for these conditions needs to be based partly on the experience in peripheral neuropathic pain conditions until further studies are done.

In spite of the increasing availability of efficient therapeutic possibilities, the treatment of neuropathic pain often remains frustrating both for the patient and the physician. Active involvement of the patient in the therapeutic decisions and the setting of realistic goals is extremely important. Although the existing evidence should guide the therapy, the physician should be flexible in the choice of treatment, especially with patients who have already failed to respond to a number of therapies. Interest in the mechanisms and treatment of chronic neuropathic pain has increased and this is likely to result in significant treatment advances in the future. Advances will make it possible to go beyond the determination of whether the treatment is effective to the identification of what treatments are most effective for which patients. Progress in basic science will lead to a greater understanding of the pathophysiological mechanisms of neuropathic pain. Important goals for clinical research are to devise methods for reliably identifying specific mechanisms in individual patients and to target treatment to them. Only when we have the tools to identify the mechanisms responsible in a particular individual and then the capacity to reverse these mechanisms, will the management of chronic neuropathic pain really advance! The goal awaits...

REFERENCES

1. WOOLF, C.J. & M.B. MAX. 2001. Mechanism-based pain diagnosis: issues for analgesic drug development. Anesthesiology **95:** 241–249.
2. MCCLESKEY, E.W. & M.S. GOLD. 1999. Ion channels of nociception. Annu. Rev. Physiol. **61:** 835–856.
3. WOOLF, C.J. & M.W. SALTER. 2000. Neuronal plasticity: increasing the gain in pain. Science **288:** 1765–1768.
4. MOGIL, J.S. *et al.* 2000. Pain genes: natural variation and transgenic mutants. Annu. Rev. Neurosci. **23:** 777–811.
5. WOOLF, C.J. *et al.* 1998. Towards a mechanism based classification of pain? Pain **77:** 227–229.
6. WOOLF, C.J. & R.J. MANNION. 1999. Neuropathic pain: aetiology, symptoms, mechanisms and management. Lancet **353:** 1959–1964.
7. CHONG, M.S. & Z.H. BAJWA. 2003. Diagnosis and treatment of neuropathic pain. J. Pain Symptom Manage. **25:** S4–S11.
8. H. MERSKEY & N. BOGDUK, Eds. 1994. Classification of Chronic Pain. 2nd ed. IASP Press. Seattle.
9. IASP (INTERNATIONAL ASSOCIATION FOR THE STUDY OF PAIN). IASP pain terminology. http://www.halcyon.com/iasp/terms-p.html.
10. CRUCCU, G. *et al.* 2004. EFNS guidelines on neuropathic pain assessment. Eur. J. Neurol. **11:** 153–162.

11. HANSSON, P. 2002. Neuropathic pain: clinical characteristics and diagnostic workup. Eur. J. Pain **6:** 47–50.
12. MEYER-ROSEBERG, K. *et al.* 2001. A comparison of the SF-36 and Nottingham Health Profile in patients with chronic neuropathic pain. Eur. J. Pain **5:** 391–403.
13. MEYER-ROSEBERG, K. *et al.* 2001. Peripheral neuropathic pain—a multidimensional burden for patients. Eur. J. Pain **5:** 379–389.
14. BOWSHER, D. 1991. Neurogenic pain syndromes and their management. Br. Med. Bull. **47:** 644–666.
15. CARTER, G.T. & B.S. GALER. 2001. Advances in the management of neuropathic pain. Phys. Med. Rehabil. Clin. North Am. **12:** 447–459.
16. SUNDERLAND, S. 1993. Brachial plexus injuries. Clin. Neurol. Neurosurg. **95:** S1–S2.
17. BOIVI, J. 1999. Central pain. *In* Textbook of Pain. P.D. Wall & R. Melzak, Eds.: 879–914. Churchill Livingstone. Edinburgh.
18. BONICA, J.J. 1991. Introduction: semantic, epidemiologic and educational issues. *In* Pain and Central Nervous System Disease: The Central Pain Syndromes. K.L. Casey, Ed.: 13–29. Raven Press. New York, NY.
19. ANDERSEN, G. *et al.* 1995. Incidence of central post-stroke pain. Pain **61:** 187–193.
20. SMITH, T.E. & M.S. CHONG. 2000. Neuropathic pain. Hosp. Med. **61:** 760–766.
21. IRVING, G. 2005. Contemporary assessment and management of neuropathic pain. Neurology **64:** S21–S27.
22. DWORKING, R.H. *et al.* 2003. Advances in neuropathic pain: diagnosis, mechanisms and treatment recommendations. Arch. Neurol. **60:** 1524–1535.
23. BENICZKY, S. *et al.* 2005. Evidence-based pharmacological treatment of neuropathic pain syndromes. J. Neural. Transm. **112:** 735–749.
24. FINNERUP, N.B. *et al.* 2001. Pain and dysaesthesia in patients with spinal cord injury: a postal survey. Spinal Cord **39:** 256–262.
25. RICHEIMER, S.H. *et al.* 1997. Utilization patterns of tricyclic antidepressants in a multidisciplinary pain clinic: a survey. Clin. J. Pain **13:** 324–329.
26. OZRA, F. *et al.* 2000. Neuropathic pain: review of mechanisms and pharmacologic management. Neurorehabilitation **14:** 15–23.
27. BOULTON, A.J.M. *et al.* 1998. Guidelines for the diagnosis and outpatient management of diabetic peripheral neuropathy. Diabet. Med. **15:** 508–514.
28. PAGE, J.C. & E.Y. CHEN. 1997. Management of painful diabetic neuropathy. A treatment algorithm. J. Am. Podiatr. Med. Assoc. **87:** 370–379.
29. PERKIN, G.D. 1999. Trigeminal neuralgia. Curr. Treat Options Neurol. **1:** 458–465.
30. NAMAKA, M. *et al.* 2004. A treatment algorithm for neuropathic pain. Clin. Ther. **26:** 951–979.
31. BERGOUIGNAN, M. 1942. Cures heureuses de neuralgies facials essentielles par le diphenylhydantoinate de soude. Rev. Laryngol. Otol. Rhinol. **63:** 34–41.
32. BEYDOUN, A. 2001. Symptomatic treatment of neuropathic pain: a focus on the role of anticonvulsants. Medsc. CME Circle Lect. http://www.medscape.com/.
33. BACKONJA, M. *et al.* 1998. Gabapentin for the symptomatic treatment of painful neuropathy in patients with diabetes mellitus: a randomized controlled trial. JAMA **280:** 1831–1836.
34. GORSON, K.C. *et al.* 1999. Gabapentin in the treatment of painful diabetic neuropathy: a placebo-controlled, double-blind, crossover trial. J. Neurol. Neurosurg. Psychiatry **66:** 251–252.

35. ROWBOTHAM, M. *et al.* 1998. Gabapentin for the treatment of postherpetic neuralgia: a randomized controlled trial. JAMA **280:** 1837–1842.
36. RICE, A.S. *et al.* 2001. Gabapentin in postherpetic neuralgia: a randomized, double-blind, placebo controlled study. Pain **94:** 215–224.
37. BONE, M. *et al.* 2002. Gabapentin in postamputation phantom limb pain: a randomized, double-blind, placebo-controlled, cross-over study. Reg. Anesth. Pain Med. **27:** 481–486.
38. PANDEY, C.K. *et al.* 2002. Gabapentin for the treatment of pain in Guillain–Barré syndrome: a double-blind, placebo-controlled, cross-over study. Anesth. Analg. **95:** 1719–1723.
39. TAI, Q. *et al.* 2002. Gabapentin in the treatment of neuropathic pain after spinal cord injury: a prospective, randomized, double-blind, crossover trial. J. Spinal Cord Med. **25:** 100–105.
40. VAN DE VUSSE, A.C. *et al.* 2004. Randomized, controlled trial of gabapentin in complex regional pain syndrome type I. BMC Neurol. **4:** 13–19.
41. MOKA, E. *et al.* 2004. The role of gabapentin as an add-on therapy in chronic neuropathic pain [abstract]. 11th International Pain Clinic WSPC, Tokyo, Abstract Book: 188.
42. WIFFEN, P.J. 2005. Gabapentin for acute and chronic pain. The Cohrane Database of Systematic Reviews **3:** Art No CD005452.
43. SERPELL, M. 2002. Gabapentin in neuropathic pain syndromes: a randomized, double-blind, placebo-controlled trial. Pain **99:** 557–566.
44. CARACENI, A. *et al.* 2004. Gabapentin for neuropathic cancer pain: a randomized, controlled trial from the gabapentin cancer pain study group. J. Clin. Oncol. **22:** 2909–2917.
45. MOKA, E. *et al.* 2004. The role of gabapentin in chronic neuropathic pain in MS patients: a 4-year experience [abstract]. 2nd International Symposium of Regional Anaesthesia and Pain Therapy, Chile.
46. ROWBOTHAM, M.C. *et al.* 1996. Lidocaine patch: double-blind, controlled study of a new treatment for post-herpetic neuralgia. Pain **65:** 39–44.
47. GALER, B.S. *et al.* 1999. Topical lidocaine patch relieves postherpetic neuralgia more effectively than a vehicle topical patch: results of an enriched enrollment study. Pain **80:** 533–538.
48. MEIER, T. *et al.* 2003. Efficacy of lidocaine patch 5% in the treatment of focal peripheral neuropathic pain syndromes: a randomized, double-blind, placebo-controlled study. Pain **106:** 151–158.
49. BARBANO, R.L. *et al.* 2004. Effectiveness, tolerability, and impact on quality of life of the 5% lidocaine patch in diabetic polyneuropathy. Arch. Neurol. **61:** 914–918.
50. ARGYRA, E. *et al.* 2005. 5% lidocaine patch in the treatment of neuropathic pain of diverse origin [abstract]. Eur. J. Pall. Care–Abstract book 9th Congress of the European Association for Palliative Care (EAPC): 80.
51. GIMBEL, J.S. *et al.* 2003. Controlled-release oxycodone for pain in diabetic neuropathy. A randomized controlled trial. Neurology **60:** 927–934.
52. WATSON, C.P. *et al.* 2003. Controlled-release oxycodone relieves neuropathic pain: a randomized controlled trial in painful diabetic neuropathy. Pain **105:** 71–78.
53. WATSON, C.P. & N. BABUL. 1998. Efficacy of oxycodone in neuropathic pain: a randomized trial in postherpetic neuralgia. Neurology **50:** 1837–1841.
54. HUSE, E. *et al.* 2001. The effect of opioids on phantom limb pain and cortical reorganization. Pain **90:** 47–55.

55. RAJA, S.N. *et al.* 2002. Opioids versus antidepressants in postherpetic neuralgia. Neurology **59:** 1015–1021.
56. MORLEY, J.S. *et al.* 2003. Low-dose methadone has an analgesic effect in neuropathic pain: a double-blind randomized controlled crossover trial. Palliative Med. **17:** 576–587.
57. ROWBOTHAM, M.C. *et al.* 2003. Oral opioid therapy for chronic peripheral and central neuropathic pain. N. Engl. J. Med. **348:** 1223–1232.
58. GILRON, I. *et al.* 2005. Morphine, gabapentin or their combination for neuropathic pain. N. Engl. J. Med. **352:** 1324–1334.
59. EISENBERG, E. *et al.* 2005. Efficacy and safety of opioid agonists in the treatment of neuropathic pain of non-malignant origin. JAMA **293:** 3043–3052.
60. BALLANTYNE, J. & J. MAO. 2003. Opioid therapy for chronic pain. N. Engl. J. Med. **349:** 1943–1953.
61. HARATI, Y. *et al.* 1998. Double-blind randomized trial of tramadol for the treatment of the pain of diabetic neuropathy. Neurology **50:** 1842–1846.
62. SINDRUP, S.H. *et al.* 1999. Tramadol relieves pain and allodynia in polyneuropathy: a randomized double-blind controlled trial. Pain **83:** 85–90.
63. BOUREAU, F. *et al.* 2003. Tramadol in post-herpetic neuralgia: a randomized double-blind placebo-controlled trial. Pain **104:** 323–331.
64. BEYDOUN, A. & M.M. BACKOGNA. 2003. Mechanistic stratification of antineuralgic agents. J. Pain Symptom Manage. **25:** S18–S30.
65. SANCHEZ, C. & J. HYTTEL. 1999. Comparison of the effects of antidepressants and their metabolites on the reuptake of biogenic amines and on receptor binding. Cell. Mol. Neurobiol. **19:** 467–489.
66. MAX, M.B. 1995. Thirteen consecutive well designed randomized trial show that antidepressants reduce pain in diabetic neuropathy and post herpetic neuralgia. Pain Forum **4:** 248–253.
67. MCQUAY, G.J. *et al.* 1996. A systematic review of antidepressants in neuropathic pain. Pain **68:** 217–227.
68. SINDRUP, S.H. & T.S. JENSEN. 1999. Efficacy of pharmacological treatments of neuropathic pain: an update and effect related to mechanism of drug action. Pain **83:** 389–400.
69. COHEN, H.W. *et al.* 2000. Excess risk of myocardial infarction in patients treated with antidepressant medication: association with use of tricyclic agents. Am. J. Med. **108:** 2–8.
70. EISENBERG, E. *et al.* 2001. Lamotrigine reduces painful diabetic neuropathy: a randomized controlled study. Neurology **57:** 505–509.
71. VESTERGAARD, K. *et al.* 2001. Lamotrigine for central poststroke pain: a randomized controlled trial. Neurology **56:** 184–190.
72. FINNERUP, N.B. *et al.* 2002. Lamotrigine in spinal cord injury pain: a randomized controlled trial. Pain **96:** 375–383.
73. SIMPSON, D.M. *et al.* 2000. A placebo controlled trial of lamotrigine for painful HIV-associated neuropathy. Neurology **54:** 2115–2119.
74. MACDONALD, J. & L.T. YOUNG. 2002. Newer antiepileptic drugs in bipolar disorder: rationale for use and role in therapy. CNS Drugs **16:** 549–562.
75. MCQUAY, H. *et al.* 1995. Antoconvulsant drugs for the management of pain: a systematic review. BMJ **311:** 1047–1052.
76. DWORKIN, R.H. *et al.* 2003. Pregabalin for the treatment of postherpetic neuralgia: a randomized placebo-controlled trial. Neurology **60:** 1274–1283.

77. ROSENSTOCK, J. *et al.* 2004. Pregabalin for the treatment of painful, diabetic, peripheral neuropathy: a double-blind, placebo controlled trial. Pain **110:** 628–638.

78. SINDRUP, S.H. & T.S. JENSEN. 2000. Pharmacologic treatment of pain in polyneuropathy. Neurology **55:** 915–920.

79. SEMENCHUK, M.R. *et al.* 2001. Double-blind, randomized, controlled trial of bupropion SR for the treatment of neuropathic pain. Neurology **57:** 1583–1588.

80. SINDRUP, S.H. *et al.* 2003. Venlafaxine versus imipramine in painful polyneuropathy: a randomized-controlled trial. Neurology **60:** 1284–1289.

81. ROWBOTHAM, M.C. *et al.* 2004. Venlafaxine-extended release in the treatment of painful diabetic neuropathy: a double-blind, placebo-controlled study. Pain **110:** 697–706.

82. TASMUTH, T. *et al.* 2002. Venlafaxine in neuropathic pain following treatment of breast cancer. Eur. J. Pain **6:** 17–24.

83. WERNICKE, J.F. *et al.* 2004. Duloxetin at doses of 60 mgr QD and 60 mgr BID is effective in treatment of diabetic neuropathic pain (DNP). [abstract] Neurology **62:** A192.

84. SEMENCHUNK, M.R. & S. SHERMAN. 2000. Effectiveness of tizanidine in neuropathic pain: an open-label study. J. Pain **1:** 285–292.

85. TAKAHASHI, H. *et al.* 1998. The NMDA-receptor antagonist ketamine abolishes neuropathic pain after epidural administration in a clinical case. Pain **75:** 391–394.

86. MACPHERSON, R.D. 2002. New directions in pain management. Drugs Today (Barc) **38:** 135–145.

87. ALVARO, M. *et al.* 1999. Transcutaneous electrostimulation: emerging treatment for diabetic neuropathic pain. Diabetes Technol. Ther. **1:** 77–80.

88. TAYLOR, R.S. *et al.* 2005. Spinal cord stimulation for chronic low back and leg pain and failed back surgery syndrome: a systematic review and analysis of prognostic factors. Spine **1:** 152–160.

89. FINNERUP, N.B. *et al.* 2005. Algorithm for neuropathic pain treatment: an evidence-based proposal. Pain [E-pub ahead of print]: 1–17.

Regulation of Dendritic Cell Differentiation by Vasoactive Intestinal Peptide

Therapeutic Applications on Autoimmunity and Transplantation

ALEJO CHORNY, ELENA GONZALEZ-REY, AND MARIO DELGADO

Institute of Parasitology and Biomedicine, CSIC, Granada, Spain

ABSTRACT: Dendritic cells (DCs) are the most potent antigen-presenting cells (APCs) involved in the defense of the body and in the maintenance of the immune tolerance. The regulation of their maturation, migration, and expression of stimulatory and costimulatory molecules has major consequences on the immune response. The endogenous factors that regulate DC function are poorly known. Vasoactive intestinal peptide (VIP) is a neuropeptide with potent anti-inflammatory actions. This anti-inflammatory profile is maintained partially through effects on DC differentiation/function. Thus, VIP has differential effects on DCs, depending on the differentiation and stimulatory states. Immature DCs treated with VIP exhibit increased CD86 expression and induce CD4$^+$ T cell proliferation. In addition, the CD4$^+$ T cells activated *in vitro* or *in vivo* by VIP-treated iDCs exhibit a Th2 phenotype. In contrast, VIP reduces both CD86 and CD80 expression on lipopolysaccharide (LPS)-stimulated DCs, and inhibits the capacity of DCs to induce *in vitro* or *in vivo* T cell proliferation. However, addition of VIP in the early states of DC differentiation results in the generation of DCs that cannot mature following inflammatory stimuli that exhibit a tolerogenic phenotype, characterized by low expression of costimulatory molecules (CD40, CD80, and CD86), low production of proinflammatory cytokines, increased production of IL-10, and capacity to induce regulatory T cells with suppressive actions. The effect of VIP on the DC-Treg axis represents an additional mechanism for their general anti-inflammatory role, particularly relevant in autoimmunity and transplantation.

KEYWORDS: dendritic cells; immune tolerance; autoimmunity; regulatory T cells

Address for correspondence: Mario Delgado, Instituto de Parasitologia y Biomedicina, CSIC, Avd. Conocimiento, PT Ciencias de la Salud, Granada 18100, Spain. Voice: 34-958-181665; fax: 34-958-181632.
e-mail: mdelgado@ipb.csic.es

Ann. N.Y. Acad. Sci. 1088: 187–194 (2006). © 2006 New York Academy of Sciences.
doi: 10.1196/annals.1366.004

INTRODUCTION

Dendritic cells (DCs) participate in the first line of defense against environmental pathogens in nonlymphoid organs, such as the skin, gastrointestinal tract, and respiratory tract. DCs act as innate immune cells capable of phagocytosis and release of proinflammatory agents, and initiate the adaptive immune response by activating antigen-specific naïve T cells.[1] Following pathogen recognition, DCs mature, acquiring the capacity to migrate to secondary lymphoid organs, where they activate naïve T cells by providing both stimulatory and costimulatory signals. Since DCs are the most potent antigen-presenting cells (APCs), the regulation of their maturation, migration, and expression of stimulatory and costimulatory molecules has major consequences on the immune response.

In addition to their classical role as sentinels of the immune response, DCs also play an important role in immune homeostasis by inducing and maintaining tolerance.[2] The maturation/activation state of DCs might be the control point for the induction of peripheral tolerance, by promoting the generation/activation of regulatory T cells (Treg). Mature DCs (mDCs) are potent APCs, enhancing T cell immunity, whereas immature DCs (iDCs) are involved in the induction of peripheral T cell tolerance.[1-3] Although the clinical use of iDCs may not be suitable in autoimmune diseases and transplantation because iDCs are likely to mature in inflammatory conditions,[4] tolerogenic DCs prevent lethal graft-versus-host disease (GVHD) in hosts transplanted with allogeneic bone marrow cells, while maintaining the graft-versus-tumor response.[5] Immunosuppressive therapy, traditionally focused on lymphocytes, has been revolutionized by targeting DCs, and the *in vitro* generation of tolerogenic DCs has become the focus of new therapies.[6]

Vasoactive intestinal peptide (VIP) is a neuropeptide released by both innervation and immune cells, particularly Th2 cells, in response to antigen stimulation and under inflammatory/autoimmune conditions.[7] VIP elicits a broad spectrum of biological functions, including immunomodulation, predominantly acting as a potent anti-inflammatory factor and a suppressive agent for Th1 responses.[7] Therefore, VIP has emerged as a promising therapeutic factor for the treatment of autoimmune/inflammatory diseases, including rheumatoid arthritis, ulcerative colitis, uveoretinitis, and experimental autoimmune encephalomyelitis.[7] Although a large body of literature focuses on its effects on macrophages and T cells, recent reports demonstrated the crucial involvement of DCs in the immunomodulatory role of VIP. In this study, we review these reports showing that differentiating, immature, and activated DCs react differently to VIP treatment leading to three subtypes of DCs with totally different immunological roles (FIG. 1).

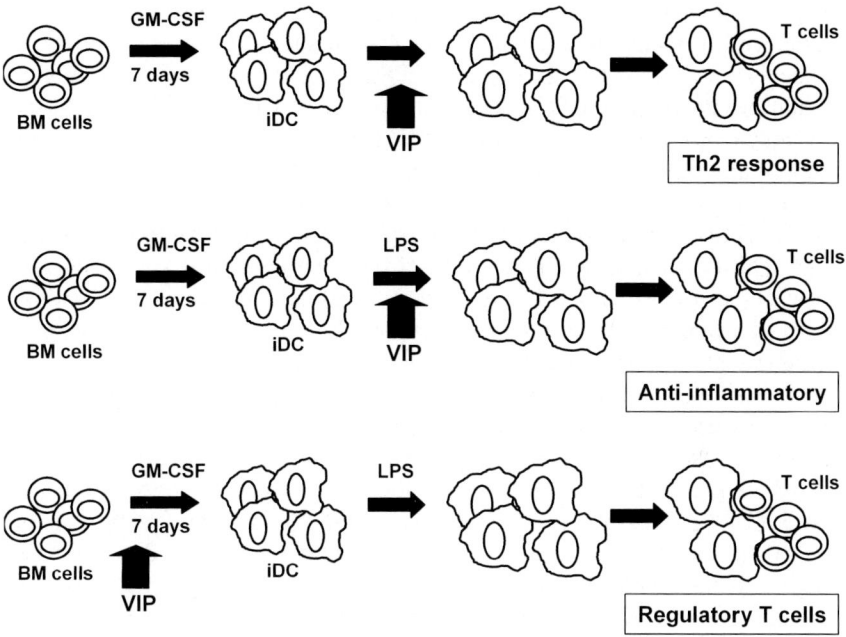

FIGURE 1. VIP differentially affects the differentiation/function of DCs. Addition of VIP during early steps of differentiation of DCs from bone marrow (BM) cells, to unstimulated iDCs or to LPS-stimulated iDCs results in three different phenotypes of DCs with very different functions.

VIP DIFFERENTIALLY REGULATES IMMATURE AND ACTIVATED DENDRITIC CELLS

Several signals are required for the activation of naïve T cells. The stimulatory signal is provided by the interaction between the MHC class II/antigenic peptide on the APCs and the TCR on T cells. The costimulatory signals are provided by interactions between the B7 family and CD40 on APCs, and CD28 and CD40L on T cells, respectively. Although all APCs express MHC class II, DCs are the only ones expressing CD80 (B7.1) and CD86 (B7.2) constitutively, which makes them the most efficient APCs for activation of naïve T cells. However, all three types of APCs, that is, DCs, macrophages, and microglia, express toll-like receptors (TLRs) involved in the recognition of pathogen-associated molecular patterns, and upregulate both stimulatory and costimulatory molecules upon encountering pathogens. One of the components of the general anti-inflammatory action of VIP is the reduction in stimulatory/costimulatory activity of DCs for antigen-specific T cells. Whereas the lipopolysaccharide (LPS) treatment of iDCs resulted in an increase in the expression of the stimulatory (MHC II) and costimulatory (CD40, CD80, CD86) molecules, VIP added at the time of LPS stimulation prevented the upregulation of CD80 and CD86 expression, but not of CD40 or MHC II.[8] As a consequence, VIP reduced the stimulatory activity of LPS-treated DCs for allogeneic and syngeneic T cells.[8] LPS-stimulated DCs induced the preferential production of the Th1-type cytokines IFNγ and IL-2. VIP treatment significantly reduced the amounts of IFNγ and IL-2 without affecting the levels of the Th2-type cytokines IL-4 and IL-5, or of the cytokines associated with certain types of regulatory T cells, that is, IL-10 and TGFβ1.[8] These results are in agreement with the previously reported anti-inflammatory activity of VIP, and with its proposed role as endogenous immune deactivators.

However, VIP had an opposite effect on iDCs. It upregulated CD86 expression, and VIP-treated iDCs acquired the capacity to stimulate the proliferation of antigen-specific T cells *in vivo* and *in vitro*.[8] Interestingly, the VIP-treated iDCs also acquired the capacity to bias the CD4$^+$ T cell response in favor of Th2 effectors.[8] This was associated *in vivo* with the predominant production of specific antibodies belonging to the IgG1 subclass, and a reduction in the IgG2a subclass. The fact that VIP induced iDCs to promote Th2 responses is in agreement with previous observations. It has previously been reported that VIP induces Th2 responses *in vivo*, preferentially protecting Th2 effectors from antigen-induced apoptosis, and promotes the *in vivo* generation of Th2 memory cells.[7,9] In addition, the role of the VIP receptor VPAC2 and of the endogenous, Th2-derived VIP for the Th1/Th2 balance *in vivo* and *in vitro* was demonstrated in a series of studies that confirmed the essential role of VIP/VPAC2 interactions in inducing and maintaining the Th2 bias.[10–12] The induction of Th2-type responses, in association with the suppression of acute, proinflammatory Th1-type responses, is in agreement with the proposed anti-inflammatory activity of the VIP.

Therefore, we propose that VIP regulates the immune response through different mechanisms. In the absence of a strong pathogenic challenge, VIP promotes Th2-type responses that could confer protection through antibody production, without eliciting acute inflammation. This might be particularly suitable for immune-privileged sites where acute inflammatory processes could lead to irreversible damage. The Th2-induced bias by VIP is probably mediated through a combination of effects on DCs, macrophages, and directly on the Th2 effectors.[7] In contrast, in the presence of strong pathogenic challenges, mimicked *in vitro* by bacterial endotoxins, the major immune function of VIP is anti-inflammatory in nature. VIP inhibits the production of cytokines and chemokines from major proinflammatory cells, that is, macrophages and CNS microglia, and reduces the capacity of DCs to stimulate T cell proliferation, primarily by preventing and/or reducing the expression of costimulatory molecules.

VIP GENERATES TOLEROGENIC DCs THAT INDUCE REGULATORY T CELLS

The induction of Ag-specific tolerance is critical for the prevention of autoimmunity and maintenance of immune tolerance. Beside their classical role as sentinels of the immune response inducing T cell reactivity, increasing evidence suggests that DCs can induce specific T cell tolerance. Although the underlying mechanisms are not fully elucidated, the capacity to induce Treg cells is an important property of tolerogenic/regulatory DCs. The *in vitro* generation of tolerogenic "designer" DCs is a desirable goal and represents the subject of intensive investigations. We have recently reported the use of VIP as a new approach to induce human and murine tolerogenic DCs with the capacity to generate CD4 and CD8 Treg cells.[13,14] The presence of VIP during the early stages of DC differentiation from human blood monocytes or from mouse bone marrow cells leads to the development of DCs that cannot mature following inflammatory stimuli. These DC_{VIPs} exhibit a tolerogenic phenotype, characterized by low expression of costimulatory molecules (CD40, CD80, and CD86), low production of proinflammatory cytokines, and increased production of IL-10. These cells do not prime T cell responses, and suppress previously primed immune responses. The stimulation of T cells with allogeneic DC_{VIP} induced CD4 and CD8 T cells that display the typical properties of Tr1-like regulatory cells, including a characteristic cytokine profile (high IL-10 and TGF-β, and little or no IFN-γ, IL-2, IL-4), intrinsic low proliferative capacity, and suppression of the Ag-specific proliferation/activation of other CD4 Th1 cells, even when Th1 cells were restimulated with mDCs.[13,14]

Although the precise mechanisms remain unknown, several possibilities may account for the generation of Treg cells by DC_{VIP}. The activation of naïve CD4 T lymphocytes requires two signals delivered by mDCs, one mediated through Ag/MHCII–TCR interaction (signal 1), and a second one mediated by interaction of costimulatory molecules, such as CD80/CD86–CD28 and CD40–CD40L. Costimulatory molecules, especially CD40, appear to be key determinants of the decision between tolerance and immunity.[15] The characteristic phenotype of DC_{VIP}, that is, high levels of MHC plus poor expression of costimulatory molecules, which deliver stimulatory but not costimulatory signals, is in agreement with their tolerance-inducing ability. In addition, the observation that DC_{VIPs} secrete IL-10 may be linked to the stability of their tolerogenic-like phenotype, since IL-10 inhibits the expression of costimulatory molecules on APCs, enriches differentiating bone marrow cells in tolerogenic DCs, and induces the generation of IL-10-producing T cells.[16]

The mechanism of Tr1-induced suppression is still controversial. For example, some evidence shows that the suppression is primarily mediated by IL-10 and TGF-β in a cell contact–independent manner, whereas others have described a cytokine-independent, cell contact–mediated mechanism.[3] Indeed,

Ag-specific IL-10-producing Tr1 cells suppress inflammation in colitis and allergic models in an IL-10-dependent manner, whereas blockade of TGF-β *in vivo* abrogates T cell–mediated suppression of severe colitis. DC_{VIP}-induced Tr1-like cells act through both soluble factors and direct cellular contact, suggesting the presence of different CD4 Treg cell subpopulations. A characteristic marker of Treg cells is the constitutive expression of CTLA4, a negative regulatory factor critical for the induction and function of Treg cells.[17] In agreement with these reports, CD4 T cells exposed to DC_{VIP} ($CD4Tr_{VIP}$) expresses high levels of CTLA4, explaining the partial dependence on cell contact for their suppressive activity. In addition, $CD4Tr_{VIP}$ expresses high levels of membrane-bound TGF-β, which has been shown to participate in the suppressive activity of Treg cells.

It has also been described that priming of naïve $CD8^+$ T cells with allogeneic DC_{VIP} reduced their proliferative and lytic activity in an Ag-dependent manner. In contrast to $DC_{controls}$, which activate CD8 T cells through the delivery of signal 1 plus signal 2, $DC_{VIP}S$ deliver a potent signal 1 and a weak signal 2 to Ag-specific $CD8^+$ T cells, resulting in anergy. The anergic state is associated with an increased number of IL-10-producing $CD8^+CD28^-$ T cells. CD8 T cells exposed to DC_{VIP} suppress syngeneic Th1 effector cells, a characteristic that seems to reside in the $CD8^+CD28^-$ population. $CD8^+CD28^-$ T cells generated in various ways can suppress CD4 T cells.[16] Although CD8 Treg with regulatory properties has received less attention than the CD4 Treg, several studies have demonstrated their importance in tolerance, and tolerogenic DCs were shown to play an essential role in the induction of CD8 Tregs.[16,18] $CD8Tr_{VIP}s$ mediated their suppressive capacity by direct cell contact with CD4 T effector cells, and increased CTLA4 expression in $CD8Tr_{VIP}s$ appears to play a major role.

Interestingly, $DC_{VIP}s$ retained their capacity to induce Treg under inflammatory conditions. This observation is particularly relevant for conditions in which ongoing Ag presentation is associated with chronic inflammation, including autoimmune diseases, allograft rejection, and GVHD. We have recently found that murine regulatory $DC_{VIP}s$ showed a prominent therapeutic action on models of rheumatoid arthritis, multiple sclerosis, and allogeneic bone marrow transplantation, even when administered after disease onset.[19,20] The *in vivo* efficacy of $DC_{VIP}s$ was antigen-specific and depends on their compatibility with the host MHC antigens. DC_{VIP} directly suppressed not only the effector functions of autoreactive T cells and *in vivo*-primed allogeneic CD4 and CD8 T cells, but also their responsiveness to *in vitro* restimulation.[13,14] Therefore, the mechanism responsible for the DC_{VIP} therapeutic effect in autoimmunity and acute GVHD involves the induction of tolerant T cells as well as direct suppression of effector T cells *in vivo*. In agreement with this hypothesis, treatment with $CD4Tr_{VIP}s$ abrogated, in a haplotype/antigen- and TGF-β/IL-10-dependent manner, the acute GVHD in bone marrow–transplanted mice and disease progression in arthritic mice.[19,20]

It has been proposed that tolerance induction by DCs requires maturation signals different from microbial or inflammatory stimuli. In steady-state conditions, VIP could represent one of the endogenous maturation signals driving the differentiation of tolerogenic DCs with a semimature phenotype. VIP is secreted in the lymphoid microenvironment, mainly by Th2 cells following antigen stimulation, and VIP levels are increased in immunopathologic conditions, such as autoimmunity and inflammation.[7] Therefore, DC_{VIPs} may represent a population of DCs that have matured to display a stable tolerogenic phenotype. Under steady-state conditions, DC_{VIPs} could be loaded with self- and commonly encountered antigens, and following migration to the lymphoid organs they could induce CD4 and CD8 Treg differentiation and tolerance. In this sense, administration of VIP on TCR-transgenic mice induced the *in vivo* emergence of DCs in draining lymph nodes with capacity to generate antigen-specific CD4 T cells with regulatory capacity.[13]

The possibility of generating human tolerogenic DC_{VIPs} opens new therapeutic avenues for the treatment of autoimmune diseases and allogeneic transplantation. In animal models the *in vitro* pulsing of tolerogenic DC_{VIPs} with self- or alloantigens, followed by *in vivo* injection, led to the differentiation of antigen-specific Treg cells. Therefore, the inclusion of tolerogenic DC_{VIPs} in future therapeutic regimens may minimize the dependence on nonspecific immunosuppressive drugs used currently for the treatment of autoimmune disorders and transplant rejection.

ACKNOWLEDGMENTS

This work was supported by grants from the Spanish Ministry of Health (PI04/0674), NIH (2RO1A047325), and Ramon Areces Foundation.

REFERENCES

1. BANCHEREAU, J., F. BRIERE, C. CAUX, *et al.* 2000. Immunobiology of dendritic cells. Annu. Rev. Immunol. **18:** 767–811.
2. STEINMAN, R.M., D. HAWINGER & M.C. NUSSENZWEIG. 2003. Tolerogenic dendritic cells. Annu. Rev. Immunol. **109:** 685–711.
3. RUTELLA, S. & R.M. LEMOLI. 2004. Regulatory T cells and tolerogenic dendritic cells: from basic biology to clinical applications. Immunol. Lett. **94:** 11–26.
4. RONCAROLO, M.C., M.K. LEVINGS & C. TRAVERARI. 2001. Differentiation of T regulatory cells by immature dendritic cells. J. Exp. Med. **193:** F5–F9.
5. MORELLI, A.E. & A.W. THOMSON. 2003. Dendritic cells: regulators of alloimmunity and opportunities for tolerance induction. Immunol. Rev. **196:** 125–146.
6. HACKSTEIN, H. & A.W. THOMSON. 2004. Dendritic cells: emerging pharmacological targets of immunosuppressive drugs. Nat. Rev. Immunol. **4:** 24–34.
7. DELGADO, M., D. POZO & D. GANEA. 2004. The significance of vasoactive intestinal peptide in immunomodulation. Pharmacol. Rev. **56:** 249–290.

8. DELGADO, M., A. REDUTA, V. SHARMA & D. GANEA. 2004. VIP/PACAP oppositely affect immature and mature dendritic cell expression of CD80/CD86 and the stimulatory activity for CD4$^+$ T cells. J. Leukoc. Biol. **75:** 1122–1130.

9. DELGADO, M., J. LECETA & D. GANEA. 2002. VIP and PACAP promote in vivo generation of memory Th2 cells. FASEB J. **16:** 1844–1846.

10. VOICE, J.K., G. DORSAM, H. LEE, et al. 2001. Allergic diathesis in transgenic mice with constitutive T cell expression of inducible VIP receptor. FASEB J. **15:** 2489–2496.

11. VOICE, J.K., A. GRINNINGER, Y. KONG, et al. 2003. Roles of vasoactive intestinal peptide (VIP) in the expression of different immune phenotypes by wild-type mice and T cell-targeted type II VIP receptor transgenic mice. J. Immunol. **170:** 308–314.

12. GOETZL, E.J., J.K. VOICE, S. SHEN, et al. 2001. Enhanced delayed-type hypersensitivity and diminished immediate type hypersensitivity in mice lacking the inducible VPAC(2) receptor for VIP. Proc. Natl. Acad. Sci. USA **98:** 13854–13859.

13. DELGADO, M., E. GONZALEZ-REY & D. GANEA. 2005. The neuropeptide vasoactive intestinal peptide generates tolerogenic dendritic cells. J. Immunol. **175:** 7311–7324.

14. GONZALEZ-REY, E., A. CHORNY, A. FERNANDEZ-MARTIN, et al. 2006. Vasoactive intestinal peptide generates human tolerogenic dendritic cells that induce CD4 and CD8 regulatory T cells. Blood **107:** 3632–3638.

15. DIEHL, L., A.T. DEN BOER, E.I. VAN DER VOORT, et al. 2000. The role of CD40 in peripheral T cell tolerance and immunity. J. Mol. Med. **78:** 363–371.

16. SATO, K., N. YAMASHITA, M. BABA & T. MATSUYAMA. 2003. Modified myeloid dendritic cells act as regulatory dendritic cells to induce anergic and regulatory T cells. Blood **101:** 3581–3589.

17. READ, S., V. MALMSTROM & F. POWRIE. 2000. Cytotoxic T lymphocyte-associated antigen 4 plays an essential role in the function of CD25$^+$CD4$^+$ regulatory cells that control intestinal inflammation. J. Exp. Med. **192:** 295–302.

18. DHODAPKAR, M.V. & R.M. STEINMAN. 2002. Antigen-bearing immature dendritic cells induce peptide-specific CD8+ regulatory T cells in vivo in humans. Blood **100:** 174–177.

19. CHORNY, A., E. GONZALEZ-REY, A. FERNANDEZ-MARTIN, et al. Vasoactive intestinal peptide induces regulatory dendritic cells with therapeutic effects on autoimmune disorders. Proc. Natl. Acad. Sci. USA **102:** 13562–13567.

20. CHORNY, A., E. GONZALEZ-REY, A. FERNANDEZ-MARTIN, et al. 2006. Vasoactive intestinal peptide induces regulatory dendritic cells that prevent acute graft-versus-host disease while maintaining the graft-versus-tumor response. Blood. **107:** 3787–3794.

Neuroendocrine Regulation of Skin Dendritic Cells

KRISTINA SEIFFERT[a] AND RICHARD D. GRANSTEIN[b]

[a]*Division of Dermatology and Cutaneous Sciences, Michigan State University, East Lansing, Michigan, USA*

[b]*Department of Dermatology, Weill Medical College of Cornell University, New York, New York, USA*

ABSTRACT: It has long been postulated that stress can affect certain skin conditions, and there is increasing experimental evidence that the neuroendocrine system can directly participate in cutaneous inflammation. Neurohormones, such as glucocorticoids and catecholamines, can reach the skin through the bloodstream after activation of the hypothalamic–pituitary–adrenal axis and the sympathetic nervous system, respectively. Multiple neuropeptides, among them calcitonin gene–related peptide, α-melanocyte stimulating hormone, pituitary adenylate cyclase–activating peptide, substance P, vasoactive intestinal peptide, and norepinephrine, may be released by cutaneous nerves or resident and infiltrating cells within the skin. Systemic neuromediators and cutaneous nerves can influence a number of target cells within the skin, among them Langerhans cells. Most of the experimental evidence to date indicates a suppressive effect of the neurohormones and neuropeptides on Langerhans cell function and cutaneous inflammation, but it has become evident lately that the timing of exposure to a stimulus is critical to the outcome of the immune response. Thus, administration of a stress hormone or exposure to a stressor before the dendritic cell (DC) encounters an antigen (Ag) may diminish the immune response toward that Ag, while a stressor may enhance immune function when acting on a maturing DC or before reexposure to the Ag. The neuroendocrine regulation of skin DCs is a complex system allowing for a quick adaptation to various stressors. Such a system, originally evolved to defend the organism against invading pathogens and maintain homeostasis, may under certain conditions become unbalanced and ultimately exacerbate cutaneous inflammation.

KEYWORDS: dendritic cell; neuropeptide; catecholamine; antigen presentation; cytokines

Address for correspondence: Richard D. Granstein, Department of Dermatology, Weill Medical College of Cornell University, 525 East 68th Street, Rm. 340, New York 10021, NY. Voice: 212-746-7274; fax: 212-746-8656.
  e-mail: rdgranst@med.cornell.edu

Ann. N.Y. Acad. Sci. 1088: 195–206 (2006). © 2006 New York Academy of Sciences.
doi: 10.1196/annals.1366.011

INTRODUCTION

It has long been postulated that stress can affect skin conditions such as atopic dermatitis, psoriasis, or acne, and there is increasing experimental evidence that the neuroendocrine system can directly participate in cutaneous inflammation.[1] Cutaneous nerves and systemic neuromediators can activate a number of target cells within the skin, among them Langerhans cells (LCs). LCs are of dendritic cell (DC) lineage and are potent initiators of immune responses.[2] On capture and processing of Ags in the periphery, LCs upregulate surface costimulatory molecules and migrate to lymphoid organs, where they can present the Ag and interact with lymphocytes. LCs are closely connected with nerve fibers in the human epidermis[3] and they express receptors for a variety of neuropeptides and neurohormones.[4–7] In the following, we will review how the LC's function can be modulated by the neuroendocrine system, paying special emphasis on mediators of the sympathetic nervous system (SNS).

THE NEUROENDOCRINE AXIS AND THE SKIN

Over the last decade there has been growing evidence that the neuroendocrine system provides mediators that can modulate immune function and the skin immune system in particular.[8,9] Both the neuroendocrine and the immune system are instrumental in adapting the organism to stressors that threaten to disturb physical or behavioral homeostasis.[10,11] An adaptive stress response is regulated by the so-called stress system, which is located in both the central nervous system (CNS) as well as the periphery. The stress system is activated in the CNS by neurosensory and blood-borne signals. Information is then relayed to the peripheral limbs of the stress system, that is, the hypothalamic–pituitary–adrenal (HPA) axis and the SNS.[12]

Activation of the HPA axis leads to release of hypophyseal corticotropin-releasing hormone (CRH), which in turn induces secretion of adrenocorticotropic hormone (ACTH) from the anterior pituitary. Circulating ACTH is the key regulator of glucocorticoid secretion by the adrenal cortex (zona fasciculata).[13] In addition to their catabolic, lipogeneic, and antireproductive effects, glucocorticoids have long been known to be potent immunosuppressors. This effect has been exploited in the therapy of many inflammatory as well as autoimmune conditions, and is still a mainstay of dermatologic therapy.

The SNS originates within the brainstem and gives rise to preganglionic efferent fibers, which travel down the spinal column and terminate in para- and prevertebral ganglia. From there, postganglionic sympathetic fibers run to the innervated tissues, where they release norepinephrine (NE) as their main neurotransmitter.[8] Among the innervated tissues are primary and secondary lymphoid organs, including the spleen, thymus, and lymph nodes,[14,15] as well as the skin. Here, sympathetic fibers travel together with sensory nerves to innervate blood vessels, sweat glands and hair follicles and appear as single nerve fibers in the dermis and epidermis.[16] Subpopulations of sympathetic neurons are able to release active substances, such as neuropeptide Y (NPY) and CRH.[8] Although NE serves as the main neurotransmitter in the periphery, the adrenal medulla contributes all of the circulating epinephrine (EPI) and some NE, which can reach the target organs through humoral circulation. Numerous studies have shown that the SNS plays a role in immunomodulation, and its effect on skin DCs will be discussed in detail below.

In addition to glucocorticoids and catecholamines, a number of neuropeptides, among them α-melanocyte-stimulating hormone (α-MSH), calcitonin gene–related peptide (CGRP), pituitary adenylate cyclase–activating peptide (PACAP), substance P (SP), and vasoactive intestinal peptide (VIP) have been shown to affect cutaneous immunity[4,5] (for review see Refs. 17 and 18). Sensory nerves, derived from dorsal root ganglion neurons, are present in all parts of the skin. Neuropeptides in the skin are released predominantly by unmyelinated afferent C-fibers.[17] But resident and infiltrating inflammatory cells in the skin are able to release neuromediators as well and, thus, directly activate target cells.[9]

GLUCOCORTICOIDS

As mentioned earlier, activation of the HPA axis has profound inhibitory effects on inflammation and immunity, as almost all cells involved in the immune response are inhibited by cortisol.[10] Studies on the immunosuppressive effect of glucocorticoids have mainly focused on their inhibition of lymphocyte function, but their influence on differentiation and function on DC has been explored as well.[19] Dexamethasone, for example, selectively downregulates the expression of costimulatory molecules on monocyte-derived DCs, inhibits their production of proinflammatory cytokines and strongly reduces their immunostimulatory properties.[20] Glucocorticoids suppress the production of IL-12 *in vitro* and *ex vivo* in antigen-presenting cells (APCs) and, thus, may skew the Th1/Th2 balance toward Th2.[21] Studies on LCs found that glucocorticoids applied to human skin *in vivo* lead to a reduction of LC number,[22] induce LC apoptosis *in situ*, and inhibit the expression of CD25, CD205, and certain costimulatory molecules.[23]

CATECHOLAMINES MODULATE THE IMMUNE FUNCTION OF CUTANEOUS DENDRITIC CELLS

Numerous studies have shown that the SNS plays a role in the modulation of immune responses.[24] Sympathetic fibers terminate in near contact with lymphocytes in the lymphoid organs,[14,15] and NE has been shown to regulate

T and B lymphocyte function *in vitro* and *in vivo*.[25] Nerve-derived NE or systemic EPI is likely to reach multiple, if not all, APC lineages. In fact, NE and EPI act on monocytes as well as DCs, where they inhibit interleukin-12 (IL-12) production through β_2-adrenergic receptors (ARs).[26,27] Because IL-12 is a potent enhancer of interferon gamma (IFN-γ) and an inhibitor of IL-4 production by T cells, suppression of IL-12 in DCs has been implicated in skewing the Th1/Th2 balance toward Th2. It is of clinical interest, though, that NE seems to have this effect only when encountering an APC that is in the early phases of Ag processings but not when acting on a naïve or "exhausted" DCs [DCs that have already secreted IL-12 and cannot be stimulated to secrete IL-12 again after a second stimulus, as defined by Langenkamp *et al*.[28]]. Maestroni[29] showed that bone marrow–derived DCs treated with NE during the first 3 h of LPS stimulation reduced their IL-12 and increased their IL-10 production, an effect that was mediated both by α_2- and β-ARs. Consequently, adoptive transfer of NE-exposed DCs by footpad injection into naïve mice resulted in a polarization toward the Th2 phenotype, when lymph node cells from these mice where reexposed to Ag at a later time point *ex vivo*. More precisely, both β_2- and α_{2A}-AR reportedly mediate IL-12 inhibition, while IL-10 stimulation is a β_2 effect.[30] NE has further been shown to inhibit the production of TNF-α and IL-1 by APCs (for review, see Ref. 31).

LCs in the skin provide the first line of defense against invading pathogens and/or sensitizing/irritating substances. The general assumption that stress can influence the manifestation and course of inflammatory skin conditions led us to investigate whether catecholamines affect LCs. In the murine model, we found that both purified LC preparations as well as LC-like cell lines express the ARs α_{1A} and β_2. *In vitro*, EPI, as well as NE and the nonspecific β-AR agonist isoproterenol, reduced the ability of unseparated epidermal cell preparations to present Ag to an Ag-specific T cell clone.[7] The same was true for highly purified LC preparations, indicating that EPI exerts its effect directly on the level of LCs and not indirectly through induction of an intermediate mediator by other epidermal cells. Furthermore, *ex vivo* pretreatment of murine epidermal cells with EPI or NE suppressed the ability of these cells to present Ag for elicitation of delayed-type hypersensitivity (DTH) when injected into previously immunized mice. This effect was blocked by the use of the β_2-adrenergic antagonist ICI 118,551 but not by the α-antagonist phentolamine, suggesting signaling through the β_2-receptor. Intradermal injection of EPI inhibited the induction of contact hypersensitivity (CHS) to epicutaneously administered haptens, whether it was administered locally at the site of challenge or at a distant site. Thus, catecholamines appear to decrease epidermal immune reactions by inhibiting Ag presentation by LCs through β_2-AR signaling. An immune-response–reducing effect of NE on the level of skin DCs is further supported by the finding that pharmacological blockade of NE release by injection of the ganglionic blocker pentolinium not only leads to an increased IFN-γ production in draining lymph nodes, but also increases the CHS in mice.[29] In addition, when β_2-ARs are blocked by administration of ICI 188,551 during the sensitization phase to FITC, the percent of CD11c+FITC+ cell (defined as LCs in that study) migration to regional lymph nodes is significantly increased and CHS is increased.[30] Of note, though, cell migration from the skin to the lymph node was assessed 24 h after administration of Ag. It is possible that this effect involves dermal DCs as well as LCs. Although Maestroni[32] described an apparent decrease in LC migration (LC defined as FITC+CD86+ cells appearing 24 h after FITC stimulation in the lymph node) and inhibition of CHS through α_{1B}-adrenergic blockade in an earlier study, he later suggested that this was probably due to locally released NE acting on β_2-ARs only.[30] Furthermore, it seems that β_2 agonists influence the migratory function of LC by increasing their chemotactic response to the chemokine CC-chemokine-ligand (CCL)-19 and CCL-21 via secretion of IL-10. Sensitization in the presence of β_2-blockade leads to an increase of IL-2 and IFN-γ production in draining lymph node cells, but does not affect IL-4, suggesting a β_2 influence on Th1 priming but no immediate Th2 shift.

THE STATE OF DC MATURATION AND THE TYPE AND AMOUNT OF AG ENCOUNTERED MAY DETERMINE THE DIRECTION OF THE IMMUNE RESPONSE

Although mediators of the SNS have mostly been shown to downregulate immune cell functions, they appear to mediate both inhibitory and stimulatory effects. In mouse peritoneal macrophages, for example, NE can augment LPS-induced production of TNF-α *via* stimulation of α_2-ARs.[8] The differences in inhibition versus enhancement of immune responses seem to depend, at least in part, on the state of DC maturation. Thus, it was shown that NE decreased migration and the CHS response when added to immature cells, but enhanced migration and CHS when added to maturing DCs 1 h after LPS stimulation.[30] When given 24 h after DC stimulation, NE had no effect. The short-acting β_2 agonist salbutamol, on the other hand, decreased DC functions when acting on immature cells and had no effect after 1 and 24 h of maturation. Thus, it is possible that β_2 receptors are quickly downregulated on DC activation and that other ARs, such as α_1, mediate the later effect. It is of interest that under certain conditions, stress can enhance immune reactions. In an *in vivo* mouse model of stress effects on CHS, previously sensitized mice were exposed to a stressor before reexposure to the Ag. This led to a significant, long-lasting increase in CHS and numbers of leukocytes at the site of Ag challenge when compared with non-stressed animals.[33,34] A different study by Flint *et al.* showed how crucial the timing of the stressor was to the outcome: When Balb/c mice were restrained before cutaneous sensitization with dinitroflourobenzene, chemical-induced ear swelling and leukocyte infiltration were diminished on challenge with the Ag. When the restraint stress was administered before the challenge, though, this immune response was enhanced.[35] The authors showed that the stress effect could be partly blocked by administration of a glucocorticoid receptor antagonist, but it is likely that catecholamines, undoubtedly released after stress, were involved at the level of cutaneous DCs. In fact, a similar experiment showed that when mice are exposed to stressors such as immobilization or overcrowding, not only was the elicitation of CHS reactions reduced, but the intensity of I-A expression and number of dendrites in epidermal sheets was also decreased,[36] indicating diminished LC function. In adrenalectomized mice, on the other hand, stress did not lead to a suppression of CHS, and epidermal sheets showed increased I-A expression as well as number of dendrites, indicating a regulating effect of epinephrine and/or glucocorticoids on the LC stress response.

Nevertheless, there is conflicting evidence in the literature as to whether stress before sensitization down- or upregulates the ensuing immune response. Viswanathan and Dhabhar[37] showed that restraint stress prior to immunization of C57Bl/6 mice with 2,4-dinitro-1-fluorobenzene (DNFB) increased the magnitude of pinnae swelling after 6 and 24 h and enhanced CD11$^+$–DC maturation and migration to regional lymph nodes. Of note, though, in this study, the authors only examined the cellular events during the initiation of an immune response, but not at the time of Ag recall as done by Flint et al.[35] In future studies, it may be important to determine whether these early cellular events could be regulatory in nature and, thus, lead to an immune suppression at recall. In another recent study, though, Dhabhar and Viswanathan[38] showed an increase in long-term DTH when C57Bl/6 mice were restrained before immunization to keyhole limpet hemocyanin (KLH). While these findings are seemingly in direct opposition to the findings by Flint et al., one has to keep in mind that the earlier study employed DNFB, a strong contact sensitizer, while the later study used KLH, a nonspecific immune stimulant that induces both a cell-mediated and a humoral response in both animals and man,[39] to elicit an immune response. Thus, it seems that not just the timing of a stressor but also the Ag encountered by the organism can influence the outcome of stress-mediated immune responses. Nevertheless, Saint-Mezard et al.[40] found that restraining BALB/c mice for 2.5 h before sensitization by DNFB leads to significant enhancement of DTH on reexposure to DNFB 5 days later. Because both the study by Saint-Mezard et al.[40] and the study by Flint et al.[35] employ the same animal model (BALB/c mice), the same type of stressor (restraint), and the same contact sensitizer (DNFB) and still have opposing outcomes (enhancement versus suppression of DTH, respectively), it is tempting to speculate that the amount of contact sensitizer used (about 10-fold higher in the latter study) may be another factor in directing stress-related immune function. Clearly, this is a field of great controversy, and future studies will have to unravel the exact mechanisms involved.

TABLE 1. Neuroendocrine mediators in the skin and their effect on circulating and epidermal dendritic cells

Neuromediator	General effect on DC	Specific effect on LC
Glucocorticoids	↓ antigen presentation, expression of CD40, CD86, CD54, MHC class II, and production of IL-1B, IL-12, p70 in MMDC[20] induces Th1 shift[21]	- ↓ number of LCs [22]
Catecholamines	↓ IL-12 production in BMDDC[27,29]; ↑ IL-10 production in BMDDC[29]; ↓ migration and CHS when added to immature DC in vitro[30]; ↑ migration and CHS when added to maturing DC in vitro[30]	- ↑ LC apoptosis [23]; - ↓ CD25, CD40, CD54, CD80, CD86, CD205 [23]; ↓ Ag presentation in vitro[7]; ↓ DTH + CHS[7]; ↑ IL-10 secretion in chemotactic response to CCL-19 and CCL-21[30]; β^2-AR blockade > ↑ migration and CHS[30]; α^{1B}-AR blockade > ↓ migration and CHS[32]
VIP/PACAP	↓ proinflammatory cytokines and chemokines, CD80, CD86[41]; VIP induces a tolerogenic phenotype in BMDDC development[42]	PACAP: ↑ IL-1β production, antigen presentation[5]; ↑ IL-10 production[5]; VIP: ↓ IL-12p40, IL-1β production, antigen presentation in vitro, DTH[4]; ↑ IL-10 production[4]
CGRP		↓ alloantigen presentation, DTH, CD86 expression[3,44]; ↓ IL-1β and IL-12 p40 (XS52 cells)[43]; ↑ IL-10 production (XS52 cells)[3,44]; promotes hapten-specific tolerance[45]
α-MSH	↓ IL-1, IL-2, IL-4, IL-6, IL-13, IFN-γ, TNF-α production and CD40, CD86, ICAM-1 expression[46]; ↑ IL-10[46]	↓ allogeneic T cell responses at 10^{-4} to 10^{-5} M, → at 10^{-6} to 10^{-11} M[48]
SP	before sensitization: ↓ CHS to DNFB[35]; ↑ CHS to DNFB[40] ↑ DTH to KLH[38]; before challenge: ↑ CHS + numbers of leukocytes at site of challenge[33-35]	↓ IA-staining intensity and number of dendrites in epidermal sheets[36]

Note: Ag = antigen; BMDDC = bone marrow-derived dendritic cells; CCL = CC-chemokine-ligand; CHS = contact hypersensitivity; DC = dendritic cells; DNFB = 2,4-dinitro-1-fluorobenzene; DTH = delayed-type hypersensitivity; LC = Langerhans cells; MDDC = monocyte-derived dendritic cells; ↓ = downregulation; ↑ = upregulation; → = no effect.

NEUROPEPTIDES DOWNREGULATE THE IMMUNE FUNCTION OF CUTANEOUS DCs

Apart from the classical neurohormones, neuropeptides may be important in regulating cutaneous DC function. VIP and PACAP, for example, have been shown to inhibit the production of proinflammatory cytokines and chemokines, and reduce the expression of the costimulatory molecules CD80 and CD86 in DCs.[41] In addition, DCs generated *in vitro* from bone marrow precursors in the presence of VIP developed a tolerogenic phenotype.[42] Our group has shown that LC immune function is downregulated by PACAP as well as VIP. *In vitro*, PACAP inhibits LPS/GM-CSF–induced stimulation of IL-1β secretion and augments IL-10 production. Furthermore, it suppresses the ability of purified LCs to present Ag to a specific T cell clone.[5] Similarly, VIP downregulates IL-12 p40 and IL-1β production by LPS-stimulated XS106 cells while augmenting the production of IL-10. VIP also inhibits the ability of highly enriched LCs to present Ag to a T cell clone, and it inhibits elicitation of a DTH response in previously immunized mice by epidermal cells enriched for LC content pulsed with Ag *in vitro*.[4]

CGRP inhibits alloantigen presentation and stimulation of a specific antigen-responsive T-T hybridoma by epidermal cells enriched for LC content.[3] Pre-treatment of epidermal cells with CGRP also inhibits the elicitation of DTH in tumor-immune mice. Upregulation of B7-2 (CD86) expression on LC is suppressed by CGRP, which might be, in part, responsible for the inhibitory effect of CGRP in the functional assay. The production of some inflammatory cytokines such as IL-1β and IL-12 p40 by LC-like cell line XS52 is down-regulated by CGRP, while induction of IL-10 is enhanced.[43,44] The functional effect of CGRP may be at least partially mediated through the induction of IL-10.[44] CGRP was also found to promote hapten-specific tolerance *in vivo* in mice; however, the cellular target of CGRP action remains undefined.[45]

Similar to VIP/PACAP and CGRP, α-MSH downregulates the production of the proinflammatory cytokines IL-1, IL-6, TNF-α, IL-2, IFN-γ, IL-4, and IL-13 as well as the expression of the costimulatory molecules CD86, CD40, and ICAM-1 on antigen-presenting DCs, while upregulating the anti-inflammatory cytokine IL-10. Because treatment of naïve mice with bone marrow–derived immature haptenized and α-MSH-pulsed DCs leads to a significant inhibition of CHS, α-MSH has been implicated in tolerance induction as well.[46] The possibility that α-MSH may exert its effects, in part, on the level of epidermal LC remains to be examined.

SP, a member of the tachykinin family of neuropeptides, is released from sensory C-fibers in the skin. Within the skin, SP promotes vasodilatation and increased vascular permeability and is recognized as one of the main neuropeptides inducing the "wheal and flare" reaction characterized by erythema, pain, and swelling.[17] It may play a role in wound healing and neoangiogenesis by inducing proliferation of endothelial and arterial smooth muscle cells, as well as fibroblasts. In contrast to most other neuropeptides (and especially CGRP, which is coreleased with SP in sensory nerve fibers), SP has been shown to have a stimulatory role on the immune system. SP is a principal mediator of "neurogenic inflammation" by enhancing T cell and mast cell proliferation and production of proinflammatory cytokines in T cells, monocytes, mast cells, endothelial cells, and keratinocytes (for review, see Ref. 47). The action of SP *in vivo* is regulated by the protease neutral endopeptidase (NEP). Radioligand binding studies show that LCs express SP receptors, but despite its generally proinflammatory function, on the level of LCs, SP seems to be without effect or to even suppress their function.[48] At high concentrations of 10^{-4} to 10^{-5} M, SP reduced allogeneic T cell responses when added early in mixed epidermal cell–lymphocyte reactions. It has no effect at lower concentration (10^{-11} to 10^{-6} M) or when added at a later time, suggesting an effect on immature LCs or early T cell activation. Nevertheless, LCs are not the only target of SP in this model system, since pretreatment of either LCs or T cells was able to inhibit the allogeneic response.

CONCLUSION

Numerous groups have attempted to isolate effects of specific transmitters of the stress system on specific cell types. While the stress hormones systemically seem to suppress cytokine secretion by several immune cells and shift the Th1/Th2 balance toward humoral immunity responses and, thus, induce as well as sustain allergic reactions,[31] they may have different local effects. The local effects depend on the organ involved, the presence or absence of antigen, the nature of the Ag, and the relative expression of particular receptor subtypes on the immune cells.[8] As mentioned earlier for APCs, the timing of exposure to the stimulus may be critical to the type of outcome that occurs. Thus, administration of a stress hormone or exposure to a stressor before the DC encounters Ag may diminish the immune response toward that Ag, while a stressor may enhance immune function when acting on a maturing DC or before reexposure to the Ag.

It is unquestionably important to define effects at the cellular level, but stress, be it emotional or physical, is always experienced by a complex organism, leading to activation of multiple interacting pathways. Indeed, the SNS, the HPA axis, and the neuropeptide system are reciprocally interconnected and engage in functionally relevant cross-talk.[8] Exposure to either catecholamines, glucocorticoids, or neuropeptides will affect numerous cell types, with varying responses. Interestingly, it has been suggested that the duration of the stressor plays a role in determining the direction of the immune response as well. Acute stress may enhance cutaneous immune function and thus be advantageous to the organism, while chronic stress may decrease it.[34] Taken together, the neuroendocrine regulation of skin DCs is a complex system in which diverse signals act on cells in distinct activation stages, ultimately allowing for a quick adaptation to various stressors. Such a system, which was originally evolved to defend the organism against invading pathogens and maintain homeostasis, may under certain circumstances become unbalanced and in appropriately exacerbate cutaneous inflammation.

REFERENCES

1. ANSEL, J.C. *et al.* 1997. Interactions of the skin and nervous system. J. Invest. Dermatol. Symp. Proc. **2:** 23–26.
2. VALLADEAU, J. & S. SAELAND. 2005. Cutaneous dendritic cells. Semin. Immunol. **17:** 273–283.
3. HOSOI, J. *et al.* 1993. Regulation of Langerhans cell function by nerves containing calcitonin gene-related peptide. Nature **363:** 159–163.
4. KODALI, S. *et al.* 2004. Vasoactive intestinal peptide modulates Langerhans cell immune function. J. Immunol. **173:** 6082–6088.
5. KODALI, S. *et al.* 2003. Pituitary adenylate cyclase-activating polypeptide inhibits cutaneous immune function. Eur. J. Immunol. **33:** 3070–3079.
6. MISERY, L. 1998. Langerhans cells in the neuro-immuno-cutaneous system. J. Neuroimmunol. **89:** 83–87.
7. SEIFFERT, K. *et al.* 2002. Catecholamines inhibit the antigen-presenting capability of epidermal Langerhans cells. J. Immunol. **168:** 6128–6135.
8. CHROUSOS, G.P. 2000. The stress response and immune function: clinical implications. The 1999 Novera H. Spector Lecture. Ann. N. Y. Acad. Sci. **917:** 38–67.
9. LUGER, T.A. 2002. Neuromediators—a crucial component of the skin immune system. J. Dermatol. Sci. **30:** 87–93.
10. CHROUSOS, G.P. 1995. The hypothalamic-pituitary-adrenal axis and immune-mediated inflammation. N. Engl. J. Med. **332:** 1351–1362.
11. CHROUSOS, G.P. & P.W. GOLD. 1992. The concepts of stress and stress system disorders. Overview of physical and behavioral homeostasis. JAMA **267:** 1244–1252.
12. ELENKOV, I.J. & G.P. CHROUSOS. 2002. Stress hormones, proinflammatory and antiinflammatory cytokines, and autoimmunity. Ann. N. Y. Acad. Sci. **966:** 290–303.
13. CHROUSOS, G.P. 1998. Stressors, stress, and neuroendocrine integration of the adaptive response. The 1997 Hans Selye Memorial Lecture. Ann. N. Y. Acad. Sci. **851:** 311–335.
14. FELTEN, D.L. *et al.* 1985. Noradrenergic and peptidergic innervation of lymphoid tissue. J. Immunol. **135:** 755s–765s.
15. MADDEN, K.S., V.M. SANDERS & D.L. FELTEN. 1995. Catecholamine influences and sympathetic neural modulation of immune responsiveness. Annu. Rev. Pharmacol. Toxicol. **35:** 417–448.
16. CHU, D. *et al.* 2003. The stucture and development of the skin. *In* Dermatology in General Medicine. I. FREEDBERG, *et al.*, Eds. McGraw-Hill New York..
17. SCHOLZEN, T. *et al.* 1998. Neuropeptides in the skin: interactions between the neuroendocrine and the skin immune systems. Exp. Dermatol. **7:** 81–96.
18. LUGER, T.A. *et al.* 2000. The role of alpha-MSH as a modulator of cutaneous inflammation. Ann. N. Y. Acad. Sci. **917:** 232–238.

19. ABE, M. & A.W. THOMSON. 2003. Influence of immunosuppressive drugs on dendritic cells. Transpl. Immunol. **11:** 357–365.
20. PAN, J. *et al.* 2001. Dexamethasone inhibits the antigen presentation of dendritic cells in MHC class II pathway. Immunol. Lett. **76:** 153–161.
21. ELENKOV, I.J., G.P. CHROUSOS & R.L. WILDER. 2000. Neuroendocrine regulation of IL-12 and TNF-alpha/IL-10 balance. Clinical implications. Ann. N. Y. Acad. Sci. **917:** 94–105.
22. ASHWORTH, J., J. BOOKER & S.M. BREATHNACH. 1988. Effects of topical corticosteroid therapy on Langerhans cell antigen presenting function in human skin. Br. J. Dermatol. **118:** 457–469.
23. HOETZENECKER, W. *et al.* 2004. Corticosteroids but not pimecrolimus affect viability, maturation and immune function of murine epidermal Langerhans cells. J. Invest. Dermatol. **122:** 673–684.
24. FELTEN, S.Y. *et al.* 1998. The role of the sympathetic nervous system in the modulation of immune responses. Adv. Pharmacol. **42:** 583–587.
25. KOHM, A.P. & V.M. SANDERS. 2001. Norepinephrine and beta 2-adrenergic receptor stimulation regulate CD4+ T and B lymphocyte function *in vitro* and *in vivo*. Pharmacol. Rev. **53:** 487–525.
26. ELENKOV, I.J. *et al.* 1996. Modulatory effects of glucocorticoids and catecholamines on human interleukin-12 and interleukin-10 production: clinical implications. Proc. Assoc. Am. Physicians. **108:** 374–381.
27. PANINA-BORDIGNON, P. *et al.* 1997. Beta2-agonists prevent Th1 development by selective inhibition of interleukin 12. J. Clin. Invest. **100:** 1513–1519.
28. LANGENKAMP, A. *et al.* 2000. Kinetics of dendritic cell activation: impact on priming of TH1, TH2 and nonpolarized T cells. Nat. Immunol. **1:** 311–316.
29. MAESTRONI, G.J. 2002. Short exposure of maturing, bone marrow-derived dendritic cells to norepinephrine: impact on kinetics of cytokine production and Th development. J. Neuroimmunol. **129:** 106–114.
30. MAESTRONI, G.J. & P. MAZZOLA. 2003. Langerhans cells beta 2-adrenoceptors: role in migration, cytokine production, Th priming and contact hypersensitivity. J. Neuroimmunol. **144:** 91–99.
31. ELENKOV, I.J. *et al.* 2000. The sympathetic nerve—an integrative interface between two supersystems: the brain and the immune system. Pharmacol. Rev. **52:** 595–638.
32. MAESTRONI, G.J. 2000. Dendritic cell migration controlled by alpha 1b-adrenergic receptors. J. Immunol. **165:** 6743–6747.
33. DHABHAR, F.S. & B.S. MCEWEN. 1996. Stress-induced enhancement of antigen-specific cell-mediated immunity. J. Immunol. **156:** 2608–2615.
34. DHABHAR, F.S. & B.S. MCEWEN. 1999. Enhancing versus suppressive effects of stress hormones on skin immune function. Proc. Natl. Acad. Sci. USA. **96:** 1059–1064.
35. FLINT, M.S. *et al.* 2001. Restraint stress applied prior to chemical sensitization modulates the development of allergic contact dermatitis differently than restraint prior to challenge. J. Neuroimmunol. **113:** 72–80.
36. HOSOI, J. *et al.* 1998. Modification of LC phenotype and suppression of contact hypersensitivity response by stress. J. Cutan. Med. Surg. **3:** 79–84.
37. VISWANATHAN, K., C. DAUGHERTY & F.S. DHABHAR. 2005. Stress as an endogenous adjuvant: augmentation of the immunization phase of cell-mediated immunity. Int. Immunol. **17:** 1059–1069.

38. DHABHAR, F.S. & K. VISWANATHAN. 2005. Short-term stress experienced at time of immunization induces a long-lasting increase in immunologic memory. Am. J. Physiol. Regul. Integr. Comp. Physiol. **289:** R738–R744.
39. RIGGS, D.R. *et al.* 2002. *In vitro* anticancer effects of a novel immunostimulant: keyhole limpet hemocyanin. J. Surg. Res. **108:** 279–284.
40. SAINT-MEZARD, P. *et al.* 2003. Psychological stress exerts an adjuvant effect on skin dendritic cell functions *in vivo*. J. Immunol. **171:** 4073–4080.
41. GANEA, D., R. RODRIGUEZ & M. DELGADO. 2003. Vasoactive intestinal peptide and pituitary adenylate cyclase-activating polypeptide: players in innate and adaptive immunity. Cell Mol. Biol. (Noisy-le-Grand) **49:** 127–142.
42. DELGADO, M., E. GONZALEZ-REY & D. GANEA. 2005. The neuropeptide vasoactive intestinal peptide generates tolerogenic dendritic cells. J. Immunol. **175:** 7311–7324.
43. TORII, H. *et al.* 1997. Regulation of cytokine expression in macrophages and the Langerhans cell-like line XS52 by calcitonin gene-related peptide. J. Leukoc. Biol. **61:** 216–223.
44. TORII, H., K. TAMAKI & R.D. GRANSTEIN. 1998. The effect of neuropeptides/hormones on Langerhans cells. J. Dermatol. Sci. **20:** 21–28.
45. KITAZAWA, T. & J.W. STREILEIN. 2000. Hapten-specific tolerance promoted by calcitonin gene-related peptide. J. Invest. Dermatol. **115:** 942–948.
46. LUGER, T.A. *et al.* 2003. New insights into the functions of alpha-MSH and related peptides in the immune system. Ann. N. Y. Acad. Sci. **994:** 133–140.
47. ANSEL, J.C. *et al.* 1996. Skin–nervous system interactions. J. Invest. Dermatol. **106:** 198–204.
48. STANIEK, V. *et al.* 1997. Binding and *in vitro* modulation of human epidermal Langerhans cell functions by substance P. Arch. Dermatol. Res. **289:** 285–291.

PPARγ, a Lipid-Activated Transcription Factor as a Regulator of Dendritic Cell Function

ISTVAN SZATMARI,[a] EVA RAJNAVOLGYI,[b] AND LASZLO NAGY[a]

[a]Department of Biochemistry and Molecular Biology, Research Center for Molecular Medicine, University of Debrecen, Medical and Health Science Center, Life Science Building, Egyetem tér 1, Debrecen, H-4010, Hungary

[b]Department of Immunology, Research Center for Molecular Medicine, University of Debrecen, Medical and Health Science Center, Life Science Building, Egyetem tér 1, Debrecen, H-4010, Hungary

ABSTRACT: In recent years it became apparent that PPARγ, besides being a key component of adipose tissue development and a target of insulin-sensitizing drugs, also has a role in immune cell differentiation and function. This receptor has been identified by us and others as a conductor of lipid handling in macrophages, and has roles also in inflammation control. Here we review recent advances on the role of this nuclear receptor in another key cell type of myeloid origin, dendritic cells (DCs). DCs are professional antigen-presenting cells having essential roles in antigen-uptake processing and presentation and in initiation of various forms of immune responses. It appears that PPARγ is expressed and is active in myeloid DCs and likely to be a regulator of DC function by altering antigen uptake, maturation, activation, migration, cytokine production, and lipid antigen presentation. Thus PPARγ is at the crossroads of lipid metabolism and innate immune response, and by studying its functions one has a unique opportunity to discern how these two seemingly distant fields (lipid metabolism and immune response) are interrelated. It is also possible that this receptor is a relevant target for pharmacological intervention in immune diseases such as chronic inflammation and autoimmune conditions.

KEYWORDS: nuclear hormone receptors; PPARγ; transcription; dendritic cells; lipid metabolism; innate immune response; CD1

Address for correspondence: Laszlo Nagy, Department of Biochemistry and Molecular Biology, Research Center for Molecular Medicine, University of Debrecen, Medical and Health Science Center, Life Science Building, Egyetem tér 1, Debrecen, H-4010, Hungary. Voice: +36-52-416-432; fax: +36-52-314-989.
e-mail: lnagy@indi.biochem.dote.hu

Ann. N.Y. Acad. Sci. 1088: 207–218 (2006). © 2006 New York Academy of Sciences.
doi: 10.1196/annals.1366.013

INTRODUCTION

The function of the immune system is tightly regulated by cytokines and by other local humoral mediators. It is well established that lipid mediators like prostaglandins and leukotrienes are very important factors for the regulation of the innate immune responses. Lipid mediators exert their effects on specific cell surface receptors, mostly GPCRs (G-protein coupled receptors); in addition lipophilic molecules can be delivered to the cell nucleus by various means and modulate the gene expression by activation of nuclear hormone receptors. One of the candidate lipid-metabolite sensors is the family of the peroxisome-proliferator-activated receptors (PPARs), which are expressed in various immune cell types.

PPARs are member of the nuclear hormone receptor superfamily of transcription factors (TABLE 1.). Their activity is regulated by lipophilic compounds (reviewed in Refs. 1 and 2). PPARs form a heterodimer with RXR (retinoic X receptor) receptors and subsequently regulate the transcription of cognate target genes. There are three isoforms of PPARs (PPARα, PPARγ, and PPARδ/β). PPARα is predominantly expressed in the liver, heart, kidney, and skeletal muscle and it has an important role in fatty acid oxidation.[3] PPARδ is ubiquitously expressed and it has a main role in utilization of fatty acids by skeletal muscle.

TABLE 1. The family of PPARs

	PPARα	**PPARγ**	**PPARβ/δ**
Expression:	*Liver, BAT*	*Adipocyte, macrophage*	*Ubiquitous*
Ligands:	Eicosanoids and fatty acids (PUFAs, oxidized FA)		
	Linoleic acid Leukotrien B4 Palmitoyl-phosphocholine	oxLDL, 15-HETE 9-, 13-HODE 15-deoxy-D12,14- prostaglandin J2	VLDL Carbacyclin
	Fibrates (Clofibrate)	TZDs (Rosiglitazone) Selective modulators	GW501516
Main roles:	*Beta-oxidation Inflammation*	*Adipogenesis Placental function Type II Diabetes Inflammation Cancer Atherosclerosis*	*Embryonic implantation Wound healing Inflammation, Cancer Osteoporosis Atherosclerosis*

Furthermore, PPARδ has been suggested to modulate the inflammatory responses of macrophages.[4] PPARγ, the focus of this review, has been initially linked to adipocyte genesis. In fact it regulates genes responsible for lipid uptake, accumulation, and storage.[1] It should be mentioned that synthetic PPARγ ligands (rosiglitazone, pioglitazone) have been used to treat type 2 diabetes.[2] Therefore this receptor is a well-established component of lipid metabolism and a drug target for metabolic diseases. Besides this well-established role in lipid metabolism, it was also reported that PPARγ is expressed in cells of monocytic origin such as macrophages and modulates the function of these cells.[5] PPARγ is part of a network of transcription factors coordinately regulating lipid uptake and cholesterol efflux in macrophages by transcriptionally regulating the scavanger receptor, D36 and the oxysterol receptor LXRα (liver X receptor α).[5,6] PPARγ ligands also have an anti-inflammatory role in monocytes/macrophages by blocking the induction of several proinflammatory cytokines.[7,8] The molecular mechanism of this trans-repression activity is poorly defined; one possible mechanism of this anti-inflammatory effect is the selective recruitment of corepressors into NFκB-responsive elements.[9]

Recently, several observations suggest that besides monocyte/macrophages a distinct myeloid cell linage, dendritic cells (DCs), also express PPARγ receptors at high levels. In this review we examine the potential roles of PPARγ in dendritic cell differentiation and function.

DCs are professional antigen-presenting cells, possessing a unique capacity to prime naive T cells.[10] Immature DCs reside in peripheral tissues and are specialized in antigen capture and processing. Upon maturation DCs undergo a process of activation, as indicated by an increased expression of MHC (major histocompatibility complex) and costimulatory molecules (CD80, CD86, and CD40) and reflected by a decreased capacity of antigen uptake and processing (FIG. 1.). Activated DCs are recruited to secondary lymphoid organs and initiate immune responses. In addition to priming antigen-specific T lymphocytes they are able to produce regulatory cytokines with the potential to polarize the immune response. In humans there are three main sources of DCs which have been used for basic research or for clinical trials: CD34+ hematopoetic stem cell–derived DCs; CD14+ monocyte-derived DCs and peripheral blood DC precursors.[11] Although their physiological relevance *in vivo* remains unclear, monocyte-derived cells are the major DC type used for *in vitro* generation of DCs. In mice, bone marrow precursors are a good source for DC generation but various DC subsets can also be directly obtained from the spleen. Although the origin of DCs is intensively investigated, the linage relationship of the various DC types is still controversial.[11] Remarkably little is known of the transcriptional events controlling the differentiation and lineage commitment of DCs and their responses to external stimuli and/or internal signals. Here we also provide an overview for the potential role of PPARγ nuclear receptor in DC development, subtype specification, and the DC's function.

Main functions of dendritic cells

immature DC:
antigen uptake by
receptor mediated endocytosis
phagocytosis and
macropinocytosis

mature (activated) DC:
antigen presentation
T cell activation

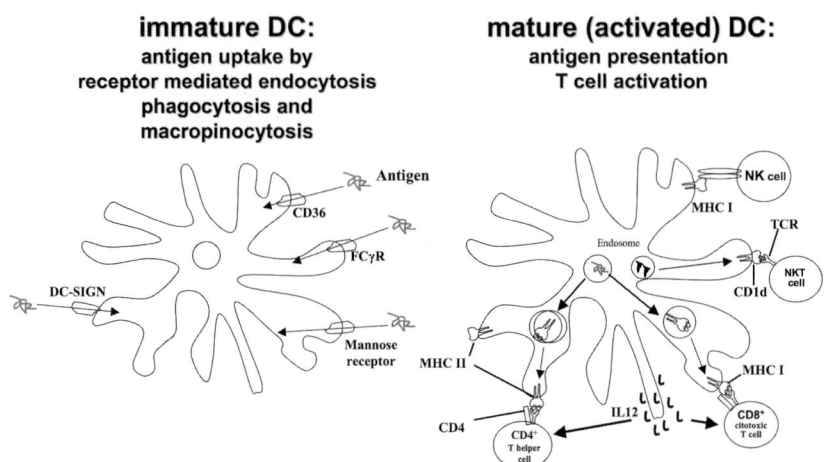

FIGURE 1. Schematic representation of dendritic cell functions.

DETECTION OF PPAR RECEPTORS DURING DENDRITIC CELL DIFFERENTIATION

PPARγ was first detected in murine spleen-derived DCs by reverse transcription polymerase chain reaction (RT-PCR) and by immunoblot.[12] According to this report PPARγ expression was more pronounced in freshly isolated cells than in activated splenic DCs. In a human monocyte-derived DC system, a DNA microarray study first indicated that the mRNA expression of PPARγ is highly upregulated in DCs when compared to freshly isolated monocytes.[13] Later this result was confirmed in several laboratories; in addition the protein product of PPARγ was also detected in human monocyte-derived DCs.[14–16] We found that besides this cytokine-induced human DC model, PPARγ is also expressed in blood-derived myeloid DCs and at least in a subset of S100-positive antigen-presenting cells of the tonsils, providing *in vivo* evidence of PPARγ-positive DCs in human peripheral lymphoid organs.[16] PPARγ was also detected in murine Langerhans cells (LCs); in addition this receptor was also found in bone-marrow-derived murine DCs.[17] Very little is known about the factors that influence the expression of PPARγ during DC development. It has been reported that hemozoin (malaria pigment)-loaded DCs express more PPARγ transcript compared to unloaded cells.[18] An intriguing question was also addressed whether the other two isoforms of PPAR receptors (α and δ) are expressed in DCs or not. It should be mentioned that both mouse and human DCs expressed an undetectable or a very low amount of PPARα.[12,14–16] In contrast, the mRNA of PPARδ was detected in monocyte-derived human or bone-marrow-derived murine DCs.[16,17] We found that administration of PPARδ activators to monocyte-derived DCs barely modify the phenotype of these cells (Ref. 16 and unpublished data) but there is no detailed study dealing with the potential role of this hormone receptor in DCs. Taken together these data imply that at least a subset of DCs is expressing the nuclear receptor. Significantly, this receptor appears to be the most tightly regulated of this family of receptors, having very little or no expression in monocytes and being robustly induced in monocyte-derived DCs.

Next we review the effects of the activation of this receptor in DCs.

ACTIVATION OF PPARγ RECEPTOR BY LIGAND TREATMENT DURING DC DIFFERENTIATION

The activation of PPARγ can be followed by detection of target gene induction. Several direct PPARγ targets have been described (CD36, FABP4, LXRα, PGAR). It was also reported that PPARγ-ligand (troglitazone or rosiglitazone)-treated human DCs expressed more CD36 compared to vehicle-treated cells.[14,15] We found that another PPARγ target, the fatty acid transporter, FABP4,[19] was also highly induced upon PPARγ ligand treatment; furthermore, this induction was abolished by the administration of a PPARγ-specific antagonist, indicating that this induction is a PPARγ-dependent event.[16] These results established that PPARγ can be activated transcriptionally in monocyte-derived DCs. It was also observed that the highest level of PPARγ expression and ligand responsiveness occurs in the first 24 h of differentiation.[16]

THE ROLE OF PPARγ ACTIVATORS ON ENDOCYTOSIS OF DCs

Endocytosis is a hallmark of immature DCs; it is therefore of importance to test whether the activation of nuclear receptors has any influence on this activity. We have observed that activation of PPARγ enhances the latex bead uptake capacity of human DCs.[16] It is important to note that monocytes also possess high capacity of latex bead uptake and PPARγ-ligand-treated DCs retain this activity. In DCs a number of cell surface receptors have been implicated in antigen uptake. One of them is CD36, which may act as a receptor also for apoptotic cell uptake and has been postulated to mediate cross-priming of cytotoxic T cells by human DCs[20] This receptor is also a known target of PPARγ.[5] We and others have examined the cell surface expression of CD36 during DC development and detected a higher expression of CD36 on PPARγ-activator-treated DCs.[14-16] However we observed that in some individuals CD36 expression divided into high and low expressors on RSG (rosiglitazone)-treated

DCs. CD36-negative cells had similar capacity as positive cells to uptake latex beads, suggesting that CD36 expression may not account for the increased uptake of latex beads in this model.[16]

MODULATION OF TH1/TH2 BALANCE BY PPARγ LIGANDS

PPARγ has an important role in the regulation of lipid metabolism;[19] it is therefore assumed that the activation of this receptor regulates mostly genes which participate in lipid metabolism. In line with this assumption, several genes, which are linked to lipid metabolism and transport (CD36, FABP4, ADRP, LXRα), have been shown to be upregulated in DCs. Besides these genes, it has been shown that genes that are important in the immunological function of DCs are also regulated by PPARγ ligand. First, it was reported that PPARγ activators reduce the level of the T-helper1 (Th1) promoting cytokine interleukin-12 (IL-12) production in murine spleen DCs.[12] These data were confirmed in human monocyte-derived DCs by showing that LPS (lipopolysaccharide) or CD40-ligand-activated DCs express less inducible IL-12 subunit upon PPARγ ligand treatment compared to untreated cells.[14] In the same report it was also shown that PPARγ-instructed mature DCs reduce the secretion of chemokines involved in Th1 cell recruitment (IP-10, RANTES [regulated on activation of normal T cell expressed and secreted]). In addition activation of PPARγ induced CD86 and decreased CD80 expression.[14] These data were later also confirmed by others.[15,16] Taken together these findings (decreased CD80/CD86 ratio, inhibition of IL-12 production by PPARγ ligand) suggest that activation of PPARγ in DCs might favor the differentiation of T cells into Th2 cytokine-producing lymphocytes. Although the reduced expression of IL-12 was confirmed by others, no one so far has been able to detect any Th2 response upon activation PPARγ in mixed leukocyte culture experiments.[15] On the contrary, it was reported that PPARγ activation prevents induction of Th2-dependent eosinophilic airway inflammation in ovalbumin-pulsed murine DCs.[17] This issue needs further investigation and clarification including genetic and *in vivo* approaches.

INTERFERENCE OF DC ACTIVATION BY PPARγ LIGANDS (PPARγ-DEPENDENT AND -INDEPENDENT EFFECTS)

Besides the reduced production of IL-12 it has been reported that PPARγ-activated cells produce less IL-15, TNFα, and IL-6, suggesting that PPARγ ligands have a general negative effect on the production of inflammatory cytokines. This is consistent with the potential anti-inflammatory role of this receptor.[15] Moreover, in that article it was also reported that PPARγ-ligand-treated cells have an impaired capacity to activate lymphocytes due

to the reduced cytokine production and impaired expression of costimulatory molecules (CD83, CD80, CD40). These data suggest that administration
of PPARγ interferes with the activation (maturation) and decreases the immunogenicity of DCs. A more detailed study indicated that these inhibitory
effects of PPARγ activators on DC activation were mediated via blocking of
NFκB and MAP kinase pathways.[21] All of these results suggest that activation
of PPARγ inhibits the immunogenicity and cytokine production of DCs. We
confirmed some of these findings, but obtained different results regarding the
T cell–activating potential of PPARγ-activated DCs.[16] We failed to detect any
decrease in the T cell–activating capacity of ligand-treated DCs; in addition we
did not detect impaired expression of CD83 upon ligand treatment. The reason
for these differences may be related to the usage of different conditions and
more importantly different doses of PPARγ ligands. It has been shown that
higher doses of PPARγ activators may induce receptor-independent inhibitory
effects.[22]

THE POTENTIAL ROLE OF PPARγ LIGAND
ON CELL MIGRATION

Upon activation, tissue resident DCs migrate into the T cell areas of draining
lymph nodes through afferent lymphatic vessels and present engulfed antigens
to T lymphocytes and initiate cellular immune responses.[10] The migration
of DCs from the periphery to the lymphoid organs represents a tightly regulated, multistep event,[23] which might be regulated by fatty acid derivatives.
Leukotriene C4 (LTC4), a known mediator of the symptoms of bronchial
asthma, and its extracellular metabolite leukotriene D4 LTD4, have been shown
to facilitate both murine and human DC chemotaxis and lymphatic migration
in an MRP1-dependent manner.[24] Using an experimental murine model of LC
migration, it was shown that activation of PPARγ specifically impairs the de-
parture of LCs from the epidermis.[25] Moreover, after intratracheal sensitization
with a fluorescein isothiocyanate (FITC)-conjugated antigen, PPARγ activation inhibits the migration of DCs from the airway mucosa to the thoracic lymph
node and profoundly reduces the priming of antigen-specific T lymphocytes
in the draining lymph nodes. These data imply that the migration of at least the
Langerhans type of DCs is negatively regulated by PPARγ activators. Interestingly TLR (toll-like receptor) ligand-stimulated human monocyte-derived
DCs which were treated with PPARγ-specific ligand also have an impaired
migratory capacity, suggesting that this effect can also be detected in human
cells.[21] It would be of interest to define the molecular mechanism of this regulation. It has been reported that PPARγ ligand treatment reduces the expression
of CCR7,[15] a key chemokine receptor involved in DC migration; downregulation of this chemokine might be responsible for the impaired migration of the
PPARγ-activated DCs.

THE ROLE OF PPARγ ACTIVATION ON LIPID
ANTIGEN PRESENTATION

CD1a is highly upregulated during monocyte-derived DC differentiation using fetal bovine serum (FBS)-containing cell-culture medium.[26] We and others have observed that addition of RSG at the initiation of DC differentiation results in marked inhibition of CD1a expression.[15,16] We have also analyzed the effect of PPARγ on the expression of the entire CD1 gene family. The CD1 locus encodes a family of conserved transmembrane proteins structurally related to MHC class I proteins.[27] We found that freshly isolated monocytes are devoid of not only CD1a expression, but also of any expression of the group I CD1s (CD1b, CD1c and CD1e). The transcript levels of these genes were strongly increased in immature DCs and, as a result of ligand treatment, the mRNA levels of these genes were much lower.[16] Unexpectedly, CD1d (group II CD1) showed a completely different expression pattern. Monocytes were CD1d-positive, but DCs expressed very low levels of CD1d mRNA, whilst RSG-treated cells retained CD1d expression.[16]

The finding that RSG-treated monocyte-derived DCs express more CD1d mRNA and protein than did untreated cells focused our attention on the physiological consequence of the increased CD1d expression on DCs. CD1d-mediated lipid presentation is indispensable for the activation and expansion of iNKT cells.[28] We reasoned that increased CD1d protein levels should translate into increased activation of iNKT cells and assessed the relative potency of DCs to induce iNKT cell proliferation in mixed leukocyte reaction (MLR). We detected a remarkable expansion of iNKT cells when the DCs were treated with PPARγ activators.[16] One may speculate on the biological consequences of increased CD1d expression and NKT cell activation. There are in vivo examples of CD1d-NKT-cell-dependent processes such as the NOD (nonobese diabetic) mouse model. In this model the expansion and differentiation of autoimmune effector T cells leads to β cell destruction and the development of type 1 diabetes. This process has been tied to both the CD1d locus and iNKT cells.[29–31] Treatment of NOD mice with PPARγ ligands substantially reduced the development of type 1 diabetes.[32] Our results are entirely consistent with the presence of a mechanism that induces activation of NKT cells in NOD mice by enhancing expression of CD1d.

THE EFFECTS OF NATURAL PPARγ AGONISTS
ON DC DEVELOPMENT

To study the potential roles of PPARγ on DC development, synthetic high-affinity PPARγ activators were applied. Another important issue is whether natural ligands of this receptor can modulate DC differentiation in a receptor-dependent manner. Although high concentrations of polyunsaturated fatty acids (PUFAs), several oxidized fatty acid species (9- and 13-HODE), and some prostaglandin derivatives can act as a PPARγ activator, the nature of PPARγ ligands *in vivo* is still controversial.[2] It has been reported that many effects of the synthetic PPARγ ligand on DCs can be mimicked by deoxy-prostaglandin J2,[15] but it is still controversial whether in living cells this ligand is really generated. There are numerous receptor-independent effects assigned to this compound in the immune system.[33] An interesting issue is whether differentiated DCs contain endogenous PPARγ activators or not. When monocyte-derived DCs were treated with PPARγ-specific antagonist (GW9662), we obtained a reduced FABP4 expression, suggesting that these cells produce a small, but detectable level of endogenous ligand activators.[16] It is not well understood what the source of these ligands could be. 15-lipoxygenase (15-LO) produces 15-HETE (15-hydroxyeicosatetraenoic acid) or 13-HODE, which are ligands or activators of PPARγ,[34] but this is still a debated issue.[35] Intriguingly, 15-LO is also induced upon DC differentiation.[36] Another (extracellular) source could be oxidized low-density lipoprotein (oxLDL) containing 9- and 13-HODE,[5] which could modulate DC differentiation from monocytes;[37] our data indicate that oxLDL is able to induce the expression of a PPARγ target gene in DCs.[16] These mechanisms require more thorough investigation including the identification of endogenous ligands/activators produced during the differentiation of DCs.

REMAINING QUESTIONS

There is an increasing amount of data on the potential role of PPARγ on DC biology (FIG. 2). Most of these studies have used pharmacological approaches, usually applying various natural or synthetic PPARγ agonists. In the future it will be important, in order to solidify the findings, to use genetic means such as gene-silencing methods to prove the receptor specificity of the described effects following treatment with the ligand. For instance it would be interesting to generate a DC-specific knockout mouse model to study the *in vivo* relevance of these receptors on antigen-presenting cells.

PPARγ activators are used in clinical practice to treat type 2 diabetes, probably with significant effect on metabolic tissues such as adipose tissue.[1] A very important question is whether these synthetic ligands really modulate *in vivo* the immune system through reprogramming of antigen-presenting cell activity. Most of the available data are on the effect of PPARγ activators *in vitro/ex vivo*. In the future it would be important to study the potential effect of ligands on the immune system *in vivo* using animal models and also to design suitable clinical studies. It is a controversial issue whether administration of PPARγ activators has a beneficial effect on the immune system. Several studies suggest that PPARγ activators have anti-inflammatory effects (including blocking DC activation) and hence these compounds can inhibit inflammation; however,

The main effects of PPARγ activators on Dendritic Cell

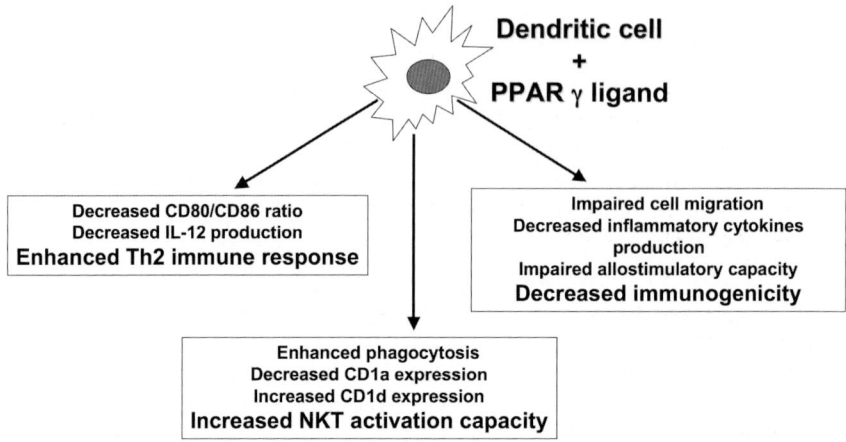

FIGURE 2. A proposed role for PPARγ ligand on the differentiation and function of dendritic cells.

occasionally they may also impair the proper immune response.[7,15] Our results suggest that activation of PPARγ in DCs leads to subtype specification of DCs and such DCs can elicit the activation of iNKT cells. Therefore *in vivo* activation of iNKT cells might have a beneficial effect against autoimmune diseases[16] Further *in vivo* and clinical study is needed to test these possibilities.

ACKNOWLEDGMENTS

The work in the authors' laboratories is supported by grants from the Hungarian National Research Fund (OTKA F038347 to IS), Ministry of Health (ETT 601/2003 to IS), and the National Office for Research and Technology (NKFP 2004 OM-00427 and RET-06/2004 to Laszlo Nagy). Laszlo Nagy is an International Scholar of the Howard Hughes Medical Institute and holds a Wellcome Trust Senior Research Fellowship in Biomedical Sciences in Central Europe.

REFERENCES

1. WILLSON, T.M., M.H. LAMBERT & S.A. KLIEWER. 2001. Peroxisome proliferator-activated receptor gamma and metabolic disease. Annu. Rev. Biochem. **70:** 341–367.
2. LEHRKE, M. & M.A. LAZAR. 2005. The many faces of PPARgamma. Cell **123:** 993–999.

3. BRAISSANT, O. *et al.* 1996. Differential expression of peroxisome proliferator-activated receptors (PPARs): tissue distribution of PPAR-alpha, -beta, and -gamma in the adult rat. Endocrinology **137:** 354–366.
4. LUQUET, S. *et al.* 2005. Roles of PPAR delta in lipid absorption and metabolism: a new target for the treatment of type 2 diabetes. Biochim. Biophys. Acta **1740:** 313–317.
5. NAGY, L. *et al.* 1998. Oxidized LDL regulates macrophage gene expression through ligand activation of PPARgamma. Cell **93:** 229–240.
6. CHAWLA, A. *et al.* 2001. A PPAR gamma-LXR-ABCA1 pathway in macrophages is involved in cholesterol efflux and atherogenesis. Mol. Cell **7:** 161–171.
7. DELERIVE, P., J.C. FRUCHART & B. STAELS. 2001. Peroxisome proliferator-activated receptors in inflammation control. J. Endocrinol. **169:** 453–459.
8. GENOLET, R., W. WAHLI & L. MICHALIK. 2004. PPARs as drug targets to modulate inflammatory responses? Curr. Drug Targets Inflamm. Allergy **3:** 361–375.
9. PASCUAL, G. *et al.* 2005. A SUMOylation-dependent pathway mediates transrepression of inflammatory response genes by PPAR-gamma. Nature **437:** 759–763.
10. BANCHEREAU, J. & R.M. STEINMAN. 1998. Dendritic cells and the control of immunity. Nature **392:** 245–252.
11. ARDAVIN, C. *et al.* 2001. Origin and differentiation of dendritic cells. Trends Immunol. **22:** 691–700.
12. FAVEEUW, C. *et al.* 2000. Peroxisome proliferator-activated receptor gamma activators inhibit interleukin-12 production in murine dendritic cells. FEBS Lett. **486:** 261–266.
13. LE NAOUR, F. *et al.* 2001. Profiling changes in gene expression during differentiation and maturation of monocyte-derived dendritic cells using both oligonucleotide microarrays and proteomics. J. Biol. Chem. **276:** 17920–17931.
14. GOSSET, P. *et al.* 2001. Peroxisome proliferator-activated receptor gamma activators affect the maturation of human monocyte-derived dendritic cells. Eur. J. Immunol. **31:** 2857–2865.
15. NENCIONI, A. *et al.* 2002. Dendritic cell immunogenicity is regulated by peroxisome proliferator-activated receptor gamma. J. Immunol. **169:** 1228–1235.
16. SZATMARI, I. *et al.* 2004. Activation of PPARgamma specifies a dendritic cell subtype capable of enhanced induction of iNKT cell expansion. Immunity **21:** 95–106.
17. HAMMAD, H. *et al.* 2004. Activation of peroxisome proliferator-activated receptor-gamma in dendritic cells inhibits the development of eosinophilic airway inflammation in a mouse model of asthma. Am. J. Pathol. **164:** 263–271.
18. SKOROKHOD, O.A. *et al.* 2004. Hemozoin (malarial pigment) inhibits differentiation and maturation of human monocyte-derived dendritic cells: a peroxisome proliferator-activated receptor-gamma-mediated effect. J. Immunol. **173:** 4066–4074.
19. TONTONOZ, P., E. HU & B.M. SPIEGELMAN. 1995. Regulation of adipocyte gene expression and differentiation by peroxisome proliferator activated receptor gamma. Curr. Opin. Genet. Dev. **5:** 571–576.
20. URBAN, B.C., N. WILLCOX & D.J. ROBERTS. 2001. A role for CD36 in the regulation of dendritic cell function. Proc. Natl. Acad. Sci. USA **98:** 8750–8755.
21. APPEL, S. *et al.* 2005. PPAR-gamma agonists inhibit toll-like receptor-mediated activation of dendritic cells via the MAP kinase and NF-kappaB pathways. Blood **106:** 3888–3894.

22. CHAWLA, A. *et al.* 2001. PPAR-gamma dependent and independent effects on macrophage-gene expression in lipid metabolism and inflammation. Nat. Med. **7:** 48–52.
23. RANDOLPH, G.J., V. ANGELI & M.A. SWARTZ. 2005. Dendritic-cell trafficking to lymph nodes through lymphatic vessels. Nat. Rev. Immunol. **5:** 617–628.
24. ROBBIANI, D.F. *et al.* 2000. The leukotriene C(4) transporter MRP1 regulates CCL19 (MIP-3beta, ELC)-dependent mobilization of dendritic cells to lymph nodes. Cell **103:** 757–768.
25. ANGELI, V. *et al.* 2003. Peroxisome proliferator-activated receptor gamma inhibits the migration of dendritic cells: consequences for the immune response. J. Immunol. **170:** 5295–5301.
26. PORCELLI, S.A. *et al.* 1998. The CD1 family of lipid antigen-presenting molecules. Immunol. Today **19:** 362–368.
27. CALABI, F. *et al.* 1989. Two classes of CD1 genes. Eur. J. Immunol. **19:** 285–292.
28. KRONENBERG, M. & L. GAPIN. 2002. The unconventional lifestyle of NKT cells. Nat. Rev. Immunol. **2:** 557–568.
29. WANG, B., Y.B. GENG & C.R. WANG. 2001. CD1-restricted NK T cells protect nonobese diabetic mice from developing diabetes. J. Exp. Med. **194:** 313–320.
30. SHI, F.D. *et al.* 2001. Germ line deletion of the CD1 locus exacerbates diabetes in the NOD mouse. Proc. Natl. Acad. Sci. USA **98:** 6777–6782.
31. CARNAUD, C. *et al.* 2001. Protection against diabetes and improved NK/NKT cell performance in NOD.NK1.1 mice congenic at the NK complex. J. Immunol. **166:** 2404–2411.
32. AUGSTEIN, P. *et al.* 2003. Prevention of autoimmune diabetes in NOD mice by troglitazone is associated with modulation of ICAM-1 expression on pancreatic islet cells and IFN-gamma expression in splenic T cells. Biochem. Biophys. Res. Commun. **304:** 378–384.
33. STRAUS, D.S. *et al.* 2000. 15-deoxy-delta 12,14-prostaglandin J2 inhibits multiple steps in the NF-kappa B signaling pathway. Proc. Natl. Acad. Sci. USA **97:** 4844–4849.
34. HUANG, J.T. *et al.* 1999. Interleukin-4-dependent production of PPAR-gamma ligands in macrophages by 12/15-lipoxygenase. Nature **400:** 378–382.
35. HSI, L.C. *et al.* 2001. 15-lipoxygenase-1 metabolites down-regulate peroxisome proliferator-activated receptor gamma via the MAPK signaling pathway. J. Biol. Chem. **276:** 34545–34552.
36. SPANBROEK, R. *et al.* 2001. IL-4 determines eicosanoid formation in dendritic cells by down-regulation of 5-lipoxygenase and up-regulation of 15-lipoxygenase 1 expression. Proc. Natl. Acad. Sci. USA **98:** 5152–5157.
37. PERRIN-COCON, L. *et al.* 2001. Oxidized low-density lipoprotein promotes mature dendritic cell transition from differentiating monocyte. J. Immunol. **167:** 3785–3791.

Roles of Glia-Derived Cytokines on Neuronal Degeneration and Regeneration

AKIO SUZUMURA, HIDEYUKI TAKEUCHI, GUIQIN ZHANG, REIKO KUNO, AND TETSUYA MIZUNO

Department of Neuroimmunology, Research Institute of Environmental Medicine, Nagoya University, Furo-cho, Chikusa, Nagoya 464-8601, Japan

ABSTRACT: Accumulation of activated microglia and reactive astrocytes is observed around degenerating neurons in various inflammatory or degenerative disorders in the central nervous system. These reactive glial cells may play either neurotoxic or neuroprotective roles. In this study, we examined the effects of glia-derived cytokines on neuronal degeneration and regeneration. Neuron-rich cultures were stimulated with supernatant of microglia and astrocytes stimulated with LPS, or a various concentrations of recombinant cytokines. Neurotoxicity was evaluated by an MTS assay. Neuronal damage was also evaluated by a frequency of dendritic beading, which was found to be an early feature of neuronal damage toward cell death. Effects of the cytokines on production of neurotrophic factors by astrocytes were also examined by RT-PCR for the expression of mRNA. Supernatant of LPS-stimulated microglia induced neuronal cell death. However, all the recombinant cytokines examined did not induce cell death, while IFNγ and TNFα induced dendrite beading, an early feature of neuronal damage. IL-1β and TNFα enhanced the production of neurotrophic factors by astrocytes. These observations suggest that glial cell–derived cytokines may synergistically function in neuronal degeneration with other toxic factors produced by activated microglia, and that some of them may also function in regeneration by inducing neurotrophic factors.

KEYWORDS: Microglia; astrocytes; neuron; degeneration; cytokines; neurotrophic factor

INTRODUCTION

Microglia and astrocytes are the main effectors of innate immune responses in the central nervous system (CNS). They are activated in pathological

Address for correspondence: Akio Suzumura, Department of Neuroimmunology, Research Institute of Environmental Medicine, Nagoya University, Furo-cho, Chikusa, Nagoya 464-8601, Japan. Voice: 81-52-789-3881; fax: 81-52-789-3885.
e-mail: suzumura@riem.nagoya-u.ac.jp

Ann. N.Y. Acad. Sci. 1088: 219–229 (2006). © 2006 New York Academy of Sciences.
doi: 10.1196/annals.1366.012

conditions, such as demyelinating and neurodegenerative diseases. The release of proinflammatory mediators, including interleukin (IL)-1,[1] IL-6,[2] tumor necrosis factor (TNF) α,[3,4] nitric oxide (NO),[5] and reactive oxygen species (ROS),[6] by microglia and astrocytes functions to exacerbate demyelinating diseases, such as multiple sclerosis (MS) and its animal model, experimental allergic encephalomyelitis (EAE). These inflammatory substances act to destroy myelin or oligodendrocytes to produce demyelinating lesions.[7,8] Proinflammatory cytokines can also cause neuronal cell death, both directly and indirectly via the induction of NO and free radicals.[9] Peroxynitrite, formed by NO- and ROS-mediated reactions, is reported to play a role in amyloid beta neurotoxicity.[10] Recently, we have shown that phosphodiesterase inhibitor, ibudilast, effectively suppresses neuronal cell death induced by activated microglia,[11] and that the protective effects of ibudilast are due to suppression of the proinflammatory mediators by activated microglia. Thus, fully activated microglia may be toxic to neurons, while activated microglia also produce neurotrophic factors (NTFs). However, the effects of each cytokines from activated microglia on neurons are still controversial.

Astrocytes provide structural, metabolic, and trophic support for neurons. Activated astrocytes, however, can secrete these inflammatory mediators to exert neurotoxic effects.[12,13] In the previous paper, we have shown that astrocytes, when activated with lipopolysaccharide (LPS) and/or IFNγ, kill neurons *in vitro* via induction of inflammatory mediators such as IL-1β and TNFα.[14] Cytosine arabinofuranoside–stimulated astrocytes increase neuronal susceptibility to glutamate.[15] These observations suggest that agents that suppress glial cell activation may be useful for the future treatment of neuroinflammatory or neurodegenerative disorders.

We have examined the effects of glial cell–derived cytokines on neuronal degeneration to examine how glial cells are involved in the pathophysiology of neuronal degeneration and regeneration. Effects of these cytokines on production of NTFs by glial cells are also examined.

MATERIALS AND METHODS

Reagents

LPS was purchased from Sigma (St. Louis, MO, USA). Recombinant murine IL-1β, IL-6, IL-10, TNFα and IFNγ were obtained from Genzyme/Techne (Minneapolis, MN, USA).

Cell Cultures

Microglia were isolated from primary mixed glial cell cultures from newborn C57/BL6 mice on the 14th day using the "shaking off" method described previously.[16] Cultures were 97%–100% pure, as determined by Fc receptor-specific immunostaining. Cultures were maintained in Dulbecco's modified Eagle's medium supplemented with 10% fetal calf serum, 5 μg/mL bovine insulin, and 0.2% glucose. Microglial cells (5×10^5) were cultured for 48 h with or without 1 μg/mL LPS. Culture supernatants (Mi-sup) were collected and stored at – 80°C until use.

Astrocytes were purified from the primary mixed glial cell cultures by three to four repetitions of trypsinization and replating. The purity of astrocytes was greater than 95% when determined by indirect immunofluorescence staining with an anti-GFAP antibody. Astrocytes were grown to confluency and cultured in serum-free medium for 3 days. Cells were then cultured for an additional 24 h with or without 10 μg/mL LPS. The cells at 24 h after stimulation were used for RNA extraction. The expression of mRNA for NGF, BDNF, GDNF, and NT-3 were analyzed by semiquantified reverse transcription polymerase chain reaction (RT-PCR), as described.[17]

Neuronal cultures were prepared from C57/BL6 mice at embryonic day 17.[11] In brief: cortices were dissected and freed of meninges. Cortical fragments were dissociated into single cells using dissociation solution (Sumitomo Bakelite, Akita, Japan), then resuspended in Neuron Medium (Sumitomo Bakelite). Primary neuronal cells were plated on 12-mm polyethyleneimine (PEI)-coated cover glass in 24-well multidishes at a density of 5×10^4 cells per well. Neuronal cells were stimulated with either supernatant of LPS-stimulated microglia or recombinant cytokines. The cytokines used for stimulation were 100 ng/mL TNF-α, IL-1-β, IL-6, IL-10, and IFN-γ.

MTS Assay

To assess neurotoxic effects of Mi-sup and each recombinant cytokines, we used Cell Titer 96 Aqueous one-solution assay (Promega, Madison, WI, USA) as described previously.[18] Purified neuronal cells (2×10^4 cells per well) were plated on 96-well culture plates and incubated at 37°C. Mi-sup and graded concentrations (0–100 ng/mL) TNF-α, IL-1-β, IL-6, IL-10, and IFN-γ (R&D Systems, Minneapolis, MN, USA) were added to culture plates up to 72 h after the 13 days *in vitro*. Absorbance at 490 nm was measured at 12, 24, 48, and 72 h after incubation in a multiple plate reader (Labsystems, Thermo BioAnalysis, Tokyo, Japan). Assays were carried out in five independent trials.

Morphological Observation

For assessment of dendritic beading, 100 ng/mL TNF-α, IL-1-β, IL-6, IL-10, or IFN-γ was added to neuronal cultures for 48 h after the 13 days *in vitro*. Cells were fixed in 4% paraformaldehyde, and permeabilized with 0.3% Triton

X-100. Then, cells were stained with mouse antimicrotubule-associated protein (MAP)-2 antibody (Chemicon) and specific binding was detected using secondary antibodies conjugated to Alexa 488 (Invitrogen). Cells were analyzed under Axioplan 2 microscope (Carl Zeiss, Göttingen, Germany). The ratio of beads-bearing neurons, which displayed at least one beading anywhere along their dendritic arbor, was calculated as a percentage of total cells in five microscopic fields.[18]

RNA Preparation and RT-PCR

Total RNA was extracted from astrocytes following the guanidinium thiocyanate method (RNeasy Mini Kit; QIAGEN). The cDNA encoding mouse NGF, BDNF, GDNF, NT-3 and NT-4 was generated by RT-PCR using SuperScript II (Invitrogen) and AmpliTaq DNA polymerase (Applied Biosystems, Branchburg, NJ), with the following primers:

NGF sense, 5'-CATGGGGGAGTTCTCAGTGT
NGF antisense, 5'-GCACCCACTCTCTCAACAGGAT
BDNF sense, 5'-GCGGCAGATAAAAAGACTGC
BDNF antisense, 5'-CTTATGAATCGCCAGCCAAT
GDNF sense, 5'-TATCCTGACCAGTTTGATGA
GDNF antisense, 5'-TCTAAAAACGACAGGTCGTC
NT-3 sense, 5'-TTTCTCGCTTATCTCCGTGGC
NT-3 antisense, 5'-AGGGTGCTCTGGTAATTTTCC
NT-4 sense, 5'-CCCTGCGTCAGTACTTCTTCGAGAC
NT-4 antisense, 5'-CTGGACGTCAGGCACGGCCTGTTC

RESULTS

Supernatant of LPS-stimulated microglia induced neuronal cell death. When the supernatant of microglia stimulated with 1 μg/mL LPS was applied to neuronal cultures, most neurons died in 24 h. After stimulation for 48 h, almost all neurons died (FIG. 1). This was confirmed by MTS assay. Viability of neurons was decreased to 48% in 24 h and 18% in 48 h, as determined by MTS assay. However, all the recombinant cytokines did not induce cell death as determined by morphological observation and MTS assay (FIG. 2), whereas 100 ng/mL IFN-γ and TNF-α were slightly toxic to neurons. Then, we examined the effects of these cytokines on morphological changes in neuronal cells. IFN-γ and TNF-α induced dendrite beadings, which were similar to those induced by low dose of Mi-sup (FIG. 3). IL-1β, IL-6 and IL-10 did not significantly affect neuronal survival and beading formation. The dendritic bead formation by these cytokines was dose-dependent. Although 10 ng/mL

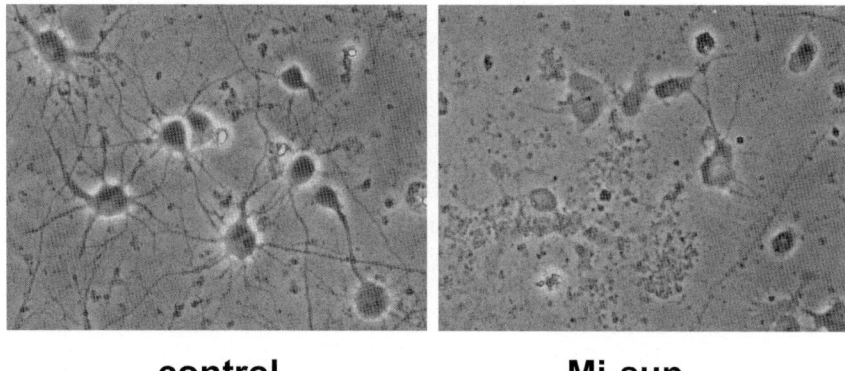

control   Mi-sup

FIGURE 1. Neurotoxicity by microglia. Neuronal culture was stimulated with supernatant of LPS-stimulated microglia (Mi-sup) for 48 h. Most of neurons died (phase contrast).

IFNγ induced dendritic beading in fewer than 10% of MAP-2-positive neurons, 100 ng/mL IFNγ induced dendritic beading in 40% of MAP-2-positve neurons after 24-h stimulation.

LPS-stimulated astrocytes also decreased neuronal survival, as determined by MTS assay and morphological observation. However, toxic effects of astrocyte-conditioned medium were much less than those for Mi-Sup (data not shown; see our previous report).[14]

When stimulated with LPS, astrocytes are induced to express NGF, BDNF, GDNF, and NT-3 mRNA. Among recombinant cytokines, IL-1β, TNF-α and IFN-γ induced mRNA expression for these NTFs in astrocytes, though the

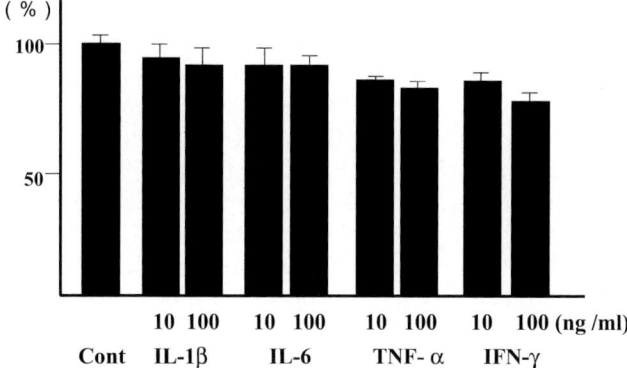

FIGURE 2. MTS assay. Neuronal cultures were stimulated with each recombinant cytokine. These cytokines by themselves did not significantly decrease viability of neurons as compared to nonstimulated cultures as a control. The columns indicate mean, and the whiskers indicate SD (n = 5).

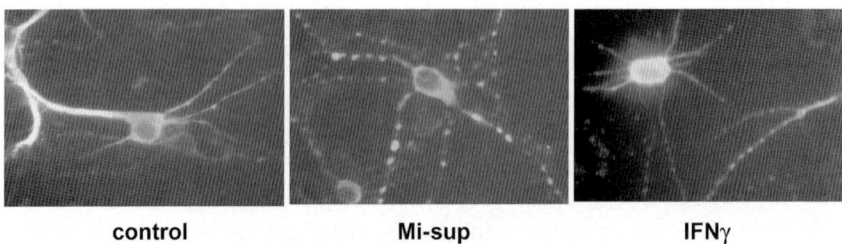

control   Mi-sup   IFNγ

FIGURE 3. Beading formation. MAP-2-positive neurons stimulated with Mi-sup or IFNγ shows dendritic beading.

induction was less than that by LPS. However, when stimulated with IL-1β and TNF-α, these cytokines synergistically increased mRNA expression for these NTFs in 12 h (FIG. 4).

DISCUSSION

In this study, we have shown that LPS-stimulated microglia and astrocytes are toxic to neurons. Although these LPS-stimulated glial cells are known to produce proinflammatory cytokines such as IL-1β, IL-6, TNFα, all these cytokines failed to induce neuronal cell death. Although TNFα has been shown to induce apoptotic cell death in neurons,[19] even a high dose of recombinant TNFα did not induce neuronal cell death in our experimental conditions. We have shown recently that the most toxic factor from activated microglia is glutamate, but not TNFα.[18] Thus, proinflammatory cytokines themselves are not so harmful to neuronal cells. However, some of these proinflammatory cytokines, such as TNFα and IFNγ, induced dendritic beading, an early feature of neuronal damage,[18] suggesting that these cytokines may be toxic in certain pathological conditions, in which other toxic stimuli disturb neuronal survival. Alternatively, because proinflammatory cytokines reportedly induce glutamate production in glial cells, glial cell–derived cytokines may synergistically function in neuronal degeneration with glutamate.[18] We have previously reported that microglia-derived TNFα work on microglia themselves in an autocrine manner to regulate its secretion of inflammatory mediators including TNFα itself.[17] Therefore, it is possible that microglia has an auto-activation system, which contributes to microglial persistent activation inducing neuronal damage.

Among proinflammatory cytokines, IFNγ was most neurotoxic as determined by dendritic bead formation. Although IFNγ is produced restrictively by immune cells such as T cells and NK cells, we have found recently that microglia produce IFNγ on stimulation with IL-12 and/or IL-18.[20] IFNγ has been shown to activate microglia to produce neurotoxic factors, including NO,

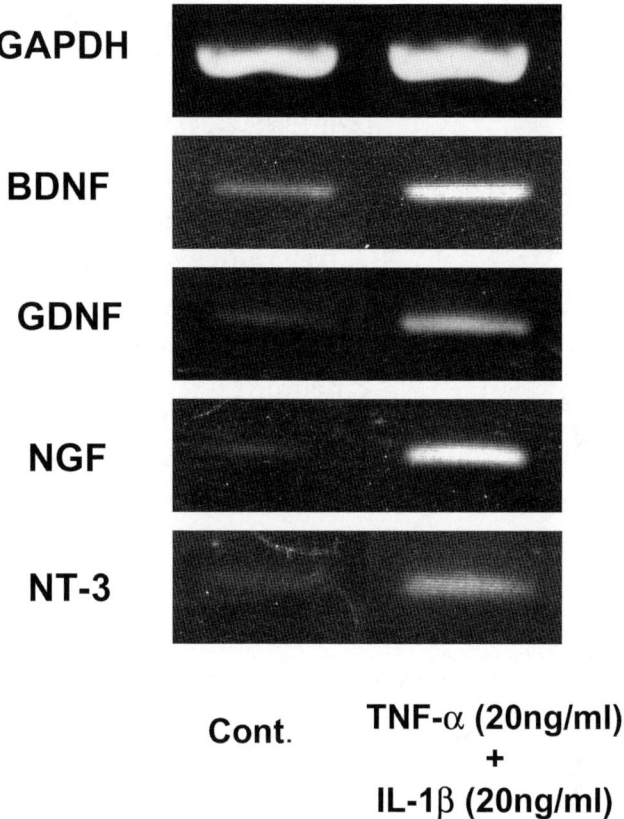

GAPDH

BDNF

GDNF

NGF

NT-3

Cont.   TNF-α (20ng/ml)
                              +
                     IL-1β (20ng/ml)

FIGURE 4. The expression of mRNA for neurotrophic factors by astrocytes. Astrocytes stimulated with TNFα and IL-1β are induced to express mRNA for BDNF, GDNF, NGF, and NT-3 in 12 h.

superoxide. IFNγ may possibly be involved in neuronal damage either directly or indirectly via activating other glial cells or macrophages.

In neurodegenerative diseases, astrocytes may rescue injured neurons by secreting NTFs. NTFs have important roles in survival of neuronal cells. NGF, BDNF, and NT-3 promote neuronal survival via tyrosine kinase receptors.[21] GDNF inhibits the expression of NO synthetase during ischemia,[22] and protects against beta-amyloid-induced apoptosis and oxidative stress.[23] Thus, the upregulation of these NTFs by glia-derived cytokines may also support neuronal cell survival.

Recent studies have shown that acute axonal loss occurs in MS and its animal model, experimental autoimmune encephalomyelitis (EAE), and that the administration of NGF has been shown to ameliorate clinical symptoms of EAE.[24,25] The mechanisms of how NGF suppresses EAE remain to be

Neuronal Degeneration by Glia-derived Cytokines

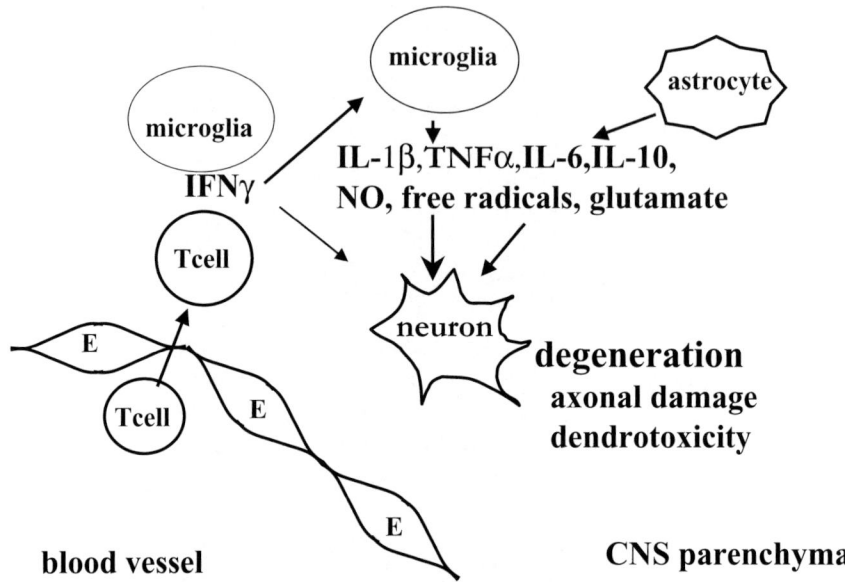

FIGURE 5. Glia-derived cytokines in neuronal degeneration. LPS-stimulated microglia and astrocytes produce proinflammatory and neurotoxic factors, and kill neurons *in vitro*. Each cytokine, however, is not potent enough to kill neurons by itself, suggesting that they may function synergistically to exert neurotoxic effects. IFNγ derived from microglia may be involved in these synergistic neurotoxic effects of glia-derived cytokines.

elucidated. Other studies suggested that NGF can act as an anti-inflammatory mediator, interfering with the functions of MHC class II–positive cells that mediate autoimmune processes in the CNS. Thus, NGF may exert its function via not only direct neuroprotection, but also by suppressive effects on glial cells. Both microglia and astrocytes express two NGF receptors, TrkA and P75, and it is reported that NGF regulates microglial survival *in vitro*, though effects of NGF on astrocytes are still unclear. In ALS (amyotrophic lateral sclerosis), it is suggested that astrocyte-derived NGFs cause neuronal apoptosis, indicating the need for of very careful consideration in therapeutic utilization.

GDNF was originally identified as a dopaminergic neurotrophin and many studies were carried out in relationship to Parkinson's disease (reviewed in Ref. 26). In MS, GDNFs reportedly contribute to the disease recovery.[27] Another report has shown that GDNF supports remyelination of regenerating axons in spinal cord injury.[28] Although the precise mechanisms of the astrocyte-derived GDNF upregulated in CNS inflammation awaits further elucidation, it is possible that glia-derived cytokines enhance astrocyte-derived GDNFs to protect neurons from harmful stimuli.

Taken altogether, glial-derived cytokines may be neurotoxic if they affect neurons directly, though each cytokine is not potent enough to kill neurons by itself. They may function synergistically with other cytokines or other toxic agents such as NO, free radicals, or glutamate (FIG. 5). However, some of these cytokines also have neurotrophic effects via activating glial cells in an autocrine or paracrine manner to produce NTFs. Thus, the fate of neurons may be determined by the balance of these toxic and protective effects of glia-derived factors.

ACKNOWLEDGMENT

This work was supported in part by the Neuroimmunological Desease Research Committee grant from the Japanese Ministry of Health, Labour, and Welfare, and a Grant-in-Aid and the 21st COE Program "Integrated Molecular Medicine for Neuronal and Neoplastic Disorders" from the Ministry of Education, Culture, Sports, Science, and Technology.

REFERENCES

1. GIULIAN, D., T.J. BAKER, L.-C.N. SHIN & L.B. LACHMAN. 1986. Interleukin 1 of the central nervous system is produced by ameboid microglia. J. Exp. Med. **164:** 594–604.
2. FREI, K., U.V. MALIPIERO, T.P. LEIST, *et al*. 1989. On the cellular source and function of interleukin 6 produced in the central nervous system in viral diseases. Eur. J. Immunol. **19:** 689–694.
3. SAWADA, M., N. KONDO, A. SUZUMURA & T. MARUNOUCHI. 1989. Production of tumor necrosis factor–alpha by microglia and astrocytes in culture. Brain Res. **491:** 394–397.
4. WOOD, P.L. 1995. Microglia as a unique cellular target in the treatment of stroke: potential neurotoxic mediators produced by activated microglia. Neurol. Res. **17:** 242–248.
5. MEDA, L., M.A. CASSATELLA, G.I. SZENDREI, *et al*. 1995. Activation of microglial cells by beta-amyloid protein and interferon-gamma. Nature **374:** 647–650.
6. TANAKA, M., A. SOTOMATSU, T. YOSHIDA, *et al*. 1994. Detection of superoxide production by activated microglia using a sensitive and specific chemiluminescence assay and microglia-mediated PC12 cell death. J. Neurochem. **63:** 266–270.
7. SELMAJ, K. & C.S. RAINE. 1988. Tumor necrosis factor mediates myelin and oligodendrocyte damage in vitro. Ann. Neurol. **23:** 339–347.
8. SELMAJ, K., C.S. RAINE, M. FAROOQ, *et al*. 1991. Cytokine cytotoxicity against oligodendrocytes. Apoptosis induced by lymphotoxin. J. Immunol. **147:** 1522–1529.
9. HU, S., P.K. PETERSON & C.C. CHAO. 1997. Cytokine–mediated neuronal apoptosis. Neurochem. International **30:** 427–431.

10. XIE, Z., M. WEI, T.E. MORGAN, et al. 2002. Peroxynitrite mediates neurotoxicity of amyloid beta-peptide1-42- and lipopolysaccharide-activated microglia. J. Neurosci. **22:** 3484–3492.

11. MIZUNO, T., T. KUROTANI, Y. KOMATSU, et al. 2004. Neuroprotective role of phosphodiesterase inhibitor ibudilast on neuronal cell death induced by activated microglia. Neuropharmacology. **46:** 404–411.

12. CHAO, C.C., S. HU, W.S. SHENG, et al. 1996. Cytokine-stimulated astrocytes damage human neurons via a nitric oxide mechanism. Glia **16:** 276–284.

13. ASCHNER, M. 1998. Astrocytes as mediators of immune and inflammatory responses in the CNS. Neurotoxicology. **19:** 269–281.

14. MIZUNO, T., R. KUNO, A. NITTA, et al. 2005. Protective effects of nicergoline against neuronal cell death induced by activated microglia and astrocytes. Brain Res. **1066:** 78–85.

15. AHLEMEYER, B., S. KOLKER, Y. ZHU, et al. 2003. Cytosine arabinofuranoside-induced activation of astrocytes increases the susceptibility of neurons to glutamate due to the release of soluble factors. Neurochem. Int. **42:** 567–581.

16. SUZUMURA, A., S.G. MEZITIS, N.K. GONATAS & D.H. SILBERBERG. 1987. MHC antigen expression on bulk isolated macrophage-microglia from newborn mouse brain: induction of Ia antigen expression by gamma-interferon. J. Neuroimmunol. **15:** 263–278.

17. KUNO, R., J. WANG, J. KAWANOKUCHI, et al. 2005. Autocrine activation of microglia by tumor necrosis factor-α. J. Neuroimmunol. **162:** 89–96.

18. TAKEUCHI, H., T. MIZUNO, G. ZHANG, et al. 2005. Neuritic beading induced by activated microglia is an early feature of neuronal dysfunction toward neuronal death by inhibition of mitochondrial respiration and axonal transport. J. Biol. Chem. **280:** 10444–10454.

19. CHAO, C.C., S.X. HU, L. EHRLICH & P.K. PETERSON. 1995. Interleukin-1 and tumor necrosis factor-α synergistically mediate neurotoxicity: involvement of nitric oxide and of N-methyl-D-aspartate receptors. Brain Behav. Immun. **9:** 355–365.

20. KAWANOKUCHI, J., T. MIZUNO, H. TAKEUCHI, et al. 2006. Production of interferon-γ by microglia. Multiple Scler. In press.

21. BARBACID, M. 1995. Structural and functional properties of the TRK family of neurotrophin receptors. Ann. N. Y. Acad. Sci. **766:** 442–458.

22. WANG, Y., S. LIN, A. CHIOU, et al. 1997. Glial cell line-derived neurotrophic factor protects against ischemia-induced injury in the cerebral cortex. J. Neurosci. **17:** 4341–4348.

23. GHRIBI, O., M.H. HERMAN, P. PRAMOONJAGO, et al. 2004. GDNF regulates the Aβ-induced endoplasmic reticulum stress response in rabbit hippocampus by inhibiting the activation of gadd 153 and the JNK and ERK kinases. Neurobiol. Dis. **16:** 417–427

24. FLUGEL, A., K. MATSUMURO, H. NEUMANN, et al. 2001. Anti-inflammatory activity of nerve growth factor in experimental autoimmune encephalomyelitis: inhibition of monocyte transendothelial migration. Eur. J. Immunol. **31:** 11–22.

25. VILLOSLADA, P., S.L. HAUSER, I. BARTKE, et al. 2000. Human nerve growth factor protects common marmosets against autoimmune encephalomyelitis by switching the balance of T helper cell type 1 and 2 cytokines within the central nervous system. J. Exp. Med. **191:** 1799–1806.

26. SIEGEL, G.J. and N.B. CHAUHAN. 2000. Neurotrophic factors in Alzheimer's and Parkinson's disease brain. Brain Res. Rev. **33:** 199–227.

27. CAGGIULA, M., A.P. BATOCCHI, G. FRISULLO, *et al.* 2005. Neurotrophic factors and clinical recovery in relapsing-remitting multiple sclerosis. Scand. J. Immunol. **62:** 176–182.
28. BLESCH, A. & M.H. TUSZYNSKI. 2003. Cellular GDNF delivery promotes growth of motor and dorsal column sensory axons after partial and complete spinal cord transections and induces remyelination. J. Comp. Neurol. **467:** 403–417.

Brain Cytokines and the 5-HT System during Poly I:C-Induced Fatigue

TOSHIHIKO KATAFUCHI, TETSUYA KONDO, SACHIKO TAKE, AND MEGUMU YOSHIMURA

Department of Integrative Physiology, Graduate School of Medical Sciences, Kyushu University, 812-8582 Fukuoka, Japan

ABSTRACT: Fatigue is evoked not only by peripheral factors, such as muscle fatigue, but also by the central nervous system (CNS). For example, it is generally known that the feeling of fatigue is greatly influenced by psychological aspects, such as motivation. However, little is known about the central mechanisms of fatigue. The clinical symptoms of chronic fatigue syndrome (CFS) are shown to include disorders in neuroendocrine, autonomic, and immune systems. On the other hand, it has been demonstrated that cytokines produced in the brain play significant roles in neural–immune interactions through their various central actions, including hypothalamo-pituitary and sympathetic activation, as well as immunosuppression. In this article, using the immunologically induced fatigue model, which was achieved by intraperitoneal (i.p.) injection of synthetic double-stranded RNAs, polyriboinosinic: polyribocytidylic acid (poly I:C) in rats, we show an involvement of brain interferon-α (IFN-α) and serotonin (5-HT) transporter (5-HTT) in the central mechanisms of fatigue. In the poly I:C-induced fatigue rats, expression of IFN-α and 5-HTT increased, while extracellular concentration of 5-HT in the medial prefrontal cortex decreased, probably on account of the enhanced expression of 5-HTT. Since the poly I:C-induced reduction of the running wheel activity was attenuated by a 5-HT$_{1A}$ receptor agonist, but not by 5-HT$_2$, 5-HT$_3$, or dopamine D$_3$ receptor agonists, it is suggested that the decrease in 5-HT actions on 5-HT$_{1A}$ receptors may at least partly contribute to the poly I:C-induced fatigue.

KEYWORDS: chronic fatigue syndrome; polyriboinosinic: polyribocytidylic acid (poly I:C); running wheel; interferon-α; serotonin transporter; 5-HT$_{1A}$ agonist

INTRODUCTION

Chronic fatigue syndrome (CFS) is characterized not only by severe fatigue, but also by impairment of autonomic, neuroendocrine, cognitive, and immune

Address for correspondence: Toshihiko Katafuchi, M.D., Ph.D., Department of Integrative Physiology, Graduate School of Medical Sciences, Kyushu University, Fukuoka, 812–8582, Japan. Voice: +81-92-642-6087; fax: +81-92-642-6093.

e-mail: kataf@physiol.med.kyushu-u.ac.jp

Ann. N.Y. Acad. Sci. 1088: 230–237 (2006). © 2006 New York Academy of Sciences.

doi: 10.1196/annals.1366.020

functions, suggesting an involvement of disorders in the neuronal–endocrine–immune interactions.[1–5] On the other hand, it is well known that cytokines produced in the brain exert various central actions, including activation of sympathetic nervous system and hypothalamic-pituitary axis, impairment of learning memory, and suppression of peripheral cellular immunity.[6,7] Therefore it is possible that brain cytokines may play a role in the pathogenesis of the CFS.

At least four types of fatigue are induced experimentally: (1) physical fatigue, such as that due to forced exercise and swimming; (2) mental fatigue; (3) environmental fatigue, such as heat exposure; and (4) immunologically induced fatigue. Of these models, the immunologically induced fatigue[8] is thought to be most closely associated with the neuronal–endocrine–immune interactions.[2] Furthermore, since it is suggested that an infection and/or reactivation of a latent virus may have a contributory role in a subset of CFS cases,[2] we decided to investigate whether fatigue is induced in rats by systemic administration of polyriboinosinic: polyribocytidylic acid (poly I:C), synthetic double-stranded RNAs that are known to mimic viral infection. To investigate brain mechanisms of fatigue in this animal model, we measured the expression of brain cytokines, such as interferon-α (IFN-α) and interleukin-1β (IL-1β). In addition, an involvement of brain 5-hydroxytryptamine (serotonin, 5-HT) system was also examined since 5-HT is implicated in the mechanisms of central fatigue after exhaustive exercise.[9]

FATIGUE INDUCED BY POLY I:C

Male Wistar rats (8–10 w) were housed individually in plastic cages with free access to food and water. Each cage contained a 30-cm-diameter running wheel that the rats could enter at any time (FIG. 1). Fatigue was assessed by decrease in total running wheel activity of each animal after intraperitoneal (i.p.) administration of poly I:C (1.0 or 3.0 mg/mL/kg) or vehicle (saline) between 9:00 AM and 10:00 PM.[10]

The averages of the total running wheel activity before treatment were about 800–1,000 wheel turns/day. The animals that were injected with poly I:C (3.0 mg/kg) showed a marked decrease in the running wheel activity compared with the saline group to about 40% of the baseline levels on day 1. The reduction of activity (60–70% of the baseline level) lasted until day 9, and then gradually recovered by day 14. The long-term depression of the voluntary running in the wheel was not directly associated with the acute-phase responses, since the rise in body temperature, serum ACTH, and catecholamine levels returned to the baseline level until the 24 h after injection.[10] Furthermore, the open field test, which can evaluate locomotor activity in the novel situation as well as anxiety, showed no differences in total distance moved, number of rearing, and length of time for center stay between poly I:C and control (saline) groups

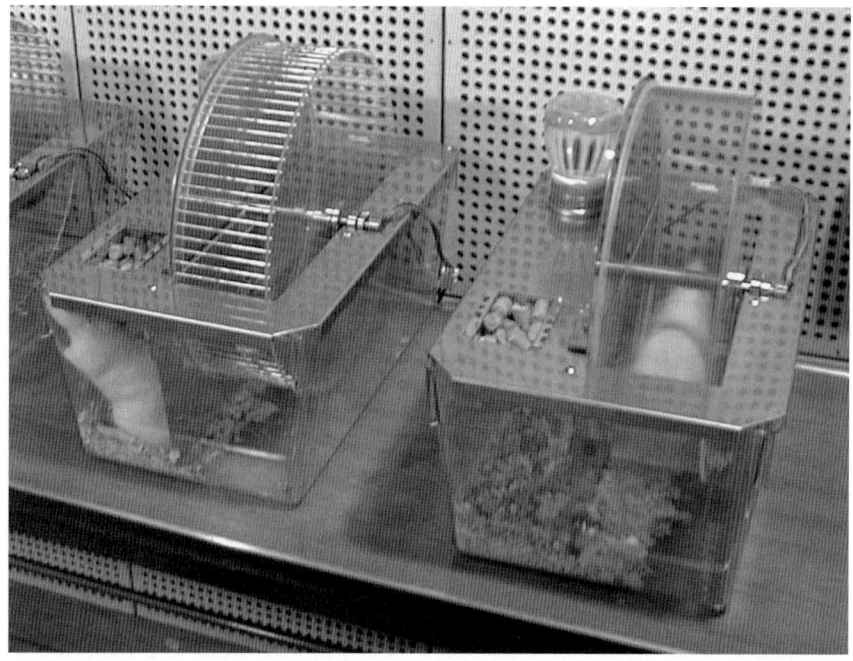

FIGURE 1. Home cage equipped with running wheel. Food and water are available *ad libitum*. Rats can enter the running wheel at any time. Wheel turns/min is continuously counted using computer software.

when performed on day 7. Thus it is strongly suggested that the decrease in running wheel activity is produced by central fatigue, but not anxiety-induced suppression or peripheral problems, such as muscle and/or joint pain.

POLY I:C-INDUCED CHANGES IN CYTOKINE mRNA EXPRESSION

Messenger RNAs (mRNAs) for IFN-α, Il-1-β, IL-6 and TNF-α in discrete regions of hypothalamic nuclei, such as medial preoptic area (MPO), lateral preoptic area (LPO), paraventricular hypothalamic nucleus (PVN), and lateral hypothalamic area (LHA), cortex, hippocampus, and cerebellum were measured quantitatively using real-time capillary RT-PCR method on day 1 and day 8 in poly I:C-injected rats. We found that the amount of both IFN-α and IL-1-β mRNAs significantly increased in the cortex and some hypothalamic nuclei, such as MPO and LPO on day 1. Although Il-1-β mRNA returned to the baseline level on day 8, an increase in IFN-α mRNA in the cortex, cerebellum, MPO, LPO, and PVN was still observed on day 8. The amounts of TNF-α and IL-6 mRNAs were not affected by poly I:C. These findings suggest that the changes in expression of IFN-α are more associated with the behavioral effect of poly I:C than that of IL-1-β, if cytokine production in the brain is involved in the mechanisms of fatigue.

The quantitative measurement of mRNAs for cytokine-related molecules, such as an inhibitor of nuclear factor κB (IκB)-β and p38 mitogen-activated protein kinase (MAPK), which are one of the IL-1-β- and IFN-α-activated transcriptional factors, respectively, was also performed on day 1 and 8 after poly I:C injection.[11] As expected, IκB-β mRNA increased only on day 1, while p38 MAPK mRNA increased both on day 1 and 8 in almost the same regions where IL-1-β and IFN-α mRNAs increased, indicating that the expression patterns of IκB-β and p38 MAPK mRNAs are very similar to those of IL-1-β and IFN-α, respectively.

POSSIBLE MECHANISMS OF IFN-α EXPRESSION IN THE BRAIN

Since we measured amounts of mRNA in the total RNA from brain tissues, the cellular origin of IFN-α is not clear. Previous studies have shown that IFN-α is detected in neurons and microglia in human brain tissues from control and neurological cases,[12,13] while astrocytes of rats and mice *in vitro* produces IFN-α/β in response to poly I:C.[14] It is also unknown how peripheral poly I:C signals the brain to induce IFN-α. Systemic injection of lipopolysaccharide (LPS) can induce fever, one of the central effects of the immune activators, through LPS itself, or peripherally and/or centrally produced cytokines by multiple routes, including (1) cerebral endothelial cells and perivascular microglial cells, (2) cells in circumventricular organs, such as the organum vasculosum of the lamina terminalis and the area postrema, which lack a functional blood–brain barrier, and (3) visceral vagal afferent nerves.[15] It has been reported that double-stranded RNAs including poly I:C are recognized by toll-like receptor (TLR) 3, which is present in the periphery and brain, to induce IFNs.[16] It is possible that the peripheral poly I:C- and LPS-induced expression of cytokines in the brain may share common pathways.

CHANGES IN 5-HTT INDUCED BY POLY I:C INJECTION

We also found that transcription of 5-HT transporter (5-HTT) increased in the hypothalamic nuclei and cortex, where IFN-α mRNA increased for more than a week after poly I:C injection. Immunoblot analysis also revealed that expression of 5-HTT increased in membrane extracts from prefrontal cortex.[11] Although *in situ* hybridization studies of 5-HTT labeled only the serotonergic cell bodies in the rat and human midbrain,[17,18] functional expression of 5-HTT mRNA in astrocytes[19] and endothelial cells[20] has been demonstrated in the rat brain by means of RT-PCR method. Since IFN-α is shown to upregulate the transcription of 5-HTT in cultured cells,[21] it is suggested that the expression of 5-HTT is enhanced by the poly I:C-induced IFN-α through its actions on astrocytes and/or endothelial cells in the respective brain regions. It has been reported that activity of 5-HTT is elevated by p38 MAPK, and this activation is abolished by suppression of p38 MAPK expression.[22] These findings are in accordance with the present results showing similar expression pattern of mRNAs for IFN-α, p38 MAPK, and 5-HTT in the brain.

To examine whether the poly I:C-induced 5-HTTs have a significant function, effects of poly I:C on extracellular 5-HT levels in the prefrontal cortex were examined using *in vivo* microdialysis technique. Within several hours after poly I:C injection, 5-HT levels started to decrease in the prefrontal cortex. A local administration of fluoxetine, a selective 5-HT reuptake inhibitor (SSRI), through a dialysis probe completely blocked the poly I:C-induced decrease in 5-HT level. Furthermore, microinjection of IFN-α into the prefrontal cortex also produced a decrease in 5-HT levels, which was again blocked by SSRI (unpublished data). It has been shown that 5-HTT expressed in astrocytes is sensitive to antidepressant drugs and contributes to the control of the extracellular 5-HT fraction in the brain; that is, 5-HT uptaken by astrocytes is inactivated through deamination by monoamine oxidase-A, then scavenged into the cerebrospinal fluid, while 5-HT uptaken by serotonergic nerve terminals is reused as a neurotransmitter.[23] These findings suggest that the functional 5-HTT overexpressed by the poly I:C-induced IFN-α in astrocytes in the prefrontal cortex scavenges 5-HT, thereby resulting in the reduction of the 5-HT levels following poly I:C injection.

BRAIN IFN-α AND FATIGUE

Since poly I:C is a strong inducer of IFN-α, it is likely that plasma IFN-α level may be elevated at least in the acute phase of poly I:C treatment. In the IFN-α-therapy-associated fatigue, which is often the dominant dose-limiting side effect, one of the causes of the fatigue is suggested to be neuromuscular fatigue, similar to that observed in patients with post-polio syndrome.[24] Since the reduction of treadmill run time to fatigue after poly I:C injection was significantly attenuated by peripheral administration of anti-IFN-α/β antibody, early fatigue induced by poly I:C may, at least partially, result from an increase in peripheral IFNs.[25] However, the persistent fatigue observed until a week after poly I:C seems to involve the central mechanisms rather than the peripheral ones for the following reasons:

First, although decrease in running wheel activity on day 1 may be due to acute sickness following poly I:C, as mentioned before, open field testing performed on day 7 suggests that a motivated activity, but not locomotor activity, has been suppressed by poly I:C. Second, it has been reported that the CFS is often accompanied by low levels of natural killer (NK) cell activity.[2,3] We have shown that the central, but not peripheral, administration of IFN-α produces a significant suppression of splenic NK cell activity through the activation of the splenic sympathetic nerve in rats.[26,27] In addition, the action site of IFN-α to induce suppression of NK activity was the MPO,[28,29] where expression of IFN-α mRNA increased on day 7 after poly I:C. It has been reported that IFN-α, but not IL-1-β and TNF-α, is elevated in cerebrospinal fluid in patients with CFS.[30] Third, brain 5-HT, which is suggested to be involved in the central mechanisms of the exercise-induced fatigue,[9] decreased in the prefrontal cortex probably because of the IFN-α-induced overexpression of 5-HTT. Finally, the poly I:C-induced fatigue was significantly attenuated by administration of 5-HT$_{1A}$ agonist, 8-hydroxy-2-(di-*n*-propylamino) tetraline (8-OH DPAT), but not 5-HT$_2$ or 5-HT$_3$ agonist.[11] These findings, taken together, suggest that the immunologically induced fatigue by poly I:C involves central mechanisms in which brain IFN-α and 5-HT system may play an important role.

It has been recently reported that in 5-HTT gene promoter polymorphism studies, the CFS patients have a significant increase in longer (L and XL) alleic variants,[31] which retain higher transcriptional activity than the short (S) allele. In addition, Narita *et al.*[31] described their preliminary observation that a selective serotonin reuptake inhibitor, fluvoxamine, was effective for about one-third of the CFS patients enough to return to work. These findings suggest that the poly I:C-induced fatigue is a useful animal model for studying central mechanisms of fatigue.

ACKNOWLEDGMENTS

This work was performed through Special Coordination Funds for Promoting Science and Technology, and Grants-in-Aid for Scientific Research (17590207) to T. K. from the Ministry of Education, Culture, Sports, Science and Technology, the Japanese Government.

REFERENCES

1. FREEMAN, R. & A.L. KOMAROFF. 1997. Does the chronic fatigue syndrome involve the autonomic nervous system? Am. J. Med. **102:** 357–364.
2. GLASER, R. & J.K. KIECOLT-GLASER. 1998. Stress-associated immune modulation: relevance to viral infections and chronic fatigue syndrome. Am. J. Med. **105:** 35S–42S.
3. WHITESIDE, T.L. & D. FRIBERG. 1998. Natural killer cells and natural killer cell activity in chronic fatigue syndrome. Am. J. Med. **105:** 27S–34S.
4. KOMAROFF, A.L. 2000. The biology of chronic fatigue syndrome [comment]. Am. J. Med. **108:** 169–171.

5. JOYCE, E. *et al.* 1996. Memory, attention, and executive function in chronic fatigue syndrome. J. Neurol. Neurosurg. Psychiatry **60:** 495–503.

6. HORI, T. *et al.,* 2001. Central cytokines: effects on peripheral immunity, inflammation and nociception. *In* Psychoneuroimmunology. R. Ader *et al.*, Eds.: 517–545. Academic Press. San Diego.

7. ROTHWELL, N.J. & S.J. HOPKINS. 1995. Cytokines and the nervous system II: actions and mechanisms of action. Trends Neurosci. **18:** 130–136.

8. CHAO, C.C. *et al.* 1992. Immunologically mediated fatigue: a murine model. Clin. Immunol. Immunopathol. **64:** 161–165.

9. YAMAMOTO, T. & E.A. NEWSHOLME. 2000. Diminished central fatigue by inhibition of the L-system transporter for the uptake of tryptophan. Brain Res. Bull. **52:** 35–38.

10. KATAFUCHI, T. *et al.* 2003. Prolonged effects of polyriboinosinic:polyribocytidylic acid on spontaneous running wheel activity and brain interferon-α mRNA in rats: a model for immunologically induced fatigue. Neuroscience **120:** 837–845.

11. KATAFUCHI, T. *et al.* 2005. Enhanced expression of brain interferon-α and serotonin transporter in immunologically induced fatigue in rats. Eur. J. Neurosci. **22:** 2817–2826.

12. AKIYAMA, H. *et al.* 1994. Expression of MRP14, 27E10, interferon-α and leukocyte common antigen by reactive microglia in postmortem human brain tissue. J. Neuroimmunol. **50:** 195–201.

13. YAMADA, T. *et al.* 1994. Immunohistochemistry using antibodies to alpha-interferon and its induced protein, MxA, in Alzheimer's and Parkinson's disease brain tissues. Neurosci. Lett. **181:** 61–64.

14. TEDESCHI, B. *et al.* 1986. Astrocytes produce interferon that enhances the expression of H-2 antigens on a subpopulation of brain cells. J. Cell Biol. **102:** 2244–2253.

15. LEDEBOER, A. *et al.* 2002. Site-specific modulation of LPS-induced fever and interleukin-1β expression in rats by interleukin-10. Am. J. Physiol. **282:** R1762–R1772.

16. ALEXOPOULOU, L. *et al.* 2001. Recognition of double-stranded RNA and activation of NF-κB by toll-like receptor 3. Nature **413:** 732–738.

17. BLAKELY, R.D. *et al.* 1991. Cloning and expression of a functional serotonin transporter from rat brain. Nature **354:** 66–70.

18. AUSTIN, M.C. *et al.* 1994. Expression of serotonin transporter messenger RNA in the human brain. J. Neurochem. **62:** 2362–2367.

19. HIRST, W.D. *et al.* 1998. Serotonin transporters in adult rat brain astrocytes revealed by [^{3}H]5-HT uptake into glial plasmalemmal vesicles. Neurochem. Int. **33:** 11–22.

20. BRUST, P. *et al.* 2000. Functional expression of the serotonin transporter in immortalized rat brain microvessel endothelial cells. J. Neurochem. **74:** 1241–1248.

21. MORIKAWA, O. *et al.* 1998. Effects of interferon-α, interferon-γ and cAMP on the transcriptional regulation of the serotonin transporter. Eur. J. Pharmacol. **349:** 317–324.

22. ZHU, C.B. *et al.* 2005. p38 MAPK activation elevates serotonin transport activity via a trafficking-independent, protein phosphatase 2A-dependent process. J. Biol. Chem. **280:** 15649–15658.

23. BEL, N. *et al.* 1997. Antidepressant drugs inhibit a glial 5-hydroxytryptamine transporter in rat brain. Eur. J. Neurosci. **9:** 1728–1738.

24. PATARCA, R. 2001. Cytokines and chronic fatigue syndrome. Ann. N. Y. Acad. Sci. **933:** 185–200.
25. DAVIS, J.M. *et al.* 1998. Immune system activation and fatigue during treadmill running: role of interferon. Med. Sci. Sports Exerc. **30:** 863–868.
26. KATAFUCHI, T. *et al.* 1993. Roles of sympathetic nervous system in the suppression of cytotoxicity of splenic natural killer cells in the rat. J. Physiol. (Lond) **465:** 343–357.
27. TAKE, S. *et al.* 1993. Central interferon-α inhibits natural killer cytotoxicity through sympathetic innervation. Am. J. Physiol. **265:** R453–R459.
28. KATAFUCHI, T. *et al.* 1993. Hypothalamic modulation of splenic natural killer cell activity in rats. J. Physiol. (Lond) **471:** 209–221.
29. TAKE, S. *et al.* 1995. Interferon-α acts at the preoptic hypothalamus to reduce natural killer cytotoxicity in rats. Am. J. Physiol. **268:** R-1406–R1410.
30. LLOYD, A. *et al.* 1991. Cytokine levels in serum and cerebrospinal fluid in patients with chronic fatigue syndrome and control subjects. J. Infect. Dis. **164:** 1023–1024.
31. NARITA, M. *et al.* 2003. Association between serotonin transporter gene polymorphism and chronic fatigue syndrome. Biochem. Biophys. Res. Commun. **311:** 264–266.

Participation of the Endocannabinoid System in the Effect of TNF-α on Hypothalamic Release of Gonadotropin-Releasing Hormone

JAVIER FERNANDEZ-SOLARI,[a] JUAN P. PRESTIFILIPPO,[a]
STEFAN R. BORNSTEIN,[b] SAMUEL M. McCANN,[a]
AND VALERIA RETTORI[a]

[a]Centro de Estudios Farmacológicos y Botánicos, Consejo Nacional de
Investigaciones Científicas y Técnicas (CEFYBO-CONICET-UBA), Paraguay
2155, (1121), Buenos Aires, Argentina

[b]Department of Medicine, Carl Gustav Carus University Hospital, University of
Dresden, 01307 Dresden, Germany

ABSTRACT: It is known that Δ^9-tetrahydrocannabinol (THC), the major
active ingredient of marijuana, can suppress reproductive function. Also,
we reported previously that the endocannabinoid, anandamide (AEA),
inhibited gonadotropin-releasing hormone (LHRH) release from medial
basal hypothalamus (MBH) of male rats incubated *in vitro* as well as
reduced plasma LH levels after i.c.v. AEA injections into the cerebral
lateral ventricle. On the other hand, it is known that during endotoxemia the hypothalamic gonadotropin axis is inhibited. Therefore, the
aim of the present study was to determine whether the effect of TNF-α,
a proinflammatory cytokine induced by lipopolysaccharide (LPS) that
inhibits LHRH release, is mediated by the activation of the endocannabinoid system. The intraperitoneal injection of LPS (5 mg/kg) as well as
the i.c.v. injection of tumor necrosis factor-α (TNF-α) (100 ng/rat) increased significantly the AEA synthesis measured *ex vivo* in MBHs removed 3 h after the treatments. To examine the possibility that TNF-α
also acted by increasing the synthesis of AEA that was released and activated the CB1-r followed by inhibition of LHRH release, we measured
the effect of TNF-α on the AEA synthase activity in MBHs incubated
in vitro. As expected, we found that TNF-α (2.9×10^{-9} M) increased
the AEA synthesis. Second, we showed that TNF-α reduced significantly
the forskolin-stimulated LHRH release and that the CB1-r antagonist
AM251 (10^{-5} M) blocked that inhibition, supporting the hypothesis that
TNF-α inhibits LHRH release, acting at least in part by activating the endocannabinoid system. Therefore, our data demonstrate a key role for the

Address for correspondence: Valeria Rettori, CEFYBO-CONICET-UBA, Paraguay 2155, (1121),
Buenos Aires, Argentina. Voice: 54-11-4508-3680; fax: 54-11-4508-3680.
e-mail: vrettori@yahoo.com

Ann. N.Y. Acad. Sci. 1088: 238–250 (2006). © 2006 New York Academy of Sciences.
doi: 10.1196/annals.1366.008

endocannabinoid system in the response of the reproductive system to inflammatory signals.

KEYWORDS: anandamide; LPS; CB1 receptor; AM251; cAMP

INTRODUCTION

It is well known that Δ^9-tetrahydrocannabinol (THC), the major active ingredient of marijuana, isolated and characterized by Gaoni and Mechoulam in 1964, can suppress reproductive function in humans, monkeys, and small rodents, such as the rat.[1–6] All previous studies, including ours,[7] indicated that the inhibitory effect of THC on the reproductive axis is exerted mainly at the hypothalamic level by inhibiting gonadotropin-releasing hormone (LHRH) release with the consequent inhibition of LH secretion by the pituitary, thereby inhibiting gonadal function. Previous *in vitro* studies performed by our group[8] showed that medial basal hypothalamic explants incubated in the presence of different concentrations of THC (10^{-11}–10^{-8} M) were without effect on basal LHRH release. However, since it was reported that catecholamines stimulate LHRH release,[9] we used this approach to evaluate the effect of THC on norepinephrine- (NE) (5×10^{-5} M) as well as dopamine (5×10^{-5} M)-stimulated LHRH release, demonstrating that THC (10^{-8} M) inhibited the stimulatory effects in both cases.

The effects of THC as well as other cannabinoids were believed to be due to a nonspecific interaction with membrane lipids, because cannabinoids are highly lipophilic. However, studies that related structure and activity of cannabinoids suggested that their actions were mediated by receptors. In fact, to date two cannabinoid receptors have been identified, cloned, and characterized: the CB-r type 1 (CB1-r) by Matsuda *et al.* in 1990,[10] expressed mainly in the central nervous system (CNS), and the CB-r type 2 (CB2-r) by Munro *et al.* in 1993,[11] mainly located on the peripheral tissues, especially in the immune system. Moreover, the current classification of cannabinoid receptors may be incomplete with the identification of a non-CB1-r and a non-CB2-r that induce responses in a variety of tissues.[12–14] Both CB1-r and CB2-r are coupled to $G_{i/o}$ proteins and respond to their ligands by inhibiting the activity of adenylyl cyclase with the consequent decrease in cAMP production.[15] The discovery of CB-rs raised the question about the existence of an endogenous CB-r agonist. The first endocannabinoid isolated and the most studied is arachidonoyl ethanolamide (anandamide, AEA).[16] After its discovery, other endogenous ligands have been identified such as 2-arachidonoyl glycerol (2-AG)[17] and 2-arachidonoyl glyceryl ether (noladin ether).[18]

The presence of CB1-r was reported in different areas of the brain.[19] In particular, we showed the presence of CB1-r in the medial basal hypothalamus (MBH) of male rats, an area that contains the neurons involved in the synthesis and release of LHRH.[20] Using double immunohistochemistry techniques we did not observe colocalization of CB1-r with LHRH neurons. The CB1-r neurons were located adjacent to the third ventricle. Having demonstrated the presence of CB1-r in the MBH, we studied the effect of the endocannabinoid, AEA, on LHRH release. We showed that AEA (10^{-9} M) decreased only by 30% the basal release of LHRH, but a greater inhibitory effect (70%) was observed on the N-methyl D-aspartic acid (NMDA)–stimulated LHRH release. The inhibitory effect of AEA was totally reversed by the specific CB1-r antagonist, AM251 (10^{-5} M), confirming the participation of the endocannabinoid system as a modulator of LHRH release in male rats. We also demonstrated that AEA (10^{-9} M) increased significantly the release of gamma-aminobutyric acid (GABA) from the MBH, but had no effect on β-endorphin release.[21] However, it was reported that AEA increased GABAergic neurotransnission by inhibiting GABA reuptake in globus pallidus.[22] Therefore, it is possible that this was the real reason we found a higher concentration of GABA in the media after the incubation of MBH with AEA rather than induced release of stored GABA. Moreover, bicuculline (10^{-4} M), a GABAergic antagonist, was capable of blocking totally the inhibitory effect of AEA on NMDA-stimulated LHRH release. However, naltrexone (10^{-6} M), an opioid receptor antagonist, did not modify the inhibitory effect of AEA.[21] These results confirmed that GABA is the inhibitory neurotransmitter that mediates the inhibition of LHRH induced by endocannabinoids, and that the opioid system is not involved in this function. Moreover, a localization of GABAergic neurons with CB1-r was also seen in the hypothalamus (personal communication, M. Herkenham, Section of Functional Neuroanatomy, National Institutes of Mental Health, Bethesda).

On the other hand, cannabinoid agonists are known to decrease neurotoxicity and AEA is able to promote anti-inflammatory responses in astrocytes via CB1 cannabinoid receptors.[23] Also, it is known that during the endotoxemia induced by lipopolysaccharide (LPS), the hypothalamic–gonadotropin axis is inhibited.[24,25] LPS seems to activate similar mechanisms in the inhibitory pathway of LHRH to those exerted by cannabinoids, principally, by increasing GABAergic activity.[26] Also it was reported that LPS increased AEA production in rat and mouse macrophages.[27,28] Moreover, it was reported that AEA inhibited nitric oxide and TNF-α production in mouse astrocytes stimulated by LPS.[29]

Therefore, the aim of the present work was to determine whether the effect of TNF-α, a proinflammatory cytokine induced by LPS that inhibits LHRH release, is mediated by the activation of the endocannabinoid system.

MATERIAL AND METHODS

Animals

Male rats of the Wistar strain (220–250 g) were kept in group cages (6 rats/ cage) in an animal room having a photoperiod of 14 h of light (05.00–19.00 h) and room temperature of 22–24°C. Animals had free access to laboratory chow and tap water. The experimental procedures reported here were approved by the Animal Care Committee of the Center of Experimental Pharmacology and Botanicals of the National Council for Research of Argentina and were carried out in accord with the Declaration of Helsinki.

In Vivo *Studies*

For the experiments with TNF-α-injected i.c.v., a cannula was implanted into the lateral cerebral ventricle of the rats, while they were anesthetized with tribromoethanol (3.5%, 1 mL/100 g animal body weight), using a stereotaxic instrument and coordinates from the atlas of Pellegrino *et al.*[30] The experiments were performed a week after the implantation of the cannulae. The MBHs were removed 3 h after the injection of TNF-α (100 ng/rat) or vehicle to measure the AEA synthase activity in the tissue. For the experiments with LPS, this drug (5 mg/kg) or vehicle was injected intraperitoneally (i.p.) and 3 h later the MBHs were removed to measure the activity of AEA synthase.

Anandamide Synthase Activity

Synthase activity in MBHs was assayed as previously described.[21] In brief, the MBHs were homogenized in 200 μL buffer Tris–HCl, 20 mM EDTA, 1 mM, pH 7.6 and centrifuged at $2{,}000 \times g$ for 15 min. Supernatant proteins (150–100 μg) were incubated in a total volume of 200 μL 5×10^{-2} M Tris–HCl (pH 9.0) with 40 μM (0.1 μCi) of [1-^{14}C] arachidonic acid (40–60 mCi‡/mmol) and 2×10^{-2} M ethanolamine for 5 min at 37°C. After evaporation, organic phases were redissolved and applied on silica gel 60 plates with concentration zone (Merck). The synthesized [^{14}C] AEA was resolved utilizing the organic layer of an ethyl acetate/hexane/acetic acid/water (100:50:20:100) mixture. After autoradiography, distribution of radioactivity on the plate was counted in a scintillation counter. The Rf values of anandamide and arachidonic acid were 0.33 and 0.78, respectively.

In Vitro *Studies*

After decapitation and removal of the brains, the MBHs were dissected by making frontal cuts just behind the optic chiasm, extending dorsally 1.0 mm, and a horizontal cut extended from this point caudally to just behind the pituitary stalk, where another frontal cut was made. Longitudinal cuts were made 1.0 mm lateral to the midline bilaterally. The hypothalami were preincubated in Krebs–Ringer bicarbonate-buffered medium (pH 7.4) containing 0.1% glucose for 15 min before replacement with fresh medium or medium containing the substances to be tested. The incubation was continued for 30 min followed by removal of the medium and storage of samples at –20°C before assays. All incubations were carried out in a Dubnoff shaker (50 cycles/min; 95% O_2/ 5% CO_2) at 37°C.

Radioimmunoassays

LHRH was measured by RIA utilizing a highly specific LHRH antiserum kindly provided by Ayala Barnea (University of Texas Southwestern Medical Center, Dallas, TX, USA). The sensitivity of the assay was 0.2 pg per tube, and the curve was linear up to 100 pg of LHRH. The intraassay coefficient of variation of the LHRH RIA ranged from 4.0% to 7.3%, and the interassay coefficient of variation was 8.9%. cAMP was measured by RIA using the anti-cAMP antibody obtained through NHPP, NIDDK, and Dr. A. F. Parlow. Intra- and interassay coefficients of variation were 8.1% and 10.5%, respectively. All samples were measured in duplicate.

Chemicals

LHRH and cAMP for iodination and standard were purchased from Peninsula Laboratories Inc., Division of Bachem (San Carlos, CA, USA). Iodine-125 for iodination was purchased from New England Nuclear™, Life Science Products (Boston, MA, USA). Forskolin, LPS, and anandamide were from Sigma Aldrich (St. Louis, MO, USA), and TNF-α was from Promega Corporation (Madison, WI, USA). AM251 [N-(piperidin-1-yl)-1-(2,4-dichlorophenyl)-5-(4-chlorophenyl)-4-methyl-1 H-pyrazole-3-carboxamide] was from Tocris™ (Ellisville, MO, USA), and ethanol from Merck (Rahway, NJ, USA).

Statistics

All data are expressed as means plus 1 SEM. Comparisons between groups were performed by using a one-way ANOVA followed by the Student-Newman-Keuls multiple comparison test for unequal replicates. Student's t test was used when comparing two groups. Differences with P values <0.05 were considered significant.

RESULTS

Effect of LPS Injected i.p. and TNF-α Injected i.c.v. on Anandamide Synthase Activity

Since it was reported that LPS stimulated AEA production in rat and mouse macrophages,[27,28] we studied the *in vivo* effect of LPS or TNF-α on the

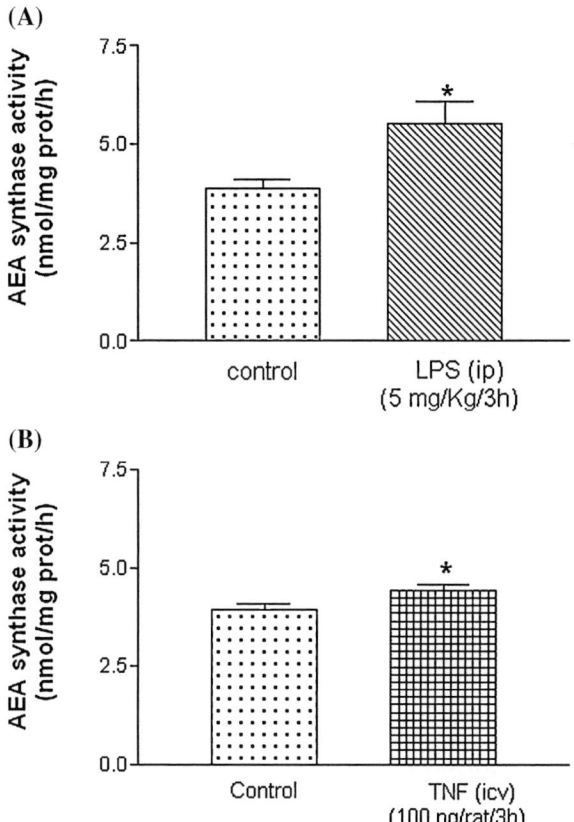

FIGURE 1. (**A**) Effect of LPS injected i.p. (5 mg/kg) on the AEA synthase activity measured *ex vivo* in MBHs extracted 3 h after injection. (**B**) Effect of TNF-α (100 ng/rat) on the AEA synthase activity measured *ex vivo* in MBHs extracted 3 h after injection (8 per group). *$P < 0.05$ vs. respective controls.

hypothalamic AEA synthase activity. The i.p. injection of LPS (5 mg/kg) (FIG. 1A) as well as the i.c.v. injection of TNF-α (100 ng/rat) (FIG. 1B) increased significantly ($P < 0.05$) the AEA synthase activity measured *ex vivo* in the MBH removed 3 h after the treatments.

Effect of TNF-α In Vitro on Anandamide Synthase Activity

In order to examine the possibility that TNF-α acted by increasing the synthesis of AEA that was released and activated the CB1-r followed by inhibition of LHRH release, we measured the effect of TNF-α on the AEA synthase activity under our experimental conditions. We found that TNF-α (2.9×10^{-9} M)

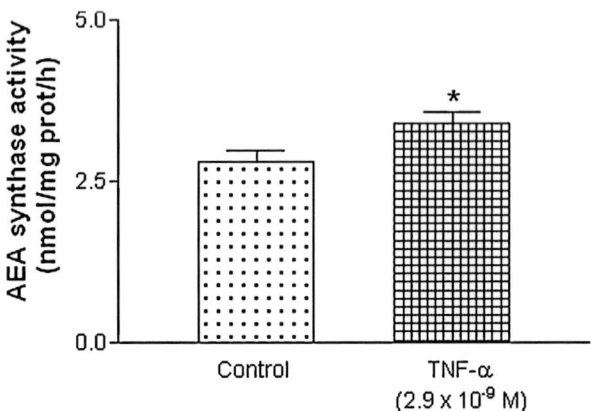

FIGURE 2. Effect of TNF-α (2.9×10^{-9} M) on AEA synthase activity in MBH (8 per group) incubated *in vitro* for 30 min. *$P < 0.05$.

in vitro increased significantly ($P < 0.05$) the AEA synthase activity (FIG. 2) suggesting that TNF-α activates the endocannabinoid system, at least in part, by increasing the production of AEA.

Effect of TNF-α on Forskolin-Stimulated cAMP Content and LHRH Release

Measurement of cAMP is a good method to determine the presence and biologic function of cannabinoid receptors, because they are coupled to Gi protein and respond by inhibiting adenylate cyclase (AC) activity. Forskolin activates AC, resulting in generation of cAMP. In addition, cAMP is the second messenger resulting from breakdown of ATP by AC that stimulates LHRH release from its neurons. Therefore, we evaluated the effect of TNF-α on the forskolin-stimulated cAMP content. cAMP content was dramatically increased (2.5-fold) by forskolin (7.6×10^{-5} M) ($P < 0.001$), and this augmentation was significantly reduced ($P < 0.001$) by TNF-α (2.9×10^{-9} M) (FIG. 3A). To investigate whether this inhibition was mediated through CB1-r, AM251, a specific antagonist of CB1-r, was added to the media. AM251 (10^{-5} M) partially but significantly ($P < 0.05$) blocked the lowering of forskolin-stimulated cAMP content induced by TNF-α. LHRH release was increased by forskolin (7.6×10^{-5} M) ($P < 0.01$) and this augmentation was significantly reduced ($P < 0.05$) by TNF-α (2.9×10^{-9}M) (FIG. 3B). AM251 (10^{-5} M) blocked ($P < 0.05$) TNF-α-induced inhibition of forskolin-stimulated LHRH release. AM251 incubated alone had no significant effect either on basal cAMP content or on basal LHRH release.

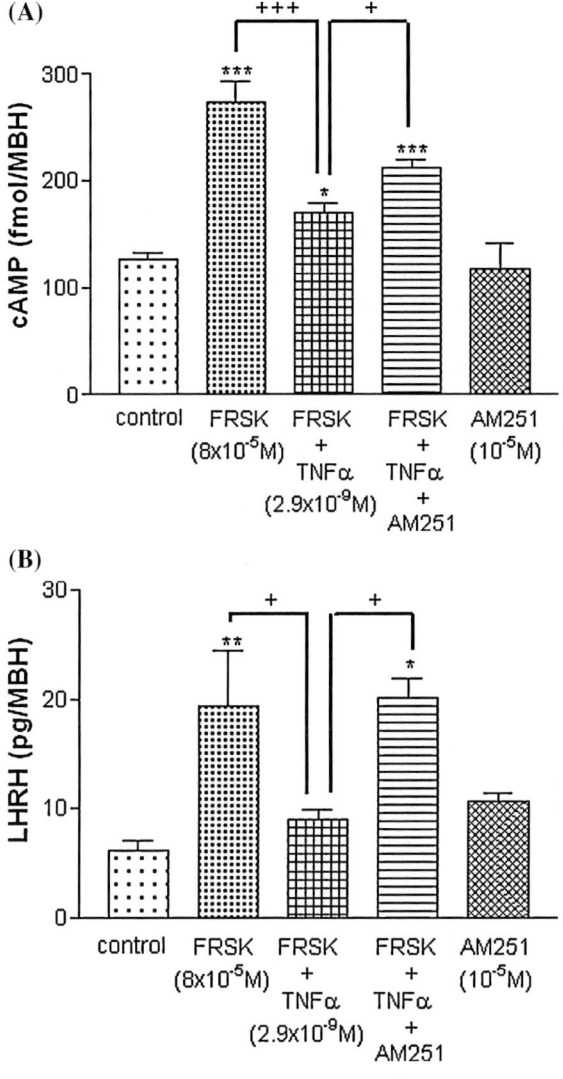

FIGURE 3. (A) Effect of forskolin (FRSK, 7.6×10^{-5} M), TNF-α (2.9×10^{-9} M) and AM251 (10^{-5} M) on cAMP content from MBH incubated *in vitro* (7 per group). *$P < 0.05$ and ***$P < 0.001$ vs. control, $^+P < 0.05$ and $^{+++}P < 0.001$ vs. FRSK + TNF-α. **(B)** Effect of forskolin (FRSK, 7.6×10^{-5} M), TNF-α (2.9×10^{-9} M) and AM251 (10^{-5} M) on LHRH release from MBH incubated *in vitro* (7 per group). *$P < 0.05$ and **$P < 0.01$ vs. control, $^+P < 0.05$ vs. FRSK + TNF-α.

DISCUSSION

The past few years have seen an increase in the number of studies examining the effects of the endocannabinoids on the cytokine biology of various cell systems.[31] Anandamide, in addition to modulating cellular responsiveness to various cytokines, was also reported to increase or decrease the production of different cytokines under varying conditions. Murine brain cortical astrocyte cultures infected with Theiler's encephalomyelitis virus produced more IL-6 in the presence of AEA.[29] Studies in human peripheral blood mononuclear cells examining a wide variety of cytokines demonstrated that AEA increased or decreased cytokine release depending upon drug concentration.[32] For example, IL-6 and IL-8 release were diminished by low doses of AEA, whereas TNF-α, INFγ, and IL-4 were inhibited at higher drug concentrations. Also, it was reported that both synthetic and endogenous cannabinoids inhibit the LPS-induced release of TNF-α from microglial cells.[33]

However, not much research was published regarding the effect of cytokines on the endocannabinoid system. It was reported that LPS increased AEA levels in mouse peritoneal macrophages by inducing AEA synthesis.[34] We demonstrated the connection between the immune and the endocannabinoid systems at the hypothalamic level by showing the increase of AEA synthase activity in MBH removed from rats injected with LPS (i.p.) or TNF-α (i.c.v.) as compared with rats receiving vehicle alone. Because TNF-α is known to be released rapidly after LPS administration[24] and mediates a number of effects attributed to LPS administration on the hypothalamic pituitary axis, we decided to work with this proinflammatory cytokine for the *in vitro* experiments. Moreover, it was reported that LPS-induced TNF-α release is controlled by the CNS.[35] We demonstrated that TNF-α (100 ng/rat) injected i.c.v. increased the AEA synthase activity measured *ex vivo* 3 h after the injections. Therefore, it is possible that LPS, through an increase in TNF-α production, activates the endocannabinoid system to inhibit the release of LHRH. To confirm this hypothesis we measured the effect of TNF-α on LHRH release from MBH incubated *in vitro*. TNF-α had no effect on the basal release of LHRH (data not shown); however, TNF-α significantly reduced the forskolin-stimulated LHRH release, and this effect was totally blocked by the CB1-r-specific blocker, AM251.

It was reported that LPS leads to the suppression of LHRH pulse generator activity through a mechanism involving TNF-α. This change was faithfully reflected in the LH secretory pattern.[36] Furthermore, we have previously demonstrated that AEA (50 ng/5 μL) injected i.c.v. reduced plasma LH levels from blood samples collected 120 min after injections[37] similarly to the reduction in LH that occurs during the endotoxemia induced by LPS in sheep.[38] These results show that the endocannabinoid system participates in neuroendocrine and immune responses. It appears that the neuroimmuno-endocannabinoid system is involved in regulating the brain–immune axis and might be exploited in future therapies for chronic diseases and immune deficiency.

In summary, in the present work we demonstrated that the LPS-induced TNF-α release increases AEA synthesis in the MBH. This augmentation of AEA production activates CB1-r, which reduces cAMP, thereby activating

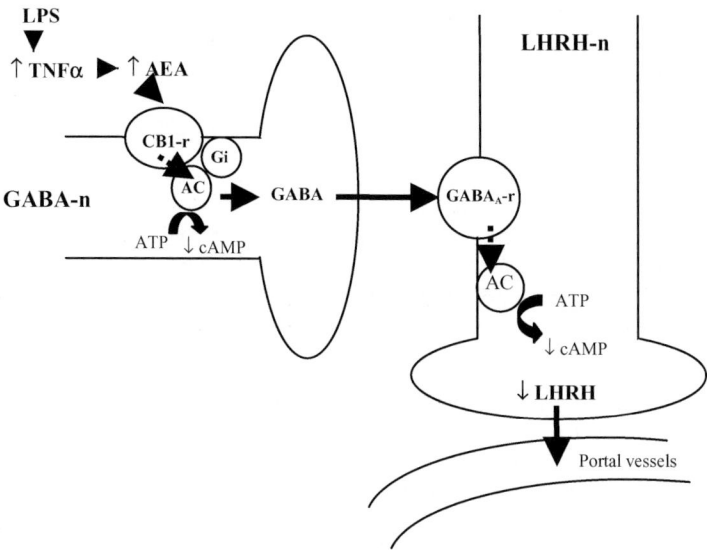

FIGURE 4. Diagrammatic representation of the postulated mechanism of action of TNF-α to suppress LHRH release by activating the endocannabinoid system. For explanation, see DISCUSSION. GABA-n, GABA neuron; GABA$_A$r, GABA$_A$ receptor; LHRH-n, LHRH neuronal terminal; AC, adenylate cyclase; Gi, guanosine triphosphate inhibitory binding protein. *Solid arrows* indicate stimulation; *dashed arrows* indicate inhibition.

GABAergic neurons that responded by increasing the release of GABA. Finally, GABA acts on GABA$_A$ receptors located on LHRH neurons to inhibit LHRH release (FIG. 4).

ACKNOWLEDGMENTS

We thank Ana Ines Casella for her administrative help. This work was supported by grants from Agencia Nacional de Promoción Científica y Tecnológica, Argentina (PICT 03-14264), BMBF-SECYT AL/TA 04-SV/027, and Deutsche Forschungsgemeinschaft (DFG) BO 1141/7-1 Grant to S.R.B.

REFERENCES

1. CICERO, T.J. & T. BADGER. 1977. Effects of alcohol on the hypothalamic-pituitary-gonadal axis in the male rat. J. Pharmacol. Exp. Ther. **201:** 427–433.
2. CICERO, T.J., K.S. NEWMAN, M. GERRITY, *et al.* 1982. Ethanol inhibits the naloxone-induced release of luteinizing hormone-releasing hormone from the hypothalamus of the male rat. Life Sci. **31:** 1587–1596.

3. MENDELSON, J.H., N.K. MELLO & J. ELLINGBOE. 1977. Effects of acute alcohol intake on pituitary-gonadal hormones in normal human males. Exp. Ther. **202:** 676–682.
4. DEES, W.L., V. RETTORI, G.P. KOZLOWSKI & S.M. McCANN. 1985. Ethanol and the pulsatile release of luteinizing hormone, follicle stimulating hormone and prolactin in ovariectomized rats. Alcohol **2:** 641–646.
5. MURPHY, L., J. GHER, R. STEGER & A. BARTKE. 1994. Effects of delta 9-tetrahydrocannabinol on copulatory behavior and neuroendocrine responses of male rats to female conspecifics. Pharmacol. Biochem. Behav. **48:** 1011–1017.
6. WENGER, T., V. RETTORI, G. SNYDER, et al. 1987. Effects of delta-9-tetrahydrocannabinol on the hypothalamic-pituitary control of luteinizing hormone and follicle-stimulating hormone secretion in adult male rats. Neuroendocrinology **46:** 488–493.
7. AYALON, D., I. NIR, T. CORDOVA, et al. 1977. Acute effect of delta1-tetrahydrocannabinol on the hypothalamo-pituitary-ovarian axis in the rat. Neuroendocrinology **23:** 31–42.
8. RETTORI, V., M.C. AGUILA, M.F. GIMENO, et al. 1990. In vitro effect of delta 9-tetrahydrocannabinol to stimulate somatostatin release and block that of luteinizing hormone-releasing hormone by suppression of the release of prostaglandin E2. Proc. Natl. Acad. Sci. USA **87:** 10063–10066.
9. NEGRO-VILAR, A., S.M. OJEDA & S.M. McCANN. 1979. Catecholaminergic modulation of luteinizing hormone-releasing hormone release by median eminence terminals in vitro. Endocrinology **104:** 1749–1757.
10. MATSUDA, L.A., S.J. LOLAIT, M.J. BROWNSTEIN, et al. 1990. Structure of a cannabinoid receptor and functional expression of the cloned cDNA. Nature **346:** 561–564.
11. MUNRO, S., K.L. THOMAS & M. ABU-SHAAR. 1993. Molecular characterization of a peripheral receptor for cannabinoids. Nature **365:** 61–65.
12. WAGNER, J.A., K. VARGA, Z. JARAI & G. KUNOS. 1999. Mesenteric vasodilatation mediated by endothelial anandamide receptor. Hypertension **33:** 429–434.
13. ZYGMUNT, P.M., D.A. ANDERSSON & E.D. HOGESTATT. 2002. Delta 9-tetrahydrocannabinol and cannabinol activate capsaicin-sensitive sensory nerves via CB1 and CB2 cannabinoid receptor-independent mechanism. J. Neurosci. **22:** 4720–4727.
14. KUNOS, G. & S. BATKAI. 2001. Novel physiologic functions of endocannabinoids as revealed through the use of mutant mice. Neurochem. Res. **26:** 1015–1021.
15. PERTWEE, R.G. 1997. Pharmacology of cannabinoid CB1 and CB2 receptors. Pharmacol Ther. **74:** 129–180.
16. DEVANE, W.A., L. HANUS, A. BREUER, et al. 1992. Isolation and structure of a brain constituent that binds to the cannabinoid receptor. Science **258:** 1946–1949.
17. DI MARZO, V. 1998. 2-arachidonoyl-glycerol as an "endocannabinoid": limelight for a formerly neglected metabolite. Biochemistry **63:** 13–21.
18. HANUS, L., S. ABU-LAFI, E. FRIDE, et al. 2001. 2-Arachidonyl glyceryl ether, an endogenous agonist of the cannabinoid CB1 receptor. Proc. Natl. Acad. Sci. USA **98:** 3662–3665.
19. MOLDRICH, G. & T. WENGER. 2000. Localization of the CB1 cannabinoid receptor in the rat brain. An immunohistochemical study. Peptides **21:** 1735–1742.
20. RETTORI, V., A. LOMNICZI, C. MOHN, et al. 2002. Mechanisms of inhibition of LHRH release by alcohol and cannabinoids. Prog. Brain. Res. **141:** 175–181.

21. FERNANDEZ-SOLARI, J., C. SCORTICATI, C. MOHN, *et al.* 2004. Alcohol inhibits luteinizing hormone-releasing hormone release by activating the endocannabinoid system. Proc. Natl. Acad. Sci. USA **101:** 3264–3268.
22. MANEUF, Y.P., J.E. NASH, A.R. CROSSMAN & J.M. BROTCHIE. 1996. Activation of the cannabinoid receptor by delta 9-tetrahydrocannabinol reduces gamma-aminobutyric acid uptake in the globus pallidus. Eur. J. Pharmacol. **308:** 161–164.
23. ORTEGA-GUTIERREZ, S., E. MOLINA-HOLGADO & C. GUAZA. 2005. Effect of anandamide uptake inhibition in the production of nitric oxide and in the release of cytokines in astrocyte cultures. Glia **52:** 163–168.
24. MCCANN, S.M., M. KIMURA, S. KARANTH, *et al.* 2000. The mechanism of action of cytokines to control the release of hypothalamic and pituitary hormones in infection. Ann. N. Y. Acad. Sci. **917:** 4–18.
25. FELEDER, C., H. JARRY, S. LEONHARDT, *et al.* 1996. Effects of endotoxin on in vitro release of LHRH and amino acid neurotransmitters by preoptic mediobasal hypothalamic fragments. Neuroimmunomodulation. **3:** 76–81.
26. FELEDER, C., D. REFOJO, H. JARRY, *et al.* 1996. Bacterial endotoxin inhibits LHRH secretion following the increased release of hypothalamic GABA levels. Different effects on amino acid neurotransmitter release. Neuroimmunomodulation **3:** 342–351.
27. MACCARRONE, M., L. DE PETROCELLIS, M. BARI, *et al.* 2001. Lipopolysaccharide downregulates fatty acid amide hydrolase expression and increases anandamide levels in human peripheral lymphocytes. Arch. Biochem. Biophys. **393:** 321–328.
28. LIU, J., S. BATKAI, P. PACHER, *et al.* 2003. Lipopolysaccharide induces anandamide synthesis in macrophages via CD14/MAPK/phosphoinositide 3-kinase/NF-kappaB independently of platelet-activating factor. J. Biol. Chem. **278:** 45034–45039.
29. MOLINA-HOLGADO, F., E. MOLINA-HOLGADO & C. GUAZA. 1998. The endogenous cannabinoid anandamide potentiates interleukin-6 production by astrocytes infected with Theiler's murine encephalomyelitis virus by a receptor-mediated pathway. FEBS Lett. **433:** 139–142.
30. PELLEGRINO, L.J., A.S. PELLEGRINO & A.J. ASHMAN. 1979. *In* A Stereotaxic Atlas of the Rat Brain, 2nd ed. Plenum Press. New York.
31. KLEIN, T.W., B. LANE, C.A. NEWTON & H. FRIEDMAN. 2000. The cannabinoid system and cytokine network. Proc. Soc. Exp. Biol. Med. **225:** 1–8.
32. BERDYSHEV, E.V., E. BOICHOT, N. GERMAIN, *et al.* 1997. Influence of fatty acid ethanolamides and delta9-tetrahydrocannabinol on cytokine and arachidonate release by mononuclear cells. Eur. J. Pharmacol. **330:** 231–240.
33. FACCHINETTI, F., E. DEL GIUDICE, S. FUREGATO, *et al.* 2003. Cannabinoids ablate release of TNFalpha in rat microglial cells stimulated with lypopolysaccharide. Glia **41:** 161–168.
34. LIU, J., S. BATKAI, P. PACHER, *et al.* 2003. Lipopolysaccharide induces anandamide synthesis in macrophages via CD14/MAPK/phosphoinositide 3-kinase/NF-kappaB independently of platelet-activating factor. J. Biol. Chem. **278:** 45034–45039.
35. MASTRONARDI, C.A., W.H. YU & S.M. MCCANN. 2001. Lipopolysaccharide-induced tumor necrosis factor-alpha release is controlled by the central nervous system. Neuroimmunomodulation **9:** 148–156.

36. YOO, M.J., M. NISHIHARA & M. TAKAHASHI. 1997. Tumor necrosis factor-α mediates endotoxin induced supression of gonadotropin-releasing hormone pulse generator activity in the rat. Endocr. J. **44:** 141–148.
37. SCORTICATI, C., J. FERNANDEZ-SOLARI, A. DE LAURENTIIS, *et al.* 2004. The inhibitory effect of anandamide on luteinizing hormone-releasing hormone secretion is reversed by estrogen. Proc. Natl. Acad. Sci. USA **101:** 11891–11896.
38. DANIEL, J.A., B.K. WHITLOCK, C.G. WAGNER & J.L. SARTIN. 2002. Regulation of the growth hormone and luteinizing hormone response to endotoxin in sheep. Domest. Anim. Endocrinol. **23:** 361–370.

Low-Grade Inflammation in Chronic Infectious Diseases

Paradigm of Periodontal Infections

NIKI M. MOUTSOPOULOS[a] AND PHOEBUS N. MADIANOS[b]

[a]*Oral Infection and Immunity Branch, National Institute of Dental and Craniofacial Research, National Institutes of Health, Bethesda, Maryland USA*

[b]*Department of Periodontology, School of Dentistry, University of Athens, Athens, Greece*

ABSTRACT: Increasing evidence implicates periodontitis, a chronic inflammatory disease of the tooth-supporting structures, as a potential risk factor for increased morbidity or mortality for several systemic conditions including cardiovascular disease (atherosclerosis, heart attack, and stroke), pregnancy complications (spontaneous preterm birth [SPB]), and diabetes mellitus. Cross-sectional, case–control, and cohort studies indicate that periodontitis may confer two- and up to sevenfold increase in the risk for cardiovascular disease and premature birth, respectively. Given the recently acquired knowledge that systemic inflammation may contribute in the pathogenesis of atherosclerosis and may predispose to premature birth, research in the field of periodontics has focused on the potential of this chronic low-grade inflammatory condition to contribute to the generation of a systemic inflammatory phenotype. Consistent with this hypothesis clinical studies demonstrate that periodontitis patients have elevated markers of systemic inflammation, such as C-reactive protein (CRP), interleukin 6 (IL-6), haptoglobin, and fibrinogen. These are higher in periodontal patients with acute myocardial infarction (AMI) than in patients with AMI alone, supporting the notion that periodontal disease is an independent contributor to systemic inflammation. In the case of adverse pregnancy outcomes, studies on fetal cord blood from SBP babies indicate a strong *in utero* IgM antibody response specific to several oral periodontal pathogens, which induces an inflammatory response at the fetal–placental unit, leading to prematurity. The importance of periodontal infections to systemic health is further strengthened by pilot intervention trials indicating that periodontal therapy may improve surrogate cardiovascular outcomes, such as endothelial function, and may reduce four- to fivefold the incidence of premature birth. Nevertheless, further research is needed to fully discern the underlying mechanisms

Address for correspondence: Phoebus N. Madianos, Department of Periodontology, School of Dentistry, University of Athens, Thivon 2, 115 27 Athens, Greece. Voice: +30-210-7461181; fax: +30-210-7461202.

e-mail: pmadian@dent.uoa.gr

Ann. N.Y. Acad. Sci. 1088: 251–264 (2006). © 2006 New York Academy of Sciences.

doi: 10.1196/annals.1366.032

by which local chronic infections can have an impact on systemic health, and in this endeavor periodontal disease may serve as an ideal disease model.

KEYWORDS: periodontitis; acute myocardial infarction (AMI)

INTRODUCTION

In the last decade, progress in molecular medicine has led us to reconsider the etiology and pathogenesis of numerous conditions. We have now come to understand that inflammation is a principal component in the development of systemic conditions previously thought to be of different etiology, such as atherosclerosis, diabetes, and adverse pregnancy outcomes.[1,2] In view of such findings, local chronic infectious conditions, which may contribute to a systemic "hyperinflammatory phenotype," are seen as potential contributors to the pathogenesis of distal inflammatory conditions. Given the nature of periodontal disease as a chronic infectious disease, its contribution to the development of systemic inflammation and disease has been the topic of extensive study and research.

The term *periodontal disease* has its origin from the Greek words *peri* (around) and *odous* (tooth)[3] and refers to a group of inflammatory conditions with bacterial etiology that target the supporting structures of the tooth. The periodontal structures include the cementum (a calcified structure of the tooth surface under the gum line), the connective tissue attachment between the tooth and the supporting bone, and the supporting osseous structures, all of which function to support the tooth. In periodontal disease, supporting tissues are destroyed and with time teeth become loose, often migrate, and eventually become lost (FIG.1). Together with the oral problems that may arise, the possibility of periodontal disease aggravating and/or causing systemic conditions, such as cardiovascular disease and adverse pregnancy outcomes, has recently attracted considerable attention.

In this report we will review the epidemiological and basic science data supporting the connection of periodontal disease to systemic health. For this we will discuss the pathogenesis of this local chronic inflammatory condition and its role in the development of systemic inflammation in the initiation of distant infection and/or inflammatory conditions and ultimately in the pathogenesis of systemic disease.

PATHOGENESIS OF PERIODONTAL DISEASE IN A NUTSHELL

Bacterial Etiology

Although periodontal disease is considered an infectious disease, there is no single bacterial species or group of microorganisms whose mere presence leads

(A)   **(B)**

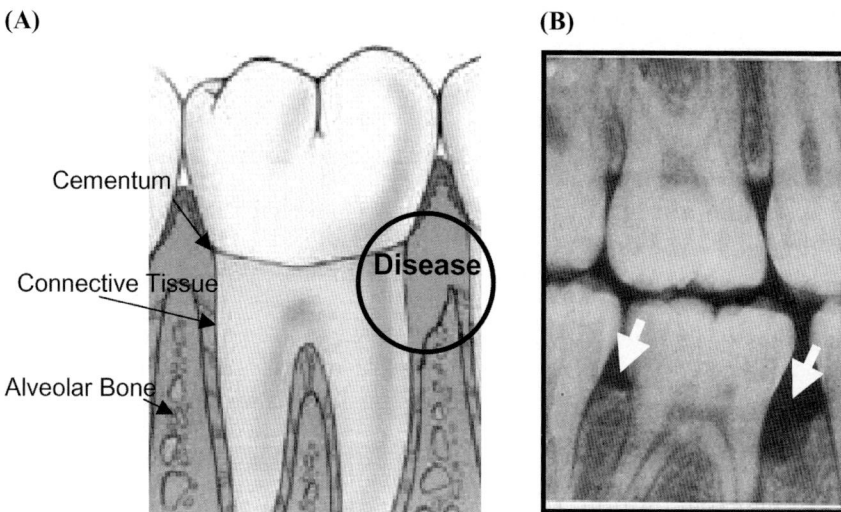

FIGURE 1. Periodontal tissues and disease destruction. (**A**) Cartoon depicts a tooth with the periodontal tissues (cementum, connective tissue, and alveolar bone) being healthy on the left side and compromised due to periodontal disease on the right side of the tooth. Tissues are labeled and *arrows* point to the corresponding areas. (**B**) Radiograph of molar teeth. Local destruction supporting alveolar bone due to periodontal disease is demonstrated by the right arrow, while bone levels are shown to be optimal by the left arrow.

to the disease, but rather a shift in the microbial ecology of the dental plaque biofilm that may account for disease progression. Dental plaque in health and in disease is a well-organized and complex multicellular ecosystem that contains over 600 different aerobic and anaerobic bacteria.[4] The composition shifts from a predominantly Gram-positive aerobic flora in health to a Gram-negative and anaerobic flora in disease. The group of bacteria that has been mostly associated with disease is referred to as the "red cluster" group and includes *Porphyromonas gingivalis, Tannerella forsythia (*formerly known as *Bacteroides forsythus),* and *Treponema denticola.*[5] Nevertheless, most of the oral organisms that are associated with disease are also present in low numbers in health, indicating that in biofilm-induced disease states, several commensal organisms appear to emerge as opportunistic pathogens to cause disease in genetically susceptible individuals.

Inflammatory Etiology

Periodontal disease is initiated by infectious agents, but disease pathogenesis and progression are immune-mediated. Histologically, periodontitis is a chronic inflammatory cell lesion, characterized by lymphocytic

(T and B cell) and monocytic infiltrate, connective tissue destruction, and bone resorption. On a molecular basis, periodontitis is mediated by increases in tissue levels of inflammatory mediators, such as interleukin-(IL-1) 1β, tumor necrosis factor-α (TNF-α), IL-6, prostaglandin E2 (PGE2), and matrix metalloproteinases (MMPs), that mediate collagen and extracellular matrix degradation and bone resorption,[6] indicating that the tissue destruction in this disease is not primarily due to infectious agents, but rather the result of a persistent but not effective inflammatory response.

The mechanisms underlying this chronic inflammation are not fully understood but are speculated to involve the deregulation of immunoregulatory pathways that are meant to "contain" inflammation after infection is cleared.[7] In periodontal disease it appears that the host overreacts to infectious stimuli by secreting increased amounts of proinflammatory cytokines, such as IL-1β, TNF-α, and IL-6, and tissue destructive mediators, such as oxygen intermediates and matrix MMPs. Hints that individual differences in cytokine secretions may contribute to periodontal susceptibility have come from data demonstrating that peripheral blood mononuclear cells from periodontitis patients secrete increased levels of proinflammatory cytokines in response to stimuli.[8] This "hyperinflammatory phenotype" has been attributed to a particular genetic background. The main focus of the studies of genetic susceptibility in periodontal disease has been the polymorphisms found in the IL-1 gene cluster, which may lead to increased cytokine production and therefore increased inflammatory destruction. A susceptible periodontitis-associated genotype (PAG) has been documented that comprises the combination of two rare alleles at separate single nucleotide polymorphisms (SNPs) in the IL-1 gene cluster (one in position −899 in the IL-1α promoter and the second at position +3954 of the IL-1β). This genotype has been correlated with the severity of chronic periodontitis, although PAG was only shown to be a significant factor in nonsmoking patients.[9] Smoking is a major risk factor for periodontal disease, estimated to be responsible for more than 50% of cases of periodontitis in the Western world[9] and appears to be a confounding periodontitis risk factor similar to the susceptible IL-1 genotype.

Together with the increased cytokine production, the persisting and at times disproportionate inflammatory response observed in periodontal disease may also be attributed to a dysfunction of mechanisms of immune resolution in this patient group. With the recent characterization of the "proresolution" lipid mediators, such as the arachidonic cascade-derived lipoxins and the omega-3-fatty acid-derived resolvins, which restrain the immune activity of phagocytes, the pathogenesis of periodontal disease, which is dominated by "uncontrolled" neutrophil-mediated destruction, may be studied under a new light. Furthermore, the observation that animal models overexpressing lipoxins are resistant to periodontal disease points to potential therapeutic potential of these compounds/pathways.[10]

LOCALIZED DISEASE WITH SYSTEMIC "SIDE EFFECTS": BACTEREMIA AND SYSTEMIC INFLAMMATION

Despite the localized nature of periodontal disease a plethora of systemic markers of this condition have been reported and speculated to contribute to systemic diseases.[11] In health, the epithelial barrier in the oral cavity together with the protective innate immune molecules inhibit oral bacteria from entering into the tissues and the bloodstream and therefore in health only small numbers of mostly facultative bacteria enter the circulation.[12] With the advent of periodontal disease it is speculated that the inflamed and ulcerated subgingival pocket epithelium forms an easy port of entry for dental plaque bacteria, many of which are Gram-negative and obligate anaerobic. Bacteremia in periodontitis has been reported after oral examination[12] and periodontal pathogens have been shown to colonize distant sites.[13] Additionally, bacterial components, such as major outer membrane proteins and endotoxins (i.e., lipopolysaccharide [LPS]), may be disseminated. Gram-negative organisms release LPS (lipopolysaccharide, endotoxin) that can trigger significant systemic inflammation. In response to the bacteremia and bacterial antigens that are systemically dispersed, white blood cells as well as tissue cells at locations where the antigens are relocated, such as endothelial cells and hepatocytes, may produce proinflammatory immune mediators. Furthermore, the locally produced proinflammatory mediators, such as IL-1β, TNF-α, IL-6, and PGE2 may "spill" into the circulation and exert systemic or distant effects. The systemic cellular and molecular markers of inflammation in periodontitis include among others an increase of the number of peripheral leukocytes and an increase in the levels of cytokines and acute-phase proteins.[14]

Peripheral Blood Leukocytes

The total number of white blood cells in the peripheral blood is a diagnostic measure of infection or inflammatory disease. In periodontitis, leukocyte counts have been shown to be slightly elevated in patients compared to healthy subjects, although not always significantly.[11] This increase in the number of leukocytes is attributed to the increase mainly of polymorphonuclear leukocytes (PMNs), which are key participants in the periodontal lesion. It has also been shown that this increase in leukocytes is aggravated by increasing severity and extent of disease, and periodontal therapy (local inflammatory control) may lead to a decrease in the number of leukocytes.[15,16]

Proinflammatory Cytokines

In health, cytokine levels in the systemic circulation are minimal and at times undetectable without the use of hypersensitive methodology. In periodontal disease, of the proinflammatory cytokines studied, levels of IL-6 have been consistently shown to increase in the periphery[11]. Furthermore, IL-6 in plasma showed a positive relation to the extent of disease. IL-6 is also a principal procoagulant cytokine and may also activate hepatocytes to produce acute-phase reactants, such as fibrinogen, plasminogen activator inhibitor 1, and CRP.

Acute-Phase Proteins

It has been long established that immune mediators originating from a site of infection or from a site of severe trauma may activate hepatocytes in the liver to produce large quantities of acute-phase proteins. The acute-phase response is characterized by fever, increased vascular permeability, and a general elevation of metabolic processes. The acute-phase reactants include C-reactive protein (CRP), serum amyloid P component, serum amyloid A protein, and alpha-1-acid glycoprotein (AGP) and possess a wide variety of functions, such as multiple proinflammatory properties and stimulation of tissue repair. It has been established in the past decade that acute-phase proteins not only appear in acute and severe disease processes, but also in longstanding, chronic conditions. For example, CRP has often been found at relatively low levels (range 0.3 to 3.0 mg/L) in subjects with chronic stomach ulcers associated with *Helicobacter pylori* and in persons with chronic lung infections. Since periodontitis is a chronic inflammatory and infectious disease, it is not surprising that CRP levels in periodontal patients have been of interest. Significantly elevated levels of CRP in periodontal patients compared to nonperiodontal controls have been shown in several studies (TABLE 1), even after adjustment of confounding factors. Levels of CRP in plasma ranged from 2–10 mg/L, consistent with the presence of a low-grade chronic inflammation. Some intervention studies have demonstrated an effect of periodontal therapy on CRP and systemic

TABLE 1. Plasma CRP levels in periodontitis patients and healthy controls

Study	Patients		Controls	
	n	Mean ± SD	n	Mean ± SD
Ebersole et al., 1997[34]	40	9.12 ± 1.61	35	2.17 ± 0.41
Fredriksson et al., 1998[35]	17	2.62 ± 2.9	38	0.87 ± 1.73
Loos et al., 2000[36]	107	2.64 ± 3.48	43	1.21 ± 1.34
Noak et al., 2001[37]	50	4.06 ± 5.55	65	1.70 ± 1.91
Glurich et al., 2002[38]	26	2.4 ± 1.89	20	1.68 ± 1.42
Craig et al., 2003[39]	44	5.78 ± 1.07	25	2.46 ± 1.44
Buhlin et al., 2003[40]	50	3.28 ± 4.64	46	1.74 ± 1.68

Adapted from Loos, 2005.[11]

cytokine levels (TABLE 2). For example, Mattila et al.[17] reported a reduction of CRP concentrations on 30 patients with chronic periodontitis; the median value at baseline was reduced from 1.05 mg/L to 0.7 mg/L after therapy and the most significant reductions were seen in patients with the highest starting CRP levels.

SYSTEMIC PERIODONTAL "SIDE EFFECTS" MAY PREDISPOSE TO CARDIOVASCULAR DISEASE

Infection is now recognized as a risk factor in the development of cardiovascular disease (CVD). The initial observations that CVD patients have higher titers of Clamydia pneumoniae[18] initiated a new way of thinking in the area of CVD pathogenesis. For oral infections, the association with CVD has been speculated to be due to the recovery of periopathogens in surgical specimens from atherosclerotic plaques. Of the atheromas studied 30% were positive by PCR for Tannerella forsythia (Bacteroides forsythus), 26% for Porphyromonas gingivalis, 18% for Actinobacillus actinomycetemcomitans, and 14% for Prevotella intermedia.[13] A pathogenic role for such bacteria in atheroma formation is also supported by the ability of oral bacteria such as Streptococcus sanguis and Porphyromonas gingivalis to induce platelet aggregation in vitro.[19]

Separate from the risks of bacteremia, the systemic inflammation induced by periodontal disease may contribute to CVD, given that inflammation plays a key role in the pathogenesis of the disease. In atherosclerotic lesions immune cells dominate, their effector molecules accelerate progression of the lesions, and activation of inflammation can elicit acute coronary syndromes. Furthermore, the markers of systemic inflammation observed in periodontal disease are known risk factors for CVD. First the levels of acute-phase proteins are associated with CVD. More than 20 prospective epidemiological studies demonstrate that slightly elevated (0.3 mg/L up to 3 mg/L) and chronically present levels of CRP (high-sensitivity CRP) are independent predictors of risk for myocardial infarction, stroke, peripheral arterial disease, and sudden cardiac death, even in apparently healthy individuals.[20] Secondly, elevated levels of IL-6 have been associated with increased risk of future myocardial infarction in healthy men.[21] Thirdly, other molecular markers elevated in periodontal disease, such as fibrinogen and the procoagulant protein von Willebrand factor,[11] may contribute to the development of thrombi.

Finally, impaired endothelial-dependent vascular dilation, an established risk factor for cardiovascular disease, is also associated with periodontal disease. A recent study[22] demonstrated significantly impaired branchial artery flow–mediated dilation in otherwise healthy, nonsmoking subjects with advanced periodontal disease compared with age-matched control subjects. The

TABLE 2. Effect of periodontal therapy on systemic inflammation

Authors	Study Type	No. of patients	Periodontal Therapy	Outcome	Conclusion
Elter et al., 2006[24]	Single masked CT	C = 22, T = 22*	nonsurgical and surgical	C: ΔCRP = 0.1mg/L; T: ΔCRP = −1mg/L; C: ΔIL-6 = −0.1 pg/L; T: ΔIL-6 = −0.6 pg/L	Therapy reduced serum IL-6 and improved endothelial function
Montebugnoli et al., 2005[41]	Single blind CT	C = 18, T = 18*	nonsurgical	C: ΔCRP = −0.01 mg/L; T: ΔCRP = −0.9 mg/L	Therapy reduced serum CRP
D'Aiuto et al., 2004[42]	Prospective CT	T = 94	nonsurgical	ΔCRP = −0.5mg/L; ΔIL-6 = −0.2 ng/L	Therapy reduced serum CRP and IL-6
Yamazaki et al., 2004[43]	Prospective CT		nonsurgical and surgical; antibiotics for 4 days after surgery	T: ΔCRP = −55.5 ng/mL	Unable to show significant decrease in CRP, IL-6 & TNF-α
Ide et al., 2003[44]	Randomized Controlled CT	C = 15, T = 24	nonsurgical	T: ΔIL-6 = −0.01 pg/mL; T: ΔTNF-α = −0.22 pg/mL; C: ΔCRP = −0.28 mg/L; C: ΔIL-1β = 0.08 pg/L; C: ΔIL-6 == −0.03 pg/L; C: ΔTNF-α = −0.19 pg/mL; T: ΔCRP = −0.14 mg/L; T: ΔIL-1β = −0.06 pg/L; T: ΔIL-6 = −0.40 pg/L; T: ΔTNF-α = −0.01 pg/L	Unable to show significant decrease in CRP, IL-1β, IL-6 & TNF-α
Iwamoto et al., 2003[45]	Prospective CT	T = 15	nonsurgical plus local antibiotic	T: ΔCRP = − 733.7 ng/mL; T: ΔTNF-α = − 0.4 pg/mL	Therapy reduced CRP and TNF-α
Mattila et al., 2002[17]	CT	T = 30	nonsurgical	T: ΔCRP = 0.35 mg/L	Therapy reduced CRP

*Test group served as control after nontreatment period.
T = therapy group; C: Control group; CT = clinical trial; ΔCRP = difference between CRP values at baseline and posttherapy; ΔIL-1β = difference between IL-1β values at baseline and posttherapy; ΔIL-6 = difference between IL-6 values at baseline and posttherapy; ΔTNF-α = difference between TNF-α values at baseline and posttherapy.

stimulation of the vascular endothelium by circulating cytokines and/or pathogens is speculated to be responsible for this "proatherogenic" phenotype. More importantly, the impaired endothelial function of patients with severe periodontitis was improved by periodontal treatment.[23,24] Periodontal treatment has been also shown to lessen other CVD risk factors, such as the levels of lipoprotein-associated phospholipase A_2 (Lp-PLA_2),[24] which hydrolyzes oxidized low-density lipoproteins (LDLs) in products with proinflammatory and proatherogenic activity.[25]

Epidemiological Data

A connection between poor oral health and atherosclerosis-induced heart disease began in the late 1980s with several case and case–control studies.[26] Stimulated by this initial association, a number of cross-sectional studies were conducted and were able to demonstrate a modest association of periodontal disease with CVD after controlling for other cardiovascular risk factors. Also, at least four studies demonstrated a positive association between periodontal disease and stroke, and one study associated periodontal disease with peripheral vascular disease.[26] In addition to the above studies linking periodontal disease with CVD outcomes, a number of studies have associated periodontal disease with CVD risk factors, such as subclinical atherosclerosis, coronary calcification, and high levels of CRP, fibrinogen, von Willebrand factor, IL-6, lipids, and endothelial function.[11,22,27] This variability in CVD outcomes from the various studies as well as the variability of periodontal disease assessments creates limitations when evaluating and comparing the data.

The highest level of existing evidence comes from longitudinal studies, given that there are no randomized controlled trials to determine the effect of periodontal disease prevention or treatment on cardiovascular events. There are now at least 16 articles published (for review see Beck and Offenbacher[28]). The results have been mixed, with 10 studies reporting positive, adjusted associations between oral status and some type of cardiovascular outcome or CRP and six studies reporting no association or nonsignificant positive trends after adjustment. The OR in the studies with significant positive results ranged from 1.2 to 3.4; however, the majority were under 2.0, indicating low-to-moderate levels of association. In fact, there has been a concern expressed about the inconsistent results among the studies reported, and there has been a great deal of discussion concerning the reasons for these differences. Some points raised have included the moderate level of the associations, lack of control for confounding, residual confounding, no measures of infection, and the wide variety of definitions used for the exposure (periodontal disease) and the outcome (cardiovascular disease).

PERIODONTAL DISEASE MAY LEAD TO ADVERSE PREGNANCY OUTCOMES

Epidemiology

The strongest data for infection-induced preterm labor exist for the association of bacterial vaginosis with premature birth.[29] For periodontal infections, the data generated thus far, from cross-sectional and prospective studies as well as from animal experiments, continue to support the hypothesis that such infections can also serve as an independent risk factor for prematurity and growth restriction. Several studies suggest a significant association between maternal periodontal disease and pregnancy complications, including premature delivery (gestational age [GA] <37 weeks), decreased fetal weight (birth weight [BW] <2,500 g), and pre-eclampsia.

The first reported human case–control study in 1996 suggested that mothers with premature, low-birth-weight babies had more severe periodontal disease than mothers with full-term deliveries and that periodontitis appeared to confer considerable risk independent of other traditional obstetric risk factors.[30] However, this investigation was a relatively small study of 124 cases and this case–control design did not permit the establishment of temporality of exposure (periodontal disease) as it relates to the outcome (preterm birth). Nonetheless, the potential magnitude of the effect of periodontal disease was surprisingly large (adjusted odds ratio [OR] 6.7, $P = 0.003$) and provided impetus for further study, prompting the conduct of cross-sectional studies to confirm this association and prospective studies to appropriately measure attributable risk. A prospective study of 1,313 mothers, conducted at the University of Alabama,[31] reported that antenatal maternal periodontitis is an independent risk factor for preterm birth and low birth weight. These investigators report that severe periodontal disease is associated with an OR = 5.2 (2.05–13.6) for preterm birth (GA<37) and OR = 7.07 (1.7–27.4) for very preterm (VPT, GA<32) deliveries, adjusting for age, race smoking, and parity. However, both studies show a biologic gradient effect in that more severe periodontal disease is associated with stronger risk for earlier-gestational-age deliveries.

Possible Mechanisms

The proposed pathogenesis of infection-induced preterm labor is the ascent of microorganisms from the cervix or vagina, with subsequent colonization of fetal membranes and decidua. Once the organisms colonize the deciduas and fetal membranes and/or invade the amniotic sac, they release LPS or other toxins. The molecular pathways eliciting this microbial effect on pregnancy have been suggested to involve microbial LPS and TLR-mediated (toll-like receptor) pathways, resulting in the release of primary inflammatory mediators,

(A)   **(B)**

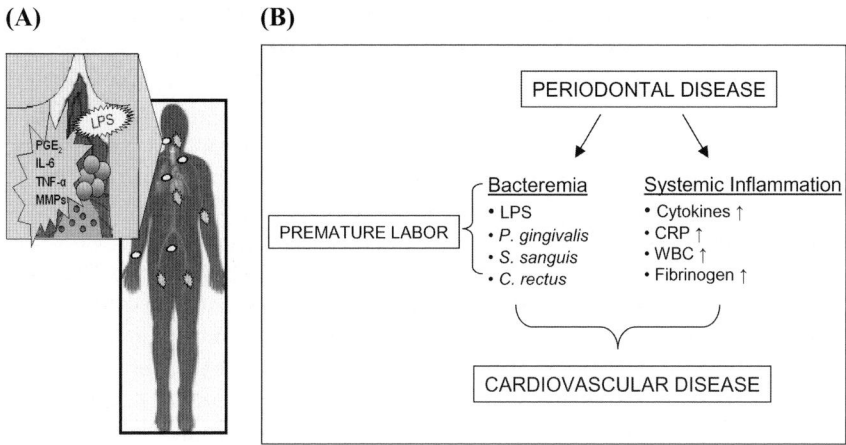

FIGURE 2. Systemic effects of periodontal disease. (**A**) Cartoon illustrates that inflammatory mediators, such as PGE2, IL-6, TNF-α, and MMP as well as infectious components, such as bacteria and LPS, present in the periodontal pocket may enter the circulation and reach distant sites. (**B**) Conceptual diagram illustrating possible mechanisms through which periodontal disease may lead to systemic disease.

such as IL-1, IL-6, TNF-α, and secondarily PGE2 (prostaglandin E2), which is capable of inducing uterine contraction and modulating placental blood flow, and in humans can mediate cervical thinning, dilation, and premature labor.[2] Inflammation of the chorioamniotic membranes can also result in MMP secretion, the breakdown of the collagenous matrix, and mechanical weakening, enhancing the likelihood of premature rupture. However, inflammatory stimuli that predispose to premature rupture of membranes and preterm labor may also have effects on the neonatal environment. Infectious exposure to the mother during pregnancy is currently believed to be a significant factor that triggers the *in utero* fetal stress that ultimately contributes to long-term growth and developmental problems. The fetal response to periodontal infections has been documented by the assessment of fetal IgM levels for 15 periodontal pathogens at birth by means of cord blood.[32] The increased prevalence of IgM seropositivity (2.9-fold increase) for one or more periopathogens in preterm versus full-term neonates demonstrates the relation of periodontal infections to prematurity. Specifically, the prevalence of positive fetal IgM to *C. rectus* and to *P. intermedia* was significantly higher for preterm neonates (20% vs. 6.3%, $P = 0.0002$ and 8.8% vs. 1.1%, $P = 0.0003$, respectively). The highest rate of prematurity was observed among those mothers without a protective IgG response, which may be capable of arresting the systemic microbial dissemination. The rate of prematurity was also higher in cases where a positive fetal IgM was coupled with a fetal inflammatory response shown by detectable CRP, or high 8-isoprostane, PGE2, or TNF-α.[33]

LOW-GRADE INFLAMMATION IN CHRONIC INFECTIOUS DISEASES AND THE PARADIGM OF PERIODONTAL INFECTIONS

We conclude that periodontal disease is a chronic infectious disease in which a persistent local inflammation is responsible for the disease pathogenesis and outcome (i.e., tissue destruction). More importantly in this disease, the systemic dissemination of infectious agents and inflammatory mediators from the oral environment may cause an elevated systemic inflammatory condition, which may contribute to the pathogenesis of distal inflammatory processes, such as the pathogenesis of CVD and the initiation of premature labor (FIG. 2). Nevertheless, the exact mechanisms through which local inflammatory conditions may contribute to systemic inflammation are not fully understood. Furthermore, the possibility of a "common genetic background" predisposing to various inflammatory conditions ("hyperinflammatory phenotype") is also a viable possibility. In this quest to understand immune-mediated disorders and their contribution/effect to systemic health, periodontal disease may serve as a uniquely appropriate model. The large prevalence of the disease, the accessibility of the oral environment for study and the presence of evidence linking this disease to systemic health all point to the fact that the paradigm of periodontal diseases may be viewed as a valuable tool for biomedical research.

REFERENCES

1. HANSSON, G.K. 2005. Inflammation, atherosclerosis, and coronary artery disease. N. Engl. J. Med. **352:** 1685–1695.
2. OFFENBACHER, S. 2004. Maternal periodontal infections, prematurity, and growth restriction. Clin. Obstet. Gynecol. **47:** 808–821; discussion, 881–882.
3. ARMITAGE, G.C. 2000. Development of a classification system for periodontal diseases and conditions. Northwest Dent. **79:** 31–35.
4. SOCRANSKY, S.S. & A.D. HAFFAJEE. 2002. Dental biofilms: difficult therapeutic targets. Periodontology 2000. **28:** 12–55.
5. SOCRANSKY, S.S. *et al.* 1998. Microbial complexes in subgingival plaque. J. Clin. Periodontol. **25:** 134–144.
6. KOLENBRANDER, P.E. 2000. Oral microbial communities: biofilms, interactions, and genetic systems. Annu. Rev. Microbiol. **54:** 413–437.
7. YAMAZAKI, K., H. YOSHIE & G.J. SEYMOUR. 2003. T cell regulation of the immune response to infection in periodontal diseases. Histol. Histopathol. **18:** 889–896.
8. SHAPIRA, L. *et al.* 1994. The secretion of PGE2, IL-1 beta, IL-6, and TNF alpha by adherent mononuclear cells from early onset periodontitis patients. J. Periodontol. **65:** 139–146.
9. TAYLOR, J.J., P.M. PRESHAW & P.T. DONALDSON. 2004. Cytokine gene polymorphism and immunoregulation in periodontal disease. Periodontology 2000 **35:** 158–182.

10. VAN DYKE, T.E. & C.N. SERHAN. 2003. Resolution of inflammation: a new paradigm for the pathogenesis of periodontal diseases. J. Dent. Res. **82:** 82–90.

11. LOOS, B.G. 2005. Systemic markers of inflammation in periodontitis. J. Periodontol. **76:** 2106–2115.

12. LI, X. *et al.* 2000. Systemic diseases caused by oral infection. Clin. Microbiol. Rev. **13:** 547–558.

13. HARASZTHY, V.I. *et al.* 2000. Identification of periodontal pathogens in atheromatous plaques. J. Periodontol. **71:** 1554–1560.

14. DANESH, J. *et al.* 1998. Association of fibrinogen, C-reactive protein, albumin, or leukocyte count with coronary heart disease: meta-analyses of prospective studies. JAMA **279:** 1477–1482.

15. CHRISTAN, C. *et al.* 2002. White blood cell count in generalized aggressive periodontitis after non-surgical therapy. J. Clin. Periodontol. **29:** 201–206.

16. FOKKEMA, S.J. *et al.* 2003. Increased release of IL-12p70 by monocytes after periodontal therapy. J. Clin. Periodontol. **30:** 1091–1096.

17. MATTILA, K. *et al.* 2002. Effect of treating periodontitis on C-reactive protein levels: a pilot study. BMC Infect. Dis. **10:** 30–33.

18. SAIKKU, P. *et al.* 1988. Serological evidence of an association of a novel *Chlamydia*, TWAR, with chronic coronary heart disease and acute myocardial infarction. Lancet **2:** 983–986.

19. HERZBERG, M.C. & M.W. WEYER. 1998. Dental plaque, platelets, and cardiovascular diseases. Ann. Periodontol. **3:** 151–160.

20. TORRES, J.L. & P.M. RIDKER. 2003. High sensitivity C-reactive protein in clinical practice. Am. Heart Hosp. J. **1:** 207–211.

21. KOH, K.K., S.H. HAN & M.J. QUON. 2005. Inflammatory markers and the metabolic syndrome: insights from therapeutic interventions. J. Am. Coll. Cardiol. **46:** 1978–1985.

22. AMAR, S. *et al.* 2003. Periodontal disease is associated with brachial artery endothelial dysfunction and systemic inflammation. Arterioscler. Thromb. Vasc. Biol. **23:** 1245–1249.

23. SEINOST, G. *et al.* 2005. Periodontal treatment improves endothelial dysfunction in patients with severe periodontitis. Am. Heart J. **149:** 1050–1054.

24. ELTER, J.E. *et al.* 2006. The effects of periodontal therapy on vascular endothelial function: a pilot trial. Am. Heart J. **151:** 47e1–47e6.

25. LOSCHE, W. *et al.* 2005. Lipoprotein-associated phospholipase A2 and plasma lipids in patients with destructive periodontal disease. J. Clin. Periodontol. **32:** 640–644.

26. SCANNAPIECO, F.A., R.B. BUSH & S. PAJU. 2003. Associations between periodontal disease and risk for atherosclerosis, cardiovascular disease, and stroke. A systematic review. Ann. Periodontol. **8:** 38–53.

27. BECK, J.D. *et al.* 2001. Relationship of periodontal disease to carotid artery intima-media wall thickness: the atherosclerosis risk in communities (ARIC) study. Arterioscler. Thromb. Vasc. Biol. **21:** 1816–1822.

28. BECK, J.D. & S. OFFENBACHER. 2005. Systemic effects of periodontitis: epidemiology of periodontal disease and cardiovascular disease. J. Periodontol. **76**(Suppl 11): 2089–2100.

29. HILLIER, S.L. *et al.* 1995. Association between bacterial vaginosis and preterm delivery of a low-birth-weight infant. The Vaginal Infections and Prematurity Study Group. N. Engl. J. Med. **333:** 1737–1742.

30. OFFENBACHER, S. *et al.* 1996. Periodontal infection as a possible risk factor for preterm low birth weight. J. Periodontol. **67:** 1103–1113.
31. JEFFCOAT, M.K. *et al.* 2003. Periodontal disease and preterm birth: results of a pilot intervention study. J. Periodontol. **74:** 1214–1218.
32. MADIANOS, P.N. *et al.* 2001. Maternal periodontitis and prematurity. Part II: maternal infection and fetal exposure. Ann. Periodontol. **6:** 175–182.
33. BOGGESS, K.A. *et al.* 2005. Fetal immune response to oral pathogens and risk of preterm birth. Am. J. Obstet. Gynecol. **193:** 1121–1126.
34. EBERSOLE, J.L. *et al.* 1997. Systemic acute-phase reactants, C-reactive protein and haptoglobin, in adult periodontitis. Clin. Exp. Immunol. **107:** 347–352.
35. FREDRIKSSON, M.I. *et al.* 1999. Effect of periodontitis and smoking on blood leukocytes and acute-phase proteins. J. Periodontol. **70:** 1355–1360.
36. LOOS, B.G. *et al.* 2000. Elevation of systemic markers related to cardiovascular diseases in the peripheral blood of periodontitis patients. J. Periodontol. **71:** 1528–1534.
37. NOACK, B. *et al.* 2001. Periodontal infections contribute to elevated systemic C-reactive protein level. J. Periodontol. **72:** 1221–1227.
38. GLURICH, I. *et al.* 2002. Systemic inflammation in cardiovascular and periodontal disease: comparative study. Clin. Diagn. Lab. Immunol. **9:** 425–432.
39. CRAIG, R.G. *et al.* 2003. Relationship of destructive periodontal disease to the acute-phase response. J. Periodontol. **74:** 1007–1016.
40. BUHLIN, K. *et al.* 2003. Risk factors for cardiovascular disease in patients with periodontitis. Eur. Heart J. **24:** 2099–2107.
41. MONTEBUGNOLI, L. *et al.* 2005. Periodontal health improves systemic inflammatory and haemostatic status in subjects with coronary heart disease. J. Clin. Periodontol. **32:** 188–192.
42. D'AIUTO, F. *et al.* 2004. Periodontitis and systemic inflammation: control of the local infection is associated with a reduction in serum inflammatory markers. J. Dent. Res. **83:** 156–160.
43. YAMAZAKI, K. *et al.* 2005. Effect of periodontal treatment on the C-reactive protein and proinflammatory cytokine levels in Japanese periodontitis patients. J. Periodontal Res. **40:** 53–58.
44. IDE, M. *et al.* 2003. Effect of treatment of chronic periodontitis on levels of serum markers of acute-phase inflammatory and vascular responses. J. Clin. Periodontol. **30:** 334–340.
45. IWAMOTO, Y. *et al.* 2003. Antimicrobial treatment decreases serum C–reactive protein, tumor necrosis factor-alpha, but not adoponectin levels in patients with chronic periodontitis. J. Periodontol. **74:** 1231–1236.

Local Amplification of Glucocorticoids by 11β-Hydroxysteroid Dehydrogenase Type 1 and Its Role in the Inflammatory Response

KAREN E. CHAPMAN,[a] AGNES COUTINHO,[a,b] MOHINI GRAY,[b]
JAMES S. GILMOUR,[a] JOHN S. SAVILL,[b] AND JONATHAN R. SECKL[a]

[a]*Endocrinology Unit, Centre for Cardiovascular Sciences, The Queen's Medical Research Institute, University of Edinburgh, 47 Little France Crescent, Edinburgh, EH16 4TJ, UK*

[b]*MRC Centre for Inflammation Research, The Queen's Medical Research Institute, University of Edinburgh, 47 Little France Crescent, Edinburgh, EH16 4TJ, UK*

ABSTRACT: Glucocorticoids are widely used to treat chronic inflammatory conditions including rheumatoid arthritis. They promote mechanisms important for normal resolution of inflammation, notably macrophage phagocytosis of leukocytes undergoing apoptosis. Prereceptor metabolism of glucocorticoids by 11β-hydroxysteroid dehydrogenase type 1 (11β-HSD1) amplifies intracellular levels of glucocorticoids by oxoreduction of intrinsically inert cortisone (in humans, 11-dehydrocorticosterone in mice) into active cortisol (corticosterone in mice) within cells expressing the enzyme. Recently, we have shown in a mouse model of acute inflammation, high expression of 11β-HSD oxoreductase but not dehydrogenase activity in cells elicited rapidly in the peritoneum by a single thioglycollate injection. 11β-HSD oxoreductase activity remained high in peritoneal cells until the inflammation resolved. *In vitro*, the 11β-HSD1 substrate, 11-dehydrocorticosterone, increased macrophage phagocytosis of apoptotic neutrophils to the same extent as corticosterone. This effect was dependent upon 11β-HSD1: these cells solely expressed the type 1 11β-HSD isozyme (not 11β-HSD2), and carbenoxolone, an 11β-HSD inhibitor, prevented the increase in phagocytosis elicited by 11-dehydrocorticosterone. Macrophages from 11β-HSD1-deficient mice failed to respond to 11-dehydrocorticosterone. *In vivo*, 11β-HSD1-deficient mice showed a delay in acquisition of macrophage phagocytic competence and had an increased number of free apoptotic neutrophils during sterile peritonitis. Importantly, in preliminary experiments, 11β-HSD1-deficient mice exhibited delayed resolution of

Address for correspondence: Karen E. Chapman, Endocrinology Unit, Centre for Cardiovascular Sciences, The Queen's Medical Research Institute, University of Edinburgh, 47 Little France Crescent, Edinburgh, EH16 4TJ, UK. Voice: 44-131-242-6736; fax: 44-131-242-6779.
e-mail: Karen.Chapman@ed.ac.uk

Ann. N.Y. Acad. Sci. 1088: 265–273 (2006). © 2006 New York Academy of Sciences.
doi: 10.1196/annals.1366.030

inflammation in experimental arthritis. These findings suggest 11β-HSD1 may be a component of mechanisms engaged early during the inflammatory response that promote its subsequent resolution.

KEYWORDS: glucocorticoid; 11β-hydroxysteroid dehydrogenase; macrophage; inflammation; arthritis

THE INFLAMMATORY RESPONSE

The acute inflammatory response, part of the innate immune system, is a beneficial defense mechanism that, upon injury, protects against invading pathogens and repairs damaged tissue. Following injury, the release of proinflammatory mediators (e.g., tumor necrosis factor-α; TNF-α) causes migration of leukocytes into damaged tissues. The first cells attracted are chiefly activated neutrophil granulocytes, phagocytic cells, which control initial infection, followed by monocytes maturing into macrophages. At the inflamed site, neutrophils undergo constitutive apoptosis, functionally isolating them from the inflammatory environment, while at the same time facilitating safe removal of their potentially histotoxic contents by macrophage phagocytosis.[1] Unlike phagocytosis of necrotic cells or invading pathogens, macrophage ingestion of apoptotic cells does not evoke a proinflammatory response.[2,3] Rather, the opposite—active anti-inflammatory and immunosuppressive responses are elicited in macrophages following phagocytosis of apoptotic cells.[4] Normally, acute inflammation rapidly resolves. However, failure to rapidly phagocytose apoptotic neutrophils allows them to undergo secondary necrosis, provoking macrophage release of proinflammatory mediators and prolonging the inflammatory response.[5,6] The sustained presence and accumulation of activated macrophages causes much of the tissue damage seen in prolonged or chronic inflammation. It is therefore crucial that mechanisms are engaged early in acute inflammation to promote the effective phagocytosis of apoptotic leukocytes to rapidly and safely resolve the response and avoid the damaging consequences of persistent inflammation.

GLUCOCORTICOIDS PROMOTE RESOLUTION OF INFLAMMATION

Glucocorticoids are potent immunomodulatory agents.[7] Endogenous glucocorticoids (predominantly cortisol in humans, corticosterone in rodents) are essential to survive the potentially lethal effects of the proinflammatory cytokines, interleukin 1 (IL-1), and TNF-α.[8] Interindividual variation in hypothalamic-pituitary-adrenal (HPA) axis activity, due to early life environmental "programming" or underlying genetic variability, profoundly influences susceptibility to inflammatory and autoimmune disease.[9-12]

Pharmacologically, glucocorticoids exert powerful immunosuppressive and anti-inflammatory effects. However, long-term glucocorticoid therapy is limited by the adverse metabolic side effects of glucocorticoids, including increased risk of cardiovascular disease,[13] insulin resistance, hypertension, and atherosclerosis, the latter in particular now considered to have a major inflammatory component.[14] Thus, under some circumstances, glucocorticoids may *exacerbate* certain "proinflammatory" disorders. Conversely, glucocorticoids are of clear and proven anti-inflammatory benefit and, since the late 1940s, have been used to treat chronic inflammatory diseases, including rheumatoid arthritis, allergy, and asthma. Clearly, the actions of glucocorticoids in regulating the immune response are complex and, importantly, their effects depend upon context—for example, in human peripheral blood mononuclear cells, glucocorticoids regulate some genes in opposite directions, depending on the activation state of the cells.[15]

Glucocorticoids both suppress the initiation of the inflammatory response and promote its subsequent resolution. The effects of glucocorticoids upon initial events are relatively well understood—they alter leukocyte distribution, reprogram cellular differentiation and regulate transcription of numerous genes in monocytes/macrophages and in granulocytes.[7,16] Many of the early suppressive effects of glucocorticoids are mediated through antagonizing the activity of the proinflammatory transcription factor, NF-κB (reviewed in Ref. 17). Less well understood are the mechanisms by which glucocorticoids promote the resolution of inflammation. Blood monocytes lack phagocytic capacity, which is acquired following differentiation into macrophages.[18] Recent work has shown that glucocorticoids reprogram monocyte differentiation into a highly phagocytic "anti-inflammatory" macrophage phenotype,[19,20] increase the capacity of individual macrophages to ingest multiple apoptotic cells,[21] and modify granulocyte apoptosis, accelerating eosinophil apoptosis while delaying neutrophil apoptosis.[22] All of these proresolution effects of glucocorticoids upon inflammation are dependent upon glucocorticoid receptor[19,21,22] and are modulated by the local (cytokine) environment.[20,23] As well as receptor density, cellular glucocorticoid action is also dependent upon intracellular availability of steroid ligand, the latter determined, in large part, by local activity of the 11β-hydroxysteroid dehydrogenase (11β-HSD) enzymes.

THE 11β-HYDROXYSTEROID DEHYDROGENASES MODULATE GLUCOCORTICOID ACTION

The 11β-HSDs interconvert active glucocorticoids (cortisol, corticosterone) and their inert 11-keto forms (cortisone, 11-dehydrocorticosterone), thereby regulating intracellular access of glucocorticoid ligand to receptors.[24] Type 2 11β-HSD (11β-HSD2) acts as a dehydrogenase *in vivo* and plays a well-defined role in mineralocorticoid target tissues, protecting mineralocorticoid receptor from inappropriate occupation by glucocorticoids,[25] and, in placenta, protecting the fetus from maternal glucocorticoids.[26] In contrast, the function of the type 1 enzyme, 11β-HSD1, has, until recently, been elusive. In most intact cells, including most primary cells examined to date, the reaction direction of 11β-HSD1 is predominantly oxoreductase (reviewed in Ref. 24), thereby regenerating active glucocorticoids within cells from the circulating pool of intrinsically inert substrate. Recent evidence has shown that the predominant oxoreductase direction of 11β-HSD1 is conferred by its co-localization and functional coupling, within the lumen of the endoplasmic reticulum, with hexose-6-phosphate dehydrogenase, which provides 11β-HSD1 with reduced NADP(H) cofactor, driving its reaction direction.[27–29] Hexose-6-phosphate dehydrogenase catalyses the first two steps of the pentose phosphate pathway and may link the activity of 11β-HSD1 to metabolic status.

Mice with a targeted disruption of the gene encoding 11β-HSD1 have been crucial in elucidating the *in vivo* relevance of this glucocorticoid-amplifying enzyme. Although circulating levels of corticosterone are maintained in these mice, they cannot reduce 11-dehydrocorticosterone to corticosterone.[30] When fasted, 11β-HSD1-deficient mice show attenuated induction of hepatic gluconeogenic enzymes,[30] consistent with blunted glucocorticoid action and suggesting that 11β-HSD1 provides a critical "boost" to glucocorticoid action following stressful stimuli. However, 11β-HSD1-deficient mice are also protected from age-associated cognitive decline[31] and from the adverse metabolic effects of glucocorticoids. They resist hyperglycemia provoked by obesity or stress[30] and show improved adipose tissue insulin sensitivity.[32] Furthermore, compared to wild-type mice fed a high-fat diet, 11β-HSD1-deficient mice gain less weight, with less lipid stored in the visceral adipose depots that, in humans, are associated with increased risk of cardiovascular disease.[32] Conversely, mice, which moderately overexpress 11β-HSD1 in adipocytes (to a similar degree to that occurring in adipose tissue of obese humans[33]), develop metabolic disease, including hypertension, central obesity, and insulin resistance.[34,35] These and other studies have focused attention on 11β-HSD1 inhibition as a potential therapy for obesity-associated metabolic and cardiovascular disease.[36,37] Several recent studies in mice using selective 11β-HSD1 inhibitors have shown considerable promise in this respect. Inhibition of 11β-HSD1 lowered blood glucose levels and improved hepatic insulin sensitivity in hyperglycemic mice.[38–40] In a mouse model of atherogenesis, inhibition of 11β-HSD1 dramatically slowed plaque progression,[40] suggesting that in this context, as with other metabolic disease, that excessive glucocorticoid action (here mediated by 11β-HSD1) contributes to the pathogenesis of cardiometabolic disease. Nevertheless, it is unclear from these experiments whether the effects of 11β-HSD1 inhibition are attributable to inhibition of the enzyme in adipose tissue and liver, associated with the documented "cardioprotective" metabolic phenotype of these mice, and/or to inhibition of activity in aortic smooth muscle or immune cells.[40] This raises the obvious question as to whether there is a role for 11β-HSD1 in the immune system, and particularly the inflammatory response, where glucocorticoids are of proven benefit. Indeed, the 1950 Nobel Prize was awarded to Philip Hench, Tadeus Reichstein, and Edward Kendall for their discovery of cortisone and its use as a treatment for rheumatoid arthritis. Of course, the intrinsically inert cortisone has to be converted to cortisol by 11β-HSD1 in order to be active.

11β-HSD1 AND THE INFLAMMATORY RESPONSE

11β-HSD1 is expressed in some, but not all, immune cells including lymphocytes[41] as well as some cells of the myeloid lineage. The level of 11β-HSD1 expression is negligible in human blood monocytes,[42,43] but is markedly induced with differentiation into dendritic cells[43] or macrophages.[42] Similarly, 11β-HSD1 is induced in the human myelomonocyte cell lines U937 and THP-1 following differentiation into macrophages.[42,44] In each case, levels of 11β-HSD1 are highly dependent upon cellular differentiation status and modulated by the cytokine environment. Thus, 11β-HSD1 expression in human monocytes is induced by the "type 2" response cytokines IL-4 and IL-13, an effect abrogated by proinflammatory IFN-γ.[42] Expression of 11β-HSD1 is maintained in immature human dendritic cells activated by proinflammatory mediators, including TNF-α or bacterial lipopolysaccharide (innate immune activating signals), whereas it is reduced following maturation by CD40 ligation (an adaptive immune activating signal).[43] Interestingly, 11β-HSD1 is not induced by proinflammatory stimuli (bacterial lipopolysaccharide, TNF-α, IL-1β) in monocytes,[42] nor regulated by bacterial lipopolysaccharide in mouse-resident peritoneal macrophages.[45] However, in a variety of cell types (notably nonimmune cells), 11β-HSD1 expression is rapidly and potently increased by TNF-α and IL-1.[46–52] Furthermore, 11β-HSD2, which inactivates glucocorticoids (albeit with a limited tissue distribution), is downregulated by the same proinflammatory mediators,[52,53] suggesting local (intracellular) regulation of glucocorticoid activity by reciprocal control of 11β-HSD isozyme expression operating in a cell-specific fashion.

We have recently shown expression of 11β-HSD1, but not 11β-HSD2, in mouse macrophages.[45] Furthermore, following an acute *in vivo* inflammatory stimulus—a single injection of thioglycollate—11β-HSD1 activity rapidly increases in cells elicited in the peritoneum, remaining high in peritoneal cells until the inflammation resolves.[45] The potential importance of this activity was shown *in vitro* where the 11β-HSD1 substrate, 11-dehydrocorticosterone, was equipotent with the active glucocorticoid, corticosterone, in promoting macrophage phagocytosis of apoptotic neutrophils. The effect of 11-dehydrocorticosterone was blocked by carbenoxolone, an inhibitor of 11β-HSD, and macrophages from 11β-HSD1-deficient mice fail to respond to 11-dehydrocorticosterone,[45] confirming the effect is due to 11β-HSD1-mediated glucocorticoid reactivation. *In vivo*, during sterile peritonitis, mice deficient in 11β-HSD1 show delayed acquisition of phagocytic competence compared to normal controls, with more free apoptotic neutrophils 2 days following injection with thioglycollate.[45] Nevertheless, the acute inflammation appears to resolve at similar times in 11β-HSD1-deficient and control mice.[45] More recently, in preliminary data obtained in a mouse model of self-resolving experimental arthritis, 11β-HSD1-deficient mice consistently show a greater degree of inflammation (redness and swelling) than control mice during the resolution phase of the model (unpublished data), during which time there is ample availability of circulating 11-dehydrocorticosterone, the substrate for 11β-HSD1. Intriguingly, recent data in humans showed that synovial inflammation (increased cellularity) in rheumatoid arthritis, but not osteoarthritis, is positively associated with cortisone reactivation, suggesting increased synovial 11β-HSD1 activity.[54] TNF-α plays a central role in the pathology of rheumatoid arthritis (reviewed in Ref. 55) and may be a key factor in the requirement for 11β-HSD1 activity for efficient resolution of arthritis-associated inflammation.

In the future, it will be important to elucidate the mechanisms underlying the involvement of 11β-HSD1 in rheumatoid arthritis compared to osteoarthritis in order to better manage these debilitating conditions. Teasing apart the role and regulation of 11β-HSD1 in these and other processes will be of prime importance in tailoring steroid therapy to the differential management of "classical" inflammatory disease and that associated with metabolic disease. Manipulation of cell-specific 11β-HSD1 activity and/or expression may provide a route to harness the beneficial anti-inflammatory actions of glucocorticoids while minimizing their adverse metabolic and cardiovascular side effects. Perhaps we are now in a position to reexamine the benefits, originally observed in the 1940s, of cortisone in the treatment of arthritis and other inflammatory conditions, in the light of our current understanding of the role of its tissue- and cell-specific reactivation by 11β-HSD1.

REFERENCES

1. SAVILL, J. *et al.* 2002. A blast from the past: clearance of apoptotic cells regulates immune responses. Nat. Rev. Immunol. **2:** 965–975.
2. MEAGHER, L.C. *et al.* 1992. Phagocytosis of apoptotic neutrophils does not induce macrophage release of thromboxane B2. J. Leukoc. Biol. **52:** 269–273.
3. FADOK, V.A. *et al.* 1998. Macrophages that have ingested apoptotic cells *in vitro* inhibit proinflammatory cytokine production through autocrine/paracrine mechanisms involving TGF-β, PGE2, and PAF. J. Clin. Invest. **101:** 890–898.
4. VOLL, R.E. *et al.* 1997. Immunosuppressive effects of apoptotic cells. Nature **390:** 350–351.

5. BOTTO, M. *et al.* 1998. Homozygous C1q deficiency causes glomerulonephritis associated with multiple apoptotic bodies. Nat. Genet. **19:** 56–59.
6. TAYLOR, P.R. *et al.* 2000. A hierarchical role for classical pathway complement proteins in the clearance of apoptotic cells *in vivo*. J. Exp. Med. **192:** 359–366.
7. MCEWEN, B.S. *et al.* 1997. The role of adrenocorticoids as modulators of immune function in health and disease: neural, endocrine and immune interactions. Brain Res. Rev. **23:** 79–133.
8. BERTINI, R., M. BIANCHI & P. GHEZZI. 1988. Adrenalectomy sensitizes mice to the lethal effects of interleukin-1 and tumor necrosis factor. J. Exp. Med. **167:** 1708–1712.
9. STERNBERG, E.M. 2001. Neuroendocrine regulation of autoimmune/inflammatory disease. J. Endocrinol. **169:** 429–435.
10. STERNBERG, E.M. *et al.* 1992. The stress response and the regulation of inflammatory disease. Ann. Intern. Med. **117:** 854–866.
11. MASON, D. 1991. Genetic variation in the stress response: susceptibility to experimental allergic encephalomyelitis and implications for human inflammatory disease. Immunol. Today **12:** 57–60.
12. SHANKS, N. *et al.* 2000. Early-life exposure to endotoxin alters hypothalamic-pituitary-adrenal function and predisposition to inflammation. Proc. Natl. Acad. Sci. USA **97:** 5645–5650.
13. WEI, L., T.M. MACDONALD & B.R. WALKER. 2004. Taking glucocorticoids by prescription is associated with subsequent cardiovascular disease. Ann. Intern. Med. **141:** 764–770.
14. ROSS, R. 1999. Atherosclerosis—an inflammatory disease. N. Engl. J. Med. **340:** 115–126.
15. GALON, J. *et al.* 2002. Gene profiling reveals unknown enhancing and suppressive actions of glucocorticoids on immune cells. FASEB J. **16:** 61–71.
16. YEAGER, M.P., P.M. GUYRE & A.U. MUNCK. 2004. Glucocorticoid regulation of the inflammatory response to injury. Acta Anaesthesiol. Scand. **48:** 799–813.
17. MCKAY, L.I. & J.A. CIDLOWSKI. 1999. Molecular control of immune/inflammatory responses: Interactions between NF-κB and steroid receptor-signaling pathways. Endocr. Rev. **20:** 435–459.
18. SAVILL, J.S. *et al.* 1989. Macrophage phagocytosis of aging neutrophils in inflammation. Programmed cell death in the neutrophil leads to its recognition by macrophages. J. Clin. Invest. **83:** 865–875.
19. GILES, K.M. *et al.* 2001. Glucocorticoid augmentation of macrophage capacity for phagocytosis of apoptotic cells is associated with reduced p130Cas expression, loss of paxillin/pyk2 phosphorylation, and high levels of active Rac. J. Immunol. **167:** 976–986.
20. HEASMAN, S.J. *et al.* 2003. Glucocorticoid-mediated regulation of granulocyte apoptosis and macrophage phagocytosis of apoptotic cells: implications for the resolution of inflammation. J. Endocrinol. **178:** 29–36.
21. LIU, Y.Q. *et al.* 1999. Glucocorticoids promote nonphlogistic phagocytosis of apoptotic leukocytes. J. Immunol. **162:** 3639–3646.
22. MEAGHER, L.C. *et al.* 1996. Opposing effects of glucocorticoids on the rate of apoptosis in neutrophilic and eosinophilic granulocytes. J. Immunol. **156:** 4422–4428.
23. HEASMAN, S.J. *et al.* 2004. Interferon-γ suppresses glucocorticoid augmentation of macrophage clearance of apoptotic cells. Eur. J. Immunol. **34:** 1752–1761.

24. SECKL, J.R. 2004. 11 β-hydroxysteroid dehydrogenases: changing glucocorticoid action. Curr. Opin. Pharmacol. **4:** 597–602.
25. EDWARDS, C.R. 1991. Lessons from licorice. N. Engl. J. Med. **325:** 1242–1243.
26. BENEDIKTSSON, R. *et al.* 1993. Glucocorticoid exposure in utero: a new model for adult hypertension. Lancet **341:** 339–341.
27. ATANASOV, A.G. *et al.* 2004. Hexose-6-phosphate dehydrogenase determines the reaction direction of 11 β-hydroxysteroid dehydrogenase type 1 as an oxoreductase. FEBS Lett. **571:** 129–133.
28. BUJALSKA, I.J. *et al.* 2005. Hexose-6-phosphate dehydrogenase confers oxoreductase activity upon 11 β-hydroxysteroid dehydrogenase type 1. J. Mol. Endocrinol. **34:** 675–684.
29. LAVERY, G.G. *et al.* 2006. Hexose-6-phosphate dehydrogenase knock-out mice lack 11 β-hydroxysteroid dehydrogenase type 1-mediated glucocorticoid generation. J. Biol. Chem. **281:** 6546–6551.
30. KOTELEVTSEV, Y. *et al.* 1997. 11β-hydroxysteroid dehydrogenase type 1 knockout mice show attenuated glucocorticoid inducible responses and resist hyperglycemia on obesity or stress. Proc. Natl. Acad. Sci. USA **94:** 14924–14929.
31. YAU, J.L. *et al.* 2001. Lack of tissue glucocorticoid reactivation in 11 β-hydroxysteroid dehydrogenase type 1 knockout mice ameliorates age-related learning impairments. Proc. Natl. Acad. Sci. USA **98:** 4716–4721.
32. MORTON, N.M. *et al.* 2004. Novel adipose tissue-mediated resistance to diet-induced visceral obesity in 11 β-hydroxysteroid dehydrogenase type 1-deficient mice. Diabetes **53:** 931–938.
33. RASK, E. *et al.* 2001. Tissue-specific dysregulation of cortisol metabolism in human obesity. J. Clin. Endocrinol. Metab. **86:** 1418–1421.
34. MASUZAKI, H. *et al.* 2001. A transgenic model of visceral obesity and the metabolic syndrome. Science **294:** 2166–2170.
35. MASUZAKI, H. *et al.* 2003. Transgenic amplification of glucocorticoid action in adipose tissue causes high blood pressure in mice. J. Clin. Invest. **112:** 83–90.
36. MASUZAKI, H. & J.S. FLIER. 2003. Tissue-specific glucocorticoid reactivating enzyme, 11 β-hydroxysteroid dehydrogenase type 1 (11 β-HSD1): a promising drug target for the treatment of metabolic syndrome. Curr. Drug Targets Immune Endocr. Metabol. Disord. **3:** 255–262.
37. THIERINGER, R. & A. HERMANOWSKI-VOSATKA. 2005. Inhibition of 11 β-HSD1 as a novel treatment for the metabolic syndrome: do glucocorticoids play a role? Expert Rev. Cardiovasc. Ther. **3:** 911–924.
38. ALBERTS, P. *et al.* 2002. Selective inhibition of 11 β-hydroxysteroid dehydrogenase type 1 decreases blood glucose concentrations in hyperglycaemic mice. Diabetologia **45:** 1528–1532.
39. ALBERTS, P. *et al.* 2003. Selective inhibition of 11 β-hydroxysteroid dehydrogenase type 1 improves hepatic insulin sensitivity in hyperglycemic mice strains. Endocrinology **144:** 4755–4762.
40. HERMANOWSKI-VOSATKA, A. *et al.* 2005. 11 β-HSD1 inhibition ameliorates metabolic syndrome and prevents progression of atherosclerosis in mice. J. Exp. Med. **202:** 517–527.
41. ZHANG, T.Y., X. DING & R.A. DAYNES. 2005. The expression of 11 β-hydroxysteroid dehydrogenase type I by lymphocytes provides a novel means for intracrine regulation of glucocorticoid activities. J. Immunol. **174:** 879–889.

42. THIERINGER, R. *et al.* 2001. 11β-hydroxysteroid dehydrogenase type 1 is induced in human monocytes upon differentiation to macrophages. J. Immunol. **167:** 30–35.

43. FREEMAN, L. *et al.* 2005. Expression of 11 β-hydroxysteroid dehydrogenase type 1 permits regulation of glucocorticoid bioavailability by human dendritic cells. Blood **106:** 2042–2049.

44. GINGRAS, M.C. & J.F. MARGOLIN. 2000. Differential expression of multiple unexpected genes during U937 cell and macrophage differentiation detected by suppressive subtractive hybridization. Exp. Hematol. **28:** 65–76.

45. GILMOUR, J.S. *et al.* Local amplification of glucocorticoids by 11ß-hydroxysteroid dehydrogenase type 1 promotes macrophage phagocytosis of apoptotic leukocytes. J. Immunol. **176:** 7605–7611.

46. ESCHER, G. *et al.* 1997. Tumor necrosis factor α and interleukin 1β enhance the cortisone/cortisol shuttle. J. Exp. Med. **186:** 189–198.

47. TOMLINSON, J.W. *et al.* 2001. Regulation of expression of 11 β-hydroxysteroid dehydrogenase type 1 in adipose tissue: tissue-specific induction by cytokines. Endocrinology **142:** 1982–1989.

48. CHARRIERE, G. *et al.* 2003. Preadipocyte conversion to macrophage. Evidence of plasticity. J. Biol. Chem. **278:** 9850–9855.

49. TETSUKA, M. *et al.* 1997. Differential expression of messenger ribonucleic acids encoding 11β-hydroxysteroid dehydrogenase types 1 and 2 in human granulosa cells. J. Clin. Endocrinol. Metab. **82:** 2006–2009.

50. TETSUKA, M. *et al.* 1999. Expression of 11β-hydroxysteroid dehydrogenase, glucocorticoid receptor, and mineralocorticoid receptor genes in rat ovary. Biol. Reprod. **60:** 330–335.

51. YONG, P.Y. *et al.* 2002. Regulation of 11 β-hydroxysteroid dehydrogenase type 1 gene expression in human ovarian surface epithelial cells by interleukin-1. Hum. Reprod. **17:** 2300–2306.

52. COOPER, M.S. *et al.* 2001. Modulation of 11 β-hydroxysteroid dehydrogenase isozymes by proinflammatory cytokines in osteoblasts: an autocrine switch from glucocorticoid inactivation to activation. J. Bone Miner. Res. **16:** 1037–1044.

53. CAI, T. *et al.* 2001. Induction of 11 β-hydroxysteroid dehydrogenase type 1 but not -2 in human aortic smooth muscle cells by inflammatory stimuli. J. Steroid Biochem. Mol. Biol. **77:** 117–122.

54. SCHMIDT, M. *et al.* 2005. Reduced capacity for the reactivation of glucocorticoids in rheumatoid arthritis synovial cells: possible role of the sympathetic nervous system? Arthritis Rheum. **52:** 1711–1720.

55. FELDMANN, M. & R.N. MAINI. 2001. Anti-TNF α therapy of rheumatoid arthritis: what have we learned? Annu. Rev. Immunol. **19:** 163–196.

Immunoneuroendocrine Interactions in Chagas Disease

ELIANE CORRÊA-DE-SANTANA, FERNANDA PINTO-MARIZ, AND WILSON SAVINO

Laboratory on Thymus Research, Department of Immunology, Oswaldo Cruz Institute, Oswaldo Cruz Foundation, Rio de Janeiro, Brazil
Inserm-Fiocruz Associated Laboratory of Immunology Rio de Janeiro, Brazil

ABSTRACT: We investigated immunoneuroendocrine interactions *in vivo* and *in vitro* following infection by *Trypanosoma cruzi*, the causative agent of Chagas disease. In a first set of experiments, we studied the hypothalamus–pituitary–adrenal axis. Nests of parasites were seen in the adrenal gland, whereas *T. cruzi*–specific PCR gene amplification product was found in both the adrenal and pituitary glands of infected mice. These endocrine glands also revealed alterations including vascular stasis, increase in the deposition of extracellular matrix (ECM), as well as T cell and macrophage infiltration. Functionally, we found a decrease in corticotrophin-releasing hormone and an increase in corticosterone contents, in hypothalamus and serum, respectively, whereas no significant changes were seen in serum adrenocortricotropic hormone of infected animals. Nevertheless, the serum levels of interleukin-6 (known to directly stimulate glucocorticoid secretion) were increased, as compared to controls. Considering the presence of T cells within the nervous tissue of chagasic animals, we performed a number of *in vitro* experiments co-culturing spleen-derived T cells from control or infected mice, with neuronal cells (being or not being directly infected *in vitro*). In particular, we looked for ECM-mediated interactions, known to affect T cell migration. We found an increase in ECM deposition in infected cultures, as compared to controls. Moreover, adhesion of T cells was enhanced when neuronal cells were infected *in vitro*, or when T cells were derived from *T. cruzi*–infected mice, events that could be abrogated with anti-ECM antibodies. Together, the data summarized above clearly reveal that neuroendocrine axes are altered in experimental Chagas disease.

KEYWORDS: *Trypanosoma cruzi*; neurons; hypothalamus; pituitary; adrenal glands; extracellular matrix; T lymphocytes

Address for correspondence: Wilson Savino, Laboratory on Thymus Research, Department of Immunology, Oswaldo Cruz Institute, Oswaldo Cruz Foundation, Ave. Brasil 4365, Manguinhos-21045-900, Rio de Janeiro, Brazil. Voice/fax: 00-55-21-3865-8101.
e-mail: savino@fiocruz.br

Ann. N.Y. Acad. Sci. 1088: 274–283 (2006). © 2006 New York Academy of Sciences.
doi: 10.1196/annals.1366.005

INTRODUCTION

Trypanosoma cruzi is the flagellate protozoan parasite that causes Chagas disease, which affects 16 to 18 million people in Latin America. Chagas disease comprises an acute phase characterized by detection of circulating parasites, followed by a chronic phase characterized by very low amounts of parasites in several tissues, such as the heart, esophagus, colon, and peripheral nervous system.[1,2] In addition, *T. cruzi* acute infection may lead to encephalitis and promotes dysfunction in the endocrine status, increasing circulating levels of corticosterone in mice.[3,4]

Herein, we summarize recent data that unravel disturbances in neuroendocrine circuits following experimental *T. cruzi* infection.

T. cruzi–or Parasite-Derived Antigens Are Present in Nervous and Endocrine Tissues

In terms of nervous tissues, parasite-derived antigens have been detected in various parts of the brain.[3] In keeping with this, we succeeded in infecting *in vitro* both neuronal cells and astrocytes after short-term co-culture with the infective flagellum-containing trypomastigote forms of the parasite (FIG. 1a).

As regards the pituitary–adrenal axis, we found nests of amastigotes (the intracellular forms of the parasite) in the adrenals (FIG. 1b), as well as parasite-derived antigens and genes in both adrenals and pituitary, as ascertained by immunohistochemistry using anti–*T. cruzi* antiserum, and RT-PCR to detect parasite-specific kinetoplast-related genes.[5] Moreover, pituitary cell lines could be infected *in vitro*, including ACTH-producing as well as GH/prolactin-secreting cells.

It should be noted that in immunocompromised animals, as exemplified by nude mice and cyclophosphamide-treated animals, various endocrine glands can be infected, including thyroid and pancreas.[6]

Inflammatory Reaction in Neuroendocrine Tissues of T. cruzi–Infected Animals: Relationship with Extracellular Matrix

The presence of an inflammatory infiltration in brain areas of *T. cruzi*–infected mice has been previously reported,[3] being particularly rich in CD8[+] T cells. We recently extended this finding, showing that both pituitary gland and adrenals of infected animals exhibit clusters of CD8[+] T cells, and to a much lesser extent, CD4[+] cells as well as macrophages.[5]

The influx of T cells toward a given target tissue is governed by a number of molecular interactions, including those mediated by chemokines as well as the migration dependent on ECM ligands and receptors.[7] In experimental

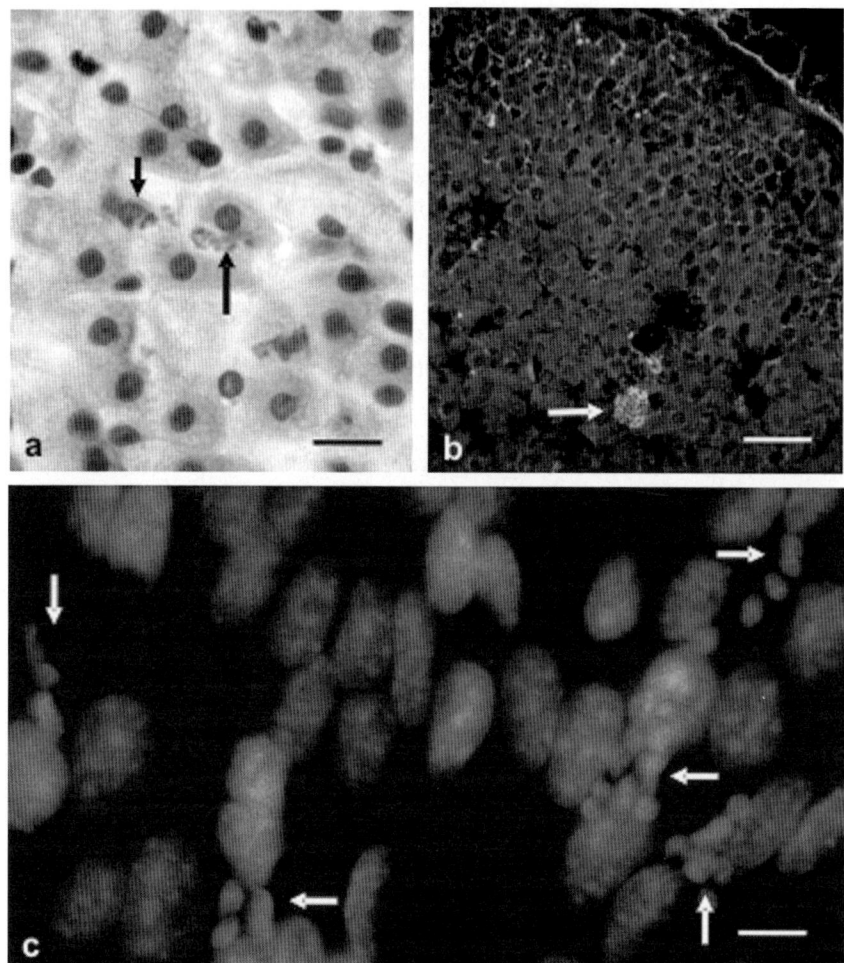

FIGURE 1. Detection of *T. cruzi* in cells from the pituitary–adrenal axis. *Panel* **a** shows one parasite nest (*black arrow*) in a paraffin section stained by hematoxylin-eosin, in the fasciculata zone of the adrenal gland. This was confirmed (*panel* **b**) by immunofluorescence (*arrows*) with anti–*T. cruzi* serum. *Panel* **c** depicts infection of the adenopituitary-derived ACTH-producing cell line. Amastigote forms of the parasite are indicated by *arrows*. Nuclei of endocrine cells were stained with DAPI.

Chagas disease, it has been shown that the carditis is accompanied by a local increase in the deposition of ECM components.[8] We have showed that the CD4$^+$ T cell–dependent autoimmune destruction of myocardial cells, seen in the chronic phase of *T. cruzi* infection,[9] could be functionally abrogated by blocking laminin-mediated interactions.[10]

We have recently showed an increase of extracellular matrix deposition (such as fibronectin and laminin) in both the adrenal and pituitary glands of infected mice, as compared to normal animals (FIG. 2a–d). *In vitro* infection of ACTH-producing cells also resulted in an enhancement of ECM production, suggesting a direct effect of the parasite and/or parasite-derived antigens upon the endocrine cells. In this respect, not only infected, but also noninfected cells exhibited such an effect on ECM upregulation. Similar findings were observed in one adenopituitary folliculo-stellate cell line (FIG. 2e, f). Accordingly, it has been shown that parasite-derived moieties are able to bind to muscle and fibroblastic cell lines, and trigger an increase in ECM production.[11]

In brain areas of infected animals, a similar increase of ECM deposition has been documented, coinciding with the inflammatory infiltrate.[3] We performed a number of *in vitro* experiments co-culturing spleen-derived T cells from control or infected mice, with neuronal cells (being directly infected or not *in vitro*). We found an increase in ECM deposition in infected cultures as compared with controls. Moreover, adhesion of T cells was enhanced when neuronal cells were infected *in vitro*, or when T cells were derived from *T. cruzi*–infected mice, and was abrogated by prior incubation of the co-cultures with anti-ECM antibodies (Pinto-Mariz *et al.*, submitted for publication). In this respect, adhesion of infection-induced activated T cells on tissue slices of brain areas, as well as penetration of these cells after passive transfer *in vivo*, could be abrogated with anti-CD49d fibronectin receptor antibody.[12]

Taken together, the findings summarized above indicate that ECM-mediated interactions are functionally relevant to drive the influx of T cells toward nervous and endocrine tissues of *T. cruzi*–infected mice.

Antineuroendocrine Tissue Autoimmunity in Chagas Disease?

Antimyocardial cell autoimmunity in Chagas disease has been known for many years,[13] and we have provided evidence incriminating a control of such autoreactivity by CD4$^+$ T cells.[9] However, there is evidence of T and B cell autoreactivity, targeting nervous as well as endocrine tissues. In murine *T. cruzi* infection, a CD4$^+$ T cell line has been reported to be able to recognize peripheral nerves.[14] Moreover, antibodies directed against cerebral gangliosides have been detected.[15] Accordingly, deposits of immunoglobulins have been documented in various brain areas of *T. cruzi*–infected mice.[3] As illustrated in FIGURE 3, both the pituitary and the adrenal glands of infected mice are also sites of immunoglobulin deposition, indicating that both nervous and endocrine tissues are recognized by autoantibodies in experimental Chagas disease. Nevertheless, which molecules are targeted in these endocrine glands remains an open field for investigation.

Normal **Infected**

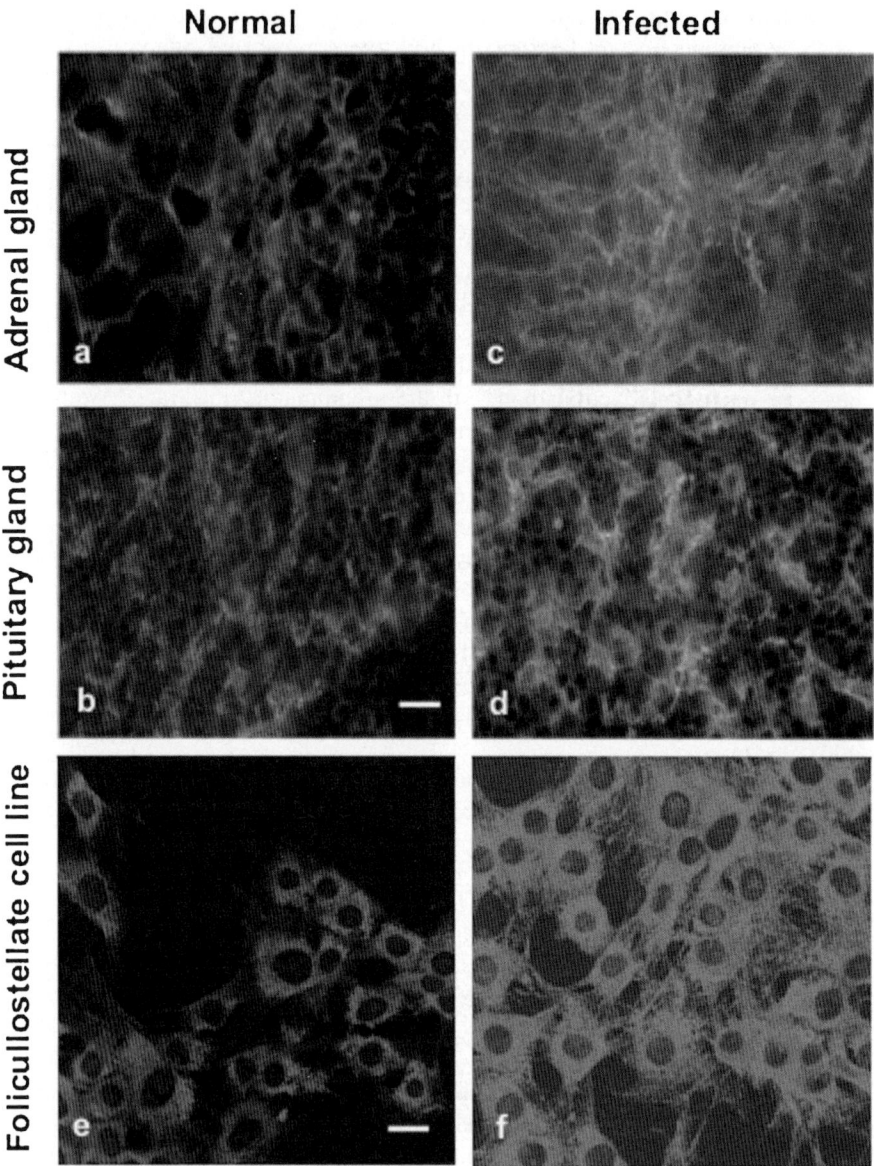

FIGURE 2. Enhancement of ECM molecules in adrenal and pituitary glands of *T. cruzi*–infected mice. Frozen sections of adrenal (*panels* **a**, **b**) and pituitary (*panels* **c**, **d**) glands were labeled with antifibronectin antibody. Deposition of the ECM molecule is clearly increased in both endocrine glands following acute infection. *In vitro* infection of the folliculo-stellate cell line (TtT-GF) with *T. cruzi* also resulted in increased ECM production, as revealed in *panels* **e**, **f** by laminin labeling. Scale bars: 20 μM (*panels* **a–d**) and 10 μM (*panels* **e–f**).

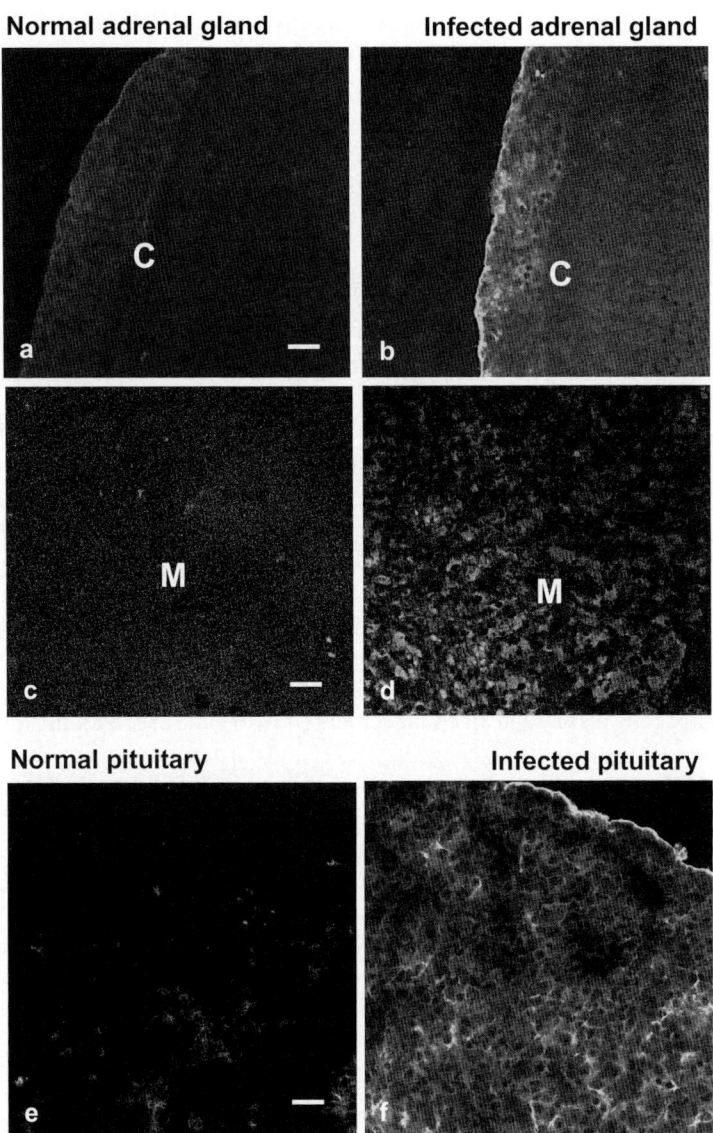

FIGURE 3. Deposition of immunoglobulins in adrenal and pituitary glands of *T. cruzi*–infected mice. Fluorescein-conjugated rat anti-mouse Ig antibody was added to frozen sections of adrenal glands from normal and infected animals. *Panels* **a** and **c** represent the detection of immunoglobulins bound in the cortex (**C**) and medulla (**M**) of normal adrenals, whereas in *panels* **b** and **d** the strong labeling reveals large amounts of autoantibodies bound to cells in the cortex (**C**) and the medulla (**M**) of infected gland. Similar differences are seen in terms of detection of autoantibodies in pituitary glands of infected mice, but not in controls (*panels* **f** and **e**, respectively). For each experiment, glands of at least five animals from each group were used. Scale bars: 20 μm

Hormonal and Cytokine Changes in the HPA Axis of T. cruzi–Infected Mice

We have previously shown that acute *T. cruzi* infection in C57BL/6 mice resulted in an increase in the serum levels of corticosterone.[4] More recently, similar data were obtained in BALB/c animals, both in the acute and chronic phases of the disease.[5] We therefore studied the HPA axis in terms of hormonal production in acutely infected mice.

We found that at the peak of parasitemia, the CRH contents in the hypothalamus were 5 times higher than controls. Interestingly, a decrease of CRH production has been reported in mice infected with the worm *Schistosoma mansoni*,[16] indicating that distinct kinds of parasites can affect hypothalamic endocrine function.

Despite the hypothalamic decrease seen in CRH contents, simultaneously with an increase of glucocorticoids in serum, circulating levels of ACTH of *T. cruzi* mice acutely infected with *T. cruzi* did not change significantly (TABLE 1). Conjointly, these findings point to an imbalance in the circuitry of the HPA axis in the course of the disease. Some pro-inflammatory cytokines may be related to such an imbalance. In particular, it is known that IL-6 is able to directly stimulate both glucocorticoid and ACTH release.[17,18] In fact, there is an increase in the serum levels of IL-6 in infected mice, in comparison with the corresponding cytokine levels in normal animals. Moreover, *in vitro* infection of ACTH-producing cells resulted in an enhancement of IL-6 gene expression.[5] Interestingly, this same cytokine is related to ACTH and corticosterone increment seen in mice infected with cytomegalovirus.[19] In this model, although the authors did find increased ACTH levels in virus-infected mice, the increased amounts in serum corticosterone remained after anti-CRH antibody treatment and was actually higher in infected CRH knockout animals.[19] Moreover, in IL-6 knockout mice, the corticosterone rise following cytomegalovirus infection, although easily detectable, was much lower than the values seen in IL-6[+/+] individuals.[20]

In *T. cruzi*–infected mice, the apparent ACTH-independent increase of glucocorticoid secretion at the adrenal cortex is likely due to an enhancement of

TABLE 1. Modulation of HPA hormone levels in *T. cruzi*–infected mice[a]

Hormone[b]	T. cruzi–infected	Controls
CRH (pg/mg of tissue)	73.7 ± 5.2	22.7 ± 8.7*
ACTH (pg/mL)	120.90 ± 66.2	99.04 ± 39.7
Corticosterone (ng/mL)	518.26 ± 82.3	201.99 ± 75.5*

[a]BALB/c mice were acutely infected with 10^5 trypomastigote forms of the *T. cruzi* Colombian strain, and sacrificed 3 weeks later, at the peak of parasitemia.

[b]Tissue CRH, as well as serum ACTH and corticosterone, were measured by radioimmunoassay. Results were compared using the unpaired Student's *t*-test, using samples of at least five animals from each experimental group. *$P < 0.005$. Modified from Ref 5.

circulating IL-1β and/or IL-6.[5] In this respect, it is noteworthy that cytokine production by endocrine cells is altered following *in vitro T. cruzi* infection, as we demonstrated for IL-6 RNA in ACTH-producing cells.[5] Moreover, as compared to controls, IL-2 production by these cells was enhanced after *in vitro T. cruzi* infection, as ascertained by cytofluorometry (FIG. 4).

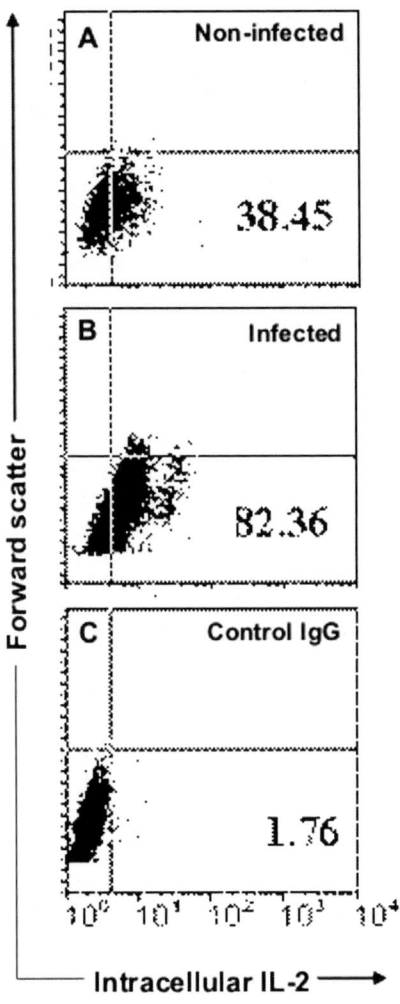

FIGURE 4. Enhancement of interleukin-2 production by ACTH-secreting cells after infection with *T. cruzi*. AtT-20 cells were stained with FITC-labeled anti–IL-2 antibody and analyzed by cytofluorometry. Panel **A** shows basal percentage of IL-2-producing cells in untreated cultures, whereas panel **B** depicts the increase in the relative numbers of IL-2+ cells after infection of cultures with *T. cruzi*. Panel **C** shows the background labeling after exposing cells to an unrelated antibody. Ten thousand events were acquired. Percentages of positive labeling correspond to the numbers appearing in each panel.

Concluding Remarks

The work summarized here demonstrates the concept that, in addition to certain brain areas and peripheral nervous tissue of the myoenteric plexus, the endocrine system, and in particular the HPA axis, can be considered as a target in Chagas disease. Moreover, similar to carditis, inflammatory infiltrates in nervous and endocrine systems are likely dependent, at least partially, on extracellular matrix-mediated interactions.

Yet determining the precise role of such neuroendocrine changes in the pathophysiology of the disease is still open to investigation.

ACKNOWLEDGMENTS

This work was partially funded with grants from Papes/Fiocruz, CNPq and Faperj (Brazil).

REFERENCES

1. HIGUCHI, M.L. *et al.* 2003. Pathophysiology of the heart in Chagas disease: current status and new developments. Cardiovasc. Res. **60:** 96–107.
2. BRENER, Z. & R.T. GAZZINELLI. 1997. Immunological control of *Trypanosoma cruzi* infection and pathogenesis of Chagas' disease. Int. Arch. Allergy Immunol. **114:** 103–110.
3. SILVA, A.A. *et al.* 1999. Chagas' disease encephalitis: intense CD8[+] lymphocytic infiltrate is restricted to the acute phase, but is not related to the presence of *Trypanosoma cruzi* antigens. Clin. Immunol. **92:** 56–66.
4. LEITE-DE-MORAES, M.C. *et al.* 1991. Studies on the thymus in Chagas' disease. II. Thymocyte subset fluctuations in *Trypanosoma cruzi*-infected mice: relationship to stress. Scand. J. Immunol. **33:** 267–275.
5. CORREA-DE-SANTANA, E. *et al.* 2006. Hypothalamus-pituitary-adrenal axis during *Trypanosoma cruzi* infection in mice. J. Neuroimmunol. **173:** 12–22.
6. CALABRESE, K.S., P.H. LAGRANGE & S.C. GONÇALVES-DA-COSTA. 1994. *Trypanosoma cruzi*: histopathology of endocrine system in immunocompromised mice. Int. J. Pathol. **75:** 453–462.
7. EPLER, J.A., R. Liu & Y. SHIMIZU. 2000. From the ECM to the cytoskeleton and back: how integrins orchestrate T cell action. Dev. Immunol. **7:** 155–170.
8. ANDRADE, S.G., J.A. GRIMAUD & S. STOCKER-GUERRET. 1989. Sequential changes of the connective matrix components of the myocardium (fibronectin and laminin) and evolution of cardiac fibrosis in mice infected with *T. cruzi*. Am. J. Trop. Med. Hyg. **40:** 252–260.
9. RIBEIRO-DOS-SANTOS, R. *et al.* 1992. Anti-CD4 abrogates rejection and reestablishes long-term tolerance to syngeneic newborn hearts grafted in mice chronically infected with *Trypanosoma cruzi*. J. Exp. Med. **175:** 29–39.
10. SILVA-BARBOSA, S.D. *et al.* 1997. Involvement of laminin and its receptor in abrogation of heart graft rejection by autoreactive T cells from *Trypanosoma cruzi*-infected mice. J. Immunol. **159:** 997–1003.

11. PINHO, R.T. *et al.* 2002. Effect of *Trypanosoma cruzi* released antigens binding to non-infected cells on anti-parasite antibody recognition and expression of extracellular matrix components. Acta Tropica **83:** 103–115.
12. ROFFE, E. *et al.* 2003. Essential role of VLA-4/VCAM-1 pathway in the establishment of CD8+ T-cell-mediated *Trypanosoma cruzi*-elicited meningoencephalitis. J. Neuroimmunol. **142:** 17–30.
13. KALIL, J. & E. CUNHA-NETO. 1996. Autoimmunity in Chagas' disease cardiopathy: fulfilling the criteria at last? Parasitol. Today **12:** 396–399.
14. HONTEBEYRIE-JOSKOWICZ, M. *et al.* 1987. L3T4+ T cells able to mediate parasite-specific delayed-type hypersensitivity play a role in the pathology of experimental Chagas' disease. Eur. J. Immunol. **17:** 1027–1033.
15. AVILA, J.L. *et al.* 1998. Increase in asialoganglioside- and monosialo-ganglioside-reactive antibodies in chronic Chagas' disease patients. Am. J. Trop. Med. Hyg. **58:** 338–342.
16. MORALES-MONTOR, J. *et al.* 2001. Altered levels of hypothalamic-pituitary–adrenocortical axis hormones in baboons and mice during the course of infection with *Schistosoma mansoni*. J. Infect. Dis. **183:** 313–320.
17. SAVINO, W. & E. ARZT. 1999. The thymus-pituitary axis: a paradigm to study immunoneuroendocrine connectivity in normal ans stress conditions. *In* Cytokines Stress and Immunity. N.P. Plotnikoff, R.E. Fatith, A.J. Murgo & R.A. Good, Eds.: 187–204. CRC Press. Boca Raton, Florida.
18. ARZT, E. *et al.* 1999. Pathophysiological role of the cytokine network in the anterior pituitary gland. Front. Neuroendocrinology **20:** 71–95.
19. SILVERMAN, M.N. *et al.* 2004. Characterization of an interleukin-6 and adrenocorticotropin-dependent, immune-to-adrenal pathway during vital infection. Endocrinology **145:** 3580–3589.
20. SILVERMAN, M.N. *et al.* 2005. Immune moduation of the hypothalamic-pituitary-adrenal (HPA) axis during viral infection. Viral Immunol. **18:** 41–78.

Thymus-Dependent T Cell Tolerance of Neuroendocrine Functions

Principles, Reflections, and Implications for Tolerogenic/Negative Self-Vaccination

VINCENT GEENEN

University of Liège, Center of Immunology (CIL), B-4000 Liège-Sart Tilman, Belgium

ABSTRACT: Under the evolutionary pressure exerted by the emergence of adaptive immunity and its inherent risk of *horror autotoxicus*, the thymus appeared some 500 million years ago as a novel lymphoid structure able to prevent autoimmunity and to orchestrate self-tolerance as a cornerstone in the physiology of the immune system. Also, the thymus plays a prominent role in T cell education to neuroendocrine principles. Some self-antigens (oxytocin, neurotensin, insulin-like growth factor 2 [IGF-2]) have been selected to be predominantly expressed in thymic epithelium and to be presented to thymus T cells for educating them to tolerate other antigens related to them. In the insulin family, *IGF2* is dominantly transcribed in cortical (c) and medullary (m) thymic epithelial cells (TECs), whereas the insulin gene (*INS*) is expressed at low level by only a few subsets of mTECs. Intrathymic transcription of both *IGF2* and *INS* is under the control of the autoimmune regulator (*Aire*) gene. The highest concentrations of IGF-2 in the thymus explain why this peptide is much more tolerated than insulin, and why tolerance to IGF-2 is so difficult to break by active immunization. The high level of tolerance to IGF-2 is correlated to the development of a tolerogenic/regulatory profile when the sequence B11-25 of IGF-2 (homologous to the autoantigen insulin B9-23) is presented to DQ8+ type 1 diabetic patients. Since subcutaneous and oral insulin does not exert any tolerogenic properties, IGF-2 and other thymus self-antigens related to type 1 diabetes (T1D) should be preferred to insulin for the design of novel specific antigen-based preventive approaches against T1D.

KEYWORDS: thymus; central tolerance; autoimmunity; self-antigens; AIRE; regulatory T cells (T_R); type 1 diabetes

Address for correspondence: Vincent Geenen, M.D., Ph.D., University of Liège Center of Immunology (CIL), Institute of Pathology CHU-B23, B-4000 Liège-Sart Tilman, Belgium. Voice: +32-43-66-25-50; fax: +32-43-66-98-59.
e-mail: vgeenen@ulg.ac.be

Ann. N.Y. Acad. Sci. 1088: 284–296 (2006). © 2006 New York Academy of Sciences.
doi: 10.1196/annals.1366.009

INTRODUCTION

Some 500 million years ago, although some rudiment of immune diversity already existed in jawless fishes (e.g., lamprey),[1] novel adaptive immunity emerged in cartilaginous fishes (e.g., shark and ray). Specialized recombination machinery in somatic lymphoid cells is the fundamental property of adaptive immunity and is responsible for the random generation of a huge diversity of immune receptors (BCRs and TCRs) able to recognize non-self antigens. The emergence of this novel form of immune defense exerted such a potent pressure that novel structures and mechanisms appeared along the paths of lymphocyte traffic to impose immunological self-tolerance, that is, the inability of the immune system to attack the host organism. Together with the generation of diversity and memory, self-tolerance is a cornerstone in physiology and homeostasis of the immune system. The progressive rise in the level of immune diversity and complexity also explains why failures of immunological self-tolerance (such as organ-specific autoimmune diseases) are more and more frequently detected in parallel with evolution, the maximum being observed in the human species. The first thymus also appeared in cartilaginous fishes concomitant with the emergence of adaptive immunity. Though some forms of tolerance induction already take place in primary hematopoietic sites (fetal liver and bone marrow), antigen-dependent B cell tolerance is predominantly due to an absence of T cell help. So, among all lymphoid structures, the thymus is the only organ specialized in the establishment of immunological self-tolerance.

The thymus crucially stands at the crossroads between the immune and neuroendocrine systems.[2] Within this organ responsible for thymopoiesis (T cell generation), the neuroendocrine system regulates the process of T cell differentiation from the very early stages. In addition, T lymphocytes undergo in the thymus a complex educative process that establishes central T cell self-tolerance of neuroendocrine principles. The thymus is a very unique place wherein these is a permanent confrontation between ancient, almost constant, neuroendocrine principles and a recent system equipped with a sophisticated machinery promoting stochastic generation of response diversity. Contrary to a previous assumption, the thymus functions throughout life and plays a fundamental role in the recovery of a competent T cell repertoire after intensive chemotherapy or during highly active antiretroviral therapy.[3,4] Finally, the thymus is an important site for the generation of self-antigen specific regulatory T cells (T_R) that suppress in the periphery the activation of self-reactive T cells that have escaped the thymus central censorship.[5,6]

DEVELOPMENTAL BIOLOGY OF THYMIC EPITHELIUM

Epithelial cells of the thymic cortex (cTEC, including thymic "nurse" cells [TNC]) and medulla (mTEC) originate from a common progenitor derived around embryonic day 11 (E11) from the endoderm of the third pharyngeal pouch.[7,8] Using lineage tracing analysis in whole embryo culture, no evidence was found for a contribution from the ectoderm of the third pharyngeal cleft. Further development of this primitive epithelial rudiment depends upon a contribution from the cephalic neural crest. Some human diseases (and animal models) include a defective thymus development, leading to primary immune deficiencies. DiGeorge's syndrome associates congenital absence (or hypoplasia) of thymus and parathyroids with defects in the heart and truncal vessels. This syndrome partly results from a migration failure of the cephalic neural crest. Mice in whom the homeobox A3 gene (*Hoxa3*) has been disrupted present thymic aplasia, parathyroid hypoplasia, and frequent defects in heart and great vessels.[9] Wild animals with immune deficiencies most closely related to DiGeorge's syndrome are "nude" mice with hairlessness and lack of thymic development resulting from defects in TECs. The "nude" phenotype is caused by mutations in the *nude* gene on murine chromosome 11 that encodes the transcription factor winged-helix nude (*whn*) or forkhead box N1 (*Foxn1*).[10] Wnt glycoproteins and dependent signaling were shown to regulate *Foxn1* expression in TECs.[11] In the absence of functional *Foxn1*, TECs are arrested at an immature progenitor stage (with expression of MTS20$^+$ and MTS24$^+$ determinants) and do not differentiate into epithelial subregions.[12] Different studies indicate that a common progenitor of TECs might exist, with a marker phenotype of MTS20$^+$ MTS24$^+$ cytokeratin 5 (K5$^+$) and K8$^+$. Once further identified, such TEC progenitor lines could be used for restoring thymus function in DiGeorge's syndrome or in immunosenescence, as well as for improving the final outcome after bone marrow and organ transplantations.

Five other transcription factors, paired box gene 1 (*Pax1*), and 9 (*Pax9*), eyes absent 1 homologue (*Eya1*), and sine oculis–related homeobox 1 homologue (*Six1*), also contribute to the ontogeny of thymic epithelium. In mice, these genes are coexpressed only in the pharyngeal endoderm and in the cephalic neural crest–derived mesenchyme (with the exception of *Pax1* and *Pax9*).[7] Important developmental signaling pathways (fibroblast growth factors [FGFs], bone morphogenetic proteins [BMP], and sonic-hedgehog homologue [Shh]) are also implicated in cell–cell interactions between thymic epithelium and mesenchymal cells, as well as the surrounding neural crest–derived mesenchyme (reviewed in Ref. 13).

From fetal liver and then bone marrow, T cell progenitors migrate into the thymus through the boundary between cortex and medulla, undergo around 20 division cycles in the outer cortex, and then differentiate after presentation of peptides by major histocompatibility complex (MHC) proteins expressed by thymic antigen-presenting cells (APCs), that is, cTECs, mTECs, dendritic cells (DCs), macrophages, and rare thymus B cells. The random rearrangement of related β then α loci generates an enormous diversity of TCRs, a great number of which are able to bind peptide/MHC ligands with high affinity and to be negatively selected. Negative selection can occur in both the cortex and the medulla,[14] though mTECs display the most complete APC competence. At the end of the differentiation process in the thymus, only ± 5% of naïve thymus T cells (thymocytes) will leave the organ in a state of self-tolerance and competence against infectious non-self antigens.

THE NEUROENDOCRINE SELF

From the investigation of the intrathymic expression of neuroendocrine-related self-peptide precursor genes, a series of specificities could be listed to define the nature of "neuroendocrine self." [15] (1) Neuroendocrine self-antigens usually correspond to peptide sequences that have been highly conserved throughout the evolution of one given family. (2) A hierarchy characterizes their expression pattern. In the neurohypophysial family, oxytocin (OT) is the dominant peptide synthesized by TEC/TNCs from different species. The binding of OT to OT receptor (OTR) expressed by pre-T cells induces a very rapid phosphorylation of focal adhesion–related kinases.[16–18] This event could play a major role in the promotion of "immunological synapses" between immature T lymphocytes and thymus APCs. Concerning the tachykinin family, neurokinin A (NKA)—but not substance P (SP)—is the peptide generated from the processing by TECs of the preprotachykinin A (*PPT-A*) gene product.[19] With regard to the insulin gene family, all members are expressed in the thymus network according to a precise hierarchy and topography: *IGF2* (cTEC/TNC and mTEC) > *IGF1* (thymic macrophages) > *INS* (mTEC).[20–23] This hierarchical pattern is significant since the tolerogenic response primarily concerns the dominant epitopes of a protein family. Contrary to (pro)insulin, the blockade of thymic IGF-mediated signaling, at the level of IGF ligands (in particular IGF-2) or IGF receptors, interferes with the early stages of T cell differentiation in fetal thymic organ cultures (FTOCs).[24] (3) Neuroendocrine precursors are not processed according to the classic model of neurosecretion, but they undergo antigenic processing for presentation by—or in association with—MHC proteins. (4) This processing differs between thymic APCs and dedicated peripheral APCs. At least for some neuroendocrine self-antigens (OT and neurotensin), such differences imply that presentation by thymic APCs is not tightly restricted by MHC alleles as much as presentation of infectious non self antigens and autoantigens by peripheral dedicated APCs (macrophages, DCs, and B cells).

During ontogeny of Balb/c mice, *OT* transcripts are detected on E13 both in thymus and brain, whereas vasopressin (*VP*) gene transcription starts on E14 in the brain and is clearly detected in the thymus only on E15.[25] The earlier *OT* expression in the thymus strongly supports the role of thymic OT in the induction of central T cell tolerance of the neurohypophysial peptides before their appearance in the hypothalamic magnocellular neurons. The expression of the neurohypophysial receptor genes (*OTR*, *V1*, *V2*, and *V3*) was investigated on murine CD4⁻ CD8⁻ T cell lines, as well as on murine T cell subsets. *OTR* transcripts are detected in CD4$^-$CD8$^-$, CD4$^+$ CD8$^+$, and CD8$^+$ cells, while a very faint *V3* expression is restricted to CD4$^+$ CD8$^+$ and CD8$^+$ cells. *V1* and *V2* expression could not be detected on any T cell subset. In FTOCs, a specific OTR antagonist increases late T cell apoptosis, confirming the involvement of OT/OTR signaling in T cell proliferation/survival.[25,26]

REGULATION OF SELF-EXPRESSION

The progressive accumulation of evidence that genes/proteins considered to be expressed only in the brain, in the neuroendocrine system, and in peripheral organs are also synthesized in the thymus finally brought into question the common view of the establishment of immunological self-tolerance and the development of organ-specific autoimmunity (completely reviewed in Ref. 27). In 1993, the term "promiscuous" was introduced to specify this unique promoter use by TECs compared to other somatic cells.[28] Another advance in the current reappraisal of the crucial role played by the thymus in preventing autoimmunity came from the identification of the gene of which mutations are responsible for the polyendocrine autoimmune disease, autoimmune polyendocrinopathy-candidiasis-ectodermal dystrophy (APECED) or autoimmune polyglandular syndrome type 1 (APS-1).[29,30] The gene *Aire* (autoimmune regulator) encodes a protein with structural and functional features suggesting a transcription factor. The generation of *Aire*$^{-/-}$ mice revealed that Aire primarily functions within TECs where its expression is maximal and where it controls transcription of genes encoding neuroendocrine self-antigens (including *Ot, Igf2, Ins2,* and *Npy*), as well as a series—but not all—tissue-restricted antigens.[31] Although Aire controls the transcription of these two neuroendocrine-related genes, *Ins2* expression is restricted to mTEC, while *Igf2* transcripts are detected in cTEC/TNCs, as well as in mTECs. The existence of epigenetic mechanisms in the Aire control of self-expression is also strongly supported by the discovery that the set of promiscuous transcripts expressed by human mTECs includes several groups of chromosomally clustered genes.[32] Such epigenetic regulation is further suggested by loss of imprinting and overexpression of *IGF2* in human mTECs.[33] Nevertheless, it remains unclear why TECs are the only somatic cells (with the exception of multipotent stem cells) to transcribe such a diversity of neuroendocrine and tissue-restricted antigens, and why this diversity seems to be correlated with the stage of TEC differentiation.

Aire promotes negative selection of self-reactive thymus T cells and, perhaps more importantly, improves the overall efficiency of antigen presentation by mTECs.[34,35] As previously mentioned, a difference between the central and peripheral mechanisms was again evidenced at this level since antigen presentation by DCs in the periphery is more efficient in the absence of Aire.[36] On the other hand, no any significant defect of the T$_R$ lineage was observed in *Aire*-deficient mice. Very interestingly, thymic Aire expression decreases and autoimmunity develops in lymphotoxin (LT) α or β receptor–deficient mice.[37] Although it is still not clear whether the LT receptor directly controls Aire expression or indirectly via regulation of mTEC development, this study illustrates the importance of lymphoepithelial crosstalk in thymus physiology. Human thymic stromal lymphopoietin (TSLP) has also been reported to induce *AIRE* expression in human DC.[38] Although helix-loop-helix transcription factors of the forkhead family (Foxn1, Foxp3, Foxo, and Foxj1) are major modulators of the immune development and responses, Aire seems to be until now the unique molecular determinant involved in the control of self-expression inside the thymus.

Altogether, those studies contributed to reevaluate the physiological importance of thymus-dependent central tolerance and "recessive" clonal deletion— as opposed to the "dominant" tolerance by T_R generation—in the prevention of autoimmunity and "horror autotoxicus" of the organism, so to speak in a conceptual view like that proposed by Ehrlich in 1901.[39] Self-tolerance homeostasis and prevention of autoimmunity by central and peripheral tolerogenic mechanisms acting synergically have, however, to be considered together as evidenced by the severe and multiple autoimmune organ deficiencies as observed in *Foxp3*- and *Foxj1*-deficient mice.[40,41]

PRESENTATION OF NEUROENDOCRINE SELF-ANTIGENS

While a vast repertoire of neuroendocrine-related and tissue-restricted self-antigens is expressed by TECs, the coupling of their thymic transcription to the MHC presentation of derived epitopes has not been extensively investigated. This point is, however, fundamental since some authors recently reported that the promiscuous gene expression of an autoantigen gene (H/Ka subunit of the gastric membrane protein H^+/K^+ ATPase) did not result in negative selection of effector self-reactive T cells.[42]

Using an immunoaffinity column prepared with a mAb to the monomorphic part of human MHC-I molecules, we identified in proteins extracted from human TEC plasma membranes a 55-kDa protein that was labeled both by anti-MHC-I and antineurophysin antibodies.[43] This membrane protein may represent a hybrid protein with a neurophysin domain (10 kDa) and a MHC-I heavy chain domain (45 kDa). Formation of such a hybrid protein could reside either at the posttranscriptional level (such as a transsplicing mechanism), or at the posttranslational level (such as the ATP-dependent binding of ubiquitin to proteins in proteolysis). The MHC-I domain would be implicated in the membrane targeting of this 55-kDa protein, while neurophysin would bind OT for presentation to thymus T cells. If this assumption were correct, this would mean that, both in the hypothalamo-neurohypophysial axis and in the thymus, the neurophysin part of the OT precursor fulfills the same function: binding of OT and transport to the surface of magnocellular neurons or TEC/TNCs. If true, this explanation would imply that the immune system has adopted during evolution a component of the neurohypophysial peptide biosynthesis for the development of tolerance to the self-antigen OT of this family. Interestingly, with regard to this hypothesis, it was recently demonstrated that a component of lipid metabolism, the binding protein apolipoprotein E, is used by the immune system for binding lipid antigens and delivering them into DC endosomal compartments containing CD1.[44] Further studies are needed to verify whether IGF-binding proteins could also be involved in the intrathymic presentation of IGF-2 to thymus T cells. This hypothesis is nevertheless plausible since several genes encoding these important components of the IGF system are transcribed in the thymus network.[22]

Cultured human TECs contain $\pm$ 5 ng neurotensin (NT) per 10^6 cells, of which 5% are associated with plasma cell membranes. HPLC analysis of immunoreactive (ir)-NT present in human TECs revealed a major peak of ir-NT corresponding to intact NT1-13. Ir-NT was not detected in the supernatant of human TEC primary cultures. Using an immunoaffinity column with an anti-MHC-I mAb, NT-related peptides were retained on the column and were eluted at basic pH just as antigens bound to MHC-I proteins.[45] The C-terminal sequence of NT includes tyrosine, leucine, and isoleucine, all residues that can be used for anchorage to most of the MHC-I alleles. Thus, NT and NT-derived C-terminal fragments could behave as natural ligands for a majority (if not all) of MHC-I alleles. This hypothesis stands in agreement with the high degree of conservation of NT-related C-terminal region throughout evolution.

DEFECTIVE CENTRAL TOLERANCE AS A PRIMARY EVENT FOR THE DEVELOPMENT OF AUTOIMMUNE ENDOCRINOPATHIES

In 1992, a defect in the process of T cell education to recognize and to tolerate the neurohypophysial self-Ag OT was hypothesized to play a pivotal role in the development of hypothalamus-specific autoimmunity and "idiopathic" diabetes insipidus.[46] As already hypothesized by Burnet in 1973, the pathogenesis of autoimmune diseases could result from the appearance of "forbidden" self-reactive effector T cell clones in the peripheral repertoire.[47] Since the thymus is the primary site for induction of self-tolerance, thorough investigation of a defective thymic censorship should provide the scientific community with important keys to understand the mechanisms underlying the development of autoimmunity. A number of abnormalities of thymic morphology and cytoarchitecture have been described for several autoimmune disorders. Apoptosis of self-reactive T cells is also defective in the thymus of NOD mice.[48] The expression of Aire is maximal in murine mTECs, but is absent in TECs of diabetic NOD mice.[49] The expression of insulin-related genes was analyzed in thymus, liver, and brain of a common animal model of type 1 diabetes (T1D), the biobreeding (BB) rat. A thymus-specific defect of *Igf2* expression was evidenced in more than 80% of diabetes-prone BB rats (BBDP).[50] This defect could explain both lymphopenia, including a lack of antigen-specific T_R cells that control autoimmune diabetes, as well as absence of central self-tolerance of insulin family in BBDP rats. Further experimental data arguing for a role the promotion of β-cell self-tolerance by thymic insulin-related peptides came from other recent experiments showing that susceptibility to diabetes was correlated with the intrathymic levels of *Ins2* expression.[51,52] As a consequence of the defective thymic censorship, self-reactive T cells bearing TCRs oriented against dominant epitopes of insulin-related peptides could continuously migrate from the thymus and enrich the peripheral pool with self-reactive T cells exhibiting a potential cytotoxic power against islet β cells. Under certain environmental influences, a molecular "bridge" could be installed between the target autoantigenic epitopes, leading to activation of the self-reactive T cell pool and subsequent β-cell destruction.

T1D (juvenile or insulin-dependent diabetes) is a chronic devastating disease resulting from an autoimmune response specifically oriented against pancreatic islet β cells, the only cells secreting insulin according to the endocrine model. In accordance with the above hypothesis, *INS* transcripts were measured at lower levels in the thymus of human fetuses with short class I variable number of tandem repeats (VNTR) alleles, a genetic trait of T1D.[53,54] A very recent study also provided evidence that both *IDDM2* alleles and *AIRE* expression could influence the level of *INS* expression in the human thymus.[55]

THEORETICAL PRINCIPLES OF "NEGATIVE SELF-VACCINATION"

The study of neuroendocrine gene expression and precursor processing in the thymus led to the identification of neuroendocrine self-peptides. With regard to insulin-related gene expression in the thymus, IGF-2 —a prominent fetal growth factor—was identified as the dominant self-peptide precursor of the insulin family expressed in the thymus from different species. This observation is in close accordance with the theory of self-recognition, which, according to F.M. Burnet, is not an inherited property but is gradually acquired in the course of fetal life. Although the tolerogenic properties of neuroendocrine self-peptides remain to be further documented, they are strongly suspected from what is known about the immunological tolerance of classic hormones. The development of specific antibodies by active immunization (i.e., experimental breakdown of self-tolerance) revealed that OT is more tolerated than VP, and that IGF-2 is also more tolerated than IGF-1, and much more than insulin. Some cases of diabetes insipidus result from an autoimmune process against VP-producing hypothalamic neurons (infundibulohypothalamitis).[56–58] Insulin is the primary autoantigen tackled by the autoimmune response observed in T1D, and the intrinsic immunogenicity of insulin might result from its very low expression in the thymus. On the contrary, autoimmunity has never been observed against OT and IGF-2. The strong tolerance of these peptides, resulting from the high expression of *OT* and *IGF2* in the thymus, may be considered as the consequence of some evolutionary pressure to protect fundamental processes, such as species reproduction and individual ontogeny, respectively.[59–61] The putative pathogenic role of "forbidden" self-reactive T cells against IGF-2 deserves to be further analyzed through immunization of $Igf2^{-/-}$ mice.[62] In this latter model, nevertheless, the absence of IGF-2 was clearly shown to decrease immunological tolerance to insulin.

Thus, while VP and insulin behave as the immunogenic autoantigens of their respective families, OT and IGF-2 may be viewed as the tolerogenic self-peptide precursors of the neurohypophysial and insulin families, respectively. In this perspective, recent experiments have shown that, compared to insulin B9-23, the presentation of the homologous peptide sequence IGF-2 B11-25 to PBMC purified from DQ8+ T1D adolescents elicits a tolerogenic/regulatory profile with a higher IL-10/IFN-γ ratio and a lower IL-4 secretion.[63] Perhaps it is now appropriate to distinguish an autoantigen from a self-antigen, in the sense that peripheral autoantigens possess "altered" peptide sequences compared to homologous thymic self-antigens. Though they are highly evolutionarily related, they are not identical and this biochemical difference could drive completely opposite immune responses (i.e., immunogenic vs. tolerogenic responses). Undoubtedly, the reevaluation of thymus-dependent central self-tolerance will lead to the design of novel strategies to cure and prevent severe autoimmune diseases (such as T1D) that constitute the heavy tribute paid by mankind, for the diversity, complexity, and efficiency of human immune defenses.

ACKNOWLEDGMENTS

Vincent Geenen is Research Director at the National Fund of Scientific Research (NFSR) of Belgium. These studies are supported by NFSR (convention 3.4508.04), Fonds Leon Fredericq (Liège University Hospital), the Walloon Region (Waleo 2 convention Tolediab), the Fonds Vaugrenier pour la Recherche en Tolerance (Geneva), and the European Union FP6 Integrated Project Euro-Thymaide (contract LSHB-CT-2003-503410).

REFERENCES

1. ALDER, M.N., I.B. ROGOZIN, L.M. IYER, *et al.* 2005. Diversity and function of adaptive immune receptors in a jawless vertebrate. Science **310:** 1970–1973.
2. GEENEN, V., F. ROBERT, H. MARTENS, *et al.* 1992. The thymic education of developing T cells in self neuroendocrine principles. J. Endocrinol. Invest. **15:** 621–629.

3. KONG, F.K., C.H. CHEN & M.D. COOPER. 1998. Thymic function can be accurately monitored by the level of recent T cell emigrants in the circulation. Immunity **18:** 514–518.
4. DOUEK, D.C., R.D. MACFARLAND, P.H. KEISER, *et al.* 1998. Changes in thymic function with age and during the treatment of HIV infection. Nature **396:** 690–695.
5. SHEVACH, E.M. 2002. CD4+ CD25+ suppressor T cells: more questions than answers. Nat. Rev. Immunol. **2:** 389–400.
6. SAKAGUSHI, S. 2004. Naturally arising CD4+ regulatory T cells for immunologic self-tolerance and negative control of immune responses. Annu. Rev. Immunol. **22:** 531–562.
7. BLACKBURN, C.C. & N.R. MANLEY. 2004. Developing a new paradigm for thymus organogenesis. Nat. Rev. Immunol. **4:** 278–289.
8. BENNETT, A.R., A. FARLEY, N.F. BLAIR, *et al.* 2002. Identification and characterization of thymic epithelial progenitor cells. Immunity **16:** 803–814.
9. MANLEY, N.R. & M.R. CAPECCHI. 1995. The role of Hoxa-3 in mouse thymus and thyroid development. Development **121:** 1989–2003.
10. NEHLS, M., D. PFEIFFER, M. SCHORPP, *et al.* 1994. New member of the winged-helix protein family disrupted in mouse and rat nude mutations. Nature **372:** 103–106.
11. BALCIUNAITE, G., M.P. KELLER, E. BALCIUNAITE, *et al.* 2002. Wnt glycoproteins regulate the expression of Foxn1, the gene defective in nude mice. Nat. Immunol. **3:** 1102–1108.
12. GILL, J., M. MALIN, G. HOLLAENDER & R. BOYD. 2002. Generation of a complete thymic microenvironment by MTS24+ thymic epithelial cells. Nat. Immunol. **3:** 635–642.
13. ANDERSON, G. & E. JENKINSON. 2001. Lymphostromal interactions in thymus development and function. Nat. Rev. Immunol. **1:** 31–40.
14. BALDWIN, K.K., B.P. TRENCHAK, J.D. ALTMAN & M.M. DAVIS. 1999. Negative selection of T cells occurs throughout thymic development. J. Immunol. **163:** 689–698.
15. GEENEN, V., F. BRILOT, I. HANSENNE & H. MARTENS. 2003. Thymus and T cells. *In* Encyclopedia of Neuroscience, 3rd Edition on CD-ROM. G. ADELMAN & B.H. SMITH, Eds.: Elsevier. New York. ISBN 0-444-51432-5.
16. GEENEN, V., J.J. LEGROS, P. FRANCHIMONT, *et al.* 1986. The neuroendocrine thymus: coexistence of oxytocin and neurophysin in the human thymus. Science **232:** 508–511.
17. GEENEN, V., J.J. LEGROS, P. FRANCHIMONT, *et al.* 1987. The thymus as a neuroendocrine organ: synthesis of oxytocin and vasopressin in human thymic epithelium. Ann. N. Y. Acad. Sci. **496:** 56–66.
18. MARTENS, H., O. KECHA, C. CHARLET-RENARD, *et al.* 1998. Neurohypophysial peptides stimulate the phosphorylation of pre-T cell focal adhesion kinases. Neuroendocrinology **67:** 282–289.
19. ERICSSON, A., V. GEENEN, F. ROBERT, *et al.* 1990. Expression of preprotachykinin-A and neuropeptide-Y messenger RNA in the thymus. Mol. Endocr. **4:** 1211–1219.
20. GEENEN, V., I. ACHOUR, F. ROBERT, *et al.* 1993. Evidence that insulin-like growth factor 2 (IGF-2) is the dominant member of the insulin superfamily. Thymus **21:** 115–127.
21. JOLICŒUR, C., D. HANAHAN & K.M. SMITH. 1994. T-cell tolerance toward a transgenic beta-cell antigen and transcription of endogenous pancreatic genes in thymus. Proc. Natl. Acad. Sci. USA **91:** 6707–6711.

22. KECHA, O., H. MARTENS, N. FRANCHIMONT, *et al.* 1999. Characterization of the insulin-like growth factor axis in the human thymus. J. Neuroendocrinol. **11:** 435–440.
23. DERBINSKI, J., A. SCHULTE, B. KYEWSKI & L. KLEIN. 2001. Promiscuous gene expression in medullary thymic epithelial cells mirrors the peripheral self. Nat. Immunol. **2:** 1032–1039.
24. KECHA, O., F. BRILOT, H. MARTENS, *et al.* 2000. Involvement of insulin-like growth factors in early T-cell development: a study using fetal thymic organ cultures. Endocrinology **141:** 1209–1217.
25. HANSENNE, I., G. RASIER, C. PEQUEUX, *et al.* 2005. Ontogenesis and functional aspects of oxytocin and vasopressin gene expression in the thymus network. J. Neuroimmunol. **158:** 67–75.
26. HANSENNE, I., G. RASIER, C. CHARLET-RENARD, *et al.* 2004. Neurohypophysial receptor gene expression by thymic T cell subsets and thymic T cell lymphoma cell lines. Clin. Dev. Immunol. **11:** 45–51.
27. KYEWSKI, B. & L. KLEIN. 2006. The central role of central tolerance. Annu. Rev. Immunol. **24:** 571–605.
28. GEENEN, V. & G. KROEMER. 1993. Multiple ways to cellular immune tolerance. Immunol. Today **14:** 573–575.
29. THE FINNISH-GERMAN APECED CONSORTIUM. 1997. An autoimmune disease, APECED, caused by mutations in a novel gene featuring two PHD-type zinc-finger domains. Nat. Genet. **17:** 399–403.
30. NAGAMINE, K., P. PETERSON, H.S. SCOTT, *et al.* 1997. Positional cloning of the APECED gene. Nat. Genet. **17:** 393–398.
31. ANDERSON, M.S., E.S. VENANZI, L. KLEIN, *et al.* 2002. Projection of an immunological self-shadow within the thymus by the Aire protein. Science **298:** 1395–1401.
32. GOTTER, J., B. BRORS, M. HERGENHAHN & B. KYEWSKI. 2004. Medullary epithelial cells of the human thymus express a highly diverse selection of tissue-specific genes colocalized in chromosomal clusters. J. Exp. Med. **199:** 155–166.
33. DERBINSKI, J., J. GÄBLER, B. BRORS, *et al.* 2005. Promiscuous gene expression in thymic epithelial cells is regulated at multiple levels. J. Exp. Med. **202:** 33–45.
34. LISTON, A., D.H. GRAY, S. LESAGE, *et al.* 2004. Gene dosage-limiting role of Aire in thymic expression, clonal deletion, and organ-specific autoimmunity. J. Exp. Med. **200:** 1015–1026.
35. ANDERSON, M.S., E.S. VENANZI, Z. CHEN, *et al.* 2005. The cellular mechanism of Aire control of T cell tolerance. Immunity **23:** 227–239.
36. RAMSEY, C., S. HASSLER, P. MARITS, *et al.* 2006. Increased antigen presenting cell-mediated T cell activation in mice and patients without the autoimmune regulator. Eur. J. Immunol. **36:** 305–317.
37. BOEHM, T., S. SCHEU, K. PFEFFER & C.C. BLEUL. 2003. Thymic medullary epithelial cell development, thymocyte emigration, and the control of autoimmunity require lympho-epithelial cross talk via LtßR. J. Exp. Med. **198:** 757–769.
38. WATANABE, N., S. HANABUCHI, V. SOUMELIS, *et al.* 2004. Human thymic stromal lymphopoietin promotes dendritic cell-mediated CD4+ T cell homeostatic expansion. Nat. Immunol. **5:** 426–434.
39. MATHIS, D. & C. BENOIST. 2004. Back to central tolerance. Immunity **20:** 509–516.
40. FONTENOT, J.D., M.A. GAVIN & A.Y. RUDENSKY. 2003. Foxp3 programs the development and function of CD4+CD25+ regulatory T cells. Nat. Immunol. **4:** 330–336.

41. LIN, L., M.S. SPOOR, A.J. GERTH, *et al.* 2004. Modulation of Th1 activation and inflammation by the NF-kappaB repressor Foxj1. Science **303:** 1017–1020.

42. ALLEN, S., S. READ, R. DIPAOLO, *et al.* 2005. Promiscuous expression of an autoantigen gene does not result in negative selection of pathogenic T cells. J. Immunol. **175:** 5759–5764.

43. GEENEN, V., E. VANDERSMISSEN, N. CORMANN-GOFFIN, *et al.* 1993. Membrane translocation and relationship with MHC class I of a human thymic neurophysin-like domain. Thymus **22:** 55–66.

44. VAN DEN ELZEN, P., S. GARG, L. LEON, *et al.* 2005. Apolipoprotein-mediated pathways of lipid antigen presentation. Nature **437:** 906–910.

45. VANNESTE, Y., A. NTODOU-THOME, E. VANDERSMISSEN, *et al.* 1996. Identification of neurotensin-related peptides in human thymic epithelial cell membranes and relationship with major histocompatibility complex class I molecules. J. Neuroimmunol. **76:** 161–166.

46. ROBERT, F.R., H. MARTENS, N. CORMANN, *et al.* 1992. The recognition of hypothalamo-neurohypophysial functions by developing T cells. Dev. Immunol. **2:** 131–140.

47. BURNET, F.M. 1973. A reassessment of the forbidden clone hypothesis of autoimmune diseases. Aust. J. Exp. Biol. Med. Sci. **50:** 1–9.

48. KISHIMOTO, H. & J. SPRENT. 2001. A defect in central tolerance in NOD mice. Nat. Immunol. **2:** 1025–1031.

49. HEINO, M., P. PETERSON, N. SILANPÄÄ, *et al.* 2000. RNA and protein expression of the murine autoimmune regulator gene (Aire) in normal, RelB-deficient and in NOD mouse. Eur. J. Immunol. **30:** 1884–1893.

50. KECHA-KAMOUN, O., I. ACHOUR, H. MARTENS, *et al.* 2001. Thymic expression of insulin-related genes in an animal model of autoimmune type 1 diabetes. Diabetes Metab. Res. Rev. **17:** 146–152.

51. CHENTOUFI, A.A. & C. POLYCHRONAKOS. 2002. Insulin expression levels in the thymus modulate insulin-specific autoreactive T-cell tolerance: the mechanism by which the *IDDM2* locus may predispose to diabetes. Diabetes **51:** 1383–1390.

52. THEBAULT-BEAUMONT, K., D. DUBOIS-LAFORGUE, P. KRIEF, *et al.* 2003. Acceleration of type 1 diabetes mellitus in proinsulin 2-deficient mice. J. Clin. Invest. **111:** 851–857.

53. VAFIADIS, P., S.T. BENNETT, J.A. TODD, *et al.* 1997. Insulin expression in human thymus is modulated by *INS* VNTR alleles at the *IDDM2* locus. Nat. Genet. **15:** 289–292.

54. PUGLIESE, A., M. ZELLER, A. Fernandez, JR., *et al.* 1997. The insulin gene is transcribed in the human thymus and transcription levels correlated with allelic variation at the *INS* VNTR-*IDDM2* susceptibility locus for type 1 diabetes. Nat. Genet. **15:** 293–297.

55. SABATER, L., X. FERRER-FRANCESCH, M. SOSPEIDRA, *et al.* 2005. Insulin alleles and autoimmune regulator (AIRE) gene both influence insulin expression in the thymus. J. Autoimmun. **25:** 312–318.

56. SCHERBAUM, W.A., G.F. BOTTAZZO, P. CZERNICHOW, *et al.* 1985. Role of autoimmunity in central diabetes insipidus. Front. Horm. Res. **13:** 232–239.

57. IMURA, H., K. NAKAO, A. SHIMATSU, *et al.* 1993. Lymphocytic infundibulo-neurohypophysitis as a cause of central diabetes insipidus. N. Engl. J. Med. **329:** 683–687.

58. De Bellis, A., A. Bizzarro & A. Bellastella. 2004. Autoimmune central diabetes insipidus. *In* Immunoendocrinology in Health and Disease. V. Geenen & G.P. Chrousos, Eds.: 439–459. Marcel Dekker. New York.
59. Martens, H., B. Goxe & V. Geenen. 1996. The thymic repertoire of neuroendocrine self-antigens: physiological implications in T-cell life and death. Immunol. Today **17:** 312–317.
60. Geenen, V. 1995. La communication cryptocrine intrathymique et la tolerance immunitaire centrale au soi neuroendocrine. Professoral thesis, University of Liège.
61. Geenen, V., O. Kecha & H. Martens. 1999. Thymic expression of neuroendocrine self-peptide precursors: role in T cell survival and self-tolerance. J. Neuroendocrinol. **10:** 811–822.
62. Hansenne, I., C. Renard-Charlet, R. Greimers & V. Geenen. 2006. Dendritic cell differentiation and immune tolerance to insulin-related peptides in *Igf2*-deficient mice. J. Immunol. **176:** 4651–4657.
63. Geenen, V., C. Louis, H. Martens & The Belgian Diabetes Registry. 2004. An insulin-like growth factor 2-derived self-antigen inducing a regulatory cytokine profile after presentation to peripheral blood mononuclear cells from DQ8+ Type 1 diabetic adolescents: preliminary design of a thymus-based tolerogenic self-vaccination. Ann. N. Y. Acad. Sci. **1037:** 59–64.

Molecular Understanding of Cytokine–Steroid Hormone Dialogue

Implications for Human Diseases

JIMENA DRUKER,[a] ANA C. LIBERMAN,[a,b] MATÍAS ACUÑA,[a]
DAMIANA GIACOMINI,[a,b] DAMIÁN REFOJO,[a,b]
SUSANA SILBERSTEIN,[a,b] MARCELO PAEZ PEREDA,[c,d]
GÜNTER K. STALLA,[d] FLORIAN HOLSBOER,[d] AND EDUARDO ARZT[a,b]

[a]*Laboratorio de Fisiología y Biología Molecular, Departamento de Fisiología y Biología Molecular y Celular, Facultad de Ciencias Exactas y Naturales (FCEN), Universidad de Buenos Aires, Ciudad Universitaria, Pabellón II, (C1428EHA), Buenos Aires, Argentina*

[b]*Members of the IFYBINE-Argentine National Research Council (CONICET) Ciudad Universitaria, Pabellón II, Buenos Aires, Argentina*

[c]*Affectis Pharmaceuticals, Kraepelinstrasse 2, 80804 Munich, Germany*

[d]*Max-Planck Institute of Psychiatry, Kraepelinstrasse 2-10, 80804 Munich, Germany*

ABSTRACT: Highly sophisticated mechanisms confer upon the immune system the capacity to respond with a certain degree of autonomy. However, the final outcome of an adaptive immune response depends on the interaction with other systems of the organism. The immune–neuroendocrine systems have an intimate cross-communication, making possible a satisfactory response to environmental changes. Part of this interaction occurs through cytokines and steroid hormones. The last step of this crosstalk is at the molecular level. In this article we will focus on the physical and functional interrelationship between cytokine signaling pathway–activated transcription factors (TFs) and steroid receptors in different cell models, where the signals triggered by cytokines and steroid hormones have major roles: (1) the ligand-dependent-activated glucocorticoid receptor (GR) influence the genetic program that specifies lineage commitment in T helper (Th) cell differentiation. How post-translational modifications of several TFs as well as nuclear hormone receptors could be implicated in the molecular crosstalk between the immune–neuroendocrine messengers is discussed. (2) glucocorticoid (GC) antagonism on the TCR-induced T cell apoptosis. (3) estrogen receptor/TGF-β family proteins molecular interaction implicated on

Address for correspondence: Dr. Eduardo Arzt, Laboratorio de Fisiología y Biología Molecular, FCEN-Universidad de Buenos Aires, Ciudad Universitaria, Pabellón II (C1428EHA), Buenos Aires, Argentina. Voice: 54-11-4576-3368; fax: 54-11-4576-3321.
e-mail: earzt@fbmc.fcen.uba.ar.

Ann. N.Y. Acad. Sci. 1088: 297–306 (2006). © 2006 New York Academy of Sciences.
doi: 10.1196/annals.1366.007

pituitary prolactinomas pathogenesis. The functional crosstalk at the molecular level between immune and steroids signals is essential to determine an integrative response to both mediators (which in the last instance results in a new gene activation/repression profile) and constitutes the ultimate integrative level of interaction between the immune and neuroendocrine systems.

KEY WORDS: glucocorticoids; cAMP; TCR; apoptosis; GATA-3; T-bet; Th1-Th2 differentiation; BMP-4; TGF-β; prolactinoma; estrogens

INTRODUCTION

The immune system is composed of a large variety of cells and molecules. It operates by a complex network of regulatory mechanisms that are able to confer on it a certain degree of autonomy. However, animal homeostasis is sustained by a group of systems that do not operate in isolation. Mutual influences between them are fundamental to make possible a satisfactory response to environmental changes. The existence of physiological interactions between the neuroendocrine and immune systems is reflected by the fact that several neuroendocrine responses occur during immune cell activation. Some of the main communicators between the immune and neuroendocrine systems are hormones and cytokines. Through these molecules cells receive information which, after processing, produces a biological response. Sustained activation of the immune system leads to an increase in both cytokine and steroid hormone blood levels. Immune responses elicit the production of soluble factors, such as tumor necrosis factor-alpha (TNF-α), interleukin (IL)-1 and IL-6, which stimulate the hypothalamus-pituitary-adrenal axis (HPA). One of the results of this activation is the elevation of circulating glucocorticoids (GCs).[1,2] Thus, a new metabolic hormonal state facilitates a homeostatic balance that limits some features of the immune reaction. The steroid receptors act both as transcription factors (TFs) themselves and as modulators of other TFs. The biological effect of cytokines and steroids is achieved by the activation of signaling cascades that elicit a specific gene expression program. Highly regulated go–stop signals between cytokines and steroid hormones are required to prevent cytokine overreaction. The ultimate level of integration of cytokine–steroid crosstalk is the molecular level.[3,4] It is widely known that the immunomodulatory actions of GCs are exerted by interfering with the proinflammatory signaling process.[4,5] Glucocorticoid receptor (GR) regulates gene transcription through DNA-dependent[6,7] and -independent mechanisms.[8–10] However, the most important anti-inflammatory effects of GCs occur independent of GR–DNA binding through direct inhibition of TF activity by a transrepression mechanism, which results in protein–protein interaction. The GR interacts with activator protein 1 (AP-1), nuclear factor-κB (NF-κB), and signal transducers and activators of transcription (STATs) that control proinflammatory gene expression.[11] GCs also play a pivotal role in the regulation of the balance between Th1/Th2 subset during the immune response.[3,12,13] This occurs by interaction with transcriptional activity of T helper (Th) 1/Th2 TFs, T box expressed in T cells (T-bet) and GATA-3. Since the transcriptional activity of steroid receptors and TFs may be regulated by posttranslational modifications,[14] how such modifications could modulate the molecular crosstalk between the immune–neuroendocrine systems will also be discussed. GCs are able to induce apoptosis in T cells but also can counteract the signals of death, leading to cell survival.[3,15] T cell apoptosis is a physiological process that facilitates immune response regulation. T cell receptor (TCR) stimulation induces apoptosis in T cells and GCs exert an antiapoptotic effect on T cell activation–induced cell death.[16–18] These molecular mechanisms will also be discussed in this article. Similar to GCs, estrogens exert several roles not only in the female reproductive system, but also in other systems. Transforming growth factor-β (TGF-β) and bone morphogenetic proteins (BMPs) transduce signals through Smad-4, a signal cotransducer. This pathway regulates the expression of proto-oncogenes that control cell proliferation. The physical and functional interaction between Smad proteins and estrogen receptor that takes place in pituitary cells[19] will be also discussed in detail.

GC INTERACTION WITH Th FACTORS

Naive Th cells differentiate into two different functional subsets known as Th1 and Th2 cells, respectively.[20,21] There are several factors that determine the fate of Th cells, the most important being cytokine environment and the presence of specific TFs, T-bet and GATA-3, which are selectively expressed in Th1 and Th2 cells, respectively.[22,23] Th1 cells secrete interferon-gamma (IFN-γ) and IL-2 and Th2 lymphocytes produce IL-4, IL-5, IL-10, and IL-13. When T-bet and GATA-3 are ectopically expressed, they increase cytokine production of their own subset[24,25] (Th1 and Th2, respectively) and at the same time inhibit the opposite subset differentiation and cytokine production.[23,25,26] Some reports have shown that GCs favor Th2 differentiation,[27,28] whereas others have shown that GCs inhibit Th2 polarization measured as Th1/2 cytokine synthesis and expression.[29,30] Above all, there is little evidence about the molecular mechanisms implicated in Th cell polarization by GCs.[31,32] Therefore, we studied the interaction between GCs, T-bet, and GATA-3. Experiments in undifferentiated splenocytes showed a strong direct inhibition of T-bet and GATA-3 expression by GCs. In addition, GCs inhibited T-bet and to a lesser degree GATA-3 transcriptional activity. We also analyzed the molecular mechanisms involved in this differential inhibition and found that transrepression was the mechanism by which GCs inhibited T-bet activity, but not GATA-3. Therefore, GCs inhibitory effect is stronger on Th1 cells, supporting the notion that a differential inhibition of T-bet and GATA-3 may be the way by which

GCs induce Th2 differentiation. As shown in the example of T-bet, NF-κB, and AP-1, GRs interact with each other by protein–protein interaction. This may be further modified by posttranslational modifications. Transcriptional activity of steroid receptors as well as several TFs may be up- or downregulated by posttranslational modifications. Proteins can be modified by phosphorylation, acetylation, prenylation and even by covalent attachment of polypeptides, such as ubiquitin and small ubiquitin-related modifier (SUMO).[14,33,34] The most widely known function of the ubiquitin system is the selective degradation of targeted proteins by proteasome machinery.[35] On the other hand, SUMO modification regulates different cellular processes including subcellular localization, transactivation activity, protein–protein interactions,[36] and in particular situations SUMO covalently modified proteins that are able to avoid ubiquitin-mediated degradation, such is the case of the inhibitor of κB (I-κB).[37,38] One of the most important mechanisms by which cytokines transduce signals that elicit specific responses in target cells involves enzymes called Janus kinases (JAKs) and TFs called signal transducers and activators of transcription, STATs.[39] Protein inhibitor of activated STAT (PIAS) proteins (SUMO E3 ligases) were originally discovered as transcriptional coregulators of JAK–STAT pathway and subsequent studies have shown that PIAS proteins are implicated in the regulation of the activity of several TFs[39–41] and steroid receptors.[42,43] GR is modified by SUMO and this covalent modification regulates the stability of the GR and potentiates its transactivation activity.[44] However, sumoylation of androgen receptor (AR) represses AR-dependent transcription.[45] Nuclear targets of many cytokine signaling pathways (STATs, AP1, NF-κB) are sumoylated as are steroid receptors,[33,39,46,47] suggesting that SUMO modification of these proteins could play a key role in steroid hormone–cytokine interaction.

GCs AND T CELL APOPTOSIS

In T cells, stimulation with either TCR or GCs induces apoptosis, and simultaneous addition of both results in cell survival.[16,17] Interestingly, cAMP, which is regulated by several neurotransmitters, such as vasoactive intestinal polypeptide (VIP), interacts with this system. cAMP inhibits apoptosis induced by TCR activation and also potentiates the apoptosis induced by GCs in the same cells, suggesting that cAMP might play an important role in adjusting T cells to the pro- and antiapoptotic stimulus.[18] cAMP also potentiates GC-induced glucocorticoid response element (GRE) activity cloned upstream of the luciferase gene. A dominant negative form of the protein kinase A (PKA) is able to block the effect of cAMP on GRE, suggesting that the effect of cAMP on GC-induced apoptosis is dependent on PKA activation. Gel shift experiments have shown that addition of cAMP enhances GR binding to GRE, a mechanism that is independent of GR concentration, as shown by the Western blot analysis of GR expression. Therefore, cAMP induces PKA, which potentiates the GR-dependent transcriptional activity and apoptosis by regulating GR binding to the DNA. Adding H89 (a pharmacological inhibitor of PKA), which reverts TCR-induced apoptosis, and CRE, oligo decoy targeting strategies indicate that cAMP inhibits TCR-induced cell death through PKA and at least partially through CREB-like TFs. TCR-induced apoptosis involves Fas ligand (FasL) induction.[48] RT-PCR analysis has also shown that cAMP inhibition of TCR-induced FasL expression is blocked by H89 and is therefore mediated by PKA, whereas GC inhibition of TCR-induced FasL expression is blocked by adding RU38486 and is therefore dependent on the GR. The inhibition exerted by GCs and cAMP on TCR-induced cell death is associated with the inhibition of NF-κB and Erk1/2 activation, and also to the blockage of the transcriptional induction of FasL expression (D. Refojo and E. Arzt, unpublished results). During stress conditions, several neurotransmitters are released. These molecules are able to regulate the levels of cAMP, so during such events a strong influence of the modulatory action of cAMP in the crosstalk at the transcriptional level between GCs and the TCR signaling pathway may take place.

CROSSTALK BETWEEN TGF-β SUPERFAMILY CYTOKINES AND STEROID HORMONES

Prolactinomas are the most frequent pituitary functional tumors in humans. Growth factors and estrogens are also known to be involved in the control of lactotroph cell proliferation. The tumorigenic action of estrogen in prolactinoma development has been shown *in vitro* as well as by clinical evidence. Members of the TGF-β superfamily also exert inhibitory effects on prolactinomas;[49,50] in addition, TGF-β inhibits c-Myc expression.[51,52] Recently, we have demonstrated that BMP-4 (a member of the TGF-β superfamily) is overexpressed in different prolactinoma models including not only dopamine 2 receptor knockout (D2R-/-) mice, but also estradiol-induced rat and human prolactinomas, as compared to normal tissue and other pituitary adenoma types.[19] BMP-4 intracellular signaling is mediated by Smad-4 and in order to study the role of BMP-4 in tumor formation in nude mice we produced GH3 clones stably transfected with a Smad-4-dominant negative construct (GH3-Smad-4dn). GH3-Smad-4dn cells formed small, lows-growing tumors that did not express c-Myc as compared to control cells, demonstrating the involvement of BMP-4 in promoting prolactinoma development. Furthermore, we have also shown that cell proliferation is upregulated by an overlapping intracellular signaling mechanism between BMP-4 and estrogens, and that their action was partially inhibited by blocking either pathways with the reciprocal antagonist. Indeed, we demonstrated by coimmunoprecipitation studies that Smad proteins physically interact with the ER.[19] When GH3 cells were treated with BMP-4, TGF-β, or 17-β-estradiol, coimmunoprecipitation of ER-α/ER-β, and Smad-4 was detected. On the contrary, coimmunoprecipitation of ER-α/ER-β and Smad-1 (a BMP-4-specific Smad-transducer protein) was detected only in the presence of BMP-4 or 17-β-estradiol, and coimmunoprecipitation of ER-α/ER-β and Smad-2 (TGF-β-specific Smad-transducer proteins) was detected only in the presence of TGF-β or 17-β-estradiol.[19] These results demonstrated that different proteins are involved in the ER/Smad complex upon stimulation. The nature of this complex may change not only the transcriptional activity of the proteins involved, but also the transcriptional regulation of the target promoters. Moreover, the crosstalk between estrogen and TGF-β/BMP-4 cytokines may be present not only in the prolactinoma cells but also in other cells, such as those of the breast and bone, in which both estrogens and the TGF-β superfamily

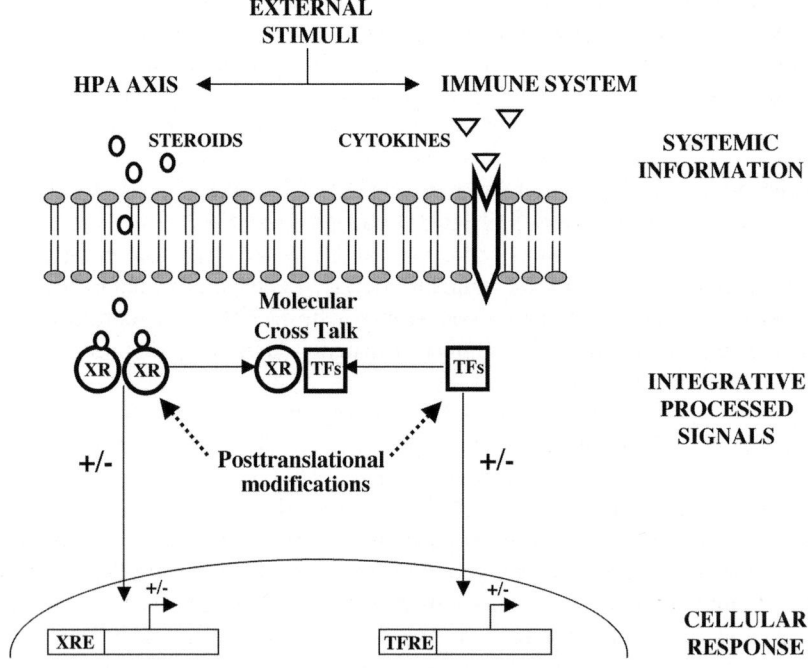

TARGET GENE EXPRESSION BALANCE

FIGURE 1. External stimuli may induce the immune system to activate the HPA axis. The result of this activation is an increase of systemic cytokines and steroid hormone levels, which are able to trigger multiple signaling cascade pathways in target cells. The cross-interaction of target proteins of these signaling pathways leads to an integrative cell response, which is reflected by a new gene activation/repression profile. Posttranslational modification of steroid receptors and TFs could be involved in the regulation of signaling crosstalk among the immune and neuroendocrine systems. XR = steroid receptors; RE = DNA response element; TFs = transcription factors.

play important roles,[53,54] implicating similar mechanisms in the progression of other diseases.

CONCLUSIONS

A coordinated functional interaction between the immune and neuroendocrine systems is essential to develop an adaptive response to environmental changes. The goal of this process is achieved by the molecular interaction of each system: cytokines and steroid hormones. As shown in FIGURE 1 the molecular crosstalk between immune and endocrine signals occurs at the cellular level, where the signaling pathways triggered by these messengers cross-interact and are mutually influenced, with functional consequences that will determine the final cell response. Inside this network, posttranslational modification of target proteins is important for signal-dependent regulation of protein activity and also for gene expression–repression profile. Increased understanding of how systemic information is integrated at cellular and molecular levels will help to elucidate the intimate cross-communication between signaling triggered by steroid hormones and cytokines in both immune and nonimmune cells. The elicited biological response achieved by each cell will result from the balance of overlapping signals released by the immune and neuroendocrine systems in response to external or internal environmental factors. Understanding how this information is integrated at the molecular level is a challenge to further dissect the complex interaction of these systems and its impact on human diseases, providing new molecular targets for pharmacological approaches.

ACKNOWLEDGMENTS

This work was supported by grants from the University of Buenos Aires, the Argentine National Research Council (CONICET), and Agencia Nacional de Promoción Científica y Tecnológica-Argentina. Jimena Druker is a recipient of a fellowship "Beca José A. Estenssoro Fundación YPF," Argentina.

REFERENCES

1. BESEDOVSKY, H.O. & A. DEL REY. 1992. Immune-neuroendocrine circuits: integrative role of cytokines. Front. Neuroendocrinol. **13:** 61–94.
2. WICK, G. *et al.* 1993. Immunoendocrine communication via the hypothalamo-pituitary-adrenal axis in autoimmune diseases. Endocr. Rev. **14:** 539–563.
3. REFOJO, D. *et al.* 2003. Integrating systemic information at the molecular level: cross-talk between steroid receptors and cytokine signaling on different target cells. Ann. N. Y. Acad. Sci. **992:** 196–204.

4. REFOJO, D. *et al.* 2001. Transcription factor-mediated molecular mechanisms involved in the functional cross-talk between cytokines and glucocorticoids. Immunol. Cell. Biol. **79:** 385–394.

5. RICCARDI, C., S. BRUSCOLI & G. MIGLIORATI. 2002. Molecular mechanisms of immunomodulatory activity of glucocorticoids. Pharmacol. Res. **45:** 361–368.

6. AUPHAN, N. *et al.* 1995. Immunosuppression by glucocorticoids: inhibition of NF-kappa B activity through induction of I kappa B synthesis. Science **270:** 286–290.

7. SCHEINMAN, R.I. *et al.* 1995. Role of transcriptional activation of I kappa B alpha in mediation of immunosuppression by glucocorticoids. Science **270:** 283–286.

8. REICHARDT, H.M. *et al.* 2001. Repression of inflammatory responses in the absence of DNA binding by the glucocorticoid receptor. EMBO J. **20:** 7168–7173.

9. CALDENHOVEN, E. *et al.* 1995. Negative cross-talk between RelA and the glucocorticoid receptor: a possible mechanism for the antiinflammatory action of glucocorticoids. Mol. Endocrinol. **9:** 401–412.

10. DE BOSSCHER, K., W. VANDEN BERGHE & G. HAEGEMAN. 2003. The interplay between the glucocorticoid receptor and nuclear factor-kappaB or activator protein-1: molecular mechanisms for gene repression. Endocr. Rev. **24:** 488–522.

11. STOCKLIN, E. *et al.* 1996. Functional interactions between Stat5 and the glucocorticoid receptor. Nature **383:** 726–728.

12. KOVALOVSKY, D. *et al.* 2000. Molecular mechanisms and Th1/Th2 pathways in corticosteroid regulation of cytokine production. J. Neuroimmunol. **109:** 23–29.

13. LIBERMAN, A.C., D. REFOJO & E. ARZT. 2003. Cytokine signaling/transcription factor cross-talk in T cell activation and Th1-Th2 differentiation. Arch. Immunol. Ther. Exp. (Warsz) **51:** 351–365.

14. MELCHIOR, F. 2000. SUMO–nonclassical ubiquitin. Annu. Rev. Cell. Dev. Biol. **16:** 591–626.

15. JAMIESON, C.A. & K.R. YAMAMOTO. 2000. Crosstalk pathway for inhibition of glucocorticoid-induced apoptosis by T cell receptor signaling. Proc. Natl. Acad. Sci. USA **97:** 7319–7324.

16. ZACHARCHUK, C.M. *et al.* 1990. Programmed T lymphocyte death. Cell activation- and steroid-induced pathways are mutually antagonistic. J. Immunol. **145:** 4037–4045.

17. ASHWELL, J.D., F.W. LU & M.S. VACCHIO. 2000. Glucocorticoids in T cell development and function. Annu. Rev. Immunol. **18:** 309–345.

18. MULLER IGAZ, L. *et al.* 2002. CRE-mediated transcriptional activation is involved in cAMP protection of T-cell receptor-induced apoptosis but not in cAMP potentiation of glucocorticoid-mediated programmed cell death. Biochim. Biophys. Acta **1542:** 139–148.

19. PAEZ-PEREDA, M. *et al.* 2003. Involvement of bone morphogenetic protein 4 (BMP-4) in pituitary prolactinoma pathogenesis through a Smad/estrogen receptor crosstalk. Proc. Natl. Acad. Sci. USA **100:** 1034–1039.

20. ABBAS, A.K., K.M. MURPHY & A. SHER. 1996. Functional diversity of helper T lymphocytes. Nature **383:** 787–793.

21. MOSMANN, T.R. & R.L. COFFMAN. 1989. TH1 and TH2 cells: different patterns of lymphokine secretion lead to different functional properties. Annu. Rev. Immunol. **7:** 145–173.

22. ZHANG, D.H. *et al.* 1997. Transcription factor GATA-3 is differentially expressed in murine Th1 and Th2 cells and controls Th2-specific expression of the interleukin-5 gene. J. Biol. Chem. **272:** 21597–21603.

23. Szabo, S.J. *et al.* 2000. A novel transcription factor, T-bet, directs Th1 lineage commitment. Cell **100**: 655–669.
24. Zheng, W. & R.A. Flavell. 1997. The transcription factor GATA-3 is necessary and sufficient for Th2 cytokine gene expression in CD4 T cells. Cell **89**: 587–596.
25. Ferber, I.A. *et al.* 1999. GATA-3 significantly downregulates IFN-gamma production from developing Th1 cells in addition to inducing IL-4 and IL-5 levels. Clin. Immunol. **91**: 134–144.
26. Ouyang, W. *et al.* 1998. Inhibition of Th1 development mediated by GATA-3 through an IL-4-independent mechanism. Immunity **9**: 745–755.
27. Miyaura, H. & M. Iwata. 2002. Direct and indirect inhibition of Th1 development by progesterone and glucocorticoids. J. Immunol. **168**: 1087–1094.
28. Blotta, M.H., R.H. DeKruyff & D.T. Umetsu. 1997. Corticosteroids inhibit IL-12 production in human monocytes and enhance their capacity to induce IL-4 synthesis in CD4+ lymphocytes. J. Immunol. **158**: 5589–5595.
29. Mori, A. *et al.* 1997. Two distinct pathways of interleukin-5 synthesis in allergen-specific human T-cell clones are suppressed by glucocorticoids. Blood **89**: 2891–2900.
30. Hu, X. *et al.* 2003. Inhibition of IFN-gamma signaling by glucocorticoids. J. Immunol. **170**: 4833–4839.
31. Jee, Y.K. *et al.* 2005. Repression of interleukin-5 transcription by the glucocorticoid receptor targets GATA3 signaling and involves histone deacetylase recruitment. J. Biol. Chem. **280**: 23243–23250.
32. Franchimont, D. *et al.* 2000. Inhibition of Th1 immune response by glucocorticoids: dexamethasone selectively inhibits IL-12-induced Stat4 phosphorylation in T lymphocytes. J. Immunol. **164**: 1768–1774.
33. Gill, G. 2004. SUMO and ubiquitin in the nucleus: different functions, similar mechanisms? Genes Dev. **18**: 2046–2059.
34. Hay, R.T. 2005. SUMO: a history of modification. Mol. Cell. **18**: 1–12.
35. Hershko, A. 2005. The ubiquitin system for protein degradation and some of its roles in the control of the cell-division cycle (Nobel lecture). Angew Chem. Int. Ed. Engl. **44**: 5932–5943.
36. Pichler, A. & F. Melchior. 2002. Ubiquitin-related modifier SUMO1 and nucleocytoplasmic transport. Traffic **3**: 381–387.
37. Desterro, J.M., M.S. Rodriguez & R.T. Hay. 1998. SUMO-1 modification of IkappaBalpha inhibits NF-kappaB activation. Mol. Cell. **2**: 233–239.
38. Hay, R.T. *et al.* 1999. Control of NF-kappa B transcriptional activation by signal induced proteolysis of I kappa B alpha. Philos. Trans. R. Soc. Lond. B Biol., Sci. **354**: 1601–1609.
39. Carbia-Nagashima, A. & E. Arzt. 2004. Intracellular proteins and mechanisms involved in the control of gp130/JAK/STAT cytokine signaling. IUBMB Life **56**: 83–88.
40. Kotaja, N. *et al.* 2002. PIAS proteins modulate transcription factors by functioning as SUMO-1 ligases. Mol. Cell. Biol. **22**: 5222–5234.
41. Jang, H.D. *et al.* 2004. PIAS3 suppresses NF-kappaB-mediated transcription by interacting with the p65/RelA subunit. J. Biol. Chem. **279**: 24873–24880.
42. Nishida, T. & H. Yasuda. 2002. PIAS1 and PIASxalpha function as SUMO-E3 ligases toward androgen receptor and repress androgen receptor-dependent transcription. J. Biol. Chem. **277**: 41311–41317.
43. Kotaja, N. *et al.* 2000. ARIP3 (androgen receptor-interacting protein 3) and other PIAS (protein inhibitor of activated STAT) proteins differ in their ability to

modulate steroid receptor-dependent transcriptional activation. Mol. Endocrinol. **14:** 1986–2000.

44. LE DREAN, Y. *et al.* 2002. Potentiation of glucocorticoid receptor transcriptional activity by sumoylation. Endocrinology **143:** 3482–3489.

45. POUKKA, H. *et al.* 2000. Covalent modification of the androgen receptor by small ubiquitin-like modifier 1 (SUMO-1). Proc. Natl. Acad. Sci. USA **97:** 14145–14150.

46. BOSSIS, G. *et al.* 2005. Down-regulation of c-Fos/c-Jun AP-1 dimer activity by sumoylation. Mol. Cell. Biol. **25:** 6964–6979.

47. GILL, G. 2005. Something about SUMO inhibits transcription. Curr. Opin. Genet. Dev. **15:** 536–541.

48. KASIBHATLA, S., L. GENESTIER & D.R. GREEN. 1999. Regulation of fas-ligand expression during activation-induced cell death in T lymphocytes via nuclear factor kappaB. J. Biol. Chem. **274:** 987–992.

49. DELIDOW, B.C. *et al.* 1991. Inhibition of prolactin gene transcription by transforming growth factor-beta in GH3 cells. Mol. Endocrinol. **5:** 1716–1722.

50. RAMSDELL, J.S. 1991. Transforming growth factor-alpha and -beta are potent and effective inhibitors of GH4 pituitary tumor cell proliferation. Endocrinology **128:** 1981–190.

51. COFFEY, R.J., JR. *et al.* 1988. Selective inhibition of growth-related gene expression in murine keratinocytes by transforming growth factor beta. Mol. Cell. Biol. **8:** 3088–3093.

52. CHEN, C.R., Y. KANG & J. MASSAGUE. 2001. Defective repression of c-myc in breast cancer cells: a loss at the core of the transforming growth factor beta growth arrest program. Proc. Natl. Acad. Sci. USA **98:** 992–999.

53. MASSAGUE, J., S.W. BLAIN & R.S. LO. 2000. TGFbeta signaling in growth control, cancer, and heritable disorders. Cell **103:** 295–309.

54. KARSENTY, G. 1999. The genetic transformation of bone biology. Genes Dev. **13:** 3037–3051.

The Role of Toll-like Receptors in the Immune–Adrenal Crosstalk

S.R. BORNSTEIN,[a] C.G. ZIEGLER,[a] A.W. KRUG,[a] W. KANCZKOWSKI,[a]
V. RETTORI,[b] S.M. McCANN,[b] M. WIRTH,[c] AND K. ZACHAROWSKI[d]

[a]Department of Anesthesiology, Heinrich Heine University,
Düsseldorf, 40225, Germany

[b]Centro de Estudios Farmacologicos y Botanicos, Consejo Nacional de
Investigaciones Cientificas y Tecnicas, 1414 Buenos Aires, Argentina

[c]Department of Urology, Carl Gustav Carus University Hospital, University of
Dresden, Dresden, Germany

[d]Department of Anaesthesiology, Heinrich Heine University, 40225 Düsseldorf,
Germany

ABSTRACT: Sepsis and septic shock remain major health concerns worldwide, and rapid activation of adrenal steroid release is a key event in the
organism's first line of defense during this form of severe illness. Toll-
like receptors (TLRs) are critical in the early immune response upon
bacterial infection, and recent data from our lab demonstrate a novel
link between the innate immune system and the adrenal stress response
mediated by TLRs. Glucocorticoids and TLRs regulate each other in
a bidirectional way. Bacterial toxins acting through TLRs directly activate adrenocortical steroid release. TLR-2 and TLR-4 are expressed in
human and mice adrenals and TLR-2 deficiency is associated with an impaired glucocorticoid response. Furthermore, TLR-2 deficiency in mice
is associated with marked cellular alterations in adrenocortical tissue.
TLR-2-deficient mice have an impaired adrenal corticosterone release
following inflammatory stress induced by bacterial cell wall compounds.
This defect appears to be associated with a decrease in systemic and intraadrenal cytokine expression. In conclusion, TLRs play a crucial role
in the immune–adrenal crosstalk. This close functional relationship needs
to be considered in the treatment of inflammatory diseases requiring an
intact adrenal stress response.

KEYWORDS: toll-like receptors; knockout; bidirectional regulation; LPA

Address for correspondence: Prof. Dr. Stefan R. Bornstein, Department of Medicine III, Carl Gustav Carus Medical School, University of Technology, Dresden, Fetscherstrasse 74, 01307 Dresden,
Germany. Voice: +49-351-458-5955; fax: +49-351-458-6398.
  e-mail: Stefan.Bornstein@uniklinikum-dresden.de

Ann. N.Y. Acad. Sci. 1088: 307–318 (2006). © 2006 New York Academy of Sciences.
doi: 10.1196/annals.1366.027

THE BIOLOGICAL IMPORTANCE
OF TOLL-LIKE RECEPTORS

Toll-like receptors (TLRs) play a crucial role in the innate immunity in mammals. Mammalian TLRs were originally found as homologues of the *Drosophila* Toll,[1] where it plays a key role in the establishment of dorsoventral polarity as well as in antifungal and antibacterial host defence. TLRs are type I transmembrane receptors that possess extracellular leucine-rich repeat domains flanked by cytoplasmatic domains. These extracellular domains can be considered as family pattern recognition receptors for the detection and response to microbial ligands. The initial host defense against bacterial infection by the innate immune system is essentially executed by these receptors. Particularly, TLR-2 and TLR-4 polymorphisms are frequent in humans. There is good evidence that impaired innate immunity mediated by TLRs is involved in sepsis and cardiovascular disease.[2-4] Several studies investigated the existence of TLR mutations in humans. TLR-2 Arg753Gln polymorphism, positively correlating with the incidence of sepsis in a white population, and a TLR-2 Arg677Trp polymorphism, correlating with the incidence of lepromatous leprosy in an Asian population, have been demonstrated.[4,5] A recent study reported a rate of nearly 10% heterozygosity for the TLR-2 Arg753Gln polymorphism,[6] suggesting clinical relevance of the TLR-2 gene during inflammation. Although the existence of a high rate of TLR-2 and TLR-4 polymorphisms in humans is shown, the role of TLR-2 and TLR-4 in the endocrine stress response during development and progression of inflammatory complications has only inadequately been investigated so far.

WHAT ARE THE FUNCTIONS OF THE DIFFERENT
MEMBERS OF THE TLR FAMILY?

To date, at least 10 members of the TLR family have been identified in humans, and several ligands recognized by TLRs have been reported. TLR-2 is expressed mainly by peripheral blood monocytes and is involved in the recognition of gram-positive bacteria and other components of different pathogens.[7] It has been shown that TLR-1 coexpressed with TLR-6 enhances the TLR-2 response.[8] TLR-4 has been implicated in lipopolysaccharide (LPS) signaling, innate immunity and inflammation. TLR-3 and 5–9 are mainly involved in the recognition of a double-stranded RNA of viruses and certain bacterial components. The role of TLR-10 remains obscure, although an expression in the spleen and lung could be documented so far. For further reading on TLR, refer to Nishimura and Naito.[9]

During the last 10 years, our lab has focused on the interaction of immune cells and their mediators with the hypothalamic-pituitary-adrenal (HPA) axis employing *in situ* hybridization, microarray analysis, immunohistochemistry, laser capture microdissection, organ perfusion, cell culture/co-culture systems, and animal models.[10–15] We have characterized the role of lymphocytes, cytokines, adipo-cytokines, and chemokines in the adrenal gland.[16–22] The nature of this immune–endocrine crosstalk is implicated in adrenal dysfunction and disease.[23–25] During inflammatory and autoimmune disorders, including sepsis, inflammatory bowel disease, and rheumatoid arthritis, immune–adrenal crosstalk becomes more critical in maintaining adequate adrenal stress response.[23,25–27]

GLUCOCORTICOIDS AND TOLL-LIKE RECEPTOR SHOW A BIDIRECTIONAL REGULATION

In addition to hypothalamic hormones, including corticotrophin-releasing hormone (CRH) and vasopressin, inflammatory cytokines such as IL-1, IL-6, and TNF-α have been identified as important modulators of the HPA axis in physiological as well as pathological situations. During inflammation, these cytokines are capable of maintaining high glucocorticoid output, suggesting a shift from neuroendocrine to immune–endocrine regulation of the adrenal during septicemia.[28] In turn, enhanced adrenal glucocorticoid release is required to prevent an uncontrolled response of inflammatory cytokines, which could result in severe damage to the cardiovascular system. Therefore, a coordinated response of the adrenal and immune system is crucial for survival during severe inflammation and sepsis.[29–31]

New data from other groups demonstrate that glucocorticoids have an influence on TLR expression. This suggests a role for glucocorticoids in the innate immune system. Although TNF-α and glucocorticoids are widely recognized as mutually antagonistic regulators of adaptive immunity and inflammation, they cooperatively regulate the components of the innate immunity like the TLR-2 expression via signal transducers and activators of transcription (STAT) and NF-κB signaling.[32] Furthermore, glucocorticoids synergistically enhance the IL-1β-induced TLR-2 expression, via upregulation of MAPK phosphatase-1 (MKP-1) expression, which, in turn, leads to the inactivation of both p38 and Jun kinase (JNK) signaling pathways, the negative regulators for TLR-2 induction.[32]

In one of our studies bidirectional action of glucocorticoids with both immunostimulatory, as well as immunosuppressive function during inflammation could be documented by gene expression profiling and reverse transcriptase polymerase chain reaction.[17] In this study, numerous newly discovered genes, playing critical roles in innate and adaptive immune responses, were found to be regulated by glucocorticoids in peripheral blood monocytes. In a global gene expression analysis, nearly 10,000 human-expressed genes were screened and 9% were considered to be down- and 12% to be upregulated by glucocorticoids. They could thus act as anti-inflammatory agents by downregulation of proinflammatory cytokines as IL-1, lymphotoxin-β, IL-1-a, IL-8, IFN-α, and IFN-β, and upregulation of others, as, for example, the transforming growth factor (TGF)-β3, IL-10, and IL10-R. Additionally, many proinflammatory ligands were downregulated, whereas anti-inflammatory soluble mediators were mostly upregulated by glucocorticoids, demonstrating their immunosuppressive and protective role against inflammation expression. Of the six major clusters analyzed, immune response–related genes and unknown genes (ESTs) were mostly regulated. The immune cluster was divided into subclusters and subcategories. Considering the great importance for glucocorticoid therapy, these observations might help to design more specific and efficient treatment strategies in the future.

DIFFERENTIAL REGULATION OF HUMAN ADRENAL STEROID RELEASE BY BACTERIAL TOXINS

Lipopolysaccharide (LPS) stimulates various levels of the HPA axis, indicative of an increase in plasma ACTH and corticosterone levels.[33] Furthermore, LPS elicits direct effects on adrenal cells. Human adrenal cells release cortisol by direct stimulation with LPS, an effect mediated via cyclooxygenase-dependent mechanisms. Thus, LPS caused a dose-dependent stimulation of basal cortisol secretion by the human adrenocortical cell line, NCI-H295R, without affecting aldosterone. Additionally, both TLRs (2/4) and their specific ligands (Pam3Cys/purified LPS and lipid A) were found to be involved in this cortisol release. LPS was also found to stimulate prostaglandin E release by these cells via Cox-2 activation.[34]

Furthermore, it is worth knowing that LPS acts specifically through the activation of TLR-4.[35] In this respect, most of the former studies using commercial LPS preparations did not notice a possible contamination with TLR-2 ligands such as lipopeptides. Thus, in our studies we confirmed by TLR-specific reporter assays that a pure LPS preparation (pLPS) solely triggered TLR-4, but was devoid of TLR-2 agonistic activity. In contrast the commercial LPS preparation (cLPS) stimulated both receptors (K.Zacharowski, unpublished data).

THE ROLE OF TLRs IN THE HPA AXIS

TLR-2/4 Could be Localized in the Human Adrenal Gland

An intact adrenal stress response is critical for a host's defense to infection.[36,37] The family of TLRs are very important in the early immune response upon bacterial infection. In addition to an immune–adrenal crosstalk mediated through secretory products of immune cells acting on adrenal cells the endocrine system may have innate immune properties itself. Unlike other non-immune cells, adrenal cells express not only cytokines and cytokine receptors,

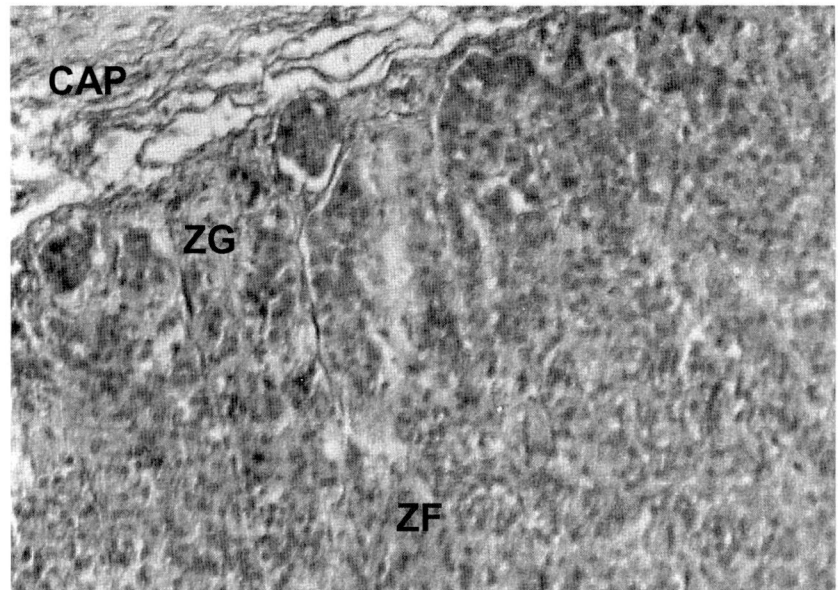

FIGURE 1. Human adrenal gland was stained with an antibody against TLR-2 (goat polyclonal S-16, Santa Cruz Biotechnology, Heidelberg, Germany). The brown staining shows DBC staining. C = capsule, ZG = zona glomerulosa, ZF = zona fasciculata.

but also major histocompatibility complex (MHC) class II molecules. Therefore, TLR-2 and TLR-4 receptors found on adrenal cells may be connected to a functional signaling system similar to the one characterized on immune cells and/or one that interacts directly with the activation of the steroid biosynthetic pathway in these cells. We could show that TLR-2/4 are expressed in the human adrenocortical cell line NCI-H295 and in human adrenal glands in the cortex, but not in the medulla[14] (FIG. 1).

Lessons Learned from TLR-2 Knockout Animals

Animal studies have shown that TLR-2-deficient mice are more susceptible to septicemia due to *Staphylococcus aureus* and *Listeria monocytogenes,* meningitis due to *Streptococcus pneumoniae,* and infection with *Mycobacterium tuberculosis,* suggesting that functional *TLR-2* polymorphisms may impair host response to a certain spectrum of microbial pathogens.

Detailed analyses show that the absence of TLR-2 in mice is associated with an enlargement of the adrenal gland and a reduction in corticosterone levels. Furthermore, plasma ACTH levels are elevated in TLR-2-deficient mice, indicating a possible impairment of the HPA axis on the level of the adrenal gland—even under basal conditions. Ultrastructural analysis from our

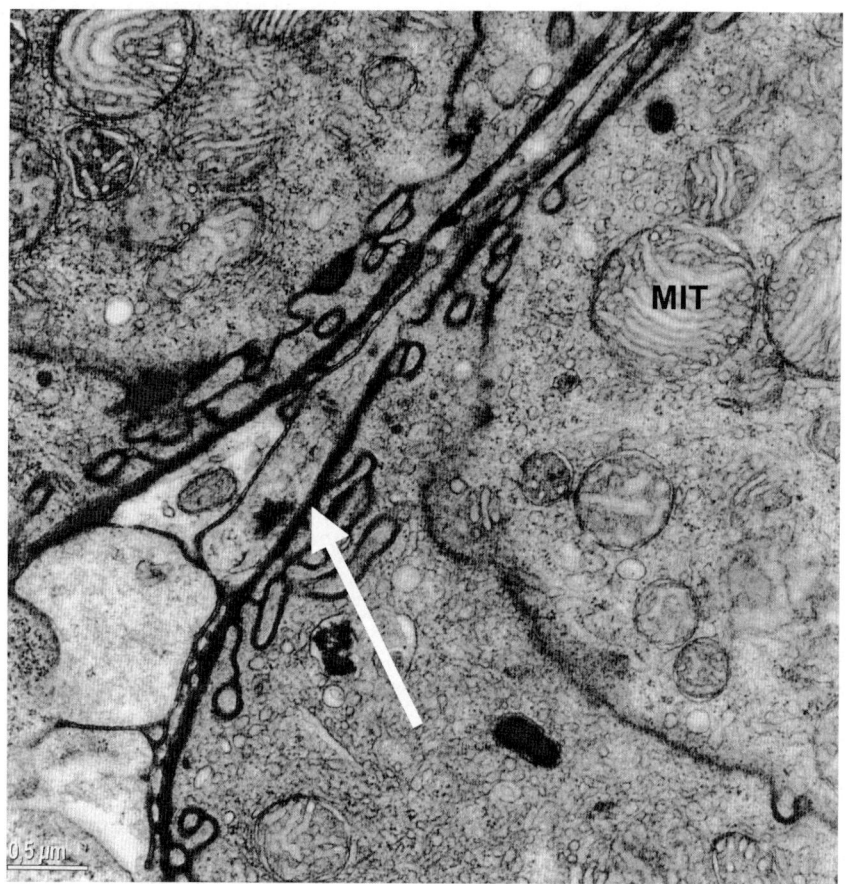

FIGURE 2. Ultrastructural image of adrenocortical cell in TLR-2-deficient animals. Cells demonstrate conspicuous alterations in membrane and mitochondrial structures in conjunction with impaired steroidogenic capacity (original magnification × 20,000). MIT = mitochondrium; *arrow* shows plasma membrane.

lab demonstrates that adrenocortical cells from TLR-2-deficient mice show marked changes of the plasma membranes with unusual interdigitations and infoldings of cell membranes (FIG. 2). This might suggest a primary defect in the adrenal function in TLR-2-deficient animals and could explain the reduction of corticosterone production.[15] Because cytokines are important in the regulation of the HPA axis, the TLR system might play a key role in the signal transduction of an adrenal stress response to inflammatory stimuli. This is in the context of the observation that mice with a targeted disruption of the TLR-2 gene are more susceptible to meningitis-induced intracranial complications. In addition, TLR-2-deficient mice have a more pronounced

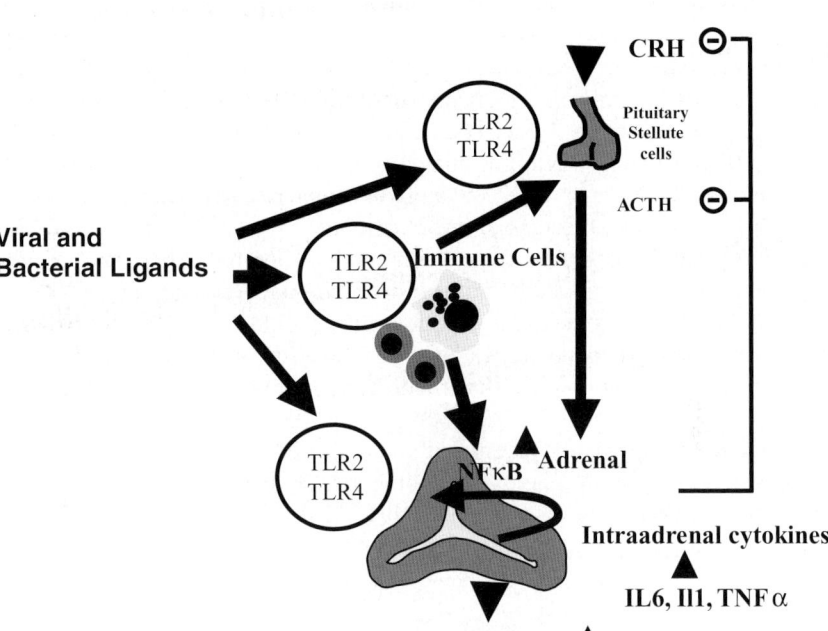

FIGURE 3. Artistic rendition of potential immune–endocrine interaction mediated by TLR-2 and TLR-4 during inflammation and sepsis. (Modified from Bornstein *et al.*[15])

reduction in body weight and a deterioration of motor impairment following experimental pneumococcal infection.[38] Similarly, TLR-2-deficient mice succumb to *M. tuberculosis* infection and are highly susceptible to *S. aureus* infection[39] compared to wild-type animals. Gram-positive bacteria such as *S. aureus* can trigger multiple organ failure and septic shock without causing endotoxemia.[40] In humans, two polymorphisms in the exon part of *TLR-2*, which attenuate receptor signaling, enhance the risk of acute severe infections, tuberculosis, and leprosy.[41]

In summary, our data demonstrate that TLR-2 and TLR-4 (R. Zacharowski, unpublished data) play important roles in the HPA axis. Thus, TLR-2 and TLR-4 constitute an important link between the immune and endocrine stress systems at both the central and peripheral levels, particularly during inflammation and sepsis (FIG. 3).

Clinical Implications

The crucial role of TLRs in the immune–adrenal crosstalk may have important clinical implications. Polymorphisms occur frequently in the TLR system in humans and it is conceivable that these individuals will have more difficulties in mounting and/or maintaining an adequate activation of the HPA axis during the severe stress of inflammation. Patients with sepsis may develop adrenocortical insufficiency and benefit from glucocorticoid therapy.[42–45] The mechanisms of adrenal impairment during sepsis and other inflammatory states still remain enigmatic and it will be of great interest to test the role of TLRs in this setting. Currently cytokine antagonists are widely used in the treatment of rheumatoid arthritis and TNF-α antagonists have been shown to downregulate TLRs in synovial tissues of these patients.[46,47] Some patients, however, fail to respond favorably to these compounds. Therefore, there may be an impaired immune–adrenal communication in conjunction with the downregulation of the TLRs in some of these patients that should be considered in future studies. On the other hand, TLR antagonists may constitute a useful tool for treating chronic inflammation states with concomitant activation of the HPA axis.

Low-grade inflammatory states with an activated HPA axis form the basis of most modern health problems, including obesity, diabetes, allergies, depression, and cardiovascular disease. Therefore, TLR antagonists may become a powerful medication for a great variety of indications in the future.

CONCLUSION

The capacity to respond to external and internal stimuli with a rapid and efficient endocrine stress response has been a critical step for survival and evolution of higher organisms. The adrenal has an astonishing capacity to adapt to physiological stressors or disease with extensive hypervascularization, zonal transformation, cellular hyperplasia, and rapid hormone release. Similar to the steroid system the toll-like family of receptors predates the animal kingdom and is remarkably preserved through the evolutionary process. TLRs and in particular TLR-2 play a fundamental role in coordinating the organisms' first line of defense. The innate immune response to endogenous and or exogenous molecules or pathways indicates tissue injury, infection, and remodeling. Therefore, a coordinated and efficient response of both systems mediated through TLR-2 and TLR-4 may have been programmed early in evolution. In this course the interactions between the innate immune system and HPA axis may be characterized by a circuit that includes (i) activation of the HPA axis and initiation of the stress response, which, in turn, has immunomodulating properties; (ii) a feedback mechanism derived from the immune system that regulates the HPA axis.

Over the past few years, it has become evident that the adrenal gland itself, as the main effector organ of the HPA axis, is a major site for both the synthesis and action of numerous cytokines. In light of the future use of TLR agonists or antagonists for a variety of inflammatory and autoimmune disorders, analyzing the adrenal function in TLR-2- and TLR-4-deficient mice[48] and human adrenal glands under normal conditions and following activation by bacterial lipids (i.e., LTA and LPS) is of great interest and has high clinical relevance.

ACKNOWLEDGMENTS

This work was supported by a DFG grant to S.R.B. (DFG BO 1141/8-1) and K.Z. (DFG ZA 243/9-1).

REFERENCES

1. MEANS, T.K., D.T. GOLENBOCK & M.J. FENTON. 2000. Structure and function of Toll-like receptor proteins. Life Sci. **68:** 241–258.
2. AGNESE, D.M., J.E. CALVANO, S.J. HAHM, *et al.* 2002. Human toll-like receptor 4 mutations but not CD14 polymorphisms are associated with an increased risk of gram-negative infections. J. Infect. Dis. **186:** 1522–1525.
3. KIECHL, S., E. LORENZ, M. REINDL, *et al.* 2002. Toll-like receptor 4 polymorphisms and atherogenesis. N. Engl. J. Med. **347:** 185–192.
4. LORENZ, E., J.P. MIRA, K.L. CORNISH, *et al.* 2000. A novel polymorphism in the toll-like receptor 2 gene and its potential association with staphylococcal infection. Infect. Immun. **68:** 6398–6401.
5. KANG, T.J., S.B. LEE & G.T. CHAE. 2002. A polymorphism in the toll-like receptor 2 is associated with IL-12 production from monocyte in lepromatous leprosy. Cytokine **20:** 56–62.
6. VON AULOCK, S., N.W. SCHRODER, S. TRAUB, *et al.* 2004. Heterozygous toll-like receptor 2 polymorphism does not affect lipoteichoic acid-induced chemokine and inflammatory responses. Infect. Immun. **72:** 1828–1831.
7. MURPHY, J.R., C.S. ANDREWS & D.Q. CRAIG. 2003. Characterization of the thermal properties of powder particles using microthermal analysis. Pharm. Res. **20:** 500–507.
8. HAJJAR, A.M., D.S. O'MAHONY, A. OZINSKY, *et al.* 2001. Cutting edge: functional interactions between toll-like receptor (TLR) 2 and TLR1 or TLR6 in response to phenol-soluble modulin. J. Immunol. **166:** 15–19.
9. NISHIMURA, M. & S. NAITO. 2005. Biol. Pharm. Bull. **28:** 886–892.
10. ZACHAROWSKI, K., P.K. CHATTERJEE & C. THIEMERMANN. 2002. Delayed preconditioning induced by lipoteichoic acid from *B. subtilis* and *S. aureus* is not blocked by administration of 5-hydroxydecanoate. Shock **17:** 19–22.
11. ZACHAROWSKI, K., R. BERKELS, A. OLBRICH, *et al.* 2001. The selective guanylate cyclase inhibitor ODQ reduces multiple organ injury in rodent models of Gram-positive and Gram-negative shock. Crit. Care Med. **29:** 1599–1608.
12. CHATTERJEE, P.K., K. ZACHAROWSKI, S. CUZZOCREA, *et al.* 2000. Inhibitors of poly (ADP-ribose) synthetase reduce renal ischemia-reperfusion injury in the anesthetized rat *in vivo*. FASEB J. **14:** 641–651.
13. ZACHAROWSKI, K., S. FRANK, M. OTTO, *et al.* 2000. Lipoteichoic acid induces delayed protection in the rat heart: a comparison with endotoxin. Arterioscler. Thromb. Vasc. Biol. **20:** 1521–1528.

14. Bornstein, S.R., R.R. Schumann, V. Rettori, *et al.* 2004. Toll-like receptor 2 and Toll-like receptor 4 expression in human adrenals. Horm. Metab. Res. **36:** 470–473.

15. Bornstein, S.R., P. Zacharowski, R.R. Schumann, *et al.* 2004. Impaired adrenal stress response in Toll-like receptor 2-deficient mice. Proc. Natl. Acad. Sci. USA **101:** 16695–16700.

16. Willenberg, H.S., G. Path, T.A. Vogeli, *et al.* 2002. Role of interleukin-6 in stress response in normal and tumorous adrenal cells and during chronic inflammation. Ann. N. Y. Acad. Sci. **966:** 304–314.

17. Galon, J., D. Franchimont, N. Hiroi, *et al.* 2002. Gene profiling reveals unknown enhancing and suppressive actions of glucocorticoids on immune cells. FASEB J. **16:** 61–71.

18. Marx, C., G.W. Wolkersdorfer & S.R. Bornstein. 1998. A new view on immune-adrenal interactions: role for Fas and Fas ligand? Neuroimmunomodulation **5:** 5–8.

19. Zouboulis, C.C., H. Seltmann, N. Hiroi, *et al.* 2002. Corticotropin-releasing hormone: an autocrine hormone that promotes lipogenesis in human sebocytes. Proc. Natl. Acad Sci USA **99:** 7148–7153.

20. Wolkersdorfer, G.W., T. Lohmann, C. Marx, *et al.* 1999. Lymphocytes stimulate dehydroepiandrosterone production through direct cellular contact with adrenal zona reticularis cells: a novel mechanism of immune-endocrine interaction. J. Clin. Endocrinol. Metab. **84:** 4220–4227.

21. Merke, D.P., S.R. Bornstein, D. Braddock & G.P. Chrousos. 1999. Adrenal lymphocytic infiltration and adrenocortical tumors in a patient with 21-hydroxylase deficiency. N. Engl. J. Med. **340:** 1121–1122.

22. Bornstein, S.R., H. Rutkowski & I. Vrezas. 2004. Cytokines and steroidogenesis. Mol. Cell Endocrinol. **215:** 135–141.

23. Bornstein, S.R. & H. Rutkowski. 2002. The adrenal hormone metabolism in the immune/inflammatory reaction. Endocr. Res. **28:** 719–728.

24. Bornstein, S.R. & M. Ehrhart-Bornstein. 2000. Basic and clinical aspects of intraadrenal regulation of steroidogenesis. Z. Rheumatol. **59**(Suppl 2): II/12–17.

25. Franchimont, D., G. Bouma, J. Galon, *et al.* 2000. Adrenal cortical activation in murine colitis adrenal cortical activation in murine colitis. Gastroenterology **119:** 1560–1568.

26. Marx, C., S. Petros, S.R. Bornstein, *et al.* 2003. Adrenocortical hormones in survivors and nonsurvivors of severe sepsis: diverse time course of dehydroepiandrosterone, dehydroepiandrosterone-sulfate, and cortisol. Crit. Care Med. **31:** 1382–1388.

27. Masi, A.T., G.P. Chrousos & S.R. Bornstein. 1999. Enigmas of adrenal androgen and glucocorticoid dissociation in premenopausal onset rheumatoid arthritis. J. Rheumatol. **26:** 247–250.

28. McEwen, B.S. & T. Seeman. 1999. Protective and damaging effects of mediators of stress. Elaborating and testing the concepts of allostasis and allostatic load. Ann. N. Y. Acad. Sci. **896:** 30–47.

29. Sapolsky, R.M., L.M. Romero & A.U. Munck. 2000. How do glucocorticoids influence stress responses? Integrating permissive, suppressive, stimulatory, and preparative actions. Endocr. Rev. **21:** 55–89.

30. Koedel, U., B. Angele, T. Rupprecht, *et al.* 2003. Toll-like receptor 2 participates in mediation of immune response in experimental pneumococcal meningitis. J. Immunol. **170:** 438–444.

31. DRENNAN, M.B., D. NICOLLE, V.J. QUESNIAUX, *et al.* 2004. Toll-like receptor 2-deficient mice succumb to Mycobacterium tuberculosis infection. Am. J. Pathol. **164:** 49–57.
32. HERMOSO, M.A., T. MATSUGUCHI, K. SMOAK & J.A. CIDLOWSKI. 2004. Glucocorticoids and tumor necrosis factor alpha cooperatively regulate toll-like receptor 2 gene expression. Mol. Cell Biol. **24:** 4743–4756.
33. GADEK-MICHALSKA, A. & J. BUGAJSKI. 2004. Role of prostaglandins and nitric oxide in the lipopolysaccharide-induced ACTH and corticosterone response. J. Physiol. Pharmacol. **55:** 663–675.
34. VAKHARIA, K. & J.P. HINSON. 2005. Lipopolysaccharide directly stimulates cortisol secretion by human adrenal cells by a cyclooxygenase-dependent mechanism. Endocrinology **146:** 1398–1402.
35. PALSSON-MCDERMOTT, E.M. & L.A. O'NEILL. 2004. Signal transduction by the lipopolysaccharide receptor, Toll-like receptor-4. Immunology **113:** 153–162.
36. CHROUSOS, G.P. 1995. The hypothalamic-pituitary-adrenal axis and immune-mediated inflammation. N. Engl. J. Med. **332:** 1351–1362.
37. BORNSTEIN, S.R. & G.P. CHROUSOS. 1999. Clinical review 104: Adrenocorticotropin (ACTH)- and non-ACTH-mediated regulation of the adrenal cortex: neural and immune inputs. J. Clin. Endocrinol. Metab. **84:** 1729–1736.
38. TAKEUCHI, O., K. HOSHINO & S. AKIRA. 2000. Cutting edge: TLR2-deficient and MyD88-deficient mice are highly susceptible to *Staphylococcus aureus* infection. J. Immunol. **165:** 5392–5396.
39. BONE, R.C. 1994. Gram-positive organisms and sepsis. Arch. Intern. Med. **154:** 26–34.
40. KIECHL, S., C.J. WIEDERMANN & J. WILLEIT. 2003. Toll-like receptor 4 and atherogenesis. Ann. Med. **35:** 164–171.
41. TEXEREAU, J., J.D. CHICHE, W. TAYLOR, *et al.* 2005. The importance of Toll-like receptor 2 polymorphisms in severe infections. Clin. Infect. Dis. **41**(Suppl 7): S408–S415.
42. BORNSTEIN, S.R. & J. BRIEGEL. 2003. A new role for glucocorticoids in septic shock: balancing the immune response. Am. J. Respir. Crit. Care Med. **167:** 485–486.
43. ANNANE, D., V. SEBILLE, C. CHARPENTIER, *et al.* 2002. Effect of treatment with low doses of hydrocortisone and fludrocortisone on mortality in patients with septic shock. JAMA **288:** 862–871.
44. COOPER, M.S. & P.M. STEWART. 2003. Corticosteroid insufficiency in acutely ill patients. N. Engl. J. Med. **348**(8): 727–734.
45. MEDURI, G.U., E.A. TOLLEY G.P. CHROUSOS & F. STENTZ. 2002. Prolonged methylprednisolone treatment suppresses systemic inflammation in patients with unresolving acute respiratory distress syndrome: evidence for inadequate endogenous glucocorticoid secretion and inflammation-induced immune cell resistance to glucocorticoids. Am. J. Respir. Crit. Care Med. **165:** 983–991.
46. ROELOFS, M.F., L.A. JOOSTEN, S. ABDOLLAHI-ROODSAZ, *et al.* 2005. The expression of toll-like receptors 3 and 7 in rheumatoid arthritis synovium is increased and costimulation of toll-like receptors 3, 4, and 7/8 results in synergistic cytokine production by dendritic cells. Arthritis Rheum. **52:** 2313–2322.
47. DE RYCKE, L., B. VANDOOREN, E. KRUITHOF, *et al.* 2005. Tumor necrosis factor alpha blockade treatment down-modulates the increased systemic and local expression of Toll-like receptor 2 and Toll-like receptor 4 in spondylarthropathy. Arthritis Rheum. **52:** 2146–58.

48. ZACHAROWSKI, K., P.A. ZACHAROWSKI, A. KOCH, *et al*. 2006. Toll-like receptor 4 plays a crucial role in the immune-adrenal response to systemic inflammatory response syndrome. Proc. Natl. Acad. Sci. USA. **103:** 6392–6397.Epub 2006 Apr. 10.

ADDITIONAL LITERATURE

BORNSTEIN,S.R. & G.P. CHROUSOS. 1999. Clinical review 104: Adrenocorticotropin (ACTH)- and non-ACTH-mediated regulation of the adrenal cortex: neural and immune inputs. J. Clin. Endocrinol. Metab **84:** 1729–1736.

CHROUSOS, G.P. 1995. The hypothalamic-pituitary-adrenal axis and immune-mediated inflammation N. Engl. J. Med. **332:** 1351–1362.

BORNSTEIN, S.R., H. RUTKOWSKI & I. VREZAS. 2004. Cytokines and steroidogenesis Mol. Cell Endocrinol. **215:** 135–141.

EHRHART-BORNSTEIN, M., J.P. HINSON, S.R. BORNSTEIN, *et al*. 1998. Intraadrenal interactions in the regulation of adrenocortical steroidogenesis Endocr. Rev. **19:** 101–143.

BORNSTEIN, S.R. 2000. Cytokines and the adrenal cortex: basic research and clinical implications. Curr Opin Endocrinol Diabetes 128–137.

BORNSTEIN, S.R. & G.P. CHROUSOS. 1999. Clinical review 104: Adrenocorticotropin (ACTH)- and non-ACTH-mediated regulation of the adrenal cortex: neural and immune inputs J. Clin. Endocrinol. Metab **84:** 1729–1736.

Adrenocortical Tumorigenesis

FELIX BEUSCHLEIN AND MARTIN REINCKE

*Medizinische Klinik–Innenstadt, Ludwig-Maximilians-University,
Munich, Germany*

ABSTRACT: Through the widespread use of imaging techniques with great sensitivity adrenal tumors are often diagnosed as an incidental finding. Although the majority of these adrenal lesions are benign and without evidence of endocrine activity or malignancy, hormone hypersecretion needs to be ruled out by specific tests. In addition to the classical forms of overt adrenocortical hypersecretion, it has become evident over the recent years that modest adrenocortical steroid autonomy as present in normokalemic primary aldosteronism and subclinical Cushing's syndrome is also associated with a significant morbidity. However, detection and differential diagnosis of these subtle changes in adrenal steroidogenesis can pose a diagnostic challenge to the clinician and is dependent on tests with reliable sensitivity and specificity. Regulation of adrenocortical development and growth, which results in clinical symptoms if disrupted, is dependent upon the distinct spatiotemporal expression of a variety of transcription factors as well as stimulation by extra-adrenal peptide hormones. Contributions to the elucidation of growth regulation of the adrenal cortex come from rare familiar syndromes associated with adrenocortical tumors, expression studies of adrenal tumor samples, *in vitro* studies on adrenocortical tumor cell lines, and mouse models displaying adrenal growth defects. In this review, we will summarize the important molecular aspects of adrenal tumorigenesis and highlight some prospects for clinical applications.

KEYWORDS: adrenal tumorigenesis; adrenocortical carcinoma; adrenocortical adenoma; adrenal incidentaloma; steroidogenesis; Cushing's syndrome; Conn's syndrome; hyperaldosteronism; p53; IGF-1; activin; inhibin

PREVALENCE AND CLINICAL PRESENTATION OF ADRENOCORTICAL TUMORS

Adrenal Tumors Diagnosed by Abdominal Imaging

The most common adrenal disorder encountered by clinicians today is the incidentally discovered adrenal mass, termed *adrenal incidentaloma*. The rate

Address for correspondence: Dr. Martin Reincke, Medizinische Klinik–Innenstadt, Klinikum der LMU München, Ziemssenstr. 1, D-80336 München, Germany. Voice: +49-89-51602100; fax: +49-89-51604428.

e-mail: martin.reincke@med.uni-muenchen.de

Ann. N.Y. Acad. Sci. 1088: 319–334 (2006). © 2006 New York Academy of Sciences.
doi: 10.1196/annals.1366.001

of detection of clinically silent adrenal masses has increased substantially over the last decades through the widespread use of modern abdominal imaging techniques. As a consequence, the management of adrenal incidentalomas has become a common clinical problem.

Recently, the National Institutes of Health Consensus Development Program convened surgeons, endocrinologists, pathologists, biostatisticians, radiologists, oncologists, and other health care professionals to address the causes, prevalence, and natural history of clinically inapparent adrenal masses, or "incidentalomas"; the appropriate evaluation and treatment of such masses.[46] The incidence of adrenal masses is dependent on the screening procedure and ranges between 1.4% and 9% in autopsy series[1,2] and 0.4% to 4% in series of abdominal CT scans.[3–5]

In the absence of a known malignancy of nonadrenal origin, the vast majority of adrenal incidentalomas are benign. Nonfunctioning cortical adenomas are the most common lesions, accounting for between 36% and 94% of cases, while hormonally active or malignant adrenocortical tumors are much less common.[6] In addition, adrenal glands are also common targets for metastatic spread of a variety of malignancies, such as lung cancer, renal cell carcinoma, melanoma, and many other tumor entities. For example, the incidence of adrenal metastases in patients with resectable non-small cell lung cancer has been estimated between 1.6%[7] and 3.5%.[8] In patients with renal cell carcinoma, 5.5% had ipsilateral adrenal metastasis at first presentation.[9] However, adrenal metastases from distant malignant tumors are the sign of general spread of disease and usually occur at multiple sites while a solitary adrenal metastasis is a rare event. Similarly, patients with renal cell carcinoma with local infiltration and ipsilateral adrenal metastasis predominately (82%) have an advanced tumor stage.[10] Thus, a single adrenal metastasis as the initial and only finding of malignant disease is an unusual clinical situation.

Adrenocortical carcinoma (ACC) is a rare but highly malignant endocrine tumor entity with a worldwide incidence of approximately two new cases per million persons per year.[11] Retrospective studies of combined surgical and medical therapy indicate an overall 5-year survival of 15–35%.[12] Overall, the long-term therapeutic results are devastating and largely dependent on tumor stage; the most severe prognostic factor is the presence of metastases. While in children ACCs are commonly functional, in elderly patients ACC tumors are usually detected at an advanced stage because of the mass effect or incidentally by radiological investigations.[13] The probability of malignancy is clearly related to the size of the tumor, as almost all lesions <3 cm are benign, whereas a diameter of >6 cm indicates a high risk of malignancy.[14] Accordingly, the proportion of malignant ACC in adrenal incidentalomas on which surgery was performed (also on the basis of tumor size) is as high as 12%.[15]

Computed tomography (CT) and magnetic resonance imaging (MRI) both have high impact in the characterization of adrenal masses. If the attenuation of a homogeneous mass with smooth border is 10 Hounsfield units or less in unenhanced CT, the diagnosis of a lipid-rich adenoma is established. Similarly, enhancement washout of more than 50% in CT at 10–15 min suggests a benign lesion.[16,17] In MRI, both rapid enhancement followed by rapid washout and signal intensity loss using opposed-phase image in chemical shift analysis also indicate the presence of an adenoma.[18,19] In contrast, adrenal carcinomas and metastases in CT scan are defined by irregular margins and inhomogeneous enhancement. Other imaging techniques, such as positron emission tomography, possibly offer additional information, such as identification of small metastases from adrenal carcinoma,[20] but have not yet been fully established in large prospective clinical studies.

Adrenocortical Tumors in Patients Presenting with Symptoms of Hormonal Excess

Although a high proportion of adrenal lesions are identified incidentally in the course of abdominal imaging procedures, overt hormonal activity translates into clinical syndromes that can raise early suspicion for the presence of functional adrenal tumors.

Primary aldosteronism has recently been recognized as the most frequent cause of secondary hypertension, occurring with a prevalence of 5% to 18% within the hypertensive population.[21–24] Only 10–30% of these patients, however, are characterized by the classical triad of hypertension, hypokalemia, and alkalosis, whereas the large majority presents with normal serum potassium, thus indicating a milder variant of this disorder.[24] Apparently, the pretest probability of hypokalemia varies between the different forms of primary hyperaldosteronism, where hypokalemia is more often found in patients with aldosterone-producing adenomas, with a reported incidence of 70–80%.[25] The aldosterone/renin ratio is currently the most recommended screening test for primary aldosteronism and application of the ratio even under antihypertensive medication is increasingly advocated.[26–29] In any case, a positive test result requires confirmation by functional testing, as the specificity of the aldosterone/renin ratio is low. Various confirmatory tests have been proposed, but an ideal test, which is simultaneously simple to perform, sensitive, and specific, is currently lacking. A common approach to confirm the diagnosis of primary aldosteronism is to demonstrate the insufficient suppression of aldosterone after oral sodium loading, acute saline infusion, or administration of captopril or fludrocortisone.[30–32] Aldosterone-producing adrenal adenomas are characterized by Autonomous aldosterone secretion independent of saline-induced renin suppression. On the basis of this principle the saline infusion test enables us to distinguish between patients with essential hypertension and those, with classical primary aldosteronism. In contrast, confirmation of the normokalemic variant of hyperaldosteronism by sodium load is not possible with an acceptable specificity and sensitivity.

Autonomous secretion of cortisol from an adrenal adenoma accounts for 9–22% of patients with Cushing's syndrome, with an annual incidence of 1.1 per million people for female and 0.1 for male.[33] Although there are only sparse data on the clinical presentation of patients with ACTH-independent Cushing's syndrome, it is likely that clinical signs and symptoms are mainly defined by the presence and extent of hypercortisolism. Thus, cushingoid habitus with truncal obesity, striae, weight gain, muscle weakness, hypertension, and abnormal glucose tolerance are hallmarks also for the clinical presentation of ACTH-independent hypercortisolism.[34] The diagnosis on adrenal Cushing's syndrome relies on the demonstration of a blunted diurnal rhythm of cortisol secretion and failure of overnight suppression by administration of low doses of dexamethasone.[35] In a recent retrospective analysis that compared the test characteristics of urinary-free cortisol, overnight low-dose dexamethasone suppression test and midnight serum cortisol, the best test characteristics were obtained for midnight serum cortisol, with a sensitivity of 92% and a specificity of 96%.[36]

Over the last decade, an increasing body of evidence has emerged demonstrating that subtle cortisol production and subsequent abnormalities in the hypothalamic-pituitary-adrenal axis are more frequent than previously thought. This entity, which has been termed *subclinical Cushing's syndrome,* has been reported to occur in 12–16% of patients with adrenal incidentalomas.[6,37,38] The diagnosis of subclinical Cushing's syndrome is less well defined than the overt form, but requires demonstration of some extent of autonomous cortisol secretion by means of elevated midnight cortisol, urinary cortisol, low baseline ACTH, and blunted increase of ACTH upon CRH stimulation.[37,39,40] A recent follow-up evaluation of patients with clinically nonfunctioning adrenal masses revealed an estimated cumulative risk for a nonsecreting adrenal incidentaloma to develop subclinical hyperfunction of 3.8% after 1 year and 6.6% after 5 years.[41] Similarly, the rate of progression from subclinical to overt Cushing's syndrome is likely to be low.[39] However, a number of recent studies have collected data on the morbidity associated with subclinical Cushing's syndrome in patients with a clinically inapparent adrenal adenoma. These studies indicate a higher cardiovascular risk profile and less favorable metabolic parameters with higher systolic blood pressure and altered glucose tolerance in patients with subclinical Cushing's syndrome.[40,42]

While benign adenomas usually maintain the expression profile of steroidogenic enzymes of the zone they originate from, steroidogenesis in malignant ACC is characterized by secretion of various steroid precursors. Although the presence of these precursors might not be associated with specific clinical symptoms,[43] half of ACCs are hormonally active and show clinical symptoms that eventually may lead to early diagnosis. As such, the concomitant occurrence of hyperandrogenism and hypercortisolism in a patient with an adrenal mass should fuel suspicion of the presence of an ACC. Similarly, in the presence of an adrenal lesion, elevated serum dehydroepiandrosterone sulfate (DHEAS) levels suggest an ACC, as benign adrenocortical tumors often exhibit low DHEAS concentrations.[44,45] In contrast, hormone concentrations are usually of limited help in predicting malignancy.

MOLECULAR ADRENAL TUMORIGENESIS

Regulation of adrenocortical growth and differentiation is a complex process that requires a diverse array of specific transcription factors and conserved signaling cascades. Clonality studies of adrenocortical tumors using X-chromosome inactivation analysis indicate monoclonal expansion of a single cell as the origin of ACC.[47,48] These findings are in good accordance with those in other forms of cancer, which are believed to originate from a single transformed cell clone in response to a series of multistep genetic alterations that result in the disruption of growth regulation. In contrast, adrenal adenomas can present as monoclonal or polyclonal tumor entities, suggesting that, in addition to tumorigenic mutations, mitogenic extra-adrenal stimuli might contribute to cellular proliferation in this benign tumor entity.[47,48]

Insulin-Like Growth Factor System

The insulin-like growth factor system is one of the best-investigated molecular pathways involved in autonomous adrenal growth. Beckwith–Wiedemann syndrome, a congenital overgrowth disorder characterized by a high risk of development of childhood tumors, is also distinguished by a high incidence of ACC.[49] The disease has been mapped to the 11p15.5 region, which harbors the IGF-II gene as well as the genes coding for insulin, H19, and p57[KIP2]. The IGF-II gene is subject to regulation by genomic imprinting, which involves methylation of specific sites within a gene that occurs at early embryologic stages and results in a stable pattern of transcriptional activation or inactivation of a given gene. In the case of IGF-II, transcripts are almost exclusively expressed from the paternal allele, indicating the importance of maternal imprinting in its transcriptional regulation. Genetic studies of adrenocortical lesions have demonstrated a variety of genetic changes resulting in IGF-II overexpression. Most common alterations consist of loss of the maternal allele, which is often accompanied by the gain of a second copy of the paternal allele through a yet unknown genetic mechanism. This process, termed *uniparental disomy*, results in the presence of two copies of the expressed IGF-II allele and, therefore, overexpression of the gene. Interestingly, two studies have identified marked elevation of IGF-II protein and mRNA levels in more than 60% of ACCs.[50,51] These findings have been recently confirmed by another study that used transcriptional profiling of a variety of adrenocortical tumors to demonstrate IGF-II overexpression in 90% of the ACCs studied.[52]

IGF-II binds two distinct receptor types, the IGF-I receptor (IGF-IR) and the IGF-II receptor (IGF-IIR). Similar to the insulin receptor, IGF-IR is a receptor tyrosine kinase composed of two heterodimeric chains that possess an intrinsic tyrosine kinase activity, and activate a variety of downstream effectors characteristically associated with this receptor family. Since overexpression of IGF-IR has been found in a substantial proportion of ACCs,[53] it is likely that locally produced IGF-II acts as an autocrine or paracrine growth factor in adrenocortical tumorigenesis. Consistent with this hypothesis, studies in transgenic mice have shown that postnatal overexpression of IGF-II is associated with an increase in adrenal weight and enhanced steroidogenesis, presumably by a direct mitogenic effect of IGF-II on adrenocortical fasciculata cells. Mice did not develop tumors, however, suggesting that IGF-II overexpression alone is not sufficient for tumorigenesis.[54] Taken together, these findings indicate that IGF-II is an important growth factor for adrenocortical cells, which is frequently co-opted by aberrant adrenocortical cells to support the development of ACC.

Tumor-Suppressor Genes

$p57^{KIP2}$, a member of the cyclin-dependent kinase inhibitor family, is another imprinted gene on chromosome 11p15.5 that, unlike IGF-II, is maternally expressed.[55] $p57^{KIP2}$ is normally involved in cell cycle arrest and cellular differentiation via its ability to bind cyclins and prevent activation of their cognate cyclin-dependent kinases.[55,56] Mice with targeted deletion of the $p57^{KIP2}$ gene exhibit some phenotypes in common with Beckwith–Wiedemann syndrome including adrenal cortical hyperplasia and cytomegaly.[57] The expression pattern, antiproliferative function, chromosomal location, and genomic imprinting of $p57^{KIP2}$ make it a candidate tumor-suppressor gene. Accordingly, low levels of $p57^{KIP2}$ mRNA, which negatively correlate with IGF-II mRNA expression, have been observed in active adult ACCs.[58] In addition, abrogation of $p57^{KIP2}$ gene expression in malignant tumors and in the human adrenocortical tumor cell line H295R is also associated with high activity of G1 cyclin–CDK complexes.[59]

Collectively, these data suggest that decreased $p57^{KIP2}$ activity participates in disruption of normal cell cycle control in adrenocortical tumors, and likely contributes to tumor proliferation in combination with increased levels of IGF-II.

The Li–Fraumeni syndrome is a rare autosomal-dominant syndrome associated with high susceptibility to a variety of cancer including ACC. The underlying genetic defect in patients with Li–Fraumeni syndrome is germline mutations in the p53 tumor-suppressor gene.[60] P53 is activated by DNA damage and hyperproliferative signals, leading to either cell cycle arrest or apoptosis, thus mediating an important cell cycle checkpoint control that effectively maintains genome integrity.[61] More than 90% of all mutations of p53 have been detected in four hypersensitive regions that lie between exons 5 and 8 of the gene, which has been mapped to human chromosome 17p13.1. Recently, mutation of Arg 377 to His has been linked to a large kindred of pediatric cases of ACC in southern Brazil.[62] Interestingly, this particular germline mutation is not associated with the usual broad spectrum of tumor types seen in Li–Fraumeni syndrome, but contributes in a tissue-specific manner to the development of pediatric ACC. Biochemical studies have suggested that this specific mutation in the tetramerization domain of the p53 protein leads to a particular pH sensitivity of the p53 complex, thus providing a potential molecular basis of the adrenal-specific loss of p53 function.[63] In addition to the familial tumor syndrome, p53 mutations have been identified in sporadic ACCs and adrenocortical tumor cell lines.[64] Taken together, these findings suggest that loss of the normal inhibitory function of the p53 tumor-suppressor protein in the cell cycle is involved in the development of ACC.

While initially identified as opposing regulators of pituitary FSH secretion,[65] both inhibin and activin have since been shown to play critical roles as paracrine and autocrine factors that regulate growth and differentiation in a number of organs including the gonads and the adrenal gland.[66] In humans, inhibin is specifically localized to the fetal zone of the developing adrenal cortex, providing speculation that the growth dynamics of the fetal zone are regulated at least in part by this hormone.[67] Like inhibin, activin has essential functions in both regulating organ development and tumor growth, where it exerts its effects by modulating cellular differentiation, survival, proliferation, and apoptosis.[68] In the human adrenal, activin has been shown to induce apoptosis specifically in cells of the fetal zone, and has been considered to be a mediator of physiological fetal zone regression.[69]

Studies on inhibin null (INH−/−) mice, which spontaneously develop activin-secreting gonadal tumors, and ACC upon gonadectomy have significantly contributed to define the role of inhibin and activin in adrenal physiology.[70] As we have demonstrated in detailed morphological and *in vitro* studies, the adrenal phenotype in INH−/− mice is indicative of an x-zone growth dysregulation. The x zone of the murine adrenal cortex is thought to be the functional equivalent of the primate fetal adrenal zone, and thus the INH−/− mouse may be considered a model of childhood adrenal cancer. Development of activin-secreting ovarian tumors in female INH−/− mice is accompanied by a decrease in adrenal weight and regression of the x zone. The ultimate cause of this regression is the distinct x-zonal expression pattern of activin receptor subunits and the intracellular mediator Smad2, which results in a particular responsiveness of the x zone to activin. As a result, activin induces apoptosis specifically in the adrenal x zone, thus preventing adrenal tumorigenesis in the presence of activin-secreting gonadal tumors. Conversely, the removal of activin-secreting ovarian tumors by surgical gonadectomy in INH−/− is followed by unopposed x-zone growth, which ultimately results in the formation of adrenal tumors.[71]

Differentiation Factors

After binding to its specific receptor (melanocortin 2 receptor, MC2-R), ACTH leads to activation of the adenylate cyclase pathway and subsequent activation of protein kinase A (PKA).[72] However, activation of other signal transduction cascades by ACTH, such as the calcium/protein kinase C pathway and the lipo-oxygenase pathway,[73] have also been described. ACTH acutely stimulates intracellular transport of cholesterol to the inner mitochondrial membrane within a few minutes by transcriptional activation of the steroidogenic acute regulatory protein (StAR), which is the rate-limiting step for steroidogenesis in the adrenal cell.[74] The rapid induction of early response genes in the *jun/fos* family suggests their participation in the acute action of ACTH to stimulate steroidogenesis.[75] Moreover, chronic stimulation with pharmacological doses of ACTH provokes a profound increase in the transcription and translation of several key steroidogenic enzymes, such as P450scc (side-chain cleavage enzyme), which in turn leads to overt hypercortisolism.[75]

Activating mutations of components of the adenylate cyclase pathway, such as G-protein–coupled receptors and guanine-triphosphate-binding proteins, have been identified in a variety of human endocrine disorders including acromegaly and toxic thyroid follicular adenomas.[76,77] In the adrenal cortex, however, activating point mutations of neither the *MC2-R* nor the α-chain of the stimulatory G-protein have been identified in benign or malignant adrenocortical tumors.[78–80] In addition, in a series of 20 cases of benign and malignant adrenocortical tumors, we have demonstrated an association between loss of constitutive heterozygosity (LOH) of the *MC2-R* gene and advanced tumor stage and a more rapid course than in ACC patients without LOH.[81] These data suggest that allelic loss of the *MC2-R* gene in adrenocortical tumors can result in loss of differentiation, a characteristic feature of human malignant neoplasms. To further define the direct effects of ACTH on adrenocortical tumor growth, we recently developed a murine tumor model using subcutaneous growth of Y6 cells.[82] Y6 cells are derivatives of the Y1 adrenocortical cell line that are ACTH resistant through the lack of MC2-R expression, but retain signaling induced by forskolin.[83] These studies demonstrated that MC2-R expression is associated with a less aggressive adrenal tumor phenotype with its antiproliferative effects being amplified through stimulation with physiological doses of ACTH. Taken together, these findings support the concept of a growth-inhibitory and thus differentiating effect of ACTH for adrenal tumors *in vivo*.

Peroxisome proliferator-activated receptor gamma (PPARγ) is a ligand-activated transcription factor and member of the nuclear hormone receptor superfamily, which is involved in a variety of physiological processes.[84] Thiazolidinediones as specific ligands for the PPARγ have been implemented into clinical practice for the treatment of type 2 diabetes mellitus. More recently, *in vitro* and preclinical *in vivo* tests have suggested that TZDs might also have favorable effects in the treatment of a variety of tumors as differentiation-inducing agents. As we and others could demonstrate, PPARγ is abundantly expressed in different adrenocortical tumor tissues including ACC. Moreover, in the human adrenocortical tumor cell NCIh295, incubation with rosiglitazone led to a decrease in cell viability in a time- and dose-dependent manner.[85,86] This decrease was paralleled by a decrease in cellular proliferation and increase in apoptosis. Interestingly, NCI h295 cells expressed higher levels of MC2-R mRNA upon treatment, while cyclin E mRNA was reduced, thus reflecting a shift toward an expression pattern found in less aggressive adrenocortical tumors *in vivo*. Taken together, these data indicate that TZDs have the potential to become an additional treatment option as differentiation-inducing agents in patients with ACC.

Molecular Pathways Involved in Benign Adrenocortical Tumor Growth and Hormonal Autonomy

The increased incidence of ACC in the context of familial tumor syndromes and expression profiling of sporadic ACCs have shed light on molecular pathways involved in adrenal carcinogenesis. In contrast, there is only limited insight into the pathogenesis of steroid and growth autonomy, specifically in benign adrenocortical adenomas. In contrast to gastrointestinal tumors, in the adrenal cortex tumors usually do not follow an adenoma–carcinoma sequence as the consequence of acquired genetic alterations. Accordingly, genetic data from comparative genomic hybridization display no common genetic hot spot between both tumor entities.[87–90] Although the different studies have demonstrated an increased frequency of DNA copy number changes in large malignant adrenocortical tumors compared with small benign tumors, there is some controversy regarding regions of consistent chromosomal aberration. However, it is clear from these profiling analyses that the molecular pathogenesis of adrenal adenomas is different from that of malignant ACCs.

The concept of illicit receptor expression in the adrenal cortex responsible for adrenocortical hyperfunction has initially been established for the rare disorder of macronodular adrenal hyperplasia.[91] However, over the last decade a growing number of patients with adrenal adenomas including Cushing's adenomas,[92] aldosterone-producing adenomas,[93] and pure androgen-producing adenomas[94–98] have been described with illicit receptor expression including GIP receptor, LH receptor, and vasopressin 1 receptor.[91] Interestingly, expression of the LH receptor has been reported in the human adrenal zona reticularis,[99] and hCG can stimulate DHEAS secretion in human fetal adrenocortical cells.[100]

Recently, it has been demonstrated that stable transfection of the GIP receptor in bovine adrenocortical cells is sufficient to induce autonomous growth and hypercortisolism after transplantation in immunodeficient mice.[101] Although these data clearly indicate that illicit receptor expression can be sufficient to induce the clinical phenotype, the initial molecular events that induce receptor expression remain unknown. Of note, several mouse models of gonadotropin-dependent adrenal tumorigenesis have been described and characterized including mice with targeted deletion of the inhibin alpha subunit,[71,102] mice with transgenic expression of simian virus 40 T-antigen under the control of the alpha inhibin promoter (Inh-Tag),[103] and various inbred mouse strains with gonadectomy-dependent adrenal tumorigenesis.[104-106] Although different with regard to the causative molecular events, these animal models share the finding of LH-dependent adrenal tumor growth and steroidogenesis with high levels of adrenal LH receptor expression.[71,107] The gonadectomy-induced elevation of LH levels is apparently crucial for the induction of LH receptor expression, which triggers formation of the adrenocortical tumors in the context of certain molecular susceptibilities, such as inhibin deficiency, Tag expression,[108] or other genetic events. Accordingly, the tumors fail to appear if the postcastration increase in gonadotropins is blocked either by treating the mice with a GnRH antagonist or by crossbreeding them to the gonadotropin-deficient hpg genetic background.[109] Expression of LH receptor and steroidogenic enzymes required for the secretion of adrenal androgens in the mouse adrenal gland is an exceptional condition, which is not found in wild-type mouse adrenal glands.[107,110,111] Interestingly, a direct functional interrelationship between LH receptor and GATA-4 with an apparent positive and reciprocal feed-forward amplification link between LH receptor and GATA-4 expression has been established in INH-Tag mice. Thus this mechanism is thought to contribute to autonomous adrenal growth and the formation of the LH-dependent adrenocortical tumors[112] and might serve as a model for other illicit receptor-expressing adrenal tumors.

ACKNOWLEDGMENT

This work was supported by a grant from the Wilhelm-Sander-Stiftung to F.B. and M.R. (2003.145.1) and a grant from the Landesstiftung Baden-Würtemberg (P-LS-ASN/5) to F.B.

REFERENCES

1. ABECASSIS, M. et al. 1985. Serendipitous adrenal masses: prevalence, significance, and management. Am. J. Surg. **149:** 783–788.
2. HEDELAND, H., G. OSTBERG & B. HOKFELT. 1968. On the prevalence of adrenocortical adenomas in an autopsy material in relation to hypertension and diabetes. Acta Med. Scand. **184:** 211–214.
3. PRINZ, R.A. et al. 1982. Incidental asymptomatic adrenal masses detected by computed tomographic scanning. Is operation required? JAMA **248:** 701–704.

4. GLAZER, H.S. *et al*. 1982. Nonfunctioning adrenal masses: incidental discovery on computed tomography. Am. J. Roentgenol. **139:** 81–85.

5. BELLDEGRUN, A. *et al*. 1986. Incidentally discovered mass of the adrenal gland. Surg. Gynecol. Obstet. **163:** 203–208.

6. KLOOS, R.T. *et al*. 1995. Incidentally discovered adrenal masses. Endocr. Rev. **16:** 460–484.

7. ETTINGHAUSEN, S.E. & M.E. BURT. 1991. Prospective evaluation of unilateral adrenal masses in patients with operable non-small-cell lung cancer. J. Clin. Oncol. **9:** 1462–1466.

8. PORTE MD, H.L. *et al*. 1998. Adrenalectomy for a solitary adrenal metastasis from lung cancer. Ann. Thorac. Surg. **65:** 331–335.

9. SIEMER, S. *et al*. 2004. Adrenal metastases in 1635 patients with renal cell carcinoma: outcome and indication for adrenalectomy. J. Urol. **171:** 2155–2159; discussion 2159.

10. ALAMDARI, F.I. & B. LJUNGBERG. 2005. Adrenal metastasis in renal cell carcinoma: a recommendation for adjustment of the TNM staging system. Scand. J. Urol. Nephrol. **39:** 277–282.

11. LIPSETT, M.B., R. HERTZ & G.T. ROSS. 1963. Clinical and pathophysiologic aspects of adrenocortical carcinoma. Am. J. Med. **35:** 374–383.

12. AHLMAN, H. *et al*. 2001. Cytotoxic treatment of adrenocortical carcinoma. World J. Surg. **25:** 927–933.

13. WOOTEN, M.D. & D.K. KING. 1993. Adrenal cortical carcinoma. Epidemiology and treatment with mitotane and a review of the literature. Cancer **72:** 3145–3155.

14. FASSNACHT, M., W. KENN & B. ALLOLIO. 2004. Adrenal tumors: how to establish malignancy? J. Endocrinol. Invest. **27:** 387–399.

15. MANTERO, F. *et al*. 2000. A survey on adrenal incidentaloma in Italy. Study Group on Adrenal Tumors of the Italian Society of Endocrinology. J. Clin. Endocrinol. Metab. **85:** 637–644.

16. KOROBKIN, M. *et al*. 1998. CT time-attenuation washout curves of adrenal adenomas and nonadenomas. AJR Am. J. Roentgenol. **170:** 747–752.

17. PENA, C.S. *et al*. 2000. Characterization of indeterminate (lipid-poor) adrenal masses: use of washout characteristics at contrast-enhanced CT. Radiology **217:** 798–802.

18. KOROBKIN, M. *et al*. 1995. Characterization of adrenal masses with chemical shift and gadolinium-enhanced MR imaging. Radiology **197:** 411–418.

19. HONIGSCHNABL, S. *et al*. 2002. How accurate is MR imaging in characterisation of adrenal masses: update of a long-term study. Eur. J. Radiol. **41:** 113–122.

20. FRILLING, A. *et al*. 2004. Importance of adrenal incidentaloma in patients with a history of malignancy. Surgery **136:** 1289–1296.

21. FARDELLA, C.E. *et al*. 2000. Primary hyperaldosteronism in essential hypertensives: prevalence, biochemical profile, and molecular biology. J. Clin. Endocrinol. Metab. **85:** 1863–1867.

22. GORDON, R.D. *et al*. 1993. How common is primary aldosteronism? Is it the most frequent cause of curable hypertension? J. Hypertens. Suppl. **11:** S310–S311.

23. LIM, P.O. *et al*. 1999. Potentially high prevalence of primary aldosteronism in a primary-care population. Lancet **353:** 40.

24. MULATERO, P. *et al*. 2004. Increased diagnosis of primary aldosteronism, including surgically correctable forms, in centers from five continents. J. Clin. Endocrinol. Metab. **89:** 1045–1050.

25. BLUMENFELD, J.D. *et al.* 1994. Diagnosis and treatment of primary hyperaldosteronism. Ann. Intern. Med. **121:** 877–885.
26. STOWASSER, M. *et al.* 2001. Diagnosis and management of primary aldosteronism. J. Renin Angiotensin Aldosterone Syst. **2:** 156–169.
27. YOUNG, W.F., JR. 2003. Minireview: primary aldosteronism—changing concepts in diagnosis and treatment. Endocrinology **144:** 2208–2213.
28. TIU, S.C. *et al.* 2005. The use of aldosterone-renin ratio as a diagnostic test for primary hyperaldosteronism and its test characteristics under different conditions of blood sampling. J. Clin. Endocrinol. Metab. **90:** 72–78.
29. SEILER, L. *et al.* 2004. Diagnosis of primary aldosteronism: value of different screening parameters and influence of antihypertensive medication. Eur. J. Endocrinol. **150:** 329–337.
30. AGHARAZII, M. *et al.* 2001. Captopril suppression versus salt loading in confirming primary aldosteronism. Hypertension **37:** 1440–1443.
31. GANGULY, A. 1998. Primary aldosteronism. N. Engl. J. Med. **339:** 1828–1834.
32. STOKES, G.S., J.C. MONAGHAN & B.A. MENNIE. 1984. Use of an intravenous sodium load in screening for primary hyperaldosteronism. Aust. N. Z. J. Med. **14:** 201–207.
33. LINDHOLM, J. *et al.* 2001. Incidence and late prognosis of Cushing's syndrome: a population-based study. J. Clin. Endocrinol. Metab. **86:** 117–123.
34. URBANIC, R.C. & J.M. GEORGE. 1981. Cushing's disease–18 years' experience. Medicine (Baltimore) **60:** 14–24.
35. PUTIGNANO, P. *et al.* 2003. Midnight salivary cortisol versus urinary free and midnight serum cortisol as screening tests for Cushing's syndrome. J. Clin. Endocrinol. Metab. **88:** 4153–4157.
36. REIMONDO, G. *et al.* 2005. Evaluation of the effectiveness of midnight serum cortisol in the diagnostic procedures for Cushing's syndrome. Eur. J. Endocrinol. **153:** 803–809.
37. REINCKE, M. *et al.* 1992. Preclinical Cushing's syndrome in adrenal "incidentalomas": comparison with adrenal Cushing's syndrome. J. Clin. Endocrinol. Metab. **75:** 826–832.
38. ROSS, N.S. 1994. Epidemiology of Cushing's syndrome and subclinical disease. Endocrinol. Metab. Clin. North Am. **23:** 539–546.
39. TERZOLO *et al.* 1998. Subclinical Cushing's syndrome in adrenal incidentaloma. Clin. Endocrinol. **48:** 89–97.
40. TERZOLO, M. *et al.* 2002. Adrenal incidentaloma: a new cause of the metabolic syndrome? J. Clin. Endocrinol. Metab. **87:** 998–1003.
41. BARZON, L. *et al.* 2002. Development of overt Cushing's syndrome in patients with adrenal incidentaloma. Eur. J. Endocrinol. **146:** 61–66.
42. TERZOLO, M. *et al.* 2005. Midnight serum cortisol as a marker of increased cardiovascular risk in patients with a clinically inapparent adrenal adenoma. Eur. J. Endocrinol. **153:** 307–315.
43. ALLOLIO, B. *et al.* 2004. Management of adrenocortical carcinoma. Clin. Endocrinol. (Oxf). **60:** 273–287.
44. OSELLA, G. *et al.* 1994. Endocrine evaluation of incidentally discovered adrenal masses (incidentalomas). J. Clin. Endocrinol. Metab. **79:** 1532–1539.
45. TERZOLO, M. *et al.* 2000. The value of dehydroepiandrosterone sulfate measurement in the differentiation between benign and malignant adrenal masses. Eur. J. Endocrinol. **142:** 611–617.

46. GRUMBACH, M.M. *et al.* 2003. Management of the clinically inapparent adrenal mass ("incidentaloma"). Ann. Intern. Med. **138:** 424–429.
47. BEUSCHLEIN, F. *et al.* 1994. Clonal composition of human adrenocortical neoplasms. Cancer Res. **54:** 4927–4932.
48. GICQUEL, C. *et al.* 1994. Clonal analysis of human adrenocortical carcinomas and secreting adenomas. Clin. Endocrinol (Oxf). **40:** 465–477.
49. WIEDEMANN, H.R. 1964. Complexe malformatif familial avec hernie ombilicale et macroglossie—un syndrome nouveau? J. Genet. Hum. **13:** 223–232.
50. GICQUEL, C. *et al.* 1994. Rearrangements at the 11p15 locus and overexpression of insulin-like growth factor-II gene in sporadic adrenocortical tumors. J. Clin. Endocrinol. Metab. **78:** 1444–1453.
51. BOULLE, N. *et al.* 1998. Increased levels of insulin-like growth factor II (IGF-II) and IGF-binding protein-2 are associated with malignancy in sporadic adrenocortical tumors. J. Clin. Endocrinol. Metab. **83:** 1713–1720.
52. GIORDANO, T.J. *et al.* 2003. Distinct transcriptional profiles of adrenocortical tumors uncovered by DNA microarray analysis. Am. J. Pathol. **162:** 521–531.
53. WEBER, M.M. *et al.* 1997. Insulin-like growth factor receptors in normal and tumorous adult human adrenocortical glands. Eur. J. Endocrinol. **136:** 296–303.
54. WEBER, M.M. *et al.* 1999. Postnatal overexpression of insulin-like growth factor II in transgenic mice is associated with adrenocortical hyperplasia and enhanced steroidogenesis. Endocrinology **140:** 1537–1543.
55. HATADA, I. & T. MUKAI. 1995. Genomic imprinting of p57KIP2, a cyclin-dependent kinase inhibitor, in mouse. Nat. Genet. **11:** 204–206.
56. MATSUOKA, S. *et al.* 1995. p57KIP2, a structurally distinct member of the p21CIP1 Cdk inhibitor family, is a candidate tumor suppressor gene. Genes Dev. **9:** 650–662.
57. ZHANG, P. *et al.* 1997. Altered cell differentiation and proliferation in mice lacking p57KIP2 indicates a role in Beckwith-Wiedemann syndrome. Nature **387:** 151–158.
58. LIU, J. *et al.* 1997. Ribonucleic acid expression of the clustered imprinted genes, p57KIP2, insulin-like growth factor II, and H19, in adrenal tumors and cultured adrenal cells. J. Clin. Endocrinol. Metab. **82:** 1766–1771.
59. BOURCIGAUX, N. *et al.* 2000. High expression of cyclin E and G1 CDK and loss of function of p57KIP2 are involved in proliferation of malignant sporadic adrenocortical tumors. J. Clin. Endocrinol. Metab. **85:** 322–330.
60. MALKIN, D. *et al.* 1990. Germ line p53 mutations in a familial syndrome of breast cancer, sarcomas, and other neoplasms. Science **250:** 1233–1238.
61. LEVINE, A.J. 1997. p53, the cellular gatekeeper for growth and division. Cell **88:** 323–331.
62. RIBEIRO, R.C. *et al.* 2001. An inherited p53 mutation that contributes in a tissue-specific manner to pediatric adrenal cortical carcinoma. Proc. Natl. Acad. Sci. USA **98:** 9330–9335.
63. DIGIAMMARINO, E.L. *et al.* 2002. A novel mechanism of tumorigenesis involving pH-dependent destabilization of a mutant p53 tetramer. Nat. Struct. Biol. **9:** 12–16.
64. REINCKE, M. *et al.* 1994. p53 mutations in human adrenocortical neoplasms: immunohistochemical and molecular studies. J. Clin. Endocrinol. Metab. **78:** 790–794.

65. VALE, W. *et al.* 1986. Purification and characterization of an FSH releasing protein from porcine ovarian follicular fluid. Nature **321:** 776–779.
66. SPENCER, S.J. *et al.* 1999. Proliferation and apoptosis in the human adrenal cortex during the fetal and perinatal periods: implications for growth and remodeling. J. Clin. Endocrinol. Metab. **84:** 1110–1115.
67. BILLIAR, R.B. *et al.* 1999. Functional capacity of fetal zone cells of the baboon fetal adrenal gland: a major source of alpha-inhibin. Biol. Reprod. **61:** 142–146.
68. CHEN, Y.G. *et al.* 2002. Regulation of cell proliferation, apoptosis, and carcinogenesis by activin. Exp. Biol. Med. (Maywood). **227:** 75–87.
69. SPENCER, S.J. *et al.* 1992. Activin and inhibin in the human adrenal gland. Regulation and differential effects in fetal and adult cells. J. Clin. Invest. **90:** 142–149.
70. MATZUK, M.M. & A. BRADLEY. 1994. Identification and analysis of tumor suppressor genes using transgenic mouse models. Semin. Cancer Biol. **5:** 37–45.
71. BEUSCHLEIN, F. *et al.* 2003. Activin induces x-zone apoptosis that inhibits luteinizing hormone-dependent adrenocortical tumor formation in inhibin-deficient mice. Mol. Cell. Biol. **23:** 3951–3964.
72. BUCKLEY, D.I. & J. RAMACHANDRAN. 1981. Characterization of corticotropin receptors on adrenocortical cells. Proc. Natl. Acad. Sci. USA **78:** 7431–7435.
73. YAMAZAKI, T. *et al.* 1996. 15-lipoxygenase metabolite(s) of arachidonic acid mediates adrenocorticotropin action in bovine adrenal steroidogenesis. Endocrinology **137:** 2670–2675.
74. LIN, D. *et al.* 1995. Role of steroidogenic acute regulatory protein in adrenal and gonadal steroidogenesis. Science **267:** 1828–1831.
75. LEHOUX, J.G., A. FLEURY & L. DUCHARME. 1998. The acute and chronic effects of adrenocorticotropin on the levels of messenger ribonucleic acid and protein of steroidogenic enzymes in rat adrenal *in vivo*. Endocrinology **139:** 3913–3922.
76. LYONS, J. *et al.* 1990. Two G protein oncogenes in human endocrine tumors. Science **249:** 655–659.
77. PARMA, J. *et al.* 1993. Somatic mutations in the thyrotropin receptor gene cause hyperfunctioning thyroid adenomas. Nature **365:** 649–651.
78. LATRONICO, A.C. *et al.* 1995. No evidence for oncogenic mutations in the adrenocorticotropin receptor gene in human adrenocortical neoplasms. J. Clin. Endocrinol. Metab. **80:** 875–877.
79. LIGHT, K. *et al.* 1995. Are activating mutations of the adrenocorticotropin receptor involved in adrenal cortical neoplasia? Life Sci. **56:** 1523–1527.
80. REINCKE, M. *et al.* 1993. No evidence for oncogenic mutations in guanine nucleotide-binding proteins of human adrenocortical neoplasms. J. Clin. Endocrinol. Metab. **77:** 1419–1422.
81. REINCKE, M. *et al.* 1997. Deletion of the adrenocorticotropin receptor gene in human adrenocortical tumors: implications for tumorigenesis. J. Clin. Endocrinol. Metab. **82:** 3054–3058.
82. ZWERMANN, O. *et al.* 2005. ACTH 1-24 inhibits proliferation of adrenocortical tumors *in vivo*. Eur. J. Endocrinol. **153:** 435–444.
83. SCHIMMER, B.P. *et al.* 1995. Adrenocorticotropin-resistant mutants of the Y1 adrenal cell line fail to express the adrenocorticotropin receptor. J. Cell. Physiol. **163:** 164–171.
84. ROSEN, E.D. & B.M. SPIEGELMAN. 2001. PPARgamma: a nuclear regulator of metabolism, differentiation, and cell growth. J. Biol. Chem. **276:** 37731–37734.

85. BETZ, M.J. *et al.* 2005. Peroxisome proliferator-activated receptor-gamma agonists suppress adrenocortical tumor cell proliferation and induce differentiation. J. Clin. Endocrinol. Metab. **90:** 3886–3896.

86. FERRUZZI, P. *et al.* 2005. Thiazolidinediones inhibit growth and invasiveness of the human adrenocortical cancer cell line H295R. J. Clin. Endocrinol. Metab. **90:** 1332–1339.

87. ZHAO, J. *et al.* 1999. Analysis of genomic alterations in sporadic adrenocortical lesions. Gain of chromosome 17 is an early event in adrenocortical tumorigenesis. Am. J. Pathol. **155:** 1039–1045.

88. DOHNA, M. *et al.* 2000. Adrenocortical carcinoma is characterized by a high frequency of chromosomal gains and high-level amplifications. Genes Chromosomes Cancer **28:** 145–152.

89. KJELLMAN, M. *et al.* 1996. Genetic aberrations in adrenocortical tumors detected using comparative genomic hybridization correlate with tumor size and malignancy. Cancer Res. **56:** 4219–4223.

90. SIDHU, S. *et al.* 2002. Comparative genomic hybridization analysis of adrenocortical tumors. J. Clin. Endocrinol. Metab. **87:** 3467–3474.

91. LACROIX, A. *et al.* 2001. Ectopic and abnormal hormone receptors in adrenal Cushing's syndrome. Endocr. Rev. **22:** 75–110.

92. ARNALDI, G. *et al.* 1998. Variable expression of the V1 vasopressin receptor modulates the phenotypic response of steroid-secreting adrenocortical tumors. J. Clin. Endocrinol. Metab. **83:** 2029–2035.

93. AMIGH, K.S. *et al.* 2005. Elevated expression of luteinizing hormone receptor in aldosterone-producing adenomas. J. Clin. Endocrinol. Metab. 2005–1298.

94. MILLINGTON, D.S. *et al.* 1976. *In vitro* synthesis of steroids by a feminising adrenocortical carcinoma: effect of prolactin and other protein hormones. Acta Endocrinol. (Copenh) **82:** 561–571.

95. DANILOWICZ, K. *et al.* 2002. Androgen-secreting adrenal adenomas. Obstet. Gynecol. **100:** 1099–1102.

96. LEINONEN, P. *et al.* 1991. Testosterone-secreting virilizing adrenal adenoma with human chorionic gonadotrophin receptors and 21-hydroxylase deficiency. Clin. Endocrinol. (Oxf) **34:** 31–35.

97. DE LANGE, W.E., J.J. PRATT & H. DOORENBOS. 1980. A gonadotrophin responsive testosterone producing adrenocortical adenoma and high gonadotrophin levels in an elderly woman. Clin. Endocrinol (Oxf) **12:** 21–28.

98. BUGALHO, M.J. *et al.* 2000. Presence of a Gs alpha mutation in an adrenal tumor expressing LH/hCG receptors and clinically associated with Cushing's syndrome. Gynecol. Endocrinol. **14:** 50–54.

99. PABON, J.E. *et al.* 1996. Novel presence of luteinizing hormone/chorionic gonadotropin receptors in human adrenal glands. J. Clin. Endocrinol. Metab. **81:** 2397–2400.

100. SERON-FERRE, M., C.C. LAWRENCE & R.B. JAFFE. 1978. Role of hCG in regulation of the fetal zone of the human fetal adrenal gland. J. Clin. Endocrinol. Metab. **46:** 834–837.

101. MAZZUCO, T.L. *et al.* 2005. Ectopic expression of the gastric inhibitory polypeptide receptor gene is a sufficient genetic event to induce benign adrenocortical tumor in a xenotransplantation model. Endocrinology **147:** 782–790.

102. MATZUK, M.M. *et al.* 1994. Development of cancer cachexia-like syndrome and adrenal tumors in inhibin-deficient mice. Proc. Natl. Acad. Sci. USA **91:** 8817–8821.

103. KANANEN, K. *et al*. 1996. Gonadectomy permits adrenocortical tumorigenesis in mice transgenic for the mouse inhibin alpha-subunit promoter/simian virus 40 T-antigen fusion gene: evidence for negative autoregulation of the inhibin alpha-subunit gene. Mol. Endocrinol. **10:** 1667–1677.
104. WOOLLEY, G.W. & C.C. LITTLE. 1945. The incidence of adrenal cortical carcinoma in gonadectomized female mice of the extreme dilution strain. II. Observation on the accessory sex organs. Cancer Res. **5:** 203–210.
105. BIELINSKA, M. *et al*. 2005. Gonadotropin-induced adrenocortical neoplasia in NU/J nude mice. Endocrinology **146:** 3975–3984.
106. BIELINSKA, M. *et al*. 2003. Mouse strain susceptibility to gonadectomy-induced adrenocortical tumor formation correlates with the expression of GATA-4 and luteinizing hormone receptor. Endocrinology **144:** 4123–4133.
107. RILIANAWATI *et al*. 1998. Direct luteinizing hormone action triggers adrenocortical tumorigenesis in castrated mice transgenic for the murine inhibin alpha-subunit promoter/simian virus 40 T-antigen fusion gene. Mol. Endocrinol. **12:** 801–809.
108. MIKOLA, M. *et al*. 2003. High levels of luteinizing hormone analog stimulate gonadal and adrenal tumorigenesis in mice transgenic for the mouse inhibin-alpha-subunit promoter/simian virus 40 T-antigen fusion gene. Oncogene **22:** 3269–3278.
109. KANANEN, K. *et al*. 1997. Suppression of gonadotropins inhibits gonadal tumorigenesis in mice transgenic for the mouse inhibin alpha-subunit promoter/simian virus 40 T-antigen fusion gene. Endocrinology **138:** 3521–3531.
110. KERO, J. *et al*. 2000. Elevated luteinizing hormone induces expression of its receptor and promotes steroidogenesis in the adrenal cortex. J. Clin. Invest. **105:** 633–641.
111. KIIVERI, S. *et al*. 1999. Reciprocal changes in the expression of transcription factors GATA-4 and GATA-6 accompany adrenocortical tumorigenesis in mice and humans. Mol. Med. **5:** 490–501.
112. RAHMAN, N.A. *et al*. 2004. Adrenocortical tumorigenesis in transgenic mice expressing the inhibin alpha-subunit promoter/simian virus 40 T-antigen transgene: relationship between ectopic expression of luteinizing hormone receptor and transcription factor GATA-4. Mol. Endocrinol. **18:** 2553–2569.

Alpha 2-Adrenergic Receptors Decrease DNA Replication and Cell Proliferation and Induce Neurite Outgrowth in Transfected Rat Pheochromocytoma Cells

G. KARKOULIAS,[a] O. MASTROGIANNI,[a] I. ILIAS,[a]
A. LYMPEROPOULOS,[b] S. TARAVIRAS,[a] N. TSOPANOGLOU,[a]
N. SITARAS,[c] AND C.S. FLORDELLIS[a]

[a]*Department of Pharmacology, School of Medicine, University of Patras-Rion, GR-26504, Greece*

[b]*Center for Translational Medicine, Department of Medicine, Thomas Jefferson University, Philadelphia, Pennsylvania 19107, USA*

[c]*Department of Pharmacology, School of Medicine, University of Athens, GR-11527, Greece*

ABSTRACT: Alpha 2-adrenergic receptors (α_2-ARs) have a widespread distribution in the central nervous system (CNS) and affect a number of biochemical and behavioral functions, including stimulation of prefrontal cortex (PFC) and cognitive function. In addition to its role as a classical neurotransmitter, norepinephrine (NE) has been recently shown to exert an important influence on the plasticity in areas of the brain where neurogenesis persists in the adult, notably the subgranular zone (SGZ) within the dentate gyrus of the hippocampus and the olfactory bulb (OB). In regulating adult neurogenesis, the noradrenergic system is functionally integrated with chronic stress and depression. Chronic stress, depression, or depletion of NE *in vivo* suppress, and antidepressant treatments induce hippocampal neurogenesis by down- or upregulating, respectively, cell proliferation. In the present study we show that α_2-AR subtypes promote the differentiation rather than cell proliferation of PC12 cells. It is conceivable that α_2-ARs might contribute neurotrophic actions *in vivo* synergistically or in permutation with other neurotrophic factors.

KEYWORDS: neuronal differentiation; α_2-adrenergic receptor; PC12 cells; neurite outgrowth

INTRODUCTION

The α_2-adrenergic receptor (α_2-AR) is a prototypical G-protein-coupled receptor (GPCR) that mediates many of the physiological actions of

Address for correspondence: Prof. C.S. Flordellis, Department of Pharmacology, School of Medicine, University of Patras-Rion, GR-26504, Greece. Voice: +30-2610-997638; fax: +30-2610-994720.
e-mail: flordell@med.upatras.gr

Ann. N.Y. Acad. Sci. 1088: 335–345 (2006). © 2006 New York Academy of Sciences.
doi: 10.1196/annals.1366.017

catecholamines and adrenergic drugs. There are three distinct subtypes (α_{2A}, α_{2B}, and α_{2C}) that differ in their ligand-binding properties, tissue distribution, chromosomal localization, regulatory mechanisms, and signal transduction pathways.[1-5]

All three subtypes are expressed in the central nervous system (CNS). Studies carried out on transgenic mice have demonstrated that central α_{2A}-ARs mediate the sedative, hypnotic, sympatholytic, and analgesic actions of α_2-agonists.[6-8] α_{2B}-AR has a restricted CNS expression mainly in the thalamus; its role is still unclear, but central α_{2B}-AR would play a role in salt-induced experimental hypertension.[9] On the other hand, the α_{2C}-AR is primarily found in the olfactory tubercles, cerebral cortex, basal ganglia, and hippocampus and is believed to exert modulatory effects on several brain functions possibly by regulating dopamine and serotonin metabolism.[10,11] Moreover, the α_{2C}-AR subtype was recently shown to participate with α_{2A}-AR in presynaptic inhibition of neurotransmitter release.[12,13]

Besides having a well-established role in neurotransmission and the regulation of sympathetic outflow,[13] α_2-ARs have recently been shown in animals *in vivo* to exert neuromodulatory and neurotrophic actions.[14,15]

Recent studies have shown that α_2-ARs influence prefrontal cortex (PFC) functions, such as cognitive performance, attention, and locomotor activity. In addition there is *in vivo* evidence indicating that α_2-ARs are implicated in adult neurogenesis exerting distinct neurotrophic influences on the hippocampus and olfactory bulb (OB).

Using clones of the rat pheochromocytoma PC12 cells transfected with α_2-AR subtypes, we have previously demonstrated *in vitro* that activation of α_2-ARs induces subtype-specific neuronal differentiation of PC12 cells and this might be indicative of a similar differentiating action of α_2-ARs *in vivo*.[16]

In the present study we show that α_{2C}-ARs induce, upon agonist-stimulation, neurite outgrowth in transfected PC12 cells, whereas they decrease DNA replication and cell proliferation. This *in vitro* effect of α_2-ARs is contrary to the effects of α_2-ARs that have been described previously *in vivo*. α_2-ARs do not exert *in vivo* differentiating actions, but stimulate progenitor cell proliferation or survival in distinct brain regions.

We speculate that α_2-ARs might exert differential effects depending on the brain region or the developmental stage, acting alone or in synergism or permutation with other neurotrophin receptors.

MATERIALS AND METHODS

Reagents

Epinephrine bitartrate, RX821002, 3-(4,5-dimethylthiazol-2-yl)-2,5-diphenyltetrazolium bromide, and monoclonal anti-α-tubulin antibody were purchased from Sigma (St. Louis, MO, USA). Nerve growth factor (NGF) was from Promega (Madison, WI, USA). Dulbecco's modified Eagle's medium (DMEM), fetal bovine serum (FBS), and horse serum were from Biochrom KG. Vitrogen 100 was obtained from Collagen Co (Fremont, CA, USA). [^{3}H] thymidine (35 Ci/mmol) was from MP Biomedicals Inc (Irvine, CA, USA). Antiperipherin antibody and horseradish peroxidase–conjugated rabbit anti-mouse antibody were from Chemicon International Inc. (Temecula, CA, USA). Enhanced chemiluminescence (ECL) reagent was from Amersham Biosciences (Piscataway, NJ, USA).

Cell Lines and Culture

The characteristics of PC12 cells stably expressing the human α$_{2C}$-AR subtype have been previously described.[17] Cells were routinely plated onto collagen-coated dishes (1% Vitrogen 100 and 0.1% bovine serum albumin) and grown in high-glucose DMEM supplemented with 10 % horse serum, 5 % fetal bovine serum, 50 μg/mL streptomycin, 100 IU/mL penicillin, 2 mM L-glutamine, 1 mM Na-pyruvate, and 20 mM NaHCO$_3$.

For the differentiation experiments, PC12 cells were plated (50,000 cells/mL) on collagen-coated culture dishes and cultured in DMEM supplemented with 1% HS and 10mM MgCl$_2$ (differentiation medium). Regulator substances were added in the differentiation medium in the presence or absence of several inhibitors. For morphological experiments, cells were visualized by phase-contrast microscopy, and representative cells were photographed. Images were prepared using the Adobe Photoshop 5.5 software.

Western Blot Analysis

PC12 cells were differentiated by treatment with epinephrine or NGF for 4 days. Cells were harvested and analyzed in SDS-PAGE as previously described.[18] Duplicate nitrocellulose blots were incubated with either antiperipherin, or anti-α-tubulin antibody. Immunostained proteins were visualized using the ECL detection system (Amersham Biosciences).

[^{3}H]-Thymidine Incorporation

PC12 cells were differentiated by treatment with epinephrine for 4 days. Proliferating (day 0) and epinephrine-treated cells were pulsed with 0.5 μCi/mL [^{3}H]-thymidine for an additional 6 h. DNA synthesis was stopped by removing the radioactive media, washing the cells with PBS, and fixing them with ice-cold methanol. Cells were then washed twice with 5% trichloroacetic acid and the acid-insoluble fractions were lysed in 0.5 N NaOH. The radioactivity was determined in a liquid scintillation counter. Each experiment included three wells in each condition tested and was repeated three times. Data at each time point were normalized to the protein level.

Cell Proliferation Assay

Cell proliferation was evaluated by 3-(4,5-dimethylthiazol-2-yl)-2,5-diphenyltetrazolium bromide (MTT) assay. PC12 cells were cultured in differentiation medium and treated or not with epinephrine for 4 days. At each time point, MTT (250 μL) solution (5 mg/mL) was added to each well and incubated for 2 h at 37°C. The blue formazan crystals were solubilized by addition of DMSO. Absorbance at 589 nm was recorded using a 96-well plate reader. Results are expressed as mean ± SE of number from cells and presented as fold increased of cell number at the beginning of experiments. Each experiment included three wells in each condition tested and was repeated at least twice.

RESULTS

The role of α_2-ARs in neuronal differentiation was studied in PC12 cells stably transfected with the human α_{2C}-AR gene. In response to chronic treatment with NGF, PC12 cells differentiate to sympathetic-like neurons with neurite outgrowth and expression of specific proteins associated with neuronal function.[19,20] Epinephrine treatment induced differentiation of PC12/α_{2C} cells, with flattening of the cell bodies and extension of cellular outgrowths, similar to the morphological changes induced by NGF (FIG. 1). Previous ligand binding, biochemical, and immunocytochemical studies have found

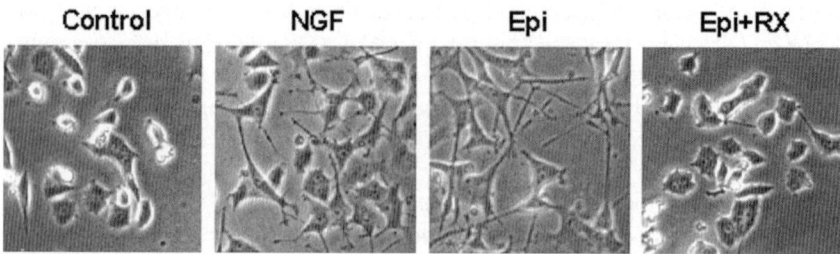

FIGURE 1. Neurite outgrowth in epinephrine-treated PC12α_2 cells. PC12 cells expressing α_{2C}-AR were cultured in differentiation medium for 4 days either without stimulation (control) or in the presence of 10 μM epinephrine or 100 ng/mL NGF. Simultaneous with the stimulation, cells were treated or not with 10 μM RX821002 for 30 min. Phase-contrast images of representative fields were taken. As shown, epinephrine induced neurite outgrowth in PC12/α_{2C} cells, similar to NGF.

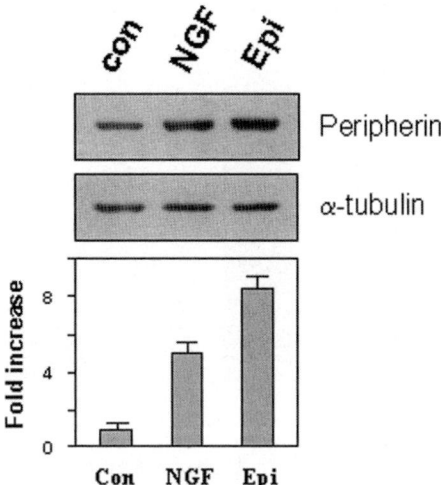

FIGURE 2. Peripherin expression in differentiating PC12α₂ cells. PC12 cells expressing α₂C-AR were cultured in differentiation medium for 4 days either without stimulation (control) or in the presence of 10 μM epinephrine or 100 ng/mL NGF. Cell lysates were immunoblotted using antibodies against peripherin and α-tubulin. Densitometric analysis was performed and data are presented as ± SE of three independent experiments.

no detectable levels of any adrenergic receptor subtype in nontransfected PC12 cells.[17,21] Moreover, the effect of epinephrine was totally abolished by pretreatment of the cells with the α₂-antagonist, RX821002, implying that the action of epinephrine was mediated by the α₂C-AR. These morphological effects were accompanied by an increase in the expression of the neurofilament protein peripherin, confirming the neuronal character of the observed morphological differentiation. Specifically, expression of peripherin was present in nondifferentiated PC12/α₂C cells, and treatment with epinephrine increased peripherin expression in levels even higher than those of NGF (FIG. 2). During terminal neuronal differentiation cells stop dividing and permanently withdraw from the cell cycle. PC12/α₂C cells were assayed for [³H]-thymidine uptake after 4 days of epinephrine treatment. As shown in FIGURE 3, treatment of PC12/α₂C cells with 10 μM epinephrine for 4 days resulted in a marked decrease in thymidine incorporation to near background levels, indicating that epinephrine treatment slows DNA synthesis. Growth arrest during epinephrine-induced neuronal differentiation was further examined by 3-(4,5-dimethylthiazol-2-yl)-2,5-diphenyltetrazolium bromide (MTT) assay. PC12 cells were cultured in differentiation medium for 4 days either without stimulation or in the presence of 10 μM epinephrine. Cells grown in differentiation medium continued to proliferate, whereas cells grown in the presence of epinephrine underwent a dramatic growth arrest (FIG. 4).

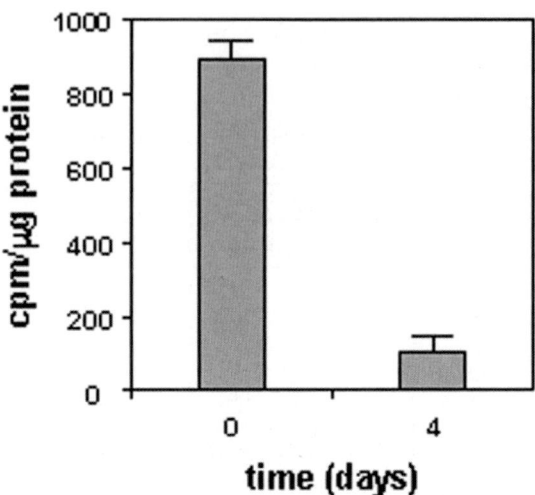

FIGURE 3. Changes in [^{3}H]-thymidine incorporation into DNA during differentiation of PC12α$_{2C}$ cells. Levels of [^{3}H]-thymidine incorporation into DNA over 6 h were measured in proliferating cells (day 0) and in epinephrine-treated PC12 cells for 4 days. Results shown are representative of three triplicate independent experiments with similar results.

DISCUSSION

Because of their widespread distribution in the CNS, α$_2$-ARs affect a number of biochemical and behavioral functions.[11,22] In particular α$_{2A/D(B)}$ and α$_{2C}$ receptor subtypes are highly expressed in hippocampus, amygdala, and neocortex, brain regions related to learning and memory and thus affect cognitive processes related to attention, learning, and memory. Thus, α$_2$-AR stimulation in PFC strengthens working memory at the cellullar and behavioral levels, whereas blocking α$_2$-ARs in PFC results in poor attention, increased distractibility, and increased impulsivity as well as induced locomotor hyperactivity, thus recreating many of the symptoms of attention deficit hyperactivity disorder (ADHD).[23,24]

In addition to its role as a classical neurotransmitter, norepinephrine (NE) has a critical influence on plasticity in areas of the brain where neurogenesis persists in the adult. Discrete regions within adult mammalian brain in several mammalian species retain the ability to form new neurons.[25,26] Among these regions are the subgranular zone (SGZ), within the dentate gyrus of the hippocampus, and the OB. The process includes proliferation of progenitors and migration into the granular cell layer in the case of hippocampus,[27] or along the rostral migratory stream to the subependymal layer of the OB,[26] where they differentiate to neural cells.[28] In this latter process progenitor cells express neuronal markers, extend neurite processes, and receive synaptic input.

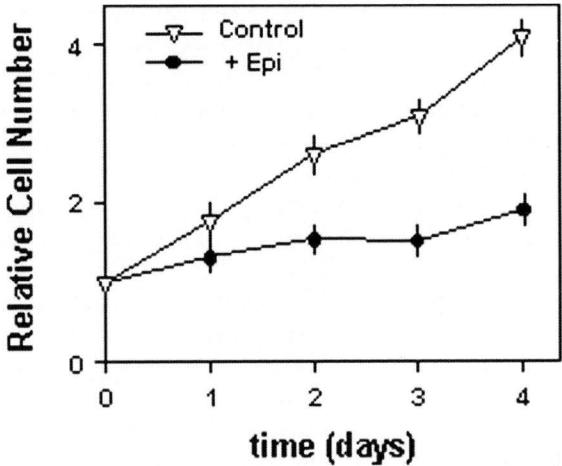

FIGURE 4. Inhibition of PC12α₂ proliferation by epinephrine. Proliferation of PC12α$_{2C}$ cells was measured in untreated cultures (control) or those grown in the presence of 10 μM epinephrine for the indicated days. Relative cell number represents the ratio of cells at a given time point to the number of cells at time 0. Data represent means ± SE of three triplicate independent experiments.

Recent studies have shown that NE exerts an important role in the regulation of adult hippocampal neurogenesis. NE depletion significantly decreases proliferation of dentate gyrus cells without affecting survival or neuronal or glial differentiation of granule cell progenitors in the adult rat hippocampus.[25] This is consistent with the substantial noradrenergic input to dentate gyrus and the effect of NE in the proliferation of neuroepithelial cells during development,[29] as well as the fact that NE system is a major target of stress and antidepressant treatments, processes that affect adult neurogenesis in hippocampus. Although it is not known whether progenitors in SGZ specifically express any of the adrenergic receptor subtypes, hippocampal neurons express several adrenergic receptor subtypes and it is possible that NE affects progenitor proliferation directly through adrenergic receptors. Alternatively, NE may act indirectly through changes in other growth factors that regulate hippocampal neurogenesis (such as the alteration in the ratio of distinct growth factors [NGF, BDNF] in hippocampus among others).[25]

The noradrenergic system is also densely innervating OB by afferents originating in the locus ceruleus. Pharmacological activation of the noradrenergic system by α₂-adrenoceptor antagonists (dexefaroxan or 5-fluoro-methoxyidazoxan- F 14413),[30] reduces deafferentation-induced neuronal death and indirectly cell proliferation in the adult mouse OB subventricular zone (SVZ) and rostral migratory stream (RMS).[26] Together these data indicate that NE might exert distinct influences on adult neurogenesis in the hippocampus and the OB. These *in vivo* data are different from the results obtained with α_2-ARs expressed in PC12 cells. We have previously demonstrated that stimulation of all three α_2-AR subtypes elicits subtype-specific morphological and molecular neuronal differentiation,[16] and in the present study we show that neurite outgrowth and expression of peripherin, a marker of the neuronal phenotype, induced by α_2-AR is associated with a decrease in DNA replication and cell proliferation.

The noradrenergic system is functionally integrated with chronic stress and depression and these three systems interact and converge in regulating adult neurogenesis. Stressful events, including psychosocial and physical stress, are the most potent factors known to elicit depression,[31] and chronic stress decreases cell proliferation and neurogenesis in the hippocampus[32] through action on excitatory pathways to the dentate gyrus,[33] whereas chronic antidepressant treatments increase BDNF mRNA levels[34] and stimulate dentate neurogenesis in hippocampus.[35] Similarly, increased hippocampal BDNF expression is observed after physical exercise and this is dependent upon noradrenergic neurotransmission.

Moreover, stress also activates the noradrenergic system and induces changes in α_2-ARs, some of which persist throughout the recovery period and might contribute to development of depression. Stress exerts a subtype-specific and time-dependent effect on α_2-AR expression. Specifically, upregulation of α_{2C}-AR in striatum and other brain areas is transient. Meanwhile, for the α_{2A}-AR, the main noradrenergic autoreceptor, a considerable decrease in its mRNA has been observed in locus ceruleus neurons after 4 weeks of chronic stress,[36] whereas at 6 weeks of chronic stress there was an upregulation of α_{2A}-AR heteroreceptors in glutamergic neurons of the lateral reticular nucleus.[37] Finally, α_{2B}-AR is persistently upregulated in the thalamic paraventricular nucleus (PVN), which regulates the hypothalamic-pituitary-adrenal (HPA) axis and temperature[38] and whose neurons project to PFC, hippocampus, and amygdala, areas important for cognition and emotion.[39]

Chronic stress, depression, or depletion of NE *in vivo* suppress and antidepressant treatments induce hippocampal neurogenesis by down- or upregulating, respectively, cell proliferation. If our findings, that α_2-AR subtypes promote the differentiation and decrease cell proliferation of PC12 cells *in vitro*, hold true also *in vivo*, it would be conceivable that epinephrine might exert neurotrophic actions *in vivo* synergistically or in permutation with other neurotrophic factors.

ACKNOWLEDGMENTS

This work was supported in part by a research grant (EPAN-Heracles, 2005) of the General Secretariat for Research and Technology of the Greek Ministry of Development.

REFERENCES

1. MACDONALD, E. *et al.* 1997. Gene targeting-homing in on alpha 2-adrenoceptor-subtype function. Trends Pharmacol. Sci. **18**: 211–219.
2. HANDY, D.E. *et al.* 1993. Diverse tissue expression of rat alpha 2-adrenergic receptor genes. Hypertension **21**: 861–865.
3. DAUNT, D.A. *et al.* 1997. Subtype-specific intracellular trafficking of alpha2-adrenergic receptors. Mol. Pharmacol. **51**: 711–720.
4. VON ZASTROW, M. *et al.* 1993. Subtype-specific differences in the intracellular sorting of G protein-coupled receptors. J. Biol. Chem. **268**: 763–766.
5. PHILIPP, M. *et al.* 2002. Physiological significance of alpha(2)-adrenergic receptor subtype diversity: one receptor is not enough. Am. J. Physiol. Regul. Integr. Comp. Physiol. **283**: R287–R295.
6. MACMILLAN, L.B. *et al.* 1996. Central hypotensive effects of the alpha2a-adrenergic receptor subtype. Science **273**: 801–803.
7. LINK, R.E. *et al.* 1996. Cardiovascular regulation in mice lacking alpha2-adrenergic receptor subtypes b and c. Science **273**: 803–805.
8. KABLE, J.W. *et al.* 2000. *In vivo* gene modification elucidates subtype-specific functions of alpha(2)-adrenergic receptors. J. Pharmacol. Exp. Ther. **293**: 1–7.
9. MAKARITSIS, K.P. *et al.* 1999. Role of the alpha2B-adrenergic receptor in the development of salt-induced hypertension. Hypertension **33**: 14–17.
10. SALLINEN, J. *et al.* 1997. Genetic alteration of alpha 2C-adrenoceptor expression in mice: influence on locomotor, hypothermic, and neurochemical effects of dexmedetomidine, a subtype-nonselective alpha 2-adrenoceptor agonist. Mol. Pharmacol. **51**: 36–46.
11. SALLINEN, J. *et al.* 1998. D-amphetamine and L-5-hydroxytryptophan-induced behaviours in mice with genetically-altered expression of the alpha2C-adrenergic receptor subtype. Neuroscience **86**: 959–965.
12. BUCHELER, M.M. *et al.* 2002. Two alpha(2)-adrenergic receptor subtypes, alpha(2A) and alpha(2C), inhibit transmitter release in the brain of gene-targeted mice. Neuroscience **109**: 819–826.
13. BREDE, M. *et al.* 2003. Differential control of adrenal and sympathetic catecholamine release by alpha 2-adrenoceptor subtypes. Mol. Endocrinol. **17**: 1640–1646.
14. LAHDESMAKI, J. *et al.* 2004. Alpha2A-adrenoceptors are important modulators of the effects of D-amphetamine on startle reactivity and brain monoamines. Neuropsychopharmacology **29**: 1282–1293.
15. MA, D. *et al.* 2005. Alpha2-adrenoceptor agonists: shedding light on neuroprotection? Br. Med. Bull. **71**: 77–92.
16. TARAVIRAS, S. *et al.* 2002. Subtype-specific neuronal differentiation of PC12 cells transfected with alpha2-adrenergic receptors. Eur. J. Cell Biol. **81**: 363–374.
17. OLLI-LAHDESMAKI, T. *et al.* 1999. Receptor subtype-induced targeting and subtype-specific internalization of human alpha(2)-adrenoceptors in PC12 cells. J. Neurosci. **19**: 9281–9288.
18. KARKOULIAS, G. *et al.* 2006. alpha(2)-Adrenergic receptors activate MAPK and Akt through a pathway involving arachidonic acid metabolism by cytochrome P450-dependent epoxygenase, matrix metalloproteinase activation and subtype-specific transactivation of EGFR. Cell Signal **18**: 729–739.

19. GREENE, L.A. 1984. The importance of both early and delayed responses in the biological actions of nerve growth factor. Trends Neurosci. **7:** 91–94.
20. PEUNOVA, N. *et al.* 1995. Nitric oxide triggers a switch to growth arrest during differentiation of neuronal cells. Nature **375:** 68–73.
21. WILLIAMS, N.G. *et al.* 1998. Differential coupling of alpha1-, alpha2-, and beta-adrenergic receptors to mitogen-activated protein kinase pathways and differentiation in transfected PC12 cells. J. Biol. Chem. **273:** 24624–24632.
22. SCHEININ, M. *et al.* 2001. Evaluation of the alpha2C-adrenoceptor as a neuropsychiatric drug target studies in transgenic mouse models. Life Sci. **68:** 2277–2285.
23. ARNSTEN, A.F. *et al.* 2005. Methylphenidate improves prefrontal cortical cognitive function through alpha2 adrenoceptor and dopamine D1 receptor actions: relevance to therapeutic effects in attention deficit hyperactivity disorder. Behav. Brain Funct. 1:2/doi. 10.1186/1744-9081-1-1-2
24. ARNSTEN, A.F. *et al.* 2005. Neurobiology of executive functions: catecholamine influences on prefrontal cortical functions. Biol. Psychiatry **57:** 1377–1384.
25. KULKARNI, V.A. *et al.* 2002. Depletion of norepinephrine decreases the proliferation, but does not influence the survival and differentiation, of granule cell progenitors in the adult rat hippocampus. Eur. J. Neurosci. **16:** 2008–2012.
26. VEYRAC, A. *et al.* 2005. Activation of noradrenergic transmission by alpha2-adrenoceptor antagonists counteracts deafferentation-induced neuronal death and cell proliferation in the adult mouse olfactory bulb. Exp. Neurol. **194:** 444–456.
27. FUCHS, E. *et al.* 2004. Alterations of neuroplasticity in depression: the hippocampus and beyond. Eur. Neuropsychopharmacol. **14:** S481–S490.
28. VAN PRAAG, H. *et al.* 2002. Functional neurogenesis in the adult hippocampus. Nature **415:** 1030–1034.
29. POPOVIK, E. *et al.* 2000. Survival and mitogenesis of neuroepithelial cells are influenced by noradrenergic but not cholinergic innervation in cultured embryonic rat neopallium. Brain Res. **853:** 227–235.
30. BAUER, S. *et al.* 2003. Effects of the alpha 2-adrenoreceptor antagonist dexefaroxan on neurogenesis in the olfactory bulb of the adult rat in vivo: selective protection against neuronal death. Neuroscience **117:** 281–291.
31. PAYKEL, E.S. 2001. Stress and affective disorders in humans. Semin. Clin. Neuropsychiatry **6:** 4–11.
32. HEINE, V.M. *et al.* 2004. Suppressed proliferation and apoptotic changes in the rat dentate gyrus after acute and chronic stress are reversible. Eur. J. Neurosci. **19:** 131–144.
33. CAMERON, H.A. *et al.* 1995. Regulation of adult neurogenesis by excitatory input and NMDA receptor activation in the dentate gyrus. J. Neurosci. **15:** 4687–4692.
34. RUSSO-NEUSTADT, A.A. *et al.* 2000. Physical activity and antidepressant treatment potentiate the expression of specific brain-derived neurotrophic factor transcripts in the rat hippocampus. Neuroscience **101:** 305–312.
35. MALBERG, J.E. *et al.* 2000. Chronic antidepressant treatment increases neurogenesis in adult rat hippocampus. J. Neurosci. **20:** 9104–9110.
36. MEYER, H. *et al.* 2000. Regulation of alpha(2A)-adrenoceptor expression by chronic stress in neurons of the brain stem. Brain Res. **880:** 147–158.

37. FLUGGE, G. *et al.* 2003. Alpha2A and alpha2C-adrenoceptor regulation in the brain: alpha2A changes persist after chronic stress. Eur. J. Neurosci. **17:** 917–928.
38. BHATNAGAR, S. *et al.* 1999. The paraventricular nucleus of the thalamus alters rhythms in core temperature and energy balance in a state-dependent manner. Brain Res. **851:** 66–75.
39. VAN DER WERF, Y.D. *et al.* 2002. The intralaminar and midline nuclei of the thalamus. Anatomical and functional evidence for participation in processes of arousal and awareness. Brain Res. Brain Res. Rev. **39:** 107–140.

Pheochromocytoma

Physiopathologic Implications and Diagnostic Evaluation

EVANGELIA ZAPANTI[a] AND IOANNIS ILIAS[b]

[a]First Department of Endocrinology, Alexandra Hospital, Athens
GR-11528, Greece

[b]Department of Pharmacology, Medical School, University of Patras, Rion
GR-26504, Greece

ABSTRACT: Pheochromocytoma (PHEO) is a chromaffin cell tumor embryologically arising from the neural crest tissue. The dominant secretory products of PHEO are catecholamines: noradrenaline (norepinephrine), adrenaline (epinephrine), and to a lesser extent dopamine. In addition to catecholamines, PHEO cells also elaborate and release several neuropeptides and inflammatory cytokines which can exert intra-adrenal and extra-adrenal systemic effects and cause characteristic clinical syndromes. In a concise review we present the intra-adrenal and extra-adrenal pathophysiologic implications of PHEO and the nuclear medicine modalities that permit functional imaging of physiological processes and help localize these tumors. The specific pathways of synthesis, metabolism, and inactivation of catecholamines (of PHEOs and paragangliomas) can be used as means to develop suitable tracers for positron emission tomography (PET) ligands. In this review we focus on imaging with PET using [^{18}F]-fluorodopamine, [^{18}F]-fluorohydroxyphenylalanine, [^{11}C]-epinephrine, or [^{11}C]-hydroxyephedrine and examine how functional imaging can often complement traditional anatomical imaging modalities and other scintigraphic techniques.

KEYWORDS: pheochromocytoma; catecholamines; pathophysiology; insulin resistance; intra-adrenal; CRH; cytokines; computed tomography; magnetic resonance imaging; radionuclide imaging; octreotide; fluorine radioisotopes; positron emission tomography

INTRODUCTION

Pheochromocytomas (PHEO's) are chromaffin cell tumors that are embryologically derived from the neural crest tissue. Cell from the neural crest

Address for correspondence: Evangelia Zapanti, 8 Saki Karagiorga, Glyfada, 16675, Athens, Greece.
e-mail: liazapanti@yahoo.gr

Ann. N.Y. Acad. Sci. 1088: 346–360 (2006). © 2006 New York Academy of Sciences.
doi: 10.1196/annals.1366.022

migrate from the thoracic region at the fifth week of gestation and settle dorsolaterally to the aorta to form the sympathetic chains. During the seventh embryonic week, neural crest precursor cells migrate into the adrenal and later differentiate into chromaffin cells in the adrenal medulla under the influence of adrenocortical steroids.[1] The term PHEO refers to the intra-adrenal tumors and its name is due to the brownish stain it gets when exposed to chromium salts (in Greek: *pheo* = dusky, *chroma* = color).[2] Although PHEO is a rare cause of hypertension, it can be potentially lethal if not diagnosed and treated adequately. Although the exact prevalence of PHEO is not precisely known, a large study of hypertensive patients screened for PHEO has revealed an incidence as high as 1.9%.[3] It has recently become apparent from autopsy series that incidentally discovered that PHEOs are more common than previously thought,[4] suggesting that the incidence of this tumor is probably underestimated.[5] It is currently believed that PHEOs account for 6.5% of adrenal tumors.[6,7] Although PHEOs are predominantly sporadic, 15%–25% of patients with apparent sporadic PHEO may be carriers of germline mutations that entail a predisposition for developing extra-adrenal and often multifocal disease.[8] In 30% of children with PHEOs, the tumors are multifocal and/or extra-adrenal. The prevalence of malignancy in sporadic adrenal PHEO has been estimated as high as 9%. At the time of diagnosis 10% of patients with PHEO present with metastatic disease.[9]

Extra-adrenally located PHEOs are called paragangliomas (PGs) and arise from paraganglia. Paraganglia are small neural crest nodules that derive from chromaffin cells located near the sympathetic and parasympathetic ganglia.[10] Most PGs are intra-abdominal, and few (15%) are extra-abdominal (mainly intrathoracic or cervical). The contribution of familial PGs to the total number of reported cases of these neoplasias varies from 10% to 50%. Approximately half of the discovered PGs are malignant. PGs are a very rare source of catecholamine secretion, and only 1% of PGs are clinically functional. One of ten sporadic PGs and 25%–50% of familial tumors can be multiple (synchronous or metachronous).[11]

SECRETORY PRODUCTS OF PHEOCHROMOCYTOMA

The dominant products of PHEO are catecholamines: noradrenaline (norepinephrine; NE), adrenalin (epinephrine; E), and to a lesser extent dopamine. Catecholamines act by binding to adrenergic receptors. There are two types of adrenergic receptors, α-adrenergic and β-adrenergic receptors, each divided in two subtypes (α1-, α2- and β1-, β2-adrenergic receptors, respectively). Generally, stimulation of α receptors by catecholamines induces vasoconstriction, whereas stimulation of β2 receptors induces vasodilation. Stimulation of β1 receptors is associated with an increase in the rate of contraction and myocardial contractile force.[12] NE increases peripheral vascular resistance with consequent increase of both systolic and diastolic blood pressure. Cardiac output and heart rate may be decreased or unaltered. Adrenaline increases cardiac output and systolic blood pressure, whereas it decreases or has no effect on diastolic blood pressure. Therefore the clinical presentation of PHEO depends on the catecholamine secreted and the type of adrenergic receptor stimulated.[13] PHEO cells may also release other peptides, some of which cause symptoms that cannot be controlled by pharmacological alpha and beta blockade only.[14] Such secretory products of PHEO include: substance P, neuropeptide Y (NPY), enkephalins, somatostatin corticotrophin-releasing hormone (CRH), adrenocorticotropin hormone (ACTH), atrial natriuretic peptide (ANP), vasointestinal peptide (VIP), parathormone, interleukin-1 (IL-1), interleukin-6 (IL-6), calcitonin gene-related peptide (CGRP) and chromogranin A.[15]

All the above secretory products of PHEO can produce intra-adrenal as well as systemic effects.

INTRA-ADRENAL EFFECTS OF PHEO

Intra-adrenal Neuroendocrine Communications

It has been shown in experiments in mammalians that a complex interaction between adrenocortical and adrenal medullary tissues exists.[1] Chromaffin cells can be found in all zones of the rat adrenal cortex; and conversely the occurrence of cortical cells in the medulla is also observed.[16–18] The proximity of cortical and medullary adrenal tissues allows paracrine interactions between the two cell types. Catecholamines have been found to exert acute and long-term stimulating effects on corticosteroid release in rats and mice,[19,20] including the control of diurnal variation of adrenal steroidogenesis. There is evidence suggesting that the sympatho-adrenomedullary system regulates adrenocortical function, in part, by increasing sensitivity to corticotropin (ACTH).[21]

However, in the normal human adrenals, catecholamines have no major effect on steroidogenesis, whereas neuropeptides secreted by adrenomedullary chromafin cells such as VIP, ANP, and vasopressin regulate adrenocortical steroid production.[21] In addition to other peptides, normal adrenal medulla can produce CRH and ACTH that may stimulate adrenal cortisol production in the absence of pituitary-driven ACTH.[1]

The presence of immune cells (lymphocytes, dendritic cells, mast cells, macrophages) has also been demonstrated within the human adrenal cortex. These cells, when activated, produce a variety of cytokines: IL-1, IL-6, and tumor necrosis factor-alpha (TNF-α) that may exert stimulating or inhibitory effects on adrenal function.[21] Particularly IL-1 and IL-6 seem to have stimulatory effects on glucocorticoid secretion in human adrenal cells,[22] whereas TNF-α exerts inhibitory indirect effects on steroidogenesis in human fetal adrenals.[23] Similarly to macrophages within the adrenal cortex, adrenocortical cells can also synthesize IL-1, IL-6, and TNF-α.[24–26] There is also evidence that cells of adrenal medulla are immunoreactive for a wide spectrum of growth factors and cytokines (IGF-1, TNF- α, IL-6).[27] All these inflammatory cytokines can modify adrenal steroid secretion and exert direct effects on growth and differentiation of adrenal cortical cells.[28,29]

Effects of PHEO Products on Adrenals

An association, although rare, between PHEO and pathological lesions of the adrenal cortex has been reported. Rarely, PHEO can cause an ectopic ACTH syndrome. In most syndromes, ACTH produced by PHEO results in bilateral adrenocortical hyperplasia. However, the coexistence of PHEO with unilateral adrenocortical adrenal hyperplasia at the same adrenal gland has been described.[30] Furthermore there is a report of an association of PHEO with an ipsilateral adrenal adenoma causing Cushing's syndrome.[31] In the medical literature, few cases of ACTH-producing PGs have been reported, of which two cases occurred in the paranasal sinus.[32] A case of ectopic ACTH syndrome caused by a cervical malignant PG producing simultaneously ACTH and IL-6 has also been reported[33] and a possible role of IL-6 in inducing ACTH production has been suggested. There is also evidence of production of IL-1 by cultured PHEO cells. According to the authors,[34] the IL-1 produced in the KAT45 cell line (a new cell line that derives spontaneously after continuous culture of a primary human PHEO also associated with Cushing's syndrome) could induce the production of CRH by tumor cells and lead to the development of Cushing's syndrome. In this case PHEO was associated with Cushing's syndrome attributable solely to ectopic production of CRH without accompanying secretion of ACTH. It has been suggested that CRH produced by PHEO, in addition to its systemic effects, could exert paracrine effects within the adrenals. In fact, CRH affected several parameters of KAT45 cell metabolism, including their proliferation rate, synthesis of catecholamines, and production of proopiomelanocortin (POMC)-derived peptides.

EXTRA-ADRENAL EFFECTS OF PHEOCHROMOCYTOMA

Effects on the Cardiovascular System

The clinical hallmark of catecholamine-secreting tumors is paroxysmal hypertension and the most commonly associated symptoms are headache, pallor (often followed by flushing), perspiration, and palpitations.[35] The classic triad of headache, sweating attacks, and tachycardia was found to have a sensitivity of 90% and specificity of 93.8%.[36] PHEOs usually secrete catecholamines either continuously or intermittently. Episodic surges of hypertension can be superimposed on a background of constant hypertension or normotension. More rarely, episodes of hypertension can alternate with episodes of normotension.[35] In general, the hypertension is paroxysmal in 48% of patients and persistent in 29%, whereas in 13% blood pressure can be normal.[37] Hypertension, however, in patients with PHEO does not correlate with circulating catecholamines.[38] The hemodynamic features of hypertension, in patients with PHEO, are similar to those in patients with essential hypertension and are characterized by an increase in peripheral vascular resistance.[39] It has been shown that in patients with PHEO, blood pressure and heart rate were significantly reduced by clonidine (a centrally acting α2-agonist that inhibits neurally mediated catecholamine release) similar to patients with essential hypertension, although plasma catecholamines were not reduced. This suggests that the sympathetic nervous system in PHEO is active and may play a role in blood pressure regulation. In fact, it has been demonstrated that in PHEO blood pressure may be normal despite high levels of plasma catecholamines, and hypertensive crises can occur without additional elevations in plasma catecholamines.[37]

The increased sympathetic activity during elevation of circulating catecholamines was suggested to be due to at least three mechanisms: the loading of sympathetic vesicles with NE, the increased sympathetic neuronal impulse frequency, and the selective desensitization of presynaptic α2-adrenergic receptors (which inhibit NE release), resulting in enhanced release of neuronal NE during nerve stimulation.[37] This operative neuronal control of blood pressure in PHEO could explain the excessive release of NE into the synaptic cleft and the precipitation of a hypertensive crisis in response to any direct or indirect stimulus to the sympathetic nervous system. Sudden massive catecholamine release can cause severe vasoconstricton and may lead to life-threatening pulmonary edema and dysrhythmias.[40] A specific catecholamine cardiomyopathy, (dilated or hypertrophic) has been documented in patients with PHEO.[15]

Association with Paraneoplastic Syndromes

PHEO can cause several paraneoplastic syndromes. Cases of PHEO associated with fever and inflammatory signs due to the production of IL-6 by PHEO cells have been reported.[41,42] IL-6 is a multifunctional molecule that plays a major role in immune and inflammatory responses as it stimulates activation and differentiation of B and T lymphocytes, induces fever, and regulates acute-phase protein synthesis, such as C-reactive protein (CRP) and fibrinogen.[43] There have been reports of adrenal and extra-adrenal tumors presenting with anemia, thrombocytosis, and hyperfibrinogenemia, which are all associated with high levels of IL-6.[44,45] Interestingly, an association of PHEO with intrahepatic cholestasis has been reported.[46] In this case the presence of IL-1 β in PHEO cells was demonstrated and probably related to the unexplained intrahepatic cholestasis.[47] PHEO cells can also produce adromedullin, a potent vasodilator peptide that belongs to the CGRP family. The expression of adromedullin is induced by hypoxia and proinflammatory cytokines. Adromedullin, in addition to having a vasodilator effect, appears to be involved in many diseases, including ischemic heart disease, inflammatory diseases, and tumor development.[48]

Effects on Carbohydrate Metabolism

Catecholamines can exert direct and indirect effects on carbohydrate metabolism. The direct effects are exerted through stimulation of adrenorecep-tors in the metabolically active tissues. The indirect effects are exerted through modulation of pancreatic hormone production.[49] The stimulation of hepatic glucose production is mediated in humans by β-adrenoreceptors and appears to be an effect of circulating catecholamines rather than the sympathetic innerva-tion of the liver.[49] Beta-adrenergic stimulation on the liver induces a prompt rise in plasma glucose, initially by enhancing glycogenolysis.[49] The most sustained effects of hepatic β-adrenergic stimulation on glucose elevation are mediated through the activation of gluconeogenesis. The effects of the sympathoadrenal system in reducing the peripheral utilization of glucose are, however, the most important of the direct effects on carbohydrate metabolism. The reduction of the peripheral glucose utilization is due largely to the inhibition of muscle glu-cose uptake and is mediated by β-adrenoreceptor stimulation.[50] The indirect effects of catecholamines are exerted by the inhibition of the production of insulin through α2-adrenergic stimulation. Although β2-adrenoreceptor stim-ulation provokes insulin release, the α2-adrenoreceptor-mediated suppressive effects of catecholamines on insulin secretion generally predominate *in vivo*.[13] Glucose intolerance in PHEO was suggested to be due to the inhibitory effect of high catecholamine levels on fasting insulin levels.[51,52] Hyperinsulinemia is also associated with PHEO,[53] suggesting that β-receptor-mediated stimulation of insulin secretion may predominate in some patients. There are also some reports suggesting a decrease in insulin sensitivity in patients with PHEO.[54] Studies with the euglycemic hyperinsulinemic clamp technique have showed that the impaired glucose metabolism in patients with PHEO was induced or exacerbated by insulin resistance entailed by the catecholamine effect.[55,56]

DIAGNOSIS OF PHEOs/PGs

Biochemical Diagnosis and Anatomical Imaging

The measurement of free plasma metanephrines has been validated as the method of choice to confirm or exclude the presence of PHEOs (for PGs biochemical means of diagnosis have not been assessed as thoroughly as for PHEO). If biochemical findings corroborate the presence of PHEO, if the presence of such a tumor seems highly probable because of positive family history (such as in multiple endocrine neoplasia 2; MEN 2), or if the clinical presentation is compatible with the eventual presence of a PHEO (such as the growth of tumors in the neck and head, features compatible with PGs), then assessment of the extent of the disease is necessary with anatomical imaging (either with computed tomography [CT] or magnetic resonance [MR]). Using CT, tumors limited to the adrenal glands with a minimum size of 0.5–1.0 cm can be detected with sensitivity of 85%–98%. Extra-adrenal tumors of at least 1.0–2.0 cm diameter can be detected with sensitivity of 77%–90% (sensitivities are lower for patients that have had previous surgery).[9,57–59] Sensitivities for MR imaging are 93%–100% for adrenal[60] and approximately 90% for extra-adrenal tumors.[61] MR imaging may be better suited for neck PGs compared to CT.[62]

Ultrasound imaging is fit mainly for the evaluation of PHEO of pregnant women or children.[63] Ultrasound and angiography are useful for evaluating neck PGs.[64]

PHEOs in patients with MEN 2 are usually exclusively intra-adrenal and secrete epinephrine. Anatomical imaging is the first (and sometimes the only) diagnostic localization modality used. Apart from cases of MEN 2, PHEOs and PGs in patients can secrete norepinephine and normetanephrine. After anatomical imaging is performed, functional (nuclear medicine) modalities are used to complement the imaging findings.

Functional Imaging

Nuclear medicine modalities can be categorized into those that are specific for the catecholamine synthesis/secretion pathway and those that are nonspecific. Functional imaging evaluation should be done first with specific functional imaging modalites and, if these turn out to be negative, nonspecific modalities should follow (FIG. 1).

Modalities Specific for the Catecholamine Synthesis/Secretion Pathway

Metaiodobenzylguanidine (MIBG) Scintigraphy

The molecule of MIBG resembles NE and shows high affinity for the NE transporter system (however, it neither binds adrenergic receptors nor is it metabolized within catecholamine processing/secreting cells). [^{123}I]-MIBG has higher sensitivity, lower radiation exposure, and enables functional imaging of better quality compared to [^{131}I]-MIBG.[65] In a large study including 75 patients with benign or malignant PHEOs, the sensitivity of [^{123}I]-MIBG was almost 90%.[66] In two other series including a smaller number of patients

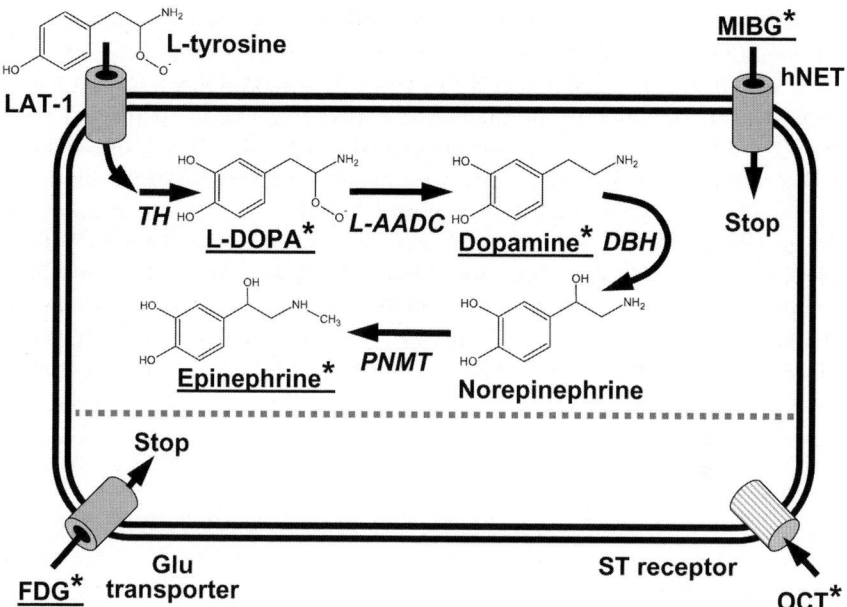

FIGURE 1. Targets for functional imaging of pheochromocytomas/paragangliomas. On the upper side are shown steps and molecules involved in the synthesis of catecholamines; these are targets for radioligands specific for such cells. On the lower side are nonspecific targets. Underlined molecules with asterisks are radiolabeled to be used for functional imaging. TH = tyrosine hydroxylase; hNET = human norepinephrine transporter (responsible for re-uptake of catecholamines); LAT-1 = large neutral aminoacid transporter; L-DOPA = L-dihydroxyphenylalanaine; L-AADC = aromatic-L-amino acid decarboxylase; DBH = dopamine beta-hydroxylase; PNMT = phenylethanolamine-N-methyltransferase; ST = somatostatin; OCT = octeotide; Glu = glucose; FDG = [^{18}F]-fluorodeoxyglocose; Stop = not metabolized further within the cells.

the sensitivity and specificity of the technique was 90%–100% and 100%, respectively.[67,68] In contrast, a sensitivity of 71% has been reported for PGs.[69]

Positron Emission Tomography

PET imaging is performed following the intravenous administration of positron-emitting radiopharmaceuticals that usually have a very short half-life. Advantages of PET include low radiation exposure and the good quality of imaging studies. Disadvantages are the high cost of production of the necessary radionuclides and equipment needed. PET for PHEOs/PGs is performed with various radioligands that target specific steps of catecholamine synthesis or reuptake pathway. PET with [^{11}C]-hydroxyephedrine exhibited a sensitivity of 90% in 10 patients with PHEOs,[70] whereas in another series including 19 patients with PHEO the sensitivity and specificity were 90% and 100%, respectively.[71] PET with [^{18}F]-fluorodopamine (DA) was performed in 18 patients with metastatic PHEO and was compared to [^{131}I]-MIBG.[72] PET with [^{18}F]-DA localized PHEOs in all patients and showed a large number of foci that were not imaged with [^{131}I]-MIBG scintigraphy.[72] In more recent studies PET with [^{18}F]-DA was shown to be superior to [^{123}I]-MIBG scintigraphy in imaging adrenal and/or benign PHEOs and PGs (Pacak *et al.*, unpublished data and Ref. 73). PET with [^{18}F]-hydroxyphenylalanine (DOPA) had 100% sensitivity and specificity in 14 patients with 17 PHEO tumors.[74] Furthermore, in 10 patients with a predisposition for PGs and PHEOs (attributed to mutations of the succinate dehydrogenase subunit D gene) PET with [^{18}F]-DOPA showed more tumors compared to MRI.[75]

Nonspecific Functional Imaging Modalities

Somatostatin Receptor Scintigraphy (SRS)

PHEOs express somatostatin receptor types 1, 2A, and 3,[76–78] and PGs also express somatostatin receptors.[77] Octreotide is a somatostatin analogue that when labeled with [^{111}In]-diethylenetriaminepentacetate (DTPA) is used for SRS.

SRS with [^{111}In]-DTPA-octreotide was positive for PHEOs larger than 1 cm that expressed somatostatin receptor type 2A ($n = 25$) and for tumors that expressed somatostatin receptor type 3 ($n = 6$).[78] In a study of patients with adrenal ($n = 32$) or metastatic phreochromcytomas ($n = 8$), the sensitivity of [^{111}In]-DTPA-octreotide was 25% and 88%, respectively.[66] SRS with [^{123}I]-tyr3- octreotide had 90%–94% sensitivity in showing PGs.[79–82] In 31 patients with PGs [^{111}In]-DTPA-octreotide was 100% sensitive,[83] whereas in another large study sensitivity and specificity were 97% and 82%, respectively.[84]

Fluorodeoxyglucose PET

Neoplasias (and those that are rapidly growing in particular) may show increased glucose uptake, thus enabling imaging with [^{18}F]-labeled deoxyglucose (FDG). The median standardized [^{18}F]-FDG uptake value (SUV) of PHEOs was shown to be 3.0 ($n = 2$), a value which is higher than that of functioning ($n = 7$; median SUV = 2.3) and that of nonfunctioning adrenal adenomas ($n = 3$; median SUV = 1.7).[85] The reported sensitivity of [^{18}F]-FDG PET in localizing adrenal or metastatic PHEOs ($n = 29$) was 72%.[86] [^{18}F]-FDG PET can be also used for imaging PGs, but to the best of our knowledge it has been implemented in case reports and small case series.[11,87,88]

Endocrine neoplasias with poorer differentiation may show low or no uptake of specific functional imaging ligands and be better imaged with [18F]-FDG PET ("flip-flop" phenomenon). This "flip-flop" phenomenon was seen in patients with PHEO that were evaluated with the tumor-specific [131I]-MIBG, [123I]-MIBG or [18F]-DA, and the nonspecific [18F]-FDG (Pacak, unpublished observations and Refs. 89 and 90). The caveat is that all tumors with high metabolic activity may show [18F]-FDG uptake, and thus it remains a nonspecific imaging modality.

Newer potential functional imaging modalities specific for the catecholamine synthesis pathway include PET with [18F]-fluorobenzylguanidine,[91] whereas newer nonspecific modalities for SRS include [99mTc]-EDDA/HYNIC-TOC for SPECT[92] and [68Ga]-DOTA-Tyr3-octreotide, [68Ga]-DOTA-Tyr3-octreotide, [64Cu]-TETA-octreotide, [18F]-FP-Gluc-TOCA, Gluc-S-Dpr([18F]FBOA)TOCA, and Cel-S-Dpr([18F]FBOA)TOCA for PET.[93-98]

CONCLUDING REMARKS

PHEOs and PGs are tumors of neuroectodermal origin that produce catecholamines and a variety of other active substances. The clinical hallmark of catecholamine-producing tumors is paroxysmal hypertension. However, the blood pressure can be persistently elevated or more rarely normal. Hypertension, in PHEO patients does not correlate with circulating catecholamines. This suggests a neuronal control of blood pressure in these patients. In addition to hypertension, PHEO can be associated with other disorders and symptoms attributable to the biologic actions of other secretory products.

Measurement of plasma metanephrines is the method of choice to confirm or exclude the presence of PHEOs. When assessment of the extent of the disease is indicated, then anatomical imaging, either with CT or MR is necessary. Although experience has been gathered in a few research centers with [18F]-FDA, [18F]-F-DOPA and [11C]-labeled radionuclides in the evaluation of PHEO and PG, it is evident that to justify their adoption more detailed studies are needed. The application of [18F]-FDA needs to be assessed in other types of tumors and it needs to be compared to [18F]-F-DOPA. The implementation of functional imaging (possibly enhanced by molecular imaging) may assist the distinction between benign and malignant tumors and permit the prediction of patient responses to therapy and eventually contribute to the elaboration of relevant patient management guidelines. Accumulated experience points to the conclusion that functional imaging can effectively influence the management of patients with chromaffin-positive and chromaffin-negative tumors, that it can predict malignant potential, and that it can be of help in monitoring treatment effect.[99]

REFERENCES

1. BORNSTEIN, M.E. *et al.* 1998. Intraadrenal interactions in the regulation of adreno-cortical steroidogenesis. Endocr. Rev. **19:** 101–143.
2. MANASSE, P. 1896. Zur Histologie und Histogenese der primaren Nierengeschwulste. Virchows Archiv. **145:** 113–157.
3. SMYTHE, G.A. *et al.* 1992. Biochemical diagnosis of pheochromocytoma by simultaneous measurement of urinary excretion of epinephrine and norepinephrine. Clin. Chem. **38:** 486–492.
4. MOTTA-RAMIREZ, G.A. *et al.* 2005. Comparison of CT findings in symptomatic and incidentally discovered pheochromocytomas. Am. J. Roentgenol. **185:** 684–688.
5. BEARD, C.M. *et al.* 1983. Occurrence of pheochromocytoma in Rochester, Minnesota, 1950 through 1979. Mayo Clin. Proc. **58:** 802–804.
6. LACK, E.E. 1997. Tumors of the Adrenal Gland and Extra-adrenal Paraganglia. Armed Forces Institute of Pathology. Washington, D.C.
7. GRUMBACH, M.M. *et al.* 2003. Management of the clinically inapparent adrenal mass ("incidentaloma"). Ann. Intern. Med. **138:** 424–429.
8. NEUMANN, H.P. *et al.* 2002. Germ-line mutations in nonsyndromic pheochromocytoma. N. Engl. J. Med. **346:** 1459–1466.
9. ILIAS, I. *et al.* 2004. Current approaches and recommended algorithm for the diagnostic localization of pheochromocytoma. J. Clin. Endocrinol. Metab. **89:** 479–491.
10. WILLIAMS, E.D. 1980. *In* Histological Typing of Endocrine Tumors: 33–39. World Health Organization. Geneva.
11. ARGIRIS, A. *et al.* 2003. PET scan assessment of chemotherapy response in metastatic paraganglioma. Am. J. Clin. Oncol. **26:** 563–566.
12. HOFFMAN, B.B. *et al.* 1990. Catecholamines and sympathomimetic agents. *In* The Pharmacologic Basis of Therapeutics. A.G. Gilman, *et al.*, Eds.: 187–220. Pergamon Press. New York.
13. BRAVO, E.L. *et al.* 1993. Pheochromocytoma. *In* Endocrine Crises. Endocrin. Metab. Clin. North Am. **22:** 329–341.
14. STEWART, A.F. *et al.* 1987. Two forms of parathyroid -like adenylate cyclase stimulating protein derived from tumours associated with humoral hypercalcemia of malignancy. J. Bone Miner. Res. **2:** 587–593.
15. FONSECA, V. *et al.* 1993. Pheochromocytoma and paraganglioma. *In* Catecholamines. Baillieres Clin. Endocrinol. Metab. **7:** 510–544.
16. FORTAK, W. *et al.* 1968. O wystepowaniu komorek chromochlonnych w korze nadnerczy szczurow bialych [On the occurrence of chromophilic cells in the adrenal cortex of white rats]. Endokrynol. Pol. **19:** 117–128.
17. KMIEC, B. 1968. Histologiczne i histochemiczne badania nad odbudowa rdzenia nadnerczy po ich enukleacji u szczurow bialych [Histologic and histochemical observations on regeneration of the adrenal medulla after enucleation in white rats]. Folia. Morphol. (Warsz) **27:** 238–245.
18. BORNSTEIN, S.R. *et al.* 1991. Morphological evidence for a close interaction of chromaffin cells with cortical cells within the adrenal gland. Cell Tissue Res. **265:** 1–9.
19. BORNSTEIN, S.R. *et al.* 1990. Effects of splanchnic nerve stimulation on the adrenal cortex may be mediated by chromaffin cells in a paracrine manner. Endocrinology **127:** 900–906.

20. EHRHART-BORNSTEIN, M. *et al.* 1991. Adrenaline stimulates cholesterol side chain cleavage cytochrome P450 mRNA accumulation in bovine adrenocortical cells. J. Endocrinol. Invest. **131:** R5–R8.
21. BORNSTEIN, S.R. *et al.* 1999. Adrenocorticotropin (ACTH)- and non-ACTH-mediated regulation of the adrenal cortex: neural and immune inputs. J. Clin. Endocrinol. Metab. **84:** 1729–1736.
22. WHITCOMB, R.W. *et al.* 1988. Monocytes stimulate cortisol production by cultured human adrenocortical cells. J. Clin. Endocrinol. Metab. **66:** 33–38.
23. VOUTILAINEN, R. 1998. Adrenocortical cells are the site of secretion and action of insulin-like growth factors and TNF. Horm. Metab. Res. **30:** 432–435.
24. GONZÁLEZ-HERNÁNDEZ, J.A. *et al.* 1995. Interleukin 1 is expressed in human adrenal gland in vivo. Possible role in a local immune-adrenal axis. Clin. Exp. Immunol . **99:** 137–141.
25. GONZÁLEZ-HERNÁNDEZ, J.A. *et al.* 1994. Interleukin-6 messenger ribonucleic acid expression in human adrenal gland in vivo: new clue to a paracrine or autocrine regulation of adrenal function. J. Clin. Endocrinol. Metab. **79:** 1492–1497.
26. GONZÁLEZ-HERNÁNDEZ, J.A. *et al.* 1996. Human adrenal cells express TNF - mRNA: evidence for a paracrine control of adrenal function. J. Clin. Endocrinol. Metab. **81:** 807–813.
27. KONTOGEORGOS, G. *et al.* 2002. Growth factors and cytokines in paragangliomas and pheochromocytomas, with special reference to sustentacular cells. Endocr. Pathol. **13:** 197–206.
28. JUDD, A.M. 1998. Cytokine expression in the rat adrenal cortex. Horm. Metab. Res. **30:** 404–410.
29. MARX, C. *et al.* 1998. Regulation of adrenocortical function by cytokines: relevance for immune-endocrine interaction. Horm. Metab. Res. **30:** 416–442.
30. EREM, C. *et al.* 2005. Pheochromocytoma combined with pre-clinical Cushing's syndrome in the same adrenal gland. J. Endocrinol. Invest. **28:** 561–565.
31. FINKENSTEDT, G. *et al.* 1999. Pheochromocytoma and subclinical Cushing's syndrome during pregnancy: diagnosis, medical pre-treatment and cure by laparoscopic unilateral adrenalectomy. J. Endocrinol. Invest. **22:** 551–557.
32. OTSUKA, F. *et al.* 2005. An extraadrenal abdominal pheochromocytoma causing ectopic ACTH syndrome. Am. J. Hypertens. **18:** 1364–1368.
33. OMURA, M. *et al.* 1994. A patient with malignant paraganglioma that simultaneously produces adrenocorticotropic hormone and interleukin-6. Cancer **74:** 1634–1639.
34. VENIHAKI, M. *et al.* 1998. KAT 45, a noradrenergic human pheochromocytoma cell line producing corticotropin- releasing hormone. Endocrinology **139:** 713–722.
35. BRAVO, E.L. *et al.* 1984. Pheochromocytoma: diagnosis, localization and management. N. Engl. J. Med. **301:** 1298–1303.
36. PLOUIN, P.F. *et al.* 1981. Le depistage du pheochromocytome: chez quels hypertendus? Etude semiologique chez 2585 hypertendus dont 11 ayant un pheochromocytome [Screening for phaeochromocytoma: in which hypertensive patients? A semiological study of 2585 patients, including 11 with phaeochromocytoma]. Nouv. Presse. Med. **10:** 869–872.
37. BRAVO, E.L. *et al.* 2003. Pheochromocytoma: state-of-the art and future prospects. Endocr. Rev. **24:** 539–553.
38. BRAVO, E.L. *et al.* 1979. Circulating and urinary catecholamines in pheochromocytoma. Diagnostic and pathophysiologic implications. N. Engl. J. Med. **301:** 682–686.

39. Bravo, E.L. *et al.* 1990. A reevaluation of the hemodynamics of pheochromocytoma. Hypertension **15** (Suppl): 128–131.
40. Sode, J. *et al.* 1967. Cardiac arrhythmias and cardiomyopathy associated with pheochromocytoma: report of three cases. Am. J. Surg. **114:** 927–931.
41. Shimizu, C. *et al.* 2001. Interleukin-6 (Il-6) producing pheochromocytoma: direct Il-6 suppression by non steroidal anti-inflammatory drugs. Clin. Endocrinol. (Oxf). **54:** 405–410.
42. Minetto, M. *et al.* 2003. Interleukin-6 producing pheoochromocytoma presenting with acute inflammatory syndrome. J. Endocrinol. Invest. **26:** 453–457.
43. Akira, S. *et al.* 1990. Biology of multifunctional cytokines: IL 6 and related molecules (IL 1 and TNF). FASEB J. **4:** 2860–2867.
44. Fukumoto, S. *et al.* 1991. Pheochromocytoma with pyrexia and marked inflammatory signs: a paraneoplastic syndrome with possible relation to interleukin-6 production. J. Clin. Endocrinol. Metab. **73:** 877–881.
45. Suzuki, K. *et al.* 1991. Interleukin-6-producing pheochromocytoma. Acta Haematologica. **85:** 217–219.
46. Chung, C.H. *et al.* 2005. Intrahepatic cholestasis as a paraneoplastic syndrome associated with pheochromocytoma. J. Endocrinol. Invest. **28:** 175–179.
47. Bornstein, S.R. *et al.* 1996. Expression of interleukin-1 in human pheochromocytoma. J. Endocrinol. Invest. **19:** 693–698.
48. Takahashi, K. 2001. Adrenomedullin from a pheochromocytoma to the eye: implications of the adrenomedullin research for endocrinology in the 21st century. Tohoku J. Exp. Med. **193:** 79–114.
49. Webber, J. *et al.* 1993. Metabolic actions of catecholamines in man. Bailliere's Clin. Endocrinol. Metab. **7:** 393–413.
50. Sacca, L. *et al.* 1982. Mechanisms of epinephrine-induced glucose intolerance in normal humans: role of the splanchnic bed. J. Clin. Invest. **69:** 284–293.
51. Turnbull, D.M. *et al.* 1980. Hormonal and metabolic studies in a patient with pheochromocytoma. J. Clin. Endocrinol. Metab. **51:** 930–933.
52. Metz, S.A. *et al.* 1978. Induction of defective insulin secretion and impaired glucose tolerance by clonidine: selective stimulation of metabolic alpha adrenergic pathways. Diabetes **27:** 554–562.
53. Lorini, R. *et al.* 1983. Pheochromocytoma and diabetes mellitus. Endocrinol. (Oxf). **19:** 275–276.
54. di Paolo, S. *et al.* 1989. Beta-adrenoreceptors desensitization may modulate catecholamine induced insulin resistance in human pheochromocytoma. Diabetes Metab. **15:** 409–415.
55. Wisner, T.D. *et al.* 2003. Improvement of insulin sensitivity after adrenalectomy in patients with pheochromocytoma. J. Clin. Endocrinol. Metab. **88:** 3632–3636.
56. Diamanti-Kandarakis, E. *et al.* 2003. Insulin resistance in pheochromocytoma improves more by surgical rather by medical treatment. Hormones (Athens) **2:** 61–66.
57. Pacak, K. *et al.* 2001. Recent advances in genetics, diagnosis, localization and treatment of pheochromocytoma. Ann. Intern. Med. **134:** 315–329.
58. Peplinski, G.R. *et al.* 1994. The predictive value of diagnostic tests for pheochromocytoma. Surgery **116:** 1101–1110.
59. Korobkin, M. *et al.* 1998. CT time-attenuation washout curves of adrenal adenomas and nonadenomas. Am. J. Roentgenol. **170:** 747–752.
60. Honigschnabl, S. *et al.* 2002. How accurate is MR imaging in characterisation of adrenal masses: update of a long-term study. Eur. J. Radiol. **41:** 113–122.

61. MANNELLI, M. *et al.* 1999. Pheochromocytoma in Italy: a multicentric retrospective study. Eur. J. Endocrinol. **142:** 619–624.
62. SADHEV, A. *et al.* 2005. CT and MR imaging of unusual locations of extra-adrenal paragangliomas (pheochromcytomas). Eur. Radiol. **15:** 85–92.
63. HIORNS, M.P. *et al.* 2001. Radiology of neuroblastoma in children. Eur. Radiol. **11:** 2071–2081.
64. ARSLAN, H. *et al.* 2000. Power Doppler scanning in the diagnosis of carotid body tumors. J. Ultrasound Med. **19:** 367–370.
65. MOZLEY, P.D. *et al.* 1994. The efficacy of iodine-123-MIBG as a screening test for pheochromocytoma. J. Nucl. Med. **35:** 1138–1144.
66. VAN DER HARST, E. *et al.* 2001. [(123)I]metaiodobenzylguanidine and [(111)In]octreotide uptake in benign and malignant pheochromocytomas. J. Clin. Endocrinol. Metab. **86:** 685–693.
67. FURUTA, N. *et al.* 1999. Diagnosis of pheochromocytoma using [123I]-compared with [131I]-metaiodobenzylguanidine scintigraphy. Int. J. Urol. **6:** 119–124.
68. KALTSAS, G. *et al.* 2001. Comparison of somatostatin analog and meta-iodobenzylguanidine radionuclides in the diagnosis and localization of advanced neuroendocrine tumors. J. Clin. Endocrinol. Metab. **86:** 895–902.
69. ERICKSON, D. *et al.* 2001. Benign paragangliomas: clinical presentation and treatment outcomes in 236 patients. J. Clin. Endocrinol. Metab. **86:** 5210–5216.
70. SHULKIN, B.L. *et al.* 1992. PET scanning with hydroxyephedrine: an approach to the localization of pheochromocytoma. J. Nucl. Med. **33:** 1125–1131.
71. TRAMPAL, C. *et al.* 2004. Pheochromocytomas: detection with 11C hydroxyephedrine PET. Radiology **230:** 423–428.
72. ILIAS, I. *et al.* 2003. Superiority of 6-[18F]-fluorodopamine positron emission tomography versus [131I]-metaiodobenzylguanidine scintigraphy in the localization of metastatic pheochromocytoma. J. Clin. Endocrinol. Metab. **88:** 4083–4087.
73. ILIAS, I. *et al.*, 2004. Comparison of 6-[18F]-fluorodopamine positron emission tomography with [123I]-metaiodobenzylguanidine and [111In]-pentetreotide scintigraphy in the localization of pheochromocytoma, ENDO: 86th Annual Meeting of the American Endocrine Society. New Orleans, LA. The Endocrine Society: 452–453.
74. HOEGERLE, S. *et al.* 2002. Pheochromocytomas: detection with 18F DOPA whole body PET–initial results. Radiology **222:** 507–512.
75. HOEGERLE, S. *et al.* 2003. 18F-DOPA positron emission tomography for the detection of glomus tumours. Eur. J. Nucl. Med. Mol. Imaging **30:** 689–694.
76. HOFLAND, L.J. *et al.* 1999. Immunohistochemical detection of somatostatin receptor subtypes sst1 and sst2A in human somatostatin receptor positive tumors. J. Clin. Endocrinol. Metab. **84:** 775–780.
77. REUBI, J.C. *et al.* 1992. *In vitro* and *in vivo* detection of somatostatin receptors in pheochromocytomas and paragangliomas. J. Clin. Endocrinol. Metab. **74:** 1082–1089.
78. MUNDSCHENK, J. *et al.* 2003. Somatostatin receptor subtypes in human pheochromocytoma: subcellular expression pattern and functional relevance for octreotide scintigraphy. J. Clin. Endocrinol. Metab. **88:** 5150–5157.
79. SCHMIDT, M. *et al.* 2002. Clinical value of somatostatin receptor imaging in patients with suspected head and neck paragangliomas. Eur. J. Nucl. Med. Mol. Imaging **29:** 1571–1580.
80. LAMBERTS, S.W. *et al.* 1990. Somatostatin-receptor imaging in the localization of endocrine tumors. N. Engl. J. Med. **323:** 1246–1249.

81. KRENNING, E.P. *et al.* 1993. Somatostatin receptor scintigraphy with [111In-DTPA-D-Phe1]- and [123I-Tyr3]-octreotide: the Rotterdam experience with more than 1000 patients. Eur. J. Nucl. Med. **20:** 716–731.
82. TELISCHI, F.F. *et al.* 2000. Octreotide scintigraphy for the detection of paragangliomas. Otolaryngol. Head Neck Surg. **122:** 358–362.
83. DUET, M. *et al.* 2003. Clinical impact of somatostatin receptor scintigraphy in the management of paragangliomas of the head and neck. J. Nucl. Med. **44:** 1767–1774.
84. BUSTILLO, A. *et al.* 2004. Octreotide scintigraphy in the head and neck. Laryngoscope **114:** 434–440.
85. MINN, H. *et al.* 2004. Imaging of adrenal incidentalomas with PET using (11)C-metomidate and (18)F-FDG. J. Nucl. Med. **45:** 972–979.
86. SHULKIN, B.L. *et al.* 1999. Pheochromocytomas: imaging with 2-[fluorine-18]fluoro-2-deoxy-D-glucose PET. Radiology **212:** 35–41.
87. MACFARLANE, D.J. *et al.* 1995. FDG PET imaging of paragangliomas of the neck: comparison with MIBG SPET. Eur. J. Nucl. Med. **22:** 1347–1350.
88. WITTEKINDT, C. *et al.* 1999. FDG PET imaging of malignant paraganglioma of the neck. Ann. Otol. Rhinol. Laryngol. **108:** 909–912.
89. EZUDDIN, S. *et al.* 2005. MIBG and FDG PET findings in a patient with malignant pheochromocytoma: a significant discrepancy. Clin. Nucl. Med. **30:** 579–581.
90. MAMEDE, M. *et al.* 2006. Discordant localization of 2-[18F]-fluoro-2-deoxy-D-glucose in 6-[18F]-fluorodopamine- and [123I]-metaiodobenzylguanidine-negative metastatic pheochromocytoma sites. Nucl. Med. Commun. **27:** 31–36.
91. BERRY, C.R. *et al.* 2002. Imaging of pheochromocytoma in 2 dogs using p-[18F] fluorobenzylguanidine. Vet. Radiol. Ultrasound **43:** 183–186.
92. PLACHCINSKA, A. *et al.* 2003. Clinical usefulness of 99mTc-EDDA/HYNIC-TOC scintigraphy in oncological diagnostics: a preliminary communication. Eur. J. Nucl. Med. Mol. Imaging **30:** 1402–1406.
93. HOFMANN, M. *et al.* 2001. Biokinetics and imaging with the somatostatin receptor PET radioligand (68)Ga-DOTATOC: preliminary data. Eur. J. Nucl. Med. **28:** 1751–1757.
94. ANDERSON, C.J. *et al.* 2001. 64Cu-TETA-octreotide as a PET imaging agent for patients with neuroendocrine tumors. J. Nucl. Med. **42:** 213–221.
95. WESTER, H.J. *et al.* 2003. PET imaging of somatostatin receptors: design, synthesis and preclinical evaluation of a novel 18F-labelled, carbohydrated analogue of octreotide. Eur. J. Nucl. Med. Mol. Imaging **30:** 117–122.
96. SCHOTTELIUS, M. *et al.* 2004. First (18)F-labeled tracer suitable for routine clinical imaging of sst receptor-expressing tumors using positron emission tomography. Clin. Cancer Res. **10:** 3593–3606.
97. KOWALSKI, J. *et al.* 2003. Evaluation of positron emission tomography imaging using [68Ga]-DOTA-D Phe(1)-Tyr(3)-Octreotide in comparison to [111In]-DTPAOC SPECT. First results in patients with neuroendocrine tumors. Mol. Imaging Biol. **5:** 42–48.
98. GABRIEL, M. *et al.* 2003. An intrapatient comparison of 99mTc-EDDA/HYNIC-TOC with 111In-DTPA-octreotide for diagnosis of somatostatin receptor-expressing tumors. J. Nucl. Med. **44:** 708–716.
99. MISKULIN, J. *et al.* 2003. Is preoperative iodine 123 meta-iodobenzylguanidine scintigraphy routinely necessary before initial adrenalectomy for pheochromocytoma? Surgery **134:** 918–922.

Beyond Heart Rate Variability

Vagal Regulation of Allostatic Systems

JULIAN F. THAYER[a] AND ESTHER STERNBERG[b]

[a]The Ohio State University, Columbus, Ohio 43210, USA

[b]The National Institutes of Health, Rockville, Maryland, USA

ABSTRACT: The autonomic nervous system (ANS) plays a role in a wide range of somatic and mental diseases. Whereas the role of the ANS in the regulation of the cardiovascular system seems evident, its role in the regulation of other systems associated with allostasis is less clear. Using a model of neurovisceral integration we describe how the ANS and parasympathetic tone in particular may be associated with the regulation of allostatic systems associated with glucose regulation, hypothalamic-pituitary-adrenal (HPA) axis function, and inflammatory processes. Decreased vagal function and heart rate variability (HRV) were shown to be associated with increased fasting glucose and hemoglobin A1c levels, increased overnight urinary cortisol, and increased proinflammatory cytokines and acute-phase proteins. All of these factors have been associated with increased allostatic load and poor health. Thus, vagal activity appears to play an inhibitory function in the regulation of allostatic systems. The prefrontal cortex and the amygdala are important central nervous system structures linked to the regulation of these allostatic systems via the vagus nerve. Finally, the identification of this neurovisceral regulatory system may help to illuminate the pathway via which psychosocial factors may influence health and disease.

KEYWORDS: heart rate variability; cortisol; glucose; inflammation; allostasis

There is growing evidence for the role of the autonomic nervous system (ANS) in a wide range of somatic and mental diseases. The ANS is generally conceived to have two major branches—the sympathetic system, associated with energy mobilization, and the parasympathetic system, associated with vegetative and restorative functions. Normally, the activity of these branches is in

Address for correspondence: Julian F. Thayer, Ph.D., Department of Psychology, The Ohio State University, 1835 Neil Avenue, Columbus, OH 43210, USA. Voice: 614-688-4966; fax: 614-688-8261.
e-mail: Thayer.39@osu.edu

Ann. N.Y. Acad. Sci. 1088: 361–372 (2006). © 2006 New York Academy of Sciences.
doi: 10.1196/annals.1366.014

dynamic balance. When this changes into a static imbalance, for example, under environmental pressures, the organism becomes vulnerable to pathology. Modern conceptions of organism function based on complexity theory hold that organism stability, adaptability, and health are maintained through variability in the dynamic relationship among system elements.[1-4] Thus, patterns of organized variability, rather than static levels, are preserved in the face of constantly changing environmental demands. One can compare this with genetic variation, which is vital in the adaptation of species. These demands can be conceived in terms of energy regulation, such that the points of relative stability represent local energy minima required by the situation. Because the system operates "far-from-equilibrium" the system is always searching for local energy minima to minimize the energy requirements of the organism. Consequentially, optimal system functioning is achieved via lability and variability in its component processes, to allow the flexible regulation of local energy expenditure. In contrast, rigid regularity is associated with mortality, morbidity, and ill health.[5,6]

A corollary of this view is that autonomic imbalance, in which one branch of the ANS dominates over the other, is associated with a lack of dynamic flexibility and health. Empirically, there is a large body of evidence to suggest that autonomic imbalance, in which typically the sympathetic system is hyperactive and the parasympathetic system is hypoactive, is associated with various pathological conditions.[7,8] In particular, when the sympathetic branch dominates for long periods of time, the energy demands on the system become excessive and ultimately cannot be met, eventuating in death. The prolonged state of alarm associated with negative emotions likewise places an excessive energy demand on the system. On the way to death, however, premature aging and disease characterize a system dominated by negative affect and autonomic imbalance.

Like many organs in the body, the heart is dually innervated. Although a wide range of physiologic factors determines heart rate (HR), the ANS is the most prominent. Importantly, when both cardiac vagal (the primary parasympathetic nerve) and sympathetic inputs are blocked pharmacologically (for example, with atropine plus propranolol, the so-called double blockade), intrinsic HR is higher than the normal resting HR.[9] This fact supports the idea that the heart is under tonic inhibitory control by parasympathetic influences. Thus, resting cardiac autonomic balance favors energy conservation by way of parasympathetic dominance over sympathetic influences. In addition, the HR time series is characterized by beat-to-beat variability over a wide range, which also implicates vagal dominance, as the sympathetic influence on the heart is too slow to produce rapid beat-to-beat changes. Low heart rate variability (HRV) is associated with increased risk of all-cause mortality, and low HRV has been proposed as a marker for disease.[10]

THE IMPORTANCE OF INHIBITION

Importantly, like the heart, sympathoexcitatory subcortical threat circuits are under tonic inhibitory control by the prefrontal cortex.[11,12] For example, the amygdala, which has outputs to autonomic, endocrine, and other physiological regulation systems, and becomes active during threat and uncertainty, is under tonic inhibitory control via gamma-aminobutyric acid (GABA)-ergic mediated projections from the prefrontal cortex.[12,13] Thus the default response to uncertainty, novelty, and threat is the sympathoexcitatory preparation for action commonly known as the fight-or-flight response. From an evolutionary perspective this represents a system that errs on the side of caution—when in doubt prepare for the worst—thus maximizing survival and adaptive responses.[14] However, in normal, modern life this response has to be tonically inhibited and this inhibition is achieved via top-down modulation from the prefrontal cortex. Thus, under conditions of uncertainty and threat the prefrontal cortex becomes hypoactive. This hypoactive state is associated with disinhibition of sympathoexcitatory circuits that are essential for energy mobilization. However, when this state is prolonged it produces the excess wear and tear on the system components that has been characterized by McEwen as allostatic load.[15] It is also important to note that psychopathological states such as anxiety, depression, posttraumatic stress disorder, and schizophrenia are associated with prefrontal hypoactivity and a lack of inhibitory neural processes as reflected in poor habituation to novel neutral stimuli, a preattentive bias for threat information, deficits in working memory and executive function, and poor affective information processing and regulation.[8] Proper functioning of inhibitory processes is vital to the preservation of the integrity of the system and therefore is vital to health. Importantly for our discussion, these inhibitory processes can be indexed by measures of vagal function such as HRV as we will illustrate below.

VAGAL FUNCTION, REGULATION OF ALLOSTATIC SYSTEMS, AND DISEASE

There are multiple measures that can be used to index activity of the vagus nerve. Resting HR, by virtue of its tonic inhibitory control via the vagus, is a simple, inexpensive, and noninvasive measure of vagal function and autonomic balance. The HR change following cessation of exercise is another measure that has been used to characterize vagal function. The decrease in HR after termination of exercise has been termed HR recovery, and standardized methods have been developed for its assessment. Measures of HRV in both the time and frequency domains have also been used successfully to index vagal activity. In the time domain, the standard deviation of the interbeat intervals

(IBI), the percentage of IBI differences greater than 50 msec, and the mean square of the successive differences in IBIs (MSD) have been shown to be useful indices of vagal activity. In the frequency domain both low-frequency (LF) and high-frequency (HF) spectral power have been used as indices of vagal activity.[10] In addition, measures of baroreflex sensitivity have also been shown to be useful indicators of vagal function. The literature linking these different indices to morbidity and mortality is extensive. Importantly, whereas there are some differences among studies, the consensus is that lower values of these indices of vagal function are associated prospectively with death and disability.[16]

For example, resting HR can be used as a rough indicator of autonomic balance, and several large studies have shown a largely linear, positive dose-response relationship between resting HR and all-cause mortality.[17] This association was independent of gender and ethnicity, and showed a threefold increase in mortality in persons with resting HR over 90 beats per min (bpm) compared to those with resting HRs of less than 60 bpm.

Vagal Regulation of Allostatic Systems

Brook and Julius[7] have detailed how autonomic imbalance in the sympathetic direction is associated with a range of metabolic, hemodynamic, trophic, and rheologic abnormalities that contribute to elevated cardiac morbidity and mortality. Although the relationship between HRV and cardiovascular morbidity and mortality may be easily comprehensible, the fact that autonomic imbalance and HRV are related to other diseases may not be as obvious. In the following we will briefly review the evidence for vagal regulation of three systems associated with physiological regulation and allostasis—glucose regulation, the hypothalamic-pituitary-adrenal (HPA) axis system, and inflammation. These systems are all critical to the wear and tear on the physiological systems associated with health and disease. As such excess wear and tear on these systems is associated with increased morbidity and mortality.

Glucose Regulation and Diabetes

Low HRV has been shown to be associated with diabetes mellitus, and decreased HRV has been shown to precede evidence of disease provided by standard clinical tests.[18] We have recently presented evidence that HRV at night is associated with fasting glucose and hemoglobin A1c (HbA1c) levels.[19] Specifically, HRV was inversely related to fasting glucose and HbA1c levels after controlling for a large number of covariates including many traditional cardiovascular disease risk factors.

In the first population-based study to examine the relationship among vagal tone, serum insulin, glucose, and diabetes, Liao *et al.* [20] investigated 154 diabetic and 1,779 nondiabetic middle-aged men and women in the ARIC study. A total of 2 min supine resting HR recordings were used to compute HF power as an index of vagal tone, whereas fasting insulin, glucose, and diagnosed diabetes were used to index diabetes and diabetes risk. Consistent with previous cross-sectional studies these researchers found that diabetics had lower vagal tone than nondiabetics after adjustment for age, race, and gender. In the nondiabetics, an inverse relationship was found between HF power, and fasting insulin and fasting glucose. However, after adjustment only the relationship between HRV and insulin remained significant. This was the first study to examine the relationship between HRV and insulin and glucose in a general population and suggests that reduced vagal tone may be involved in the pathogenesis of diabetes.

Singh *et al.* [21] examined the relationship between HRV and blood glucose levels in 1,919 men and women from the Framingham Heart Study (FHS). The first 2 h of ambulatory HR recordings were used to calculate a number of time and frequency domain indices of HRV. Fasting glucose levels were used to classify individuals as having normal or impaired fasting glucose, as well as to identify those with diabetes (in addition to those with diabetic diagnosis). Several indices of HRV including LF and HF power were inversely associated with fasting glucose levels and were significantly reduced in diabetics and those with impaired fasting glucose compared to those with normal fasting glucose levels. The association between reduced HRV and diabetes remained significant after adjustment for age, gender, HR, BMI, antihypertensive and cardiac medications, blood pressure, smoking, and alcohol and coffee consumption.

The prospective association between autonomic dysfunction, indexed by high HR and low HRV, and the development of diabetes was examined by Carnethon *et al.* [22] in 8,185 middle-aged men and women from the ARIC study. During the 8-year follow-up period 1,063 persons developed type 2 diabetes. Compared to those in the highest quartile of LF power, those in the lowest quartile had a 1.2-fold greater risk of developing diabetes after adjustment for age, race, gender, study center, education, alcohol use, smoking, heart disease, physical activity, and BMI. Those with HR in the highest quartile had 1.6 greater risk of diabetes than those in the lowest HR quartile with similar results for analyses restricted to those with normal fasting glucose.

The association between fasting glucose and HR recovery was investigated in 5,190 healthy men and women enrolled in the Lipids Research Clinics Prevalence study.[23] Exercise testing was done and the HR drop 2 min after exercise cessation was examined using a cutoff of < 42 bpm as an indication of an abnormal response. Fasting glucose was an independent predictor of an abnormal HR recovery response across diabetic and nondiabetic participants and remained a significant predictor after controlling for age, gender, BMI, resting HR, resting blood pressure, anti-hypertensive treatment, cholesterol, education, and alcohol consumption. Over the 12-year follow-up abnormal HR recovery was a significant predictor of all-cause mortality across the range of fasting glucose levels and the combination of abnormal HR recovery and impaired fasting glucose was associated with a 2.4 greater risk of mortality.

Taken together these studies suggest a significant relationship between vagal function and energy regulation as indexed by glucose regulation. These results have clear implications for the excess energy demands placed upon the system that characterizes allostatic load. Another related energy regulation system involves glucocorticoids such as cortisol. We will briefly review some evidence for the role of vagal function in cortisol regulation in the next section.

The HPA Axis

We have recently investigated the relationship between vagal function and HPA axis regulation in a large study of healthy men. In this study we examined the well-known relationship between alcohol consumption and HPA axis function and the modulatory role that the vagus might play in this relationship.[24] We found that apparently healthy adult men that drank more than 20 g of alcohol per day had significantly higher levels of urinary cortisol as well as significantly lower levels of HRV than men that drank less than 20 g of alcohol per day. The higher alcohol-use group also had significantly higher blood pressure and more self-reported sleep problems compared to the lower alcohol-use group. Urinary cortisol levels were positively correlated with alcohol use, and inversely associated with HRV even after controlling for a wide range of covariates and potential confounders. Importantly, these relationships among alcohol use, cortisol, and HRV were greatly altered in the high-alcohol-use group. Cortisol and alcohol use were no longer related in the high-use group and the inverse relationship between cortisol and HRV was greatly attenuated and no longer significant. Thus, in the high-alcohol-use group evidence for HPA axis dysregulation was found.

The observed relationship between cortisol and HRV suggests that the appropriate regulation of the HPA axis depends in part on the ANS and parasympathetic influences in particular. Thus the observed inverse relationship may suggest a negative feedback mechanism by which cortisol output is modulated by the ANS. Clearly the HPA axis and the ANS are related as components of an internal regulation system.[4,25,26] However, as cogently described by Benarroch, this internal regulation system is regulated by a set of neural structures which he has termed the central autonomic network (CAN).[25,26] The CAN includes a number of structures throughout the neuraxis including the prefrontal cortex and the amygdala. The overlap of the CAN with the network hypothesized to be involved in the inhibitory control of the HPA axis is therefore not surprising.[27,28] Moreover, given that peripheral measures such as cortisol and HRV are associated with activity of the amygdala and the prefrontal cortex, respectively, the observed inverse relationship between cortisol and HRV may reflect the inhibitory influence of the prefrontal cortex on the amygdala which has been reported in both animal and human studies.[12,29]

The attenuated negative association between cortisol and HRV found in the high drinking group may reflect a breakdown of the "functional connectivity" between the PFC and the amygdala that has been reported in healthy subjects in two recent neuroimaging studies of the serotonin transporter gene as well as the breakdown of such connectivity with certain polymorphisms.[30,31] Alcoholism has been associated with dysregulated serotonin function such that alcoholics have decreased levels of serotonin, and enhanced serotonin has been associated with decreased alcohol intake.[32–34] These findings become even more relevant when one notes that cortisol is associated with enhanced serotonin reuptake and thus lower levels of serotonin.[35,36] Moreover, we have recently reported that decreased brain serotonin levels induced by tryptophan depletion are associated with reduced HRV in remitted depressed patients with a history of suicidal ideation.[37] Thus elevated levels of cortisol, whether induced by alcohol use, stress, or genetics, may act via altered serotonin levels to alter the functional connectivity between the PFC and the amygdala.

Very recent studies in epilepsy have also found evidence for impaired inhibitory control of the HPA axis.[28] Moreover, these authors provided a particularly informative analysis of the deficient inhibitory control. In particular they noted that the amygdala is a target region for control of the HPA axis due in part to the high concentration of CRH neurons in the extended amygdala. They further noted that the amygdala receives large inputs from the vagus nerve which might serve to modulate the CRH neurons and thus contribute to the feedback control of the HPA axis. In addition they and others[12,13,29,38,39] have noted that the prefrontal cortex exerts inhibitory control on the amygdala and thus might be a site of relevance to the impaired inhibitory control seen in a wide range of disorders including epilepsy, depression, and alcohol abuse. This inhibitory control appears to be at least partly vagally mediated as well as a result of common central nervous system circuits and thus is consistent with the neurovisceral integration model, which stresses the importance of the parasympathetic nervous system in providing negative feedback on sympathoexcitatory stress responses.[12,29]

These results are consistent with the idea that the vagus nerve is involved in the regulation of the HPA axis. Of course, cortisol is a potent anti-inflammatory agent and associations between the HPA axis and inflammation are well known. Of particular importance, recent research suggests an association between vagal function and inflammatory processes as well.

Inflammation

Vagal function and HRV have been associated with immune dysfunction and inflammation, which have been implicated in a wide range of conditions such as aging, cardiovascular disease, diabetes, osteoporosis, arthritis, Alzheimer's disease, periodontal disease, and certain types of cancer as well as a decline in muscle strength and increased frailty and disability.[40,41] The common mechanism seems to involve excess proinflammatory cytokines such as tumor necrosis factor, interleuken- 1 and -6, and C-reactive protein (CRP). Importantly, increased parasympathetic tone and acetylcholine (the primary parasympathetic neurotransmitter) have been shown to attenuate release of these proinflammatory cytokines, and sympathetic hyperactivity is associated with their increased production.[42–44]

Inflammation is now thought to play a major role in cardiovascular disease.[45] Importantly, evidence linking decreased vagal function with increased inflammation is quickly accumulating. Tracey[44] has described the cholinergic anti-inflammatory pathway in which acetylcholine and vagal function tonically inhibits release of proinflammatory cytokines. Clinical evidence in humans is just now starting to become available. In a study of 121 women with coronary heart disease 24-h recordings of HR were collected and several inflammatory markers examined.[46] Both time and frequency domain indices of HRV were inversely associated with interleukin- 6 (IL-6) levels after controlling for age, menopausal status, BMI, smoking, education level, diabetes, and cardiac rehabilitation participation. In a sample of 643 middle-aged and elderly men and women increased HR and reduced HRV were found to be significant independent predictors of white blood cell (WBC) count and CRP levels after controlling for age and gender.[47] Our group has also found an association between vagally mediated HRV and several inflammatory markers.[48] In a sample of 613 men and women 24-h MSD was inversely associated with WBC and CRP even after controlling for a large number of potential covariates including sympathetic nervous system activity as indexed by norepinephrine.

Stress, Negative Emotions, and Vagal Function

Although the idea is not new,[49] several recent reviews have provided strong evidence linking negative affective states and dispositions to disease and ill health.[2,41,50–53] All of these reviews implicate altered ANS function and decreased parasympathetic activity as a possible mediator in this link. For example, low HRV is consistent with the cardiac symptoms of panic anxiety as well as with its psychological expressions in poor attentional control and emotion regulation, and behavioral inflexibility.[1,2] Similar reductions in HRV have been found in depression,[54] generalized anxiety disorder,[55] and posttraumatic stress disorder.[56] Many of these affective states and dispositions have been associated with increased allostatic load as indexed by excess proinflammatory cytokines, excess cortisol, and poor glucose regulation.

In summary, we have tried to briefly provide evidence for the role of the ANS, and vagal function in particular, in the regulation of allostatic processes that modulate the wear and tear on the system that can lead to morbidity and mortality. Vagal function was shown to be associated with glucose regulation, HPA axis function, and inflammatory processes. The central nervous system concomitants of such regulation are comprised of a set of neural structures that include the prefrontal cortex and the amygdala. Importantly, identification of this neurovisceral regulatory system may elucidate a pathway via which psychosocial factors may "get under the skin" to confer risk for a wide range of disorders associated with death and disability.

REFERENCES

1. FRIEDMAN, B.H. & J.F. THAYER. 1998. Anxiety and autonomic flexibility: a cardiovascular approach. Biol. Psychol. **49:** 303–323.
2. FRIEDMAN, B.H. & J.F. THAYER. 1998. Autonomic balance revisited: panic anxiety and heart rate variability. J. Psychosom. Res. **44:** 133–151.
3. THAYER, J.F. & B.H. FRIEDMAN. 1997. The heart of anxiety: a dynamical systems approach. *In* The (Non) Expression of Emotions in Health and Disease. A. Vingerhoets, Ed.: 39–49. Springer Verlag. Amsterdam.
4. THAYER, J.F. & R.D. LANE. 2000. A model of neurovisceral integration in emotion regulation and dysregulation. J. Affect. Disord. **61:** 201–216.
5. LIPSITZ, L.A. & A.L. GOLDBERGER. 1992. Loss of complexity and aging—potential applications of fractals and chaos theory to senescence. J. Am. Med. Assoc. **267:** 1806–1809.
6. PENG, C.K., S.V. BULDYREV, J.M. HAUSDORFF, *et al.* 1994. Non-equilibrium dynamics as an indispensable characteristic of a healthy biological system. Integr. Physiol. Behav. Sci. **29:** 283–293.
7. BROOK, R.D. & S. JULIUS. 2000. Autonomic imbalance, hypertension, and cardiovascular risk. Am. J. Hypertens. **13:** 112S–122S.
8. THAYER, J.F. & B.H. FRIEDMAN. 2004. A neurovisceral integration model of health disparities in aging. *In* Critical Perspectives on Racial and Ethnic Differences in Health in Late Life. N.B. Anderson, R.A. Bulato & B. Cohen, Eds.: 567–603. The National Academies Press.Washington, DC.
9. JOSE, A.D. & D. COLLISON. 1970. The normal range and determinants of the intrinsic heart rate in man. Cardiovasc. Res. **4:** 160–167.
10. TASK FORCE OF THE EUROPEAN SOCIETY OF CARDIOLOGY AND THE NORTH AMERICAN SOCIETY OF PACING ELECTROPHYSIOLOGY. 1996. Heart rate variability: standards of measurement, physiological interpretation, and clinical use. Circulation **93:** 1043–1065.
11. AMAT, J., M.V. BARATTA, E. PAUL, *et al.* 2005. Medial prefrontal cortex determines how stressor controllability affects behavior and dorsal raphe nucleus. Nat. Neurosci. **8:** 365–371.

12. THAYER, J.F. 2006. On The importance of inhibition: central and peripheral manifestations of nonlinear inhibitory processes in neural systems. Dose Response **4:** 2–21.
13. DAVIDSON, R.J. 2000. The functional neuroanatomy of affective style. *In* Cognitive Neuroscience of Emotion. R.D. Lane & L. Nadel, Eds.:106–128. Oxford University Press. New York.
14. LEDOUX, J. 1996. The Emotional Brain. Simon and Schuster. New York.
15. MCEWEN, B.S. 1998. Protective and damaging effects of stress mediators. N. Engl. J. Med. **338:** 171–179.
16. THAYER, J.F. & R.D. LANE. The role of vagal function in the risk for cardiovascular disease and mortality. Biol. Psychol. In press.
17. HABIB, G.B. 1999. Reappraisal of heart rate as a risk factor in the general population. Eur. Heart J. Suppl. **1:** H2–H10.
18. ZIEGLER, D., D. LAUDE, F. AKILA & J.L. ELGHOZI. 2001. Time and frequency domain estimation of early diabetic cardiovascular autonomic neuropathy. Clin. Auton. Res. **11:** 369–376.
19. THAYER, J.F. & J.E. FISCHER. 2005a. Heart rate variability during sleep is inversely associated with glycosylated haemoglobin and fasting glucose in apparently healthy adults [abstract]. Psychosom. Med. **67:** S4.
20. LIAO, D., J. CAI, F.L. BRANCATI, *et al.* 1995. Association of vagal tone with serum insulin, glucose, and diabetes mellitus: the ARIC study. Diabetes Res. Clin. Pract. **30:** 211–221.
21. SINGH, J.P., M.G. LARSON, C.J. O'DONNELL, *et al.* 2000. Association of hyperglycemia with reduced heart rate variability (the Framingham Heart Study). Am. J. Cardiol. **86:** 309–312.
22. CARNETHON, M.R., S.H. GOLDEN, A.R. FOLSOM, *et al.* 2003. Prospective investigation of autonomic nervous system function and the development of type 2 diabetes: the atherosclerosis risk in communities study, 1987–1998. Circulation **107:** 2190–2195.
23. PANZER, C., M.S. LAUER, A. BRIEKE, *et al.* 2002. Association of fasting plasma glucose with heart rate recovery in healthy adults—a population-based study. Diabetes **51:** 803–807.
24. THAYER, J.F., M. HALL, J.J. SOLLERS 3rd & J.E. FISCHER. 2006. Alcohol use, urinary cortisol, and heart rate variability in apparently healthy men: evidence for impaired inhibitory control of the HPA axis in heavy drinkers. Int. J. Psychophysiol. **59:** 244–250.
25. BENARROCH, E.E. 1993. The central autonomic network: functional organization, dysfunction, and perspective. Mayo Clin. Proc. **68:** 988–1001.
26. BENARROCH, E.E. 1997. The central autonomic network. *In* Clinical Autonomic Disorders, 2nd ed. P.A. Low, Ed.: 17–23. Lippincott-Raven. Philadelphia.
27. DIORIO, D., V. VIAU & M.J. MEANEY. 1993. The role of the medial prefrontal cortex (cingulate gyrus) in the regulation of the hypothalamic-pituitary-adrenal response to stress. J. Neurosci. **13:** 3839–3847.
28. ZOBEL, A., J. WELLMER, S. SCHULZE-RAUSCHENBACH, *et al.* 2004. Impairment of inhibitory control of the hypothalamic pituitary adrenocortical system in epilepsy. Eur. Arch. Psychiatry Clin. Neurosci. **254:** 303–311.
29. THAYER, J.F. & J.F. BROSSCHOT. 2005. Psychosomatics and psychopathology: looking up and down from the brain. Psychoneuroendocrinology **30:** 1050–1058.
30. HEINZ, A. *et al.* 2005. Amygdala-prefrontal coupling depends on a genetic variation of the serotonin transporter. Nat. Neurosci. **8:** 20–21.

31. PEZAWAS, L. *et al.* 2005. 5-HTTLPR polymorphism impacts human cingulate-amygdala interactions: a genetic susceptibility mechanism for depression. Nat. Neurosci. **8:** 828–834.

32. ANTHENELLI, R.M., R.A. MAXWELL, T.D. GERACIOTI & R. HAUGER. 2001. Stress hormone dysregulation at rest and after serotonergic stimulation among alcohol-dependent men with extended abstinence and controls. Alcohol. Clin. Exp. Res. **25:** 692–703.

33. MANUCK, S.B., J.R. KAPLAN & F.E. LOTRICH. 2005. Brain serotonin and aggressive disposition in humans and non-human primates. *In* Handbook on the Biology of Aggression. R.J. Nelson, Ed.: 65–113. Oxford University Press. New York.

34. MCBRIDE, W.J. & T.K. LI. 1998. Animal models of alcoholism: neurobiology of high-alcohol-drinking behavior in rodents. Crit. Rev. Neurobiol. **12:** 339–369.

35. TAFET, G.E., M. TOISTER-ACHITUV & M. SHINITZKY. 2001. Enhancement of serotonin uptake by cortisol: a possible link between stress and depression. Cogn. Affect. Behav. Neurosci. **1:** 96–104.

36. TAFET, G.E., V.P. IDOYAGA-VARGAS, D.P. ABULAFIA, *et al.* 2001. Correlation between cortisol level and serotonin uptake in patients with chronic stress and depression. Cogn. Affect. Behav. Neurosci. **1:** 388–393.

37. BOOIJ, L., C.A. SWENNE, J.F. BROSSCHOT, *et al.* 2006. Tryptophan depletion affects heart rate variability and impulsivity in remitted depressed patients with a history of suicidal ideation. Biol. Psychiatry. 2006 Apr 5 [E-pub ahead of print].

38. DAVIDSON, R.J. 2002. Anxiety and affective style: role of prefrontal cortex and amygdala. Biol. Psychiatry **51:** 68–80.

39. DREVETS W.C. 1999. Prefrontal cortical-amygdalar metabolism in major depression. Ann. N. Y. Acad. Sci. **877:** 614–637.

40. ERSHLER, W. & E. KELLER. 2000. Age-associated increased interleukin-6 gene expression, late life diseases, and frailty. Annu. Rev. Med. **51:** 245–270.

41. KIECOLT-GLASER, J.K., L. McGuire, T.F. ROBLES & R. GLASER. 2002. Emotions, morbidity, and mortality: new perspectives from psychoneuroimmunology. Annu. Rev. Psychol. **53:** 83–107.

42. DAS, U.N. 2000. Beneficial effect(s) of n-3 fatty acids in cardiovascular disease: but, why and how? Prostaglandins Leukot. Essent. Fatty Acids **63:** 351–362.

43. MAIER, S.F. & L.R. WATKINS. 1998. Cytokines for psychologists: implications of bi-directional immune-to-brain communication for understanding behavior, mood, and cognition. Psychol. Rev. **105:** 83–107.

44. TRACEY, K.J. 2002. The inflammatory reflex. Nature **420:** 853–859.

45. RIDKER, P.M.. 2001. High-sensitivity C-reactive protein—potential adjunct for global risk assessment in the primary prevention of cardiovascular disease. Circulation **103:** 1813–1818.

46. JANSZKY, I., M. ERICSON, M. LEKANDER, *et al.* 2004. Inflammatory markers and heart rate variability in women with coronary heart disease. J. Intern. Med. **256:** 421–428.

47. SAJADIEH, A., O.W. NIELSEN, V. RASMUSSEN, *et al.* 2004. Increased heart rate and reduced heart-rate variability are associated with subclinical inflammation in middle-aged and elderly subjects with no apparent heart disease. Eur. Heart J. **25:** 363–370.

48. THAYER, J.F. & J.E. FISCHER. 2005b. Evidence for the cholinergic anti-inflammatory pathway in healthy human adults. [abstract]. Psychosom. Med. **67:** S8.

49. STERNBERG, E.M. 1997. Emotions and disease: from balance of humors to balance of molecules. Nat. Med. **3:** 264–267.

50. KRANTZ, D.S. & M.K. MCCENEY. 2002. Effects of psychological and social factors on organic disease: a critical assessment of research on coronary heart disease. Annu. Rev. Psychol. **53:** 341–369.
51. MUSSELMAN, D.L., D.L. EVANS & C.B. NEMEROFF. 1998. The relationship of depression to cardiovascular disease. Arch. Gen. Psychiatry **55:** 580–592.
52. ROZANSKI, A., J.A. BLUMENTHAL& J. KAPLAN. 1999. Impact of psychological factors on the pathogenesis of cardiovascular disease and implications for therapy. Circulation **99:** 2192–2217.
53. VERRIER, R.L.& M.A. MITTLEMAN. 2000. The impact of emotions on the heart. Prog. Brain Res. **122:** 369–380.
54. THAYER, J.F., M. SMITH, L.A. ROSSY, *et al.* 1998. Heart period variability and depressive symptoms: gender differences. Biol. Psychiatry **44:** 304–306.
55. THAYER, J.F., B.H. FRIEDMAN & T.D. Borkovec. 1996. Autonomic characteristics of generalized anxiety disorder and worry. Biol. Psychiatry **39:** 255–266.
56. COHEN, H., M.A. MATAR, Z. KAPLAN & M. KOTLER. 1999. Power spectral analysis of heart rate variability in psychiatry. Psychother. Psychosom. **68:** 59–66.

Interleukin-6

A Cytokine and/or a Major Modulator of the Response to Somatic Stress

GEORGE MASTORAKOS[a] AND IOANNIS ILIAS[b]

[a]Endocrine Unit, Second Department of Obstetrics and Gynecology, Medical School, University of Athens, Athens, Greece

[b]Department of Pharmacology, Medical School, University of Patras, Rion, Greece

ABSTRACT: The hypothalamic-pituitary-adrenal (HPA) axis and the proinflammatory cytokines (and interleukin-6 [IL-6] in particular) are enmeshed in the response to somatic stress, either in health or in acute or chronic disease. Usually IL-6 is elevated in states of septic (such as sepsis) or aseptic inflammation (such as rheumatoid arthritis). Exercise is a form of somatic stress. Local tissue IL-6 elevation is noted during shorter and less intense exercise, whereas brief peripheral IL-6 "bursts" are observed with longer and more intense exercise. Therapeutic interventions that target IL-6 or its soluble receptor are currently assessed, with an emphasis on autoimmune diseases and inflammatory conditions.

KEYWORDS: interleukin-6 secretion; hypothalamus; hypothalamo–hypophyseal system; pituitary-adrenal system; stress/blood/etiology/immunology

INTRODUCTION

Stress is the state to which an organism is led because of external or internal forces (stressors) that threaten to alter its dynamic equilibrium (homeostasis). After a certain stress threshold has been surpassed, the stress system in the brain is activated along with its peripheral components, the hypothalamic-pituitary-adrenal (HPA) axis and the autonomic sympathetic system. To cope with stress, behavioral and physical responses ("somatic stress," characterized by higher heart rate, higher breathing rate, and greater muscle tension) are elicited.[1]

Address for correspondence: Dr. George Mastorakos at 3, Neofytou Vamva Street, Athens, GR-10674, Greece. Voice: +30-210-3636230; fax: +30-210-3636229.
e-mail: mastorak@mail.kapatel.gr

Ann. N.Y. Acad. Sci. 1088: 373–381 (2006). © 2006 New York Academy of Sciences.
doi: 10.1196/annals.1366.021

THE STRESS RESPONSE

The HPA Axis

Parvocellular neurons of the paraventricular nucleus in the hypothalamus secrete corticotropin-releasing hormone (a 41–amino acid neuropeptide; CRH) into the hypophyseal portal system. CRH stimulates the secretion of corticotropin (ACTH) from the pituitary corticotroph cells. ACTH is transported via the systemic circulation to the adrenal cortex, stimulating the synthesis and release of cortisol and adrenal androgens. Cortisol is enmeshed in a negative feedback loop with both CRH and ACTH. Furthermore, cortisol, as well as synthetic glucocorticoids, affect in many ways the immune/inflammatory (I/I) response, leading mainly to inhibition of the production and traffic of leukocytes and inflammatory mediators.[2]

Proinflammatory Cytokines

Monocytes secrete cytokines that enhance inflammation (the so-called proinflammatory cytokines: interleukin [IL]-1, IL-6, and tumor necrosis factor alpha [TNF-α]) in a cascade-like mode at inflammatory sites. These cytokines stimulate their own secretion; furthermore, IL-1 and TNF-α stimulate the secretion of IL-6, whereas the latter inhibits the secretion of both IL-1 and TNF-α.[3] Cytokines are large molecules that would not be expected to cross the blood–brain barrier; nevertheless, passage has been documented either under normal conditions (at the organum vasculosum of the lamina terminalis) or under pathologic states (such as in infection or inflammation).[3]

ENDOGENOUS IL-6 AND THE HPA AXIS IN HEALTH

IL-6 and the HPA Axis

In *in vitro* experimental studies IL-1 was found to be more potent than IL-6 or TNF-α in stimulating the HPA axis.[4] Furthermore, both IL-6 and its receptor are expressed in the adrenal glands; *in vitro* adrenal culture studies have shown that IL-6 may regulate steroidogenesis locally in the adrenal glands, possibly acting as a long-term regulator of the stress response.[5] In mice, the effect of IL-6 on the adrenal response is more pronounced in females than males.[6] IL-6 given once at 3 μg/kg (but not at 0.3 μg/kg) in healthy humans suppressed corticosteroid-binding globulin, which determines cortisol bioavailability.[7]

Exercise, the HPA Axis and Cytokines

Exercise causes multiple adaptive modifications to human physiology. Thus, it can be assimilated to a stress phenomenon.[1] Exercise stimulates the HPA axis.[8] Furthermore, plasma IL-6 secretion is stimulated during strenuous treadmill testing in humans.[9] The exercise-stimulated IL-6 correlates well with plasma catecholamines,[9] while the administration of glucocorticoids attenuates the rise in IL-6 but has no effect on plasma catecholamine levels.[9] On the other hand, exercise/stress-induced endogenous glucocorticoids during strenuous exercise at 100% maximal oxygen utilization suppress IL-1-β and TNF-α, but have no effect on IL-6 production.[10] Yet, strenuous—but less intense—exercise has different effects of shorter duration on IL-6 and cortisol. In a relevant study eight healthy males underwent exhaustive physical exercise combined with reduced energy intake and sleep deprivation for 7 days (this level of exercise accounts for continuous exercise at 35% maximal oxygen utilization). At this level of exercise both plasma IL-6 and cortisol increased on days 2 to 4, but IL-6 became undetectable and cortisol reverted to normal levels by day 7.[11] Interestingly, in a recent microdialysis study of the trapezius muscle in six healthy volunteers that underwent 20-min-long low-force exercise, local interstitial IL-6 rose markedly,[12] although these high interstitial IL-6 levels were not reflected in peripheral IL-6 levels.[12] Thus, IL-6 may rise—at least locally—during shorter and less intense exercise and show brief peripheral "bursts" with longer and more intense exercise.

Exercise and Vasopressin

In an elegant research work Smoak *et al.* studied five male and five female healthy volunteers during treadmill exercise testing after pretreatment with CRH; the response of corticotropin to exercise was not abolished, suggesting a stimulating effect of a factor other than CRH.[13] That factor is presumably antidiuretic hormone or vasopressin (AVP), the other major secretagogue of the HPA axis. Vasopressin-secreting cells in the median eminence and the suprachiasmatic nucleus express IL-6, whereas CRH-secreting cells in the median eminence express both IL-6 and AVP.[14] Thus, AVP is secreted following the same stimuli that lead to IL-6 secretion.[15] In addition, studies further presented, have proposed IL-6 as a potent stimulus of AVP secretion.

Strenuous exercise may lead to disturbances in AVP secretion. In a study summarizing the effects of endurance exercise from reports worldwide, of 2,135 athletes that participated in such events, 3.5% developed hyponatremia and gained weight at the end of their participation.[16] These are attributed, in part, to the syndrome of inappropriate antidiuretic hormone secretion (SIADH) (excess fluid ingestion and failure of mobilization of nonosmotically active sodium may also be implicated).[16] In the following section we present further results of studies that link the HPA axis with IL-6 and SIADH.

ENDOGENOUS IL-6 AND THE HPA AXIS IN DISEASE

Aseptic Situations

In patients with untreated rheumatoid arthritis, plasma IL-6 levels show a distinct diurnal variation and a slight increase compared to control subjects. Moreover, in patients with rheumatoid arthritis, IL-6 has a positive temporal correlation with ACTH and cortisol (preceding them by 1 and 2 h, respectively), whereas cortisol has a negative temporal correlation with IL-6 (with cortisol preceding by a 5-h lag time). Nevertheless, neither 24-h time-integrated plasma ACTH and cortisol, nor free cortisol in urine or plasma ACTH and cortisol responses to ovine CRH are different between patients with rheumatoid arthritis and control subjects. Thus, in patients with rheumatoid arthritis, the overall status of the HPA axis is inappropriately normal, regardless of high IL-6 levels, with cortisol being unable to restrain the inflammatory process.[17,18] As expected, in patients with active rheumatoid arthritis and no previous history of glucocorticoid treatment, plasma IL-6 is positively correlated with serum C-reactive protein.[19]

In addition, in a study of patients with untreated newly diagnosed sarcoidosis (a T lymphocyte–associated autoimmune disease), we have shown that the IL-6 response to treadmill exercise increased as compared to controls, whereas the cortisol response was similar to that of controls, indicating that the HPA axis in these patients does not readily respond to increased IL-6 levels.[20]

Various degrees of dysregulation in the HPA axis have been observed in patients with fibromyalgia. In particular, CRH administration in patients provokes a higher ACTH response compared to subjects with low back pain [21] or healthy controls.[22,23] In other studies, the ACTH response to CRH compared to healthy controls was not significantly different, but the cortisol response was lower (along with lower 24-h baseline urine cortisol).[24] It has been suggested that failure of adequate HPA responses to stressors may predispose to this disease.[25,26] Interestingly, patients with long-standing fibromyalgia show elevated peripheral blood cytokines, including IL-1, IL-6, and TNF-α; hyperalgesia is attributed to interaction with cytokine receptors on glial cells.[27]

Another aspect of the IL-6–HPA axis association regards IL-6 stimulation by AVP secretion. IL-6 given intravenously (i.v.) to humans stimulates AVP secretion.[28] In a study in which recombinant IL-6 was administered i.v. to six human subjects in doses ranging from 0.3 μg/kg to 30 μg/kg, maximal plasma ACTH and cortisol responses were noted regardless of the dose administered (suggesting that the amount of the cytokine used was at the plateau section of the dose-response curve); AVP was also elevated (at a 2-h time lag), with IL-6 doses higher than 3 μg/kg. The latter finding suggested that IL-6 activates magnocellular vasopressin-secreting neurons.[28]

To further assess the association of IL-6 with AVP secretion we studied their profiles in children with SIADH after head injury.[29] In this study, time-integrated serum IL-6 was positively correlated with time-integrated AVP secretion. This quantitative correlation suggests that IL-6 is involved either directly or indirectly with the pathogenesis of SIADH.[29,30]

Septic Inflammation

In a model of chronic septic inflammation, patients with African trypanoso-miasis (sleeping sickness) show impaired adrenocortical function (secondary adrenal insufficiency) despite markedly elevated IL-6 and TNF-α levels before therapy.[33] On the other hand, in a model of acute septic inflammation, endotoxin given i.v. to healthy males (at doses resulting in levels lower than those observed during acute infectious disease) resulted in a rapid increase in serum IL-6 and TNF-α within 2 h. The IL-6/TNF-α ratio was positively correlated with the ratio of serum cortisol/dehydroepiandrosterone.[34] Protozoan or viral infections in mice lead to IL-6 elevation that is not always accompanied by high corticotropin levels.[35,36] Nevertheless, in humans with sepsis IL-6 is elevated,[31,32] along with high cortisol and macrophage migration inhibitory factor.[37] Thus, it seems that the IL-6/HPA axis response shows differences in adapting between chronic and acute septic inflammation. Their inappropriately low or normal response to chronic septic inflammation parallels that observed in chronic aseptic situations, such as chronic autoimmune diseases.

EXOGENOUS IL-6 AND THE HPA AXIS

When recombinant IL-6 was administered i.v. to five human subjects at a dose of 30 μg/kg/day for 7 days, plasma ACTH and cortisol were markedly elevated on day 1, with ACTH levels dropping to normal levels and cortisol remaining high by day 7.[38] In a subsequent study recombinant IL-6 (0.3 to 30 μg/kg) was administered i.v. to humans, and maximal plasma ACTH and cortisol responses were noted regardless of the dose administered.[28]

In 12 healthy volunteers the infusion of IL-6 at physiological doses (30 μg/h) increased plasma cortisol and induced neutrocytosis and lymphopenia, resembling the pattern observed during intense exercise.[39] It has been suggested that muscle-induced IL-6 is implicated in exercise-induced leukocyte trafficking.[39]

PHARMACOLOGIC INTERVENTIONS—PERSPECTIVES

Glucocorticoids have differential actions depending on dosage, which may be attributed to the implication of different glucocorticoid receptor types: type 1 (high affinity or mineralocorticoid receptors) is mainly activational, whereas type 2 (low affinity or glucocorticoid receptors) can be activational or inhibitory.[3] The administration of a single p.o. pharmacological dose (80 mg) of hydrocortisone in six healthy volunteers suppressed the *ex vivo* lipopolysaccharide-induced IL-1-β, TNF-α, and IL-6 production in their whole blood.[10] The administration of a single physiological (20 mg) dose of hydrocortisone suppressed only TNF-α production.[10]

Although it has been proposed that the inhibitory effect that IL-6 exerts on IL-1 and TNF-α can be beneficial in patients with septic shock,[3] no preclinical or clinical trials have been attempted with it. In preclinical trials in mice the concomitant administration of anti-IL-6 antibodies and antibodies targeted against soluble IL-6 receptors prevented effectively systemic inflammation.[40]

Tocilizumab, a humanized monoclonal antibody against IL-6, has been given i.v. every 4 weeks, thrice at 4 mg/kg and 8 mg/kg doses (in 164 adults) or at 2 mg/kg to 8 mg/kg (in 18 children) in phase 1 and 2 clinical trials of patients with rheumatoid arthritis. The results were promising: most patients showed good responses according to the American College of Rheumatology improvement criteria.[41,42] Avimers, a new class of protein-binding molecules that are smaller than antibodies, have been effectively used to block IL-6 in mice, and may hold a therapeutic potential.[43,44]

REFERENCES

1. MASTORAKOS, G. *et al.* 2005. Exercise and the stress system. Hormones (Athens, Greece) **4:** 73–89.
2. CHROUSOS, G.P. 1995. The hypothalamic-pituitary-adrenal axis and immune-mediated inflammation. N. Engl. J. Med. **332:** 1351–1362.
3. O'CONNOR, T.M. *et al.* 2000. The stress response and the hypothalamic-pituitary-adrenal axis: from molecule to melancholia. QJM **93:** 323–333.
4. BASEDOVSKY, H.O. *et al.* 2000. The cytokine-HPA axis feedback circuit. Z. Rheumatol. **59** (Suppl 2): 26–30.
5. PATH, G. *et al.* 1997. Interleukin-6 and the interleukin-6 receptor in the human adrenal gland: expression and effects on steroidogenesis. J. Clin. Endocrinol. Metab. **82:** 2343–2349.
6. BETHIN, K.E. *et al.* 2000. Interleukin-6 is an essential, corticotropin-releasing hormone-independent stimulator of the adrenal axis during immune system activation. Proc. Natl. Acad. Sci. USA **97:** 9317–9322.
7. TSIGOS, C. *et al.* 1998. Prolonged suppression of corticosteroid-binding globulin by recombinant human interleukin-6 in man. J. Clin. Endocrinol. Metab. **83:** 3379.

8. MASTORAKOS, G. *et al.* 2005. Exercise as a stress model and the interplay between the hypothalamus-pituitary-adrenal and the hypothalamus-pituitary-thyroid axes. Horm. Metab. Res. **37:** 577–584.
9. PAPANICOLAOU, D.A. *et al.* 1996. Exercise stimulates interleukin-6 secretion: inhibition by glucocorticoids and correlation with catecholamines. Am. J. Physiol. **271:** E601–E605.
10. DERIJK, R. *et al.* 1997. Exercise and circadian rhythm-induced variations in plasma cortisol differentially regulate interleukin-1 beta (IL-1 beta), IL-6, and tumor necrosis factor-alpha (TNF alpha) production in humans: high sensitivity of TNF alpha and resistance of IL-6. J. Clin. Endocrinol. Metab. **82:** 2182–2191.
11. GUNDERSEN, Y. *et al.* 2006. Seven days' around the clock exhaustive physical exertion combined with energy depletion and sleep deprivation primes circulating leukocytes. Eur. J. Appl. Physiol. 10.1007/s00421-0150-8 [doi].
12. ROSENDAL, L. *et al.* 2005. Increase in interstitial interleukin-6 of human skeletal muscle with repetitive low-force exercise. J. Appl. Physiol. **98:** 477–481.
13. SMOAK, B. *et al.* 1991. Corticotropin-releasing hormone is not the sole factor mediating exercise-induced adrenocorticotropin release in humans. J. Clin. Endocrinol. Metab. **73:** 302–306.
14. GONZALEZ-HERNANDEZ, T. *et al.* 2006. Interleukin-6 and nitric oxide synthase expression in the vasopressin and corticotrophin-releasing factor systems of the rat hypothalamus. J. Histochem. Cytochem. **54:** 427–441.
15. GHORBEL, M.T. *et al.* 2003. Microarray analysis reveals interleukin-6 as a novel secretory product of the hypothalamo-neurohypophyseal system. J. Biol. Chem. **278:** 19280–19285.
16. NOAKES, T.D. *et al.* 2005. Three independent biological mechanisms cause exercise-associated hyponatremia: evidence from 2,135 weighed competitive athletic performances. Proc. Natl. Acad. Sci. USA **102:** 18550–18555.
17. CROFFORD, L.J. *et al.* 1997. Circadian relationships between interleukin (IL)-6 and hypothalamic-pituitary-adrenal axis hormones: failure of IL-6 to cause sustained hypercortisolism in patients with early untreated rheumatoid arthritis. J. Clin. Endocrinol. Metab. **82:** 1279–1283.
18. MASTORAKOS, G. *et al.* 2000. Relationship between interleukin-6 (IL-6) and hypothalamic-pituitary-adrenal axis hormones in rheumatoid arthritis. Z. Rheumatol. **59**(Suppl 2): 75–79.
19. BOSS, B. *et al.* 2000. Correlation of IL-6 with the classical humoral disease activity parameters, ESR and CRP and with serum cortisol, reflecting the activity of the HPA axis in active rheumatoid arthritis. Z. Rheumatol. **59** (Suppl 2): 62–64.
20. MASTORAKOS, G. *et al.* 1998. Interleukin 6 changes during cardiopulmonary exercise test in sarcoidosis patients and controls [abstract]. The Endocrine Society's 80th Annual Meeting, New Orleans, June 24–27: 431.
21. GRIEP, E.N. *et al.* 1998. Function of the hypothalamic-pituitary-adrenal axis in patients with fibromyalgia and low back pain. J. Rheumatol. Suppl. **25:** 1374–1381.
22. RIEDEL, W. *et al.* 1998. Secretory pattern of GH, TSH, thyroid hormones, ACTH, cortisol, FSH, and LH in patients with fibromyalgia syndrome following systemic injection of the relevant hypothalamic-releasing hormones. Z. Rheumatol. **57** (Suppl 2): 81–87.
23. GRIEP, E.N. *et al.* 1993. Altered reactivity of the hypothalamic-pituitary-adrenal axis in the primary fibromyalgia syndrome. J. Rheumatol. **20:** 469–474.

24. CROFFORD, L.J. *et al.* 1994. Hypothalamic-pituitary-adrenal axis perturbations in patients with fibromyalgia. Arthritis Rheum. **37:** 1583–1592.
25. MCBETH, J. *et al.* 2005. Hypothalamic-pituitary-adrenal stress axis function and the relationship with chronic widespread pain and its antecedents. Arthritis Res. Ther. **7:** R992–R1000.
26. TSIGOS, C. *et al.* 2002. Hypothalamic-pituitary-adrenal axis, neuroendocrine factors and stress. J. Psychosom. Res. **53:** 865–871.
27. THOMPSON, M.E. *et al.* 2003. Fibromyalgia, hepatitis C infection, and the cytokine connection. Curr. Pain Headache Rep. **7:** 342–347.
28. MASTORAKOS, G. *et al.* 1994. Hypothalamic-pituitary-adrenal axis activation and stimulation of systemic vasopressin secretion by recombinant interleukin-6 in humans: potential implications for the syndrome of inappropriate vasopressin secretion. J. Clin. Endocrinol. Metab. **79:** 934–939.
29. GIONIS, D. *et al.* 2003. Hypothalamic-pituitary-adrenal axis and interleukin-6 activity in children with head trauma and syndrome of inappropriate secretion of antidiuretic hormone. J. Pediatr. Endocrinol. Metab. **16:** 49–54.
30. MOSES, A.M. 1994. Comments on some clinical implications of the release of adrenocorticotropin and vasopressin by interleukin-6 and other cytokines. J. Clin. Endocrinol. Metab. **79:** 932–933.
31. HARRIS, M.C. *et al.* 1994. Cytokine elevations in critically ill infants with sepsis and necrotizing enterocolitis. J. Pediatr. **124:** 105–111.
32. STRATAKIS, C.A. *et al.* 1994. Interleukin-6 elevation in critically ill infants with sepsis and necrotizing enterocolitis. J. Pediatr. **125:** 504.
33. REINCKE, M. *et al.* 1994. Impairment of adrenocortical function associated with increased plasma tumor necrosis factor-alpha and interleukin-6 concentrations in African trypanosomiasis. Neuroimmunomodulation **1:** 14–22.
34. STRAUB, R.H. *et al.* 2002. The endotoxin-induced increase of cytokines is followed by an increase of cortisol relative to dehydroepiandrosterone (DHEA) in healthy male subjects. J. Endocrinol. **175:** 467–474.
35. SILVERMAN, M.N. *et al.* 2004. Characterization of an interleukin-6- and adrenocorticotropin-dependent, immune-to-adrenal pathway during viral infection. Endocrinology **145:** 3580–3589.
36. CORREA-DE-SANTANA, E. *et al.* 2006. Hypothalamus-pituitary-adrenal axis during *Trypanosoma cruzi* acute infection in mice. J. Neuroimmunol. **173:** 12–22.
37. BEISHUIZEN, A. *et al.* 2001. Macrophage migration inhibitory factor and hypothalamo-pituitary-adrenal function during critical illness. J. Clin. Endocrinol. Metab. **86:** 2811–2816.
38. MASTORAKOS, G. *et al.* 1993. Recombinant interleukin-6 activates the hypothalamic-pituitary-adrenal axis in humans. J. Clin. Endocrinol. Metab. **77:** 1690–1694.
39. STEENSBERG, A. *et al.* 2003. IL-6 enhances plasma IL-1ra, IL-10, and cortisol in humans. Am. J. Physiol. Endocrinol. Metab. **285:** E433–E437.
40. PALLUA, N. *et al.* 2003. Pathogenic role of interleukin-6 in the development of sepsis. Part II: significance of anti-interleukin-6 and anti-soluble interleukin-6 receptor-alpha antibodies in a standardized murine contact burn model. Crit. Care Med. **31:** 1495–1501.
41. NISHIMOTO, N. 2006. Interleukin-6 in rheumatoid arthritis. Curr. Opin. Rheumatol. **18:** 277–281.
42. WOO, P. *et al.* 2005. Open label phase II trial of single, ascending doses of MRA in Caucasian children with severe systemic juvenile idiopathic arthritis: proof

of principle of the efficacy of IL-6 receptor blockade in this type of arthritis and demonstration of prolonged clinical improvement. Arthritis Res. Ther. **7:** R1281–R1288.

43. SILVERMAN, J. *et al.* 2005. Multivalent avimer proteins evolved by exon shuffling of a family of human receptor domains. Nat. Biotechnol. **23:** 1556–1561.

44. JEONG, K.J. *et al.* 2005. Avimers hold their own. Nat. Biotechnol. **23:** 1493–1494.

The Role of Stress in the Clinical Expression of Thyroid Autoimmunity

AGATHOCLES TSATSOULIS

Department of Endocrinology, University of Ioannina 45110, Ioannina, Greece

ABSTRACT: During stress, activation of the hypothalamic-pituitary-adrenal axis and the sympathoadrenal system leads to increased secretion of glucocorticoids and catecholamines, respectively, in order to maintain homeostasis. Recent evidence suggests that stress hormones, acting on antigen-presenting immune cells, may influence the differentiation of bipotential T helper (Th) cells away from Th1 and toward a Th2 phenotype. This results in suppression of cellular immunity and potentiation of humoral immunity. Thyroid autoimmunity is clinically expressed as Hashimoto's thyroiditis (HT) and its variants (sporadic or postpartum thyroiditis) or as Grave's disease (GD). The different phenotypic expression of thyroid autoimmunity is largely dependent on the balance of Th1 versus Th2 immune response. A predominantly Th1-mediated immune activity may promote apoptotic pathways on thyroid follicular cells leading to thyroid cell destruction and HT. Conversely, predominance of Th2-mediated immune response may induce antigen-specific B lymphocytes to produce anti-TSH receptor (TSHr) antibodies causing GD. The weight of evidence from epidemiological and case–control studies supports an association between stress and GD. On the other hand, there is little information available on the effect of stress on HT, but there is evidence for an increase in postpartum thyroiditis, following the cellular immune suppressive effect of pregnancy. Whether stress has a causative effect on GD remains elusive. Circumstantial evidence supports the hypothesis that stress may influence the clinical expression of thyroid autoimmunity in susceptible individuals favoring the development of GD by shifting the Th1–Th2 balance away for Th1 and toward Th2. Conversely, recovery from stress or the immune suppressive effect of pregnancy may induce a Th2 to Th1 "return shift" leading to autoimmune (sporadic) or postpartum thyroiditis, respectively.

KEYWORDS: stress; autoimmunity; Grave's disease; autoimmune thyroiditis

Address for correspondence: Agathocles Tsatsoulis, M.D., Ph.D., F.R.C.P., Department of Endocrinology, University of Ioannina 45110, Ioannina, Greece. Voice: +3026510-99625; fax: +3026510-46617.

e-mail: atsatsou@cc.uoi.gr

Ann. N.Y. Acad. Sci. 1088: 382–395 (2006). © 2006 New York Academy of Sciences.
doi: 10.1196/annals.1366.015

INTRODUCTION

Stress has a significant effect on the immune system through neuroendocrine pathways. During stress, the hypothalamic-pituitary-adrenal (HPA) axis, together with the sympathoadrenal system, is activated, resulting in systemic elevations in glucocorticoids and catecholamines, respectively. Both systems act in concert to maintain the internal milieu or homeostasis.[1] It has long been thought that stress hormones, and in particular glucocorticoids, exert a general immune suppressive effect. However, it is becoming clear that stress, through its effector pathways, has a differential effect on immune response, suppressing cellular and potentiating humoral immunity.[2,3]

Thyroid autoimmunity may be clinically expressed as chronic autoimmune or Hashimoto's thyroiditis (HT) and its variants (postpartum/sporadic thyroiditis) or as Graves' disease (GD) and atrophic thyroiditis. Recent evidence suggests that the phenotypic expression of thyroid autoimmunity toward one or the other clinical entity is largely dependent on the pattern of immune response that predominates at a given time.[4,5] The aim of this article is to provide evidence from experimental and clinical research in support of the hypothesis that stress may influence the clinical expression of thyroid autoimmunity.

TH1–TH2 BALANCE AND IMMUNE RESPONSE

The type of immune response is regulated by antigen-presenting cells (APCs), including dendritic cells (DCs), macrophages, and natural killer (NK) cells, which are components of innate immunity. These cells present (auto) antigens in conjunction with major histocompatibility complex (MHC) molecules and costimulatory signals to T helper (Th) cells, which express CD4$^+$ surface antigens. The CD4$^+$ Th cells are further subdivided into two subtypes, Th1 and Th2 cells, which are components of adaptive immunity. Th1 cells primarily secrete type 1 cytokines including interleukin-2 (IL-2), interferon-γ (IFN-γ), and tumor necrosis factor-α (TNF-α) which activate cellular immunity leading to tissue damage. On the other hand, Th2 cells secrete type 2 cytokines, primarily interleukin-4 (IL-4), IL-5, and IL-10 and provide help to antigen-specific B lymphocytes to produce antibodies involved in humoral immunity.[6,7] Precursor CD4$^+$ Th cells are thus bipotential and their differentiation toward Th1 or Th2 subtypes is dependent on the kind of signals they receive from APCs during antigen presentation. Thus, IL-12 produced by activated macrophages or DCs acting in concert with NK cell-derived IFN-γ on naïve CD4+Th cells, induce Th1, whereas IL-4 and IL-10 promote Th2 differentiation. Furthermore, Th1 and Th2 effector arms of immune response are mutually inhibitory. Type 1 cytokines inhibit Th2, and type 2 cytokines inhibit Th1 response.[8,9]

STRESS HORMONES AND TH1–TH2 BALANCE

Effect of Glucocorticoids and Catecholamines

Glucocorticoids, at levels achieved during stress, suppress cellular and potentiate humoral immunity. Glucocorticoids, acting through their cytoplasmic/nuclear receptors on APCs, suppress the production of IL-12, the main inducer of Th1 responses and downregulate the expression of IL-12 receptors on T and NK cells. Glucocorticoids also appear to upregulate the production of IL-4 and IL-10 by Th2 cells. This could be the result of a direct effect of glucocorticoids on T cells and/or the result of blocking the restraining effect of IL-12 and IFN-γ on Th2 cells.[10–13]

In a similar manner, the two major catecholamines, epinephrine and norepinephrine, acting on APCs through β2-adrenergic receptors (ARs) suppress the production of IL-12, thus inhibiting the differentiation of Th1 cells while promoting Th2 cell differentiation.[10] In addition, catecholamines appear to inhibit the production of TNF-α and, at the same time, to potentiate the production of IL-10 by APCs.[14,15] Furthermore β2-ARs are expressed only on Th1 cells and not on Th2 cells, and this may provide an additional explanation for the differential effect of catecholamines on Th1–Th2 balance. Thus, β2-AR agonists inhibit IFN-γ production by Th1 cells, but do not affect IL-4 production by Th2 cells.[16] In conclusion, both glucocorticoids and catecholamines by downregulating type 1 and upregulating type 2 cytokine secretion may cause selective suppression of cellular immunity and a shift toward Th2-mediated humoral immunity.

Local CRH–Mast Cell–Histamine Axis

Apart from the central hypothalamic corticotrophin-releasing hormone (CRH) that influences the type of immune response indirectly, through activation of the HPA axis, CRH is also secreted locally at peripheral sites, (peripheral or immune CRH) and may influence the immune system directly through local modulatory actions.[1,17] It appears that mast cells are the targets of immune CRH, clusters of which are found in periarterial sympathetic plexuses and plexuses of nerve fibers within lymphoid parenchyma. Peripheral CRH activates mast cells via a CRH type 1 receptor–dependent mechanism, leading to the release of histamine and other contents of the mast cell granules. In turn, histamine acting through the H1 receptor may induce acute inflammation and allergic reactions, while through activation of H2 receptor may induce suppression of Th1 activity and a Th2 shift.[18,19] Thus, the activation of the CRH–mast cell–histamine axis, through stimulation of H2 receptors, might shift the Th1–Th2 balance toward a Th2 phenotype.

Adrenal DHEA and Th1–Th2 Balance

Dehydroepiandrosterone (DHEA) is produced by the adrenal glands and is found in the plasma mainly as its sulfated derivative, DHEAS. As one of the effectors of the HPA axis, DHEA supports the body's adaptive stress response and may be involved in immune regulation. Circumstantial evidence suggests that DHEA is involved in immune homeostasis by promoting Th1 and inhibiting Th2-type responses.[20] During acute stress, a dissociation of DHEA from cortisol release is observed in that the secretion of DHEA is decreased.[21] This implies that under stressful conditions, the reduced DHEA secretion may allow a shift away from Th1 toward Th2-type activity.[20]

Oxidative Stress and Th1–Th2 Balance

Glutathione (GSH) in its reduced form is the single most important regulatory antioxidant in cells. As it is oxidized, it becomes oxidized glutathione (GSSG), and the intracellular ratio of GSH:GSSG is a useful measure of the cell's overall antioxidant status.[22] Studies in mice by Peterson *et al.* have shown that depletion of GSH from APCs *in vivo* results in lower Th1 activity and higher Th2 activity, whereas GSH repletion had the opposite effect.[23] Along the same lines, Murata *et al.* showed that macrophages with most of their GSH in the reduced form are effectively type 1 cells capable of inducing Th1 differentiation, whereas macrophages with mostly GSSG are effectively type 2 cells and could induce Th2 responses.[24] It appears therefore that immune response can have Th1 or Th2 character depending on the relative antioxidant status of the APCs directing this process. The same group also demonstrated that high GSH inside the macrophage supports gene activity that leads to secretion of IL-12, the major Th1-polarizing cytokine. Furthermore, exposure of the macrophage to INF-γ tends to raise its GSH, thereby reinforcing its orientation toward type 1. Conversely, exposure of the macrophage to IL-4 lowers its GSH and steers it toward type 2 activity.[25]

It can be concluded that antioxidant status at the level of APCs and their microenvironment can markedly affect the ultimate pattern of immune response. Thus conditions associated with increased oxidative stress may deplete APCs of antioxidants and influence their phenotypic orientation toward Th2-type response.

TH1–TH2 BALANCE AND DIFFERENTIAL EXPRESSION OF THYROID AUTOIMMUNITY

Autoimmune thyroid disease (AITD), the most common organ-specific autoimmune condition, may be clinically expressed as chronic autoimmune thyroiditis or HT and its variants postpartum and sporadic thyroiditis, GD, and

Basedow and others.[32] These early reports were followed by epidemiological observations of an increase in the incidence of GD during every major war, a condition named "Krieqsbasedow."[34] Indeed, the incidence of GD in Denmark increased fourfold in 1942 compared with 1940. Hospital admissions for thyrotoxicosis in occupied Scandinavian countries increased five- to sixfold during the 1939–1945 war and returned to normal rates after the war.[34] A recent evidence for this association was the fivefold increase in GD as opposed to toxic nodular goiter (TNG), observed during the civil war in former Yugoslavia.[35] Earlier studies failed to show an increase in antithyroid drug use during the civil unrest in Northern Ireland [36] or an increase in stressful life events in consecutive thyrotoxic patients attending an outpatients' clinic.[37] However, these reports can be criticized for failing to distinguish between GD and other causes of thyrotoxicosis. Following these early clinical observations, a number of formal case–control studies and population-based surveys using self-rated questionnaires have examined the effect of stress on the onset or the clinical course of Graves' thyrotoxicosis.

Effect of Stress on the Onset of GD

The first large population-based case–control study that established an association between stressful life events and the onset of GD was from Sweden. Using a self-rated questionnaire, 208 patients with newly diagnosed GD were found to have more negative life events and higher negative life event scores in the year preceding the diagnosis than 372 matched controls.[38] The association of stressful life events with the onset of GD was subsequently confirmed by several other case–control studies in different ethnic populations.[39–41] One of these studies from Japan reported an association of stress with GD in women but not men.[42] These studies have been criticized because of their retrospective nature, the influence of recall bias, and the fact that thyrotoxicosis itself might manifest with anxiety and negative emotional events, raising the question of distinguishing between cause and effect.[43,44] This problem was partially addressed by a more recent study.[45] The authors have compared patients with GD, patients with TNG, and healthy controls, to correct for the effect of thyrotoxicosis. A significant increase in the number of negative life events was found in the GD patients compared to TNG or normal controls.[45] This finding supports the view that stress precipitates autoimmune as opposed to non-autoimmune hyperthyroidism.

Effect of Stress on the Clinical Course of GD

In contrast to studies on the onset of GD, few studies have examined the effect of stress on its clinical course. In a retrospective study, treatment with a benzodiazepine, in addition to antithyroid drug therapy, reduced the relapse rate from 74% in untreated patients to 29% in treated patients, suggesting that stress management was effective in improving the prognosis of GD.[46] Two prospective case–control studies also suggest that stress has a negative impact on the outcome of GD. A study from Japan investigated the association between the short-term outcome of patients with newly diagnosed GD, assessed 12 months after the start of antithyroid drug therapy, and stressful life events. The authors reported that "daily stresses" at 6 months after beginning therapy were associated with continued hyperthyroid state 12 months later.[47] This effect was seen only in women, however, as the number of males in the study was too small to reach a significant effect. In a more recent study it was shown that in GD daily stresses and some personality traits were related to the relapse rate after antithyroid drug treatment, and that stress scores correlated with the titer of anti-TSHr antibodies after the cessation of antithyroid drugs.[48]

Effect of Stress on GD: Case Reports

Apart from the epidemiological observations and case–control studies discussed above, there are also some clinical case reports that support a possible relationship between stress and the onset or outcome of GD. Thus, Misaki et al. reported three cases of Graves' hyperthyroidism occurring after partial thyroidectomy for papillary carcinoma.[49] The authors suggested that surgical stress might alter immune homeostasis converting preclinical GD into full-blown hyperthyroidism. A relationship between stress with the onset and clinical course of GD has also been reported in children. Mortillo and Gardner reported four children in whom a "separation" event was related to the onset or relapse of GD.[50] We have reported five patients who developed mild autoimmune hyperthyroidism following major stressful life events including bereavement, job loss, stress at work, and major surgery.[51] In each case the hyperthyroidism followed a short course (up to 6 months) on a small dose of antithyroid medication and went into remission as the stress situation resolved.

Stress and HT

In contrast to GD, few studies have examined the possible association between stress and HT. Two case–control studies evaluated the role of stressful events in HT or postpartum thyroiditis. They concluded that stress was not a trigger in either condition.[52,53] The onset and clinical course of HT are often insidious and the diagnosis may be delayed until the patients develop overt hypothyroidism, making it difficult to assess the role of stress in the onset and course of the disease. A recent population study also did not find a relationship between stressful life events and the presence of anti-TPO antibodies in euthyroid women.[54]

In summary, the weight of evidence from the epidemiological observations, and clinical case–control studies suggests an association between stress and GD but not with HT. However, the biologic mechanisms underlying the association of stress with GD remain uncertain.

ROLE OF STRESS IN THE CLINICAL EXPRESSION OF THYROID AUTOIMMUNITY: A UNIFYING HYPOTHESIS

Evidence from animal studies and certain clinical observations suggest that a hyperactive or hypoactive stress system may be associated with decreased or increased vulnerability to different types of autoimmune diseases.[55] Thus, Fisher rats that have a hyperactive stress system exhibit resistance to experimentally induced Th1-mediated autoimmune diseases, such as rheumatoid arthritis, uveitis, and experimental allergic encephalomyelitis. Conversely, Lewis rats, which have a hypoactive HPA axis, are prone to develop Th1-mediated autoimmune conditions.[55]

Another experiment of nature with changes in the Th1–Th2 balance is pregnancy and the postpartum period. Pregnancy results in suppression of Th1-mediated cellular immune activity and preservation or enhancement of Th2-mediated humoral immunity. In the third trimester of pregnancy, Th1-type cytokines such as IFN-γ and IL-2 decline and Th2 cytokines, particularly IL-4, increase.[56] This shift appears to permit the histoincompatible fetal–placental unit to avoid rejection by a cell-mediated immune attack by the mother.

The above immune changes develop in parallel with a marked increase in glucocorticoid levels together with increases in estrogen and progesterone. These hormones suppress cell-mediated and enhance humoral immune responses, as discussed earlier. The changes in the hormonal milieu may explain why pregnant women experience remission of Th1-mediated autoimmune diseases such as rheumatoid arthritis, multiple sclerosis, type 1 diabetes and autoimmune thyroiditis, and aggravation of Th2-mediated autoimmunity such as lupus glumerulonephritis.[55,56] Post partum, the hormonal milieu abruptly changes, with glucocorticoids, estrogens, and progesterone decreasing to subnormal levels, allowing a prompt recovery of cell-mediated immune function.[56,57] This Th2 to Th1 "return shift" in the puerperium might explain the outbreak of postpartum thyroiditis and other Th1-mediated autoimmune conditions. Analogous clinical situations associated with a decreased stress system activity are seen during the period that follows cure from Cushing's syndrome or discontinuation of glucocorticoid therapy.[1,55] These situations have been associated with increased susceptibility to Th1-mediated immune disorders. This might also include the period that follows cessation of chronic stress or a rebound reaction upon relief of various stressors.

On the other hand, GD is reported to be associated with allergic rhinitis, and Th2-predominant conditions are frequently associated with allergic diseases.[58]

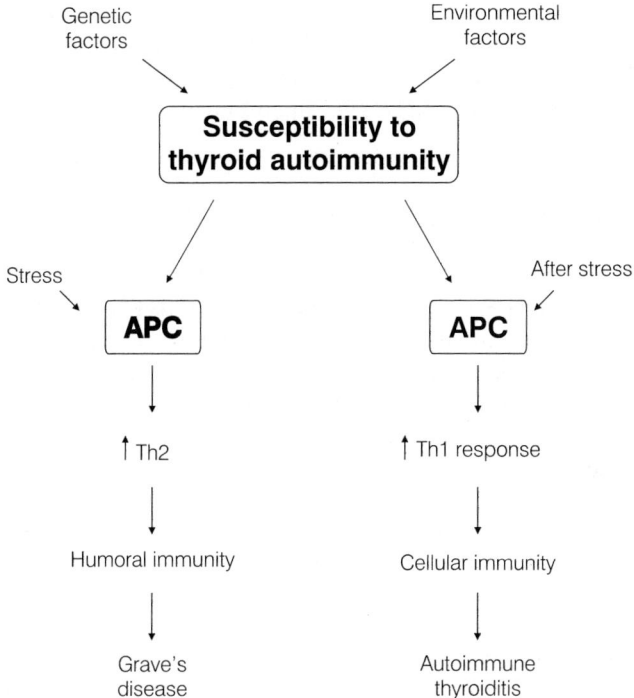

FIGURE 2. Role of stress in the clinical expression of AITD.

Further support for the importance of the Th2 pathway in GD comes from work showing that recurrence after antithyroid drug therapy is more likely after attacks of allergic rhinitis and elevated IgE levels, which is a marker of Th2 activity.[59] Moreover, humanized anti-CD52 monoclonal antibody therapy for multiple sclerosis, which causes the immune response to change from the Th1 to Th2 phenotype, was reported to trigger the development of GD.[60]

In light of the information currently available, the following hypothesis for the role of stress in the clinical expression of thyroid autoimmunity is proposed (FIG. 2). Genetic and environmental factors may induce an aberrant immune response against thyroid autoantigens and render an individual susceptible to develop thyroid autoimmunity. The potential for the APCs to activate differentiation of precursor Th cells toward Th1- or Th2-type cells is an important branch point toward the development of cell-mediated or humoral immunity, respectively. If such an individual is under stress, the stress hormones will influence the APC to steer the balance toward a Th2-type activity. Effector Th2 cells and type 2 cytokines will induce antigen-specific B lymphocytes to produce anti-TSHr antibodies. The parallel suppression of Th1-effector pathway will protect thyroid cells from immune attack. Under these circumstances, the clinical outcome is GD. Conversely, if a susceptible individual is recovering from a stress response or the immune suppressive effect of pregnancy, a rebound reaction may create the potential for APCs to activate the Th1-mediated pathway, leading to cellular immunity and destruction of thyroid follicular cells. The likely outcome then will be autoimmune (sporadic) or postpartum thyroiditis, respectively.

CONCLUSION

Circumstantial evidence suggests that the AITD HT, and GD manifest a different immune phenotype. HT is predominantly a Th1-mediated autoimmune disease, whereas GD has a predominant Th2 phenotype. There is strong evidence from epidemiologic and clinical studies supporting an association between stress and GD, but there are few reports on the relationship of stress with HT. However, whether stress has a causative effect on GD is not yet clear. It is likely that in susceptible individuals, stress hormones influence the clinical expression of thyroid autoimmunity toward the development of GD by suppressing cellular immunity and potentiating humoral immunity. Recovery from stress, through a rebound effect, may favor the development of autoimmune thyroiditis. This is, however, a working hypothesis based on circumstantial evidence and further clarification is required.

REFERENCES

1. CHROUSOS, G.P. 1998. Stressors, stress and neuroendocrine integration of the adaptive response. The 1997 Hans Selye memorial lecture. Ann. N. Y. Acad. Sci. **851:** 311–335.
2. ELENKOV, I.J. & G.P. CHROUSOS. 1999. Stress hormones, Th1/Th2 patterns, pro/anti-inflammatory cytokines and susceptibility to disease. Trends Endocrinol. Metab. **10:** 359–368.
3. ROOK, G.A.W. 1999. Glucocorticoids and immune function. Bail. Clin. Endocrinol. Metab. **13:** 567–581.
4. WEETMAN, A.P. 2004. Cellular immune responses in autoimmune thyroid disease. Clin. Endocrinol. (Oxf.) **61:** 405–413.
5. FOUNTOULAKIS, S. & A. TSATSOULIS. 2004. On the pathogenesis of autoimmune thyroid disease: a unifying hypothesis. Clin. Endocrinol. (Oxf.) **60:** 397–409.
6. MOSMANN, T.R. & S. SAD. 1996. The expanding universe of T-cell subsets: Th1, Th2 and more. Immunol. Today. **17:** 138–146.
7. ABBAS, A.K., W.K.M. MURPHY & A. SHER. 1996. Functional diversity of helper T-lymphocytes. Nature **383:** 787–795.
8. FEARON, D.T. & R.M. LOCKSLEY. 1996. The instructive role of innate immunity in the acquired immune response. Science **272:** 50–53.
9. TRINCHIERI, G. 1995. Interleukin-12: a proinflammatory cytokine with immunoregulatory functions that bridge innate resistance and antigen-specific adaptive immunity. Annu. Rev. Immunol. **13:** 251–276.

10. ELENKOV, I.J., D.A. PAPANIKOLAOU, R.L. WILDER & G.P. CHROUSOS. 1996. Modulatory effects of glucocorticoids and catecholamines on human interleukin-12 and interleukin-10 production: clinical implications. Proc. Assoc. Am. Physicians **108:** 374–381.
11. BLOTTA, M.H., R.H. DEKRUYFF & D.T. UMETSU. 1997. Corticosteroids inhibit IL-12 production in human monocytes and enhance their capacity to induce IL-4 synthesis in DC4$^+$ lymphocytes. J. Immunol. **158:** 5589–5595.
12. WU, C.Y., K. WANG, J.F. MC DYER & R.A. SEDER. 1998. Prostaglandin E$_2$ and dexamethasone inhibit IL-12 receptor expression and IL-12 responsiveness. J. Immunol. **161:** 2723–2730.
13. RAMIERZ, F., D.J. FOWELL, M. SIMMONDS & D. MASON. 1996. Glucocorticoids promote a Th2 cytokine response by CD$_4$$^+$ T-cells *in vitro*. J. Immunol. **150:** 2406–2412.
14. PANINA-BORDIGNON, P., D. MAZZEO, P.D. LUCIA, *et al.* 1997. Beta 2-agonists prevent Th1 development by selective inhibition of interleukin-12. J. Clin. Invest. **100:** 1513–1519.
15. HASKO, G., C. SZABO, Z.H. NEMETH, *et al.* 1998. Stimulation of beta-adrenoceptors inhibits endotoxin-induced IL-12 production in normal and IL-10 deficient mice. J. Neuroimmunol. **88:** 57–61.
16. SANDERS, V.M., R.A. BAKER, D.S. RAMER-QUINN, *et al.* 1997. Differential expression of the beta 2-adrenergic receptor by Th1 and Th2 clones: implications for cytokine production and B-cell help. J. Immunol. **158:** 4200–4210.
17. KARALIS, K., H. SANO, I. REDWINE, *et al.* 1991. Autocrine or paracrine inflammatory actions of corticotropin-releasing hormone *in vivo*. Science **254:** 421–423.
18. WEBSTER, E.L., D.J. TORPY, I.J. ELENKOV & G.P. CHROUSOS. 1998. Corticotropin-releasing hormone and inflammation. Ann. N. Y Acad. Sci. **840:** 21–23.
19. ELENKOV, I.J., WEBSTER, D.A. PAPANIKOLAOU, *et al.* 1998. Histamine potently suppresses human IL-12 and stimulates IL-10 production via H$_2$ receptors. J. Immunol. **161:** 2586–2593.
20. SCHWARTZ, K.E. 2002. Autoimmunity, dehydroepiandrosterone (DHEA), and stress. J. Adolesc. Health **305:** 37–43.
21. PARKER, L.N., E.R. LEVIN & E.T. LIFRAK. 1985. Evidence for adrenocortical adaptation to severe illness. J. Clin. Endocrinol. Metab. **60:** 947–952.
22. KIDD, P.M. 1997. Glutathione: systemic protectant against oxidative and free radical damage. Altern. Med Rev. **2:** 155–176.
23. PETERSON, J.D., L.A. HERZENBERG, K. VASQUEZ & C. WALTENBAUGH. 1998. Glutathione levels in antigen-presenting cells modulate Th1 versus Th2 response patterns. Proc. Nat. Acad. Sci. USA **95:** 3071–3076.
24. MURATA, Y., T. SHIMAMURA & J. HAMURO. 2002. The polarization of Th1/Th2 balance is dependent on the intracellular thiol redox status of macrophages due to distinctive cytokine production. Int. Immunol. **14:** 201–212.
25. MURATA, Y., T. SHIMAMURA, T. TAGAMI, *et al.* 2002. The skewing to Th1 induced by lentinan is directed through the distinctive cytokine production by macrophages with elevated intracellular glutathione content. Int. Immunopharmacol. **2:** 673–689.
26. PEARCE, E.N., A.P. FARWELL & L.E. BRAVERMAN. 2003. Current concepts: thyroiditis. N. Engl. J. Med. **348:** 2640–2655.
27. ROURA–MIR, C., M. CATALF M. SOSPEDRA, *et al.* 1997. Single-cell analysis of intrathyroidal lymphocytes shows differential cytokine expression in Hashimoto's and Graves' disease. Eur. J. Immunol. **27:** 3290–3302.

28. KOTANI, T., Y. ARATAKE, K. HIRAI, et al. 1995. Apoptosis in thyroid tissue from patients with Hashimoto's thyroiditis. Autoimmunity **20:** 231–236.
29. HEUER, M., G. AUST, S. ODE-HAIM & W.A. SCHERBAUM. 1996. Different cytokine mRNA profile in Graves' disease, Hashimoto's thyroiditis and in autoimmune thyroid disorders determined by quantitative reverse transcriptase polymerase chain reaction (RT-PCR). Thyroid **6:** 97–105.
30. ORGIAZZI, J. 2000. Anti-TSH receptor antibodies in clinical practice. Endocrinol. Metabol. Clin. N. Am. **29:** 339–355.
31. RUWHOF, C. & H.A. DREXHAGE. 2001. Iodine and thyroid autoimmune disease in animal models. Thyroid **11:** 427–436.
32. BRETZ, J.D. & J.R. BAKER, JR. 2001. Apoptosis and autoimmune thyroid disease: following a TRAIL to thyroid destruction? Clin. Endocrinol (Oxf.) **55:** 1–11.
33. ROSCH, P.J. 1993. Stressful life events and Graves' disease. Lancet **341:** 566–567.
34. GORMAN, C.A. 1990. A critical review of the role of stress in hyperthyroidism *In* The Thyroid Gland, Environment and Autoimmunity. H.A. Drexhage, J.T.M. de Vijlder & W.M. Wiersinga, Eds.: 191–200. Elsevier Science Publishers. Amsterdam.
35. PAUNKOVIC, N., J. PAUNKOVIC, O. PAVLOVIC & Z. PAUNKOVIC. 1998. The significant increase in incidence of Graves' disease in eastern Serbia during the civil war in the former Yugoslavia (1992 to 1995). Thyroid **8:** 37–41.
36. HADDEN, D.R. & D.G. NC DEVITT. 1974. Environmental stress and thyrotoxicosis: absence of association. Lancet **ii:** 577–578.
37. GRAY, J. & R. HOFFNBERG. 1985. Thyrotoxicosis and stress. Q. J. Med **54:** 153–160.
38. WINSA, B., H. ADAMI, R. BERGSTROM, et al. 1991. Stressful life events and Graves' disease. Lancet **338:** 1475–1479.
39. SOVINO, N., M.E. GIRELLI, M. BOSCATO, et al. 1993. Life events in the pathogenesis of Graves' disease. A controlled study. Acta Endocrinol. (Copenh.) **128:** 293–296.
40. KUNG, A.W.. 1995. Life events, daily stresses and coping in patients with Graves' disease. Clin. Endocrinol. (Oxf.) **42:** 303–308.
41. RADOSAVLJEVIC, V.R., S.M. JANKOVIC & J.M. MARINKOVIC. 1996. Stressful life events in the pathogenesis of Graves' disease. Eur. J. Endocrinol. **134:** 699–701.
42. YOSHIUCHI, K., H. KUMANO, S. NOMURA, et al. 1998. Stressful life events and smoking were associated with Graves' disease in women, but not in men. Psychosom. Med. **60:** 182–185.
43. CHIOVATO, L. & A. PINCHERA. 1996. Stressful life events and Graves' disease. Eur. J. Endocrinol. **134:** 680–682.
44. DAYAN, C.M.. 2001. Stressful life events and Graves' disease revisited. Clin. Endocrinol. (Oxf.) **55:** 13–14.
45. MATOS-SANTOS, A., E.L. NOBILE, J.G.E. COSTA, et al. 2001. Relationship between the number and impact of stressful life events and the onset of Graves' disease and toxic nodular goitre. Clin. Endocrinol. (Oxf.) **55:** 15–19.
46. BENVENGA, S.. 1996. Benzodiazepines and remission of Graves' disease. Thyroid **6:** 659–660.
47. YOSHIUCHI, K., H. KUMANO, S. NOMURA, et al. 1998. Psychosocial factors influencing the short-term outcome of antithyroid drug therapy in Graves' disease. Psychosom. Med. **60:** 592–596.
48. FUKAO, A., J. TAKAMATSU, J.Y. MURAKAMI, et al. 2001. The relationship of psychological factors to the prognosis of hyperthyroidism in antithyroid drug-treated patients with Graves' disease. Clin. Endocrinol. (Oxf.) **58:** 550–555.

49. MISAKI, I., M. IWATA, K. KASAGI, *et al*. 2000. Hyperthyroid Graves' disease after hemithyroidectomy for papillary carcinoma: report of three cases. Endocr. J. **47:** 191–195.
50. MORILLO, E. & L.I. GARDNER. 1979. Bereavement as an antecedent factor in thyrotoxicosis of childhood: four case studies with survey of possible metabolic pathways. Psychosom. Med. **41:** 545–555.
51. TSATSOULIS, A. & K. PANTELI. 1996. Stress-induced mild thyrotoxicosis. Eur. J. Int. Med. **7:** 247–250.
52. MARTINDUPAN, R.C. 1998. Triggering role of stress and pregnancy in the occurrence of 98 cases of Graves' disease compared to 95 cases of Hashimoto's thyroiditis and 97 cases of thyroid nodules. Ann. Endocrinol. (Paris) **59:** 107–112.
53. ORETTI, R.C., B. HARRIS, J.H. LAZARUS, *et al*. 2003. Is there an association between life events, postnatal depression and thyroid dysfunction in thyroid antibody positive women? Int. J. Soc. Psychiatry **49:** 70–76.
54. STREDER, I.G.A., M.F. PRUMMEL, J.G.P. TIJSSEEN, *et al*. 2005. Stress is not associated with thyroid peroxidase autoantibodies in euthyroid women. Brain Behav. Immunity. **19:** 203–206.
55. WILDER, R.L. 1995. Neuroendocrine–immune system interactions and autoimmunity. Ann. Rev. Immunol. **83:** 307–338.
56. ELENKOV, I.J., J. HOFFMAN & R.L. WILDER. 1997. Does differential neuroendocrine control of cytokine production govern the expression of autoimmune diseases in pregnancy and the postpartum period? Mol. Med. Today **3:** 379–383.
57. MULLER, A.F., H.A. DREXHAGE & A. BERGHOUT. 2001. Postpartum thyroiditis and autoimmune thyroiditis in women of childbearing age: recent insights and consequences for antenatal and postnatal care. Endocr. Reviews **22:** 605–630.
58. AMINO, N., Y. HIDAKA, T. TAKANO, *et al*. 2003. Association of seasonal allergic rhinitis is high in Graves' disease and low in painless thyroiditis. Thyroid **13:** 811–814.
59. SATO, A., Y. TAKEMURA, T. TAMADA, *et al*. 1999. A possible role of immunoglobulin E in patients with hyperthyroid Graves' disease. J. Clin. Endocrinol. Metabol. **84:** 3602–3605.
60. COLES, A.J., M. WING, S. SMITH, *et al*. 1999. Pulsed monoclonal antibody treatment and autoimmune thyroid disease in multiple sclerosis. Lancet **354:** 1691–1965.

Annexin 1, Glucocorticoids, and the Neuroendocrine–Immune Interface

JULIA C. BUCKINGHAM,[a] CHRISTOPHER D. JOHN,[a] EGLE SOLITO,[a]
TANYA TIERNEY,[a] RODERICK J. FLOWER,[b] HELEN CHRISTIAN,[c]
AND JOHN MORRIS[c]

[a]Division of Neuroscience and Mental Health, Imperial College London,
Hammersmith Campus, Du Cane Road, London W12 0NN, UK

[b]Department of Biochemical Pharmacology, The William Harvey Research
Institute, London EC1M 6BQ, UK

[c]Department of Human Anatomy and Genetics, The University of Oxford,
South Parks Road, Oxford OX1 3QX, UK

ABSTRACT: Annexin 1 (ANXA1) was originally identified as a mediator
of the anti-inflammatory actions of glucocorticoids (GCs) in the host defense system. Subsequent work confirmed and extended these findings
and also showed that the protein fulfills a wider brief and serves as a
signaling intermediate in a number of systems. ANXA1 thus contributes
to the regulation of processes as diverse as cell migration, cell growth
and differentiation, apoptosis, vesicle fusion, lipid metabolism, and cytokine expression. Here we consider the role of ANXA1 in the neuroendocrine system, particularly the hypothalamo-pituitary-adrenocortical
(HPA) axis. Evidence is presented that ANXA1 plays a critical role in
effecting the negative feedback effects of GCs on the release of corticotrophin (ACTH) and its hypothalamic-releasing hormones and that it
is particularly pertinent to the early-onset actions of the steroids that are
mediated via a nongenomic mechanism. The paracrine/juxtacrine mode
of ANXA1 action is discussed in detail, with particular reference to the
significance of the secondary processing of ANXA1, the processes that
control the intracellular and transmembrane trafficking of the protein
of the molecule and the mechanism of ANXA1 action on its target cells.
In addition, the role of ANXA1 in the perinatal programming of the HPA
axis is discussed.

KEYWORDS: annexin 1; HPA axis; glucocorticoids; cytokines

Address for correspondence: Julia C. Buckingham, Division of Neuroscience and Mental Health,
Imperial College London, Hammersmith Campus, Du Cane Road, London W12 0NN. Voice: 44-208-
383-8034; fax: 44-208-383-8032.
e-mail: j.buckingham@imperial.ac.uk

Ann. N.Y. Acad. Sci. 1088: 396–409 (2006). © 2006 New York Academy of Sciences.
doi: 10.1196/annals.1366.002

INTRODUCTION

Annexin 1 (ANXA1, formerly known as lipocortin 1) is a 37-kDa member of the annexin superfamily of Ca^{2+} and phospholipid binding proteins. Members of this family show a high degree of structural homology, with each including four (or 8 in the case of ANXA6) repeated units of some 70 amino acids within the core and C-terminal regions; these units confer the Ca^{2+} and phospholipid binding properties of the proteins. The N-terminal region of each family member is, however, unique and is considered to confer the biological specificity of the individual proteins. The basic structure of ANXA1 is shown in FIGURE 1. Crystallography studies indicate that the four repeated sequences are arranged around a pore, giving the protein a "doughnut" appearance. The N-terminal domain is embedded within the pore at low Ca^{2+} concentrations, but elevations in $[Ca^{2+}]$ expose this region and may thereby influence the biological activity of the protein.[1] The gene encoding ANXA1 is well characterized in rodents (rat and mouse) and man[2–4] (FIG. 1). Although the gene is multiexonic in structure, no spliced variants have been described to date. Sequence analysis has, however, revealed multiple potential sites for secondary processing, including tyrosine, serine, and threonine phosphorylation, acetylation, and lipidation. The protein may thus exist in multiple forms.

ANXA1 was first identified as a glucocorticoid (GC)-inducible protein in rat peritoneal macrophages and was heralded as a potential mediator of the powerful anti-inflammatory actions of these steroid hormones. Subsequent studies have confirmed that ANXA1 does indeed contribute to the anti-inflammatory actions of GCs. These studies have also revealed that the protein fulfills wider brief as in intra- and intercellular signaling molecule and that it is concerned with processes as diverse as cell growth and differentiation, apoptosis, vesicle

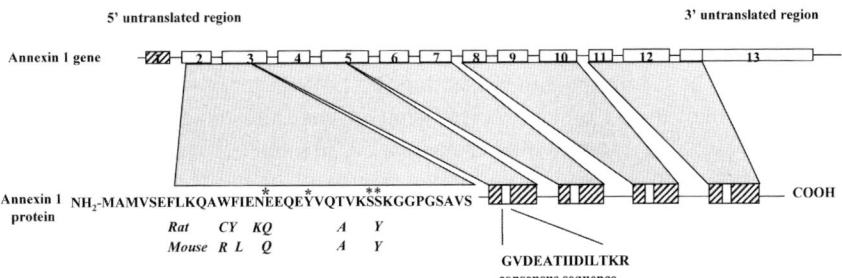

FIGURE 1. Schematic diagram to show the structure of the human annexin 1 gene and protein. Note that the N-terminal includes potential sites for phosphorylation (*) and that each of the four repeats in the core domain includes a 17–amino acid consensus sequence, which is critical to Ca^{2+} binding. Differences in the N-terminal amino acid sequence of the rat and mouse proteins are indicated in *italics*. (Reprinted by permission from *Endocrinology*[8]).

fusion, endocytosis, exocytosis, and neuroprotection. Work in our laboratory has focused on the role of ANXA1 in the neuroendocrine system, particularly in relation to the negative feedback actions of GCs within the hypothalamo-pituitary-adrenocortical (HPA) axis.

EXPRESSION AND FUNCTION OF ANXA1 IN THE HPA AXIS

Localization

ANXA1 is expressed in abundance in the anterior pituitary gland, where it is localized specifically to the S100-positive folliculostellate cells.[5,6] It is also found in lesser amounts in the hypothalamus, hippocampus, and other parts of the brain.[7] Within the hypothalamus, ANXA1 is concentrated in the median eminence and the supraoptic and paraventricular nuclei.[5] It is particularly prevalent in the ependymal cells lining the third ventricle and in activated glial cells but is not detectable in hypothalamic neurons.

Functional Studies

GCs act within the brain and pituitary gland to maintain the blood levels of GCs within appropriate limits by modulating the secretion of corticotrophin (ACTH) and its hypothalamic-releasing hormones, corticotrophin-releasing hormone (CRH) and arginine vasopressin (AVP). The actions of the steroids are complex and, in addition to acting at several different sites (e.g., pituitary gland, hypothalamus, hippocampus, ventral tegmental area), they also act via several different molecular mechanisms. GCs thus exert effects that are slow in onset (>2 h) and are characterized by suppression of the genes encoding ACTH, CRH, and AVP. In addition, they exert more immediate effects (onset 15–60 min) that inhibit the release of preformed hormone into the blood stream.

The early-onset actions of GCs within the HPA axis can be readily demonstrated in the rat and other species using *in vivo* and *in vitro* experimental systems. Thus, for example, the release of ACTH and corticosterone induced by stressors, such as restraint, endotoxin treatment, or surgical intervention, is readily suppressed by administration of GCs 15 min–1 h before the onset of stress. Similarly, *in vitro*, the stimulus-evoked release of ACTH and CRH/AVP from pituitary and hypothalamic tissue is inhibited by inclusion of GCs in the medium 15 min–1 h prior to addition of a secretagogue. Using these experimental models, we have identified an important role for ANXA1 in mediating the "early-onset" actions of GC in both the pituitary gland and the hypothalamus. We have thus shown that the inhibitory effects of GCs on the stress-induced release of ACTH and corticosterone *in vivo* are mimicked by intracerebroventricular (i.c.v.) injection of human recombinant ANXA1 (hrANXA1) or peptides

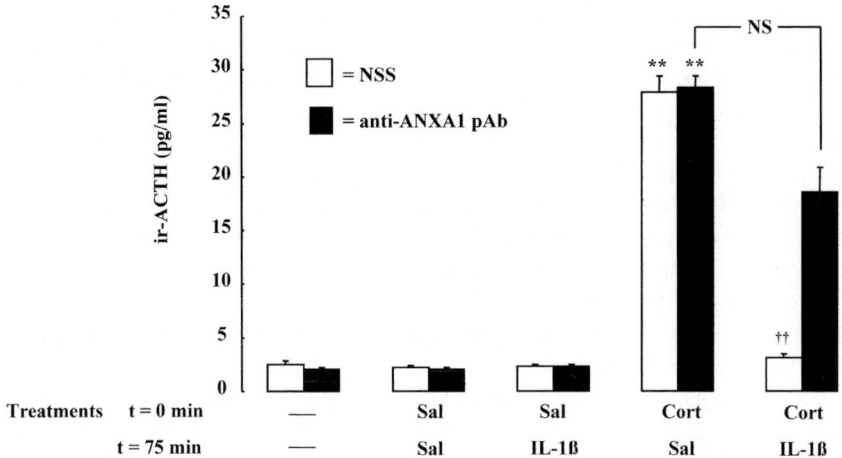

FIGURE 2. Reversal of the inhibitory effects of corticosterone on the IL-1β-stimulated release of ACTH in adult male rats by administration of an antiannexin 1 polyclonal antiserum raised in sheep against $ANXA1_{Ac2-26}$. Corticosterone 500 μg/kg, i.p in a volume of 1 mL/kg; IL-1β 10 ng/rat in a volume of 3μL, i.c.v. Controls received equivalent volumes of the sterile saline (Sal) vehicle. Antiannexin 1 antiserum (anti-ANXA1 pAb) 1mL/kg, s.c. or nonimmune sheep serum (NSS, control) 1mL/kg, s.c. was administered 15 min before the steroid. Values represent mean ± SEM ($n = 6$–7). **$P < 0.01$ versus Sal–Sal treated control; †† $P < 0.01$ versus Sal–IL-1-β treated group; NS = not significant ($P > 0.05$). (ANOVA plus Scheffé's test).

derived from its N terminus and antagonized specifically by central (i.c.v.) or peripheral subcutaneous (s.c.) administration of neutralizing anti-ANXA1 antisera (FIG. 2). Similarly *in vitro*, hrANXA1 mimics the inhibitory effects of GCs on the release of CRH and ACTH from rodent (rat or mouse) hypothalamic and pituitary tissue, respectively. Furthermore, the effects of the steroids are specifically reversed by neutralizing anti-ANXA1 antisera or antisense oligodeoxynucleotides (ODNs) directed specifically against ANXA1 mRNA.[8–10] Interestingly, *in vivo,* ANXA1 appears to play a particularly important role in modulating the HPA responses to inflammatory stimuli.[10,11] Similarly, at the hypothalamic level, ANXA1 is particularly effective in suppressing the CRH responses to proinflammatory cytokines *in vitro*.[11]

MECHANISM OF ANNEXIN 1 ACTION WITHIN THE HPA AXIS

The Paracrine/Juxtacrine Hypothesis

Studies involving cell fractionation techniques and electron microscopic immunohistochemistry have shown that ANXA1 is distributed between three cellular compartments, namely, the cytoplasm, within the membranes of cell organelles, and in association with the plasma membrane, where a proportion of the protein is localized to the outer cell surface.[6,7] Early work in our laboratory revealed that GCs regulate both the synthesis and the cellular disposition of ANXA1 in the anterior pituitary gland and the hypothalamus.[9,11] GCs thus induce *de novo* ANXA1 synthesis in these tissues and cause the translocation of the protein from the cytoplasm to the outer cell membrane, where it is retained by a Ca^{2+}-dependent mechanism. The transfer of cytoplasmic ANXA1 to the cell surface is apparent within 15 min of GC contact both *in vivo* and *in vitro*. By contrast, the induction of ANXA1 synthesis is slow in onset (>2 h) and appears to serve primarily as a mechanism for replenishing the diminished cytoplasmic pool of the protein.[7]

The findings that ANXA1 is not expressed by CRH/AVP neurons or corticotrophs, but is present in the nonendocrine cells adjacent to them, together with evidence that the protein is promptly translocated to the cell surface by GCs, led us to propose that ANXA1 acts via paracrine/juxtacrine mechanism to mediate the inhibitory effects of the steroids on CRH/AVP and ACTH release. Several lines of evidence support this hypothesis. Firstly, specific, high-affinity (Kd $= 14 \pm 3$ nM), proteinaceous ANXA1 binding sites are expressed on the cell surface of the corticotrophs and other endocrine cells in the anterior pituitary gland.[12] Secondly, enzymatic destruction of these sites ablates ANXA1 binding and the antisecretory effects of both GCs and ANXA1 on ACTH secretion in primary cultures of rat pituitary tissue, suggesting that these sites play an important role in mediating ANXA1 actions.[12] Thirdly, immunogold labeling has revealed that ANXA1 release occurs at focal points on the FS cell membranes, particularly at loci where the stellar projections of the cells make close contact with the endocrine cells[13] (FIG. 3). Finally, drugs that prevent the GC-induced translocation of ANXA1 to the cell membrane (e.g., PKC inhibitors, ATP-sensitive K^+ channel openers) overcome the acute inhibitory effects of GCs on ACTH secretion in *in vitro* models.[14,15]

Confirmation that ANXA1 serves as cell–cell mediator of GC action in the pituitary gland was provided by studies on a co-culture system comprising two cell lines, viz., murine corticotroph (AtT20, clone D1) and murine FS (TtTGF). TtT/GF cells express ANXA1 in abundance and readily translocate the protein to the cell surface in response to a GC challenge.[16] By contrast, while specific ANXA1 binding sites are readily detected on the cell surface of the AtT20 D1 cells by FACS analysis, the cell line does not express ANXA1 mRNA or protein as detected by RT-PCR and Western blot analysis. These two cell lines thus mirror the pattern of expression of ANXA1 and ANXA1 binding observed *in vivo* and, thus, provide a useful model for exploration of ANXA1 biology. When cultured alone, the AtT20 D1 cells are unresponsive to GCs but respond readily to ANXA1 and peptides derived from it. The CRH-induced release of ACTH from the cells is thus unaffected by the inclusion of

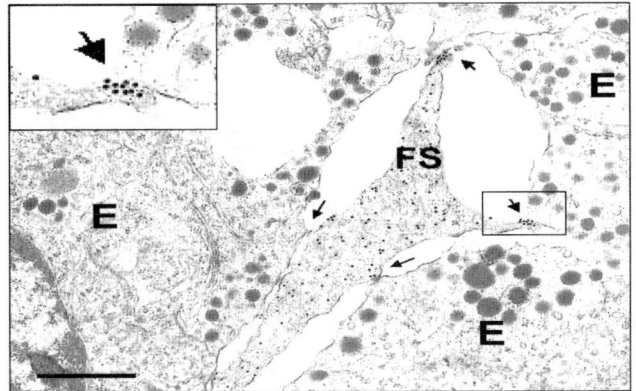

FIGURE 3. Electron micrograph showing immunogold detection of annexin 1 in a folliculostellate cell adjacent to three endocrine (E) cells in freeze-substituted mouse anterior pituitary tissue. Gold particles (15 nm) are scattered over the cytoplasm and adjacent to the plasma membrane of the cell; they are also localized on the FS cell surface at the ends of the processes contacting endocrine cells (see enlarged *inset*). *Arrows* indicate intercellular junctions. *Scale bar:* 1 μm. (Reprinted by permission from *Endocrinology*[13]).

dexamethasone in the incubation medium, but is readily blocked by ANXA1 and ANXA1$_{Ac2-26}$. However, when co-cultured with TtT/GF cells, the AtT20 D1 cells respond to dexamethasone with a marked reduction in CRH-induced ACTH release; furthermore, the magnitude of the response to dexamethasone is proportional to the ratio of TtT/GF to AtT20 D1 cells in culture (FIG. 4). The importance of ANXA1 in mediating this action of dexamethasone was confirmed by antisense studies that showed clearly that the effects of the steroid were ablated by antisense ODNs directed against ANXA1 mRNA but not by corresponding sense- or antisense sequences.[16]

Translocation of ANXA1 to the Cell Surface

The amino acid sequence of ANXA1 does not include a signal sequence. Consequently, the protein is not packaged into vesicles by the Golgi system for release by exocytosis, and its translocation to the cell membrane is unaffected by drugs that interfere with various steps within the exocytotic pathway (e.g., nocodazole, brefeldin A).[7] Early studies indicated that the association of ANXA1 with membranes is strongly influenced by the phosphorylation status of the molecule.[17] Accordingly, we examined the potential role of phosphorylation in the GC-induced translocation of ANXA1 to cell membrane. Our initial studies indicated that cell surface ANXA1 is phosphorylated on both serine and tyrosine residues.[14,18] However, while blockade of PKC-dependent serine phosphorylation prevents the GC-induced translocation of ANXA1 to the

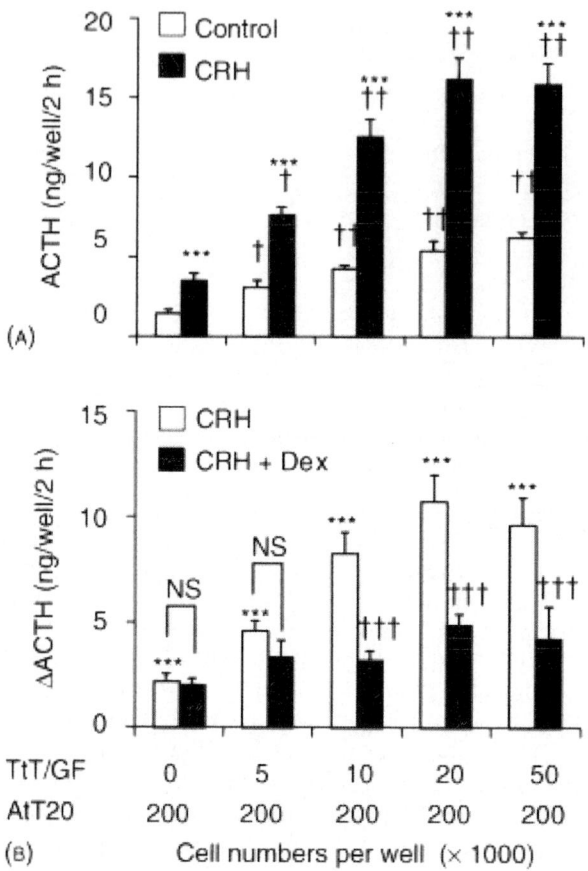

FIGURE 4. Effects of corticotrophin-releasing hormone (CRH 1 μm) and dexamethasone (Dex 100 nm) on the secretion of adrenocorticotrophic hormone (ACTH) by AtT20 D1 cells (200,000 per well) cultured alone and in the presence of increasing numbers of TtT/GF cells (5,000–50,000 cells per well). (**A**) basal and CRH-stimulated release of ACTH. ***P < 0.001 basal versus CRH. †P < 0.05, ††P < 0.01 co-cultures versus AtT20 D1 cells alone. (**B**) The effects of Dex on CRH-stimulated ACTH release; Dex had no effect on basal ACTH release (data not shown). ***P < 0.001 Basal versus CRH. †††P < 0.001 CRH + Dex versus corresponding group treated with CRH alone. Data shown are mean ± SEM of six wells per group. Statistical analysis was carried out by ANOVA and Tukey's *post hoc* test. The data shown are representative of three separate experiments. (Reprinted by permission from the *Journal of Neuroendocrinology*[16]).

cell surface of primary FS cells,[14] inhibition of tyrosine phosphorylation does not.[18] Together these data suggest that serine but not tyrosine phosphorylation is critical to the GC-induced transfer of ANXA1 across the cell membrane. Further evidence to support a role for serine phosphorylation emerged from studies on a human FS cell line (PDFS). Work on this line also demonstrated that the actions of GCs are mediated via the glucocorticoid receptor but that downstream signaling is effected by a nongenomic mechanism that uses PI3 kinase and MAP kinase as well as PKC.[19] The ANXA1 sequence includes multiple serine phosphorylation sites; and we are therefore exploiting site-directed mutagenesis and green fluorescent protein (GFP) tagging to determine the relative importance of each. Our initial data suggest that serine-27 is important in this regard, but other sites, particularly serine-5, may also have a significant role. In addition, they have identified a potential role for protein lipidation in the signaling cascade.[20]

The mechanism by which phosphorylated ANXA1 traverses the membrane is poorly understood. Double-labeling immunohistochemistry has shown that ANXA1 co-localizes with an ATP binding cassette (ABC) transporter protein (ABCA1) at focal points in the membrane of primary and transformed (TtT/GF) FS cells, thus raising the possibility that this protein may be important in this regard.[21] This hypothesis was supported by the evidence that glyburide, which blocks ABCA1, inhibits not only the GC-induced exportation of ANXA1 in FS cells and primary pituitary tissue, but also the ANXA1-dependent inhibitory effects of dexamethasone on ACTH release from pituitary tissue.[21] However, doubts regarding the role of ABCA1 have emerged, as Tangiers lymphocytes, which lack the ability to traffic ABCA1 to the cell membrane, readily export ANXA1 in response to a steroid challenge. This unexpected finding could be explained by the development of a compensatory mechanism. However, glyburide is not specific to ABCA1, but also opens ATP-sensitive K^+ channels (K^+_{ATP} channels). These channels are expressed by FS cells. Moreover, the K^+_{ATP} channel blockers, chromokalim and minoxidil, induce the translocation of ANXA1 to the cell surface of TtT/GF cells in a concentration-dependent manner; furthermore, their effects are blocked by glyburide and other K^+_{ATP} channel openers. Thus, while the role of ABCA1 is uncertain, it seems likely that K^+_{ATP} channels contribute to the signaling mechanism involved in the membrane translocation of ANXA1.

Actions of ANXA1 on Endocrine Cells

As discussed above, there is good evidence that ANXA1 acts via specific membrane-bound receptors on the corticotrophs and other pituitary endocrine cells to suppress pituitary hormone release.[12] The nature of these receptors is ill-defined, but data from other systems have raised the possibility that formyl peptide receptors (FPRs) may be important in this regard.[22] In humans, three members of this G-protein-coupled family of receptors have been characterized, namely, FPR, FPR-L1, and FPR-L2. Furthermore, ANXA1 and certain peptides derived from it have been shown to bind to both FPR and FPR-L1. However, in rodents the family is more extensive with eight or possibly nine family members. The majority are poorly characterized, but Fpr1 and

Fpr-rs1/Fpr-rs2 are mooted to be the murine equivalents of the human FPR and FPR-L1. We have recently shown that Fpr1 is not expressed in the mouse or rat pituitary gland and that Fpr1 gene deletion does not affect the capacity of ANXA1 or dexamethasone to suppress ACTH release from murine pituitary tissue. Other members of the FPR family are, however, found in the murine anterior pituitary gland. Furthermore, the inhibitory effects of dexamethasone and ANXA1 on ACTH release are mimicked by lipoxin A4, a lipid mediator purported to be an endogenous ligand of FPR-L1, and by high concentrations of the bacterial peptide, formyl-methione-leucine-proline (fMLF), which shows low affinity for FPR-L1. These findings, together with evidence that the effects of GCs, ANXA1, fMLF, and lipoxin A4 on ACTH release are blocked by N-Boc-MLP, an analogue of fMLP, which shows antagonist activity at both FPR and FPR-L1, supports the premise that a member of the FPR family contributes to the regulatory actions of ANXA1 on ACTH release. The signaling mechanism downstream of the receptor is largely unexplored. However, other data suggest that ANXA1 disrupts signaling at a point distal to the formation of cyclic AMP and the entry of Ca^{2+} and that, while the protein readily suppresses adenylyl cyclase-dependent secretagogue signaling, it does not affect phospholipase C-driven exocytosis.[8–10,14,23]

The sequences within the ANXA1 molecule that are required for the inhibition of peptide release have been explored using peptide analogues.[14] Removal of the third and fourth repeat units of the core ($ANXA1_{1-188}$) has no effect on either the potency or the efficacy of the protein in the pituitary gland. However, additional loss of the second repeat and much of the first repeat ($ANXA1_{1-50}$) results in a significant loss of potency but not efficacy. $ANXA1_{Ac2-26}$ shows a marked reduction in both potency and efficacy, and shorter N-terminal sequences (e.g., $ANXA1_{Ac2-12}$, $ANXA1_{Ac13-26}$) are without effect.[18] These data support the premise that the N-terminal plays an essential role in the manifestation of ANXA1 action, as also does our finding that neutralizing antisera directed specifically against the N-terminal domain attenuate the inhibitory effects of GCs on ACTH release *in vivo* (FIG. 2). However, they also reveal marked differences in the activity profile and potency ratios of the peptides studied in this and other systems (e.g., models of inflammation; see FIG. 5), where, for example, $ANXA1_{1-188}$ is less potent than the parent molecule ($ANXA1_{1-346}$) and $ANXA1_{Ac2-26}$ displays full efficacy.[24] Taken together, these data raise the possibility that two or more receptor subtypes mediate the actions of ANXA1 in the body, a view that is consistent with a role for two or more members of the FPR family.

EARLY LIFE PROGRAMMING OF THE ANXA1 SYSTEM

The ontogeny of ANXA1 expression in the developing fetus/neonate has not been studied in detail. However, striking tissue-specific changes in ANXA1

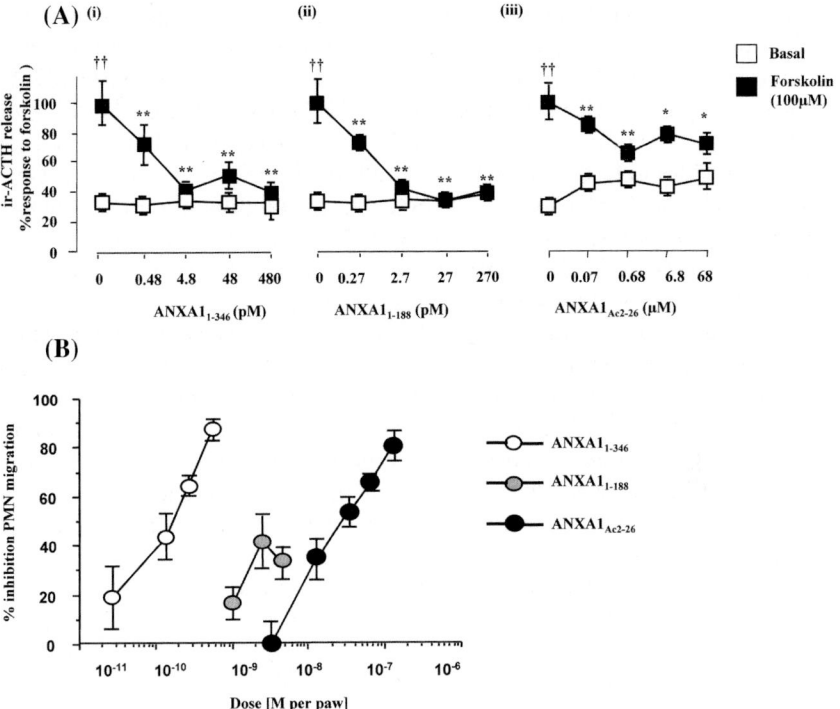

FIGURE 5. Comparison of the biological activity of full-length human recombinant annexin 1 (hrANXA1$_{1-346}$), a truncated protein (ANXA1$_{1-188}$), and an N-terminal peptide (ANXA1$_{Ac2-26}$) on (*a*) pituitary function and (*b*) in a model of inflammation. (**A**) demonstrates the inhibitory effects of graded concentrations of (i) ANXA1$_{1-346}$, (ii) ANXA1$_{1-188}$, and (iii) ANXA1$_{Ac2-26}$ on the release of ir-ACTH from rat anterior pituitary segments in *in vitro* data. Mean ± SEM (*n* = 6) are expressed as percentage of the secretory response to forskolin alone (100 μM). *$P < 0.05$, **$P < 0.01$ versus forskolin alone group (ANOVA and Duncan's multiple range test). (**B**) demonstrates the effects of the peptides *in vivo* on the IL-1β-induced migration of neutrophils into a mouse air pouch migration (elicited by *in vivo* injection of IL-1-β into a small air pouch in the mouse). ANXA1 protein/peptides were co-injected with IL-1-β; the data are expressed as the mean ± SEM, *n*-4–10. Note (*a*) that in the pituitary gland, ANXA1$_{1-364}$ and ANXA1$_{1-188}$ are roughly equipotent, whereas in the air pouch model ANXA1$_{1-346}$ is approximately two orders of magnitude more potent than ANXA1$_{1-188}$, (*b*) that ANXA1$_{Ac2-26}$ shows the full efficacy of the parent protein in the air pouch model but not in the pituitary gland, where at best it produces a 60% inhibition of peptide release and (*c*) that while ANXA1$_{Ac2-26}$ is less potent than the parent protein in both models, the potency difference is considerably greater in the pituitary gland. (Reprinted by permission from *Trends in Endocrinology and Metabolism*[24]).

expression occur in the neonate at the time of the stress hyporesponsive period (SHRP). In particular, ANXA1 expression in the anterior pituitary gland and hippocampus is raised (vs. adult) while thymic ANXA1 is reduced.[25] Complementary functional experiments suggest that the upregulation of ANXA1 in the neuroendocrine system may be an important factor in the maintenance of the quiescent state of the HPA axis during this period. ANXA1 may thus serve to protect the developing organism from the potentially harmful effects of overexposure to GCs at this time.[25] The regulatory effects of ANXA1 on AVP from the hypothalamus appear to be particularly important in this regard as, in addition to facilitating the inhibitory actions of GCs in the release of CRH/AVP and ACTH from the hypothalamus and pituitary gland, respectively, ANXA1 exerts a tonic inhibitory effect on AVP release at this stage and thereby quenches that stimulatory effects of interleukin IL-1α, IL-1β, and IL-6 on the release of the peptide.[25]

Interestingly, administration of very low doses of dexamethasone to dams via the drinking water in late gestation (E16–19) or post partum (day 1–7) causes tissue-specific changes in ANXA1 expression in the brain and pituitary gland of the offspring that persist into adulthood.[26] Furthermore, ANXA1-dependent GC feedback is blunted in animals exposed to exogenous GCs in the perinatal period, apparently because the GC-induced translocation of ANXA1 to cell surface is compromised.[26] These and other (unpublished) data raise the possibility that ANXA1 contributes to the disturbances in HPA function and associated pathologies that are evident in adults rats treated with GCs at critical stages of development.

CONCLUSIONS

Since its discovery in 1979, ANXA1 has been shown to play a diverse role as a signaling molecule in a number of physiological and pathophysiological systems, including the neuroendocrine system as discussed in this article. Our data suggest that ANXA1 acts via a paracrine/juxtacrine mechanism to suppress the release of ACTH and its hypothalamic-releasing hormones (FIG. 6). New technologies now pave the way for important new insights to the mechanisms which regulate the secondary processing and trafficking of ANXA1, to the physiological significance of these processes, and to the molecular mechanisms of ANXA1 action. The knowledge that emerges from these studies should provide new insight into the role of this protein in health and disease and may ultimately lead to the therapeutic exploitation of ANXA1-mimietics.

ACKNOWLEDGMENTS

Our work on ANXA1 has been generously supported by the Wellcome Trust, BBSRC, MRC, GSK, and the Society for Endocrinology.

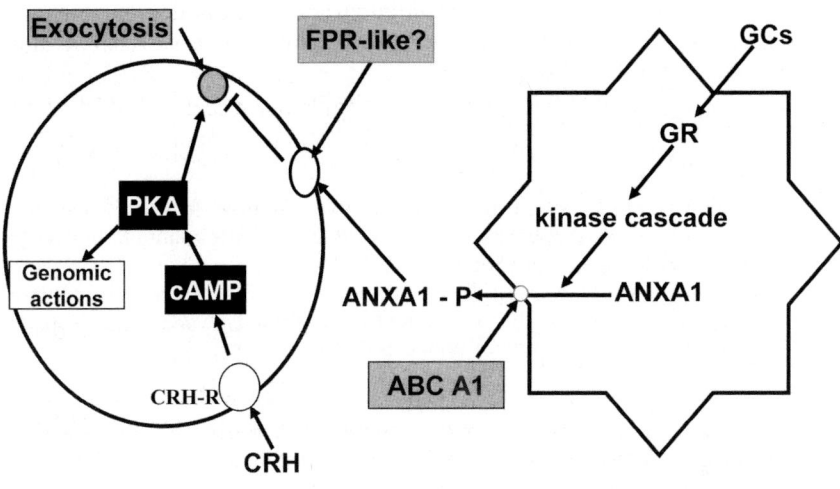

FIGURE 6. Schematic diagram illustrating the proposed mechanism by which ANXA1 produced and stored in folliculostellate cells acts as paracrine/juxtacrine mediator of the early inhibitory effects of GCs on the release of ACTH from the corticotrophs. CRH = corticotrophin-releasing hormone; CRH-R = corticotrophin-releasing hormone receptor; PKA = protein kinase A; GC = glucocorticoid; GR = glucocorticoid receptor; ANXA1 = annexin 1; ANXA1–P = serine-phosphorylated ANXA1; ABC A1–ATP binding cassette protein A1, the putative ANXA1 transporter; FPR-like = formyl peptide receptor like, the putative ANXA1 receptor. (Reprinted by permission from *Trends in Endocrinology and Metabolism*[24]).

REFERENCES

1. ROSENGARTH, A. & H. LUECKE. 2003. A calcium-driven conformational switch of the N-terminal and core domains of annexin A1. J. Mol. Biol. **326:** 1317–1325.
2. HORLICK, K.R. *et al.* 1991. Mouse lipocortin I gene structure and chromosomal assignment: gene duplication and the origins of a gene family. Genomics **10:** 365–374.
3. KOVACIC, R.T. *et al.* 1991. Correlation of gene and protein structure of rat and human lipocortin I. Biochemistry **30:** 9015–9021.
4. WALLNER, B.P. *et al.* 1986. Cloning and expression of human lipocortin, a phospholipase A2 inhibitor with potential anti-inflammatory activity. Nature **320:** 77–81.
5. SMITH, T., R.J. FLOWER & J.C. BUCKINGHAM. 1993. Lipocortins 1, 2 and 5 in the central nervous system and pituitary gland of the rat: selective induction by dexamethasone of lipocortin 1 in the anterior pituitary gland. Mol. Neuropharmacol. **3:** 45–55.
6. TRAVERSO, V. *et al.* 1999. Lipocortin 1 (annexin 1): a candidate paracrine agent localized in pituitary folliculo-stellate cells. Endocrinology **140:** 4330–4338.

7. PHILIP, J.G., R.J. FLOWER & J.C. BUCKINGHAM. 1997. Glucocorticoids modulate the cellular disposition of lipocortin 1 in the rat brain *in vivo* and *in vitro*. Neuroreport **8:** 1871–1876.

8. TAYLOR, A.D. *et al.* 1997. An antisense oligodeoxynucleotide to lipocortin 1 reverses the inhibitory actions of dexamethasone on the release of adreno-corticotropin from rat pituitary tissue *in vitro*. Endocrinology **138:** 2909–2918.

9. TAYLOR, A.D. *et al.* 1993. Lipocortin 1 mediates an early inhibitory action of glucocorticoids on the secretion of ACTH by the rat anterior pituitary gland *in vitro*. Neuroendocrinology **58:** 430–439.

10. TAYLOR, A.D., R.J. FLOWER & J.C. BUCKINGHAM. 1995. Dexamethasone inhibits the release of TSH from the rat anterior pituitary gland *in vitro* by mechanisms dependent on *de novo* protein synthesis and lipocortin 1. J. Endocrinol. **147:** 533–544.

11. LOXLEY, H.D. *et al.* 1993. Modulation of the hypothalamo-pituitary-adrenocortical responses to cytokines in the rat by lipocortin 1 and glucocorticoids: a role for lipocortin 1 in the feedback inhibition of CRF-41 release? Neuroendocrinology **57:** 801–814.

12. CHRISTIAN, H.C. *et al.* 1997. Characterization and localization of lipocortin 1-binding sites on rat anterior pituitary cells by fluorescence-activated cell analysis/sorting and electron microscopy. Endocrinology **138:** 5341–5351.

13. CHAPMAN, L.P. *et al.* 2002. Externalization of annexin I from a folliculo-stellate-like cell line. Endocrinology **147:** 4330–4338.

14. JOHN, C. *et al.* 2002. Annexin 1-dependent actions of glucocorticoids in the anterior pituitary gland: roles of the N-terminal domain and protein kinase C. Endocrinology **143:** 3060–3070.

15. PAYNE, J.P. *et al.* 2005. Modulators of the SUR2B/Kir6.1 ATP-sensitive K+ channel regulate annexin 1 release in the TtT/GF folliculostellate cell line. Endocrine Abstracts **9:** OC22.

16. TIERNEY, T. *et al.* 2003. Evidence from studies on co-cultures of TtT/GF and AtT20 cells that Annexin 1 acts as a paracrine or juxtacrine mediator of the early inhibitory effects of glucocorticoids on ACTH release. J. Neuroendocrinol. **15:** 1134–1143.

17. CREUTZ, C.E. *et al.* 1987. Identification of chromaffin granule-binding proteins. Relationship of the chromobindins to calelectrin, synhibin, and the tyrosine kinase substrates p35 and p36. J. Biol. Chem. **262:** 1860–1868.

18. JOHN, C.D. *et al.* 2003. Kinase-dependent regulation of the secretion of thyrotrophin and luteinizing hormone by glucocorticoids and annexin 1 peptides. J. Neuroendocrinol. **15:** 946–957.

19. SOLITO, E. *et al.* 2003. Dexamethasone induces rapid serine-phosphorylation and membrane translocation of annexin 1 in a human folliculostellate cell line via a novel nongenomic mechanism involving the glucocorticoid receptor, protein kinase C, phosphatidylinositol 3-kinase, and mitogen-activated protein kinase. Endocrinology **144:** 1164–1174.

20. SOLITO, E. *et al.* 2006. Post translational modification plays an essential role in the translocation of annexin A1 from the cytoplasm to the cell surface. FASEB J. **20:** 1498–1500.

21. CHAPMAN, L.P. *et al.* 2003. Evidence for a role of the ATP-binding cassette transporter A1 (ABCA1) in the externalisation of annexin 1 from pituitary folliculostellate cells. Endocrinology **144:** 1062–1073.

22. GERKE, V. & S.E. MOSS. 2002. Annexins: from structure to function. Physiol. Rev. **82:** 331–371.

23. TAYLOR, A.D. *et al.* 2000. Annexin 1 (lipocortin 1) mediates the glucocorticoid inhibition of cyclic adenosine 3′,5′-monophosphate-stimulated prolactin secretion. Endocrinology **141:** 2209–2219.

24. JOHN, C.D. *et al.* 2004. Annexin 1 and the regulation of endocrine function. Trends Endocrinol. Metab. **15:** 103–109.

25. BUCKINGHAM, J.C. & R.J. FLOWER. 1997. Lipocortin-1: a second messenger of glucocorticoid action in the hypothalamo-pituitary-adrenocortical axis. Mol. Med. Today **3:** 196–302.

26. THEOGARAJ, E. *et al.* 2005. Perinatal glucocorticoid treatment produces molecular, functional, and morphological changes in the anterior pituitary gland of the adult male rat. Endocrinology **146:** 4804–4813.

Index of Contributors

Acuña, M., 297–306
Alexaki, V.-I., 139–152
Argyra, E., 164–186
Arzt, E., 297–306

Basso, A.S., 116–131
Beuschlein, F., 319–334
Bornstein, S.R., 238–250, 307–318
Britto, L.R.G., 116–131
Buckingham, J.C., 396–409

Castanas, E., 139–152
Chapman, K.E., 265–273
Charalampopoulos, I., 139–152
Chorny, A., 187–194
Christian, H., 396–409
Chrousos, G.P., xiii–xiv, xvi–xix
Corrêa-de-Santana, E., 274–283
Costa-Pinto, F.A., 116–131
Coutinho, A., 265–273

Dardenne, M., 153–163
De Laurentiis A., 1–11
de Sá-Rocha, L.C., 116–131
Delgado, M., 187–194
Dermitzaki, E., 139–152
Druker, J., 297–306

Fernandez-Solari, J., 238–250
Flordellis, C.S., 335–345
Flower, R.J, 396–409
Forsythe, P., 65–77

Geenen, V., 284–296
Giacomini, D., 297–306
Gilmour, J.S., 265–273
Gonzalez-Rey, E., 187–194
Granstein, R.D., 195–206
Gravanis, A., 139–152
Gray, M., 265–273

Holsboer, F., 297–306

Ilias, I., 335–345, 346–360, 373–381

John, C.D., 396–409
Johnson, E.O., 41–51

Kalogeromitros, D., 78–99
Kaltsas, G.A., xv, xvi–xix
Kanczkowski, W., 307–318
Karkoulias, G., 335–345
Katafuchi, T., 230–237
Kondo, T., 230–237
Koon, H.W., 23–40
Kostandi, M., 41–51
Krug, A.W., 307–318
Kuno, R., 219–229

Lasaridis, I., 139–152
Liberman, A.C., 297–306
Lymperopoulos, A., 335–345

Madianos, P.N., 251–264
Mantzoukis, D., 132–138
Margioris, A.N., 139–152
Mastorakos, G., xvi–xix, 373–381
Mastrogianni, O., 335–345
McCann, S.M., 1–11, 238–250, 307–318
Minas, V., 139–152
Mizuno, T., 219–229
Moka E., 164–186
Morris, J., 396–409
Moutsopoulos, H.M., 41–51
Moutsopoulos, N.M., 251–264

Nagy, L., 207–218

Palermo-Neto, J., 116–131
Pereda, M.P., 297–306
Pinto-Mariz, F., 274–283
Pothoulakis, C., 23–40
Prestifilippo, J.P., 238–250
Psarra, A.M.G., 12–22

Rajnavolgyi E., 207–218
Refojo, D., 297–306
Reincke, M., 319–334
Rettori, V., 1–11, 238–250, 307–318
Routsias, J.G., 52–64
Russo, M., 116–131

Saade N., 153–163
Safieh-Garabedian, B., 153–163
Savill, J.S., 265–273
Savino, W., 274–283
Seckl, J.R., 265–273
Seiffert, K., 195–206
Sekeris, C.E., 12–22
Siafaka, I., 164–186
Silberstein, S., 297–306
Sitaras, N., 335–345
Solakidi, S., 12–22
Solito, E., 396–409
Stalla, G.K., 297–306
Sternberg, E., 361–372
Stournaras, C., 139–152
Suzumura, A., 219–229
Szatmari, I., 207–218

Take, S., 230–237
Takeuchi, H., 219–229

Taraviras, S., 335–345
Tassios, Y., 100–115
Thayer, J.F., 361–372
Theoharides, T.C., 78–99
Tierney, T., 396–409
Tsatsanis, C., 139–152
Tsatsoulis, A., 382–395
Tsitoura, D.C., 100–115
Tsopanoglou, N., 335–345
Tzioufas, A.G., 52–64

Vadalouca, A., 164–186
Vardouli, L., 139–152
Vassilopoulos, D., 132–138
Vig, R.S., 65–77
Vliagoftis, H., 65–77
Vrachnou, E., 164–186

Wirth, M., 307–318

Yoshimura, M., 230–237

Zacharowski, K., 307–318
Zapanti, E., 346–360
Zhang, G., 219–229
Ziegler, C.G., 307–318

This volume may circulate for 1 week.

Renewals may be made in person or by phone: X6-6050; from outside dial 746-6050. No VMX renewals please. Fines are charged for overdue items. Please renew promptly. Thank you.

Date Due	Date Returned